Pediatric Rotations

Nancy Liao • John Mahan
Sanghamitra Misra • Rebecca Scherzer
Jocelyn Schiller
Editors

Pediatric Rotations

A Quick Guide for Medical Students

Springer

Editors
Nancy Liao
Pediatrics
Nationwide Children's Hospital/The Ohio State University College of Medicine
Columbus, OH, USA

John Mahan
Pediatrics
Nationwide Children's Hospital/The Ohio State University College of Medicine
Columbus, OH, USA

Sanghamitra Misra
Pediatrics
Texas Children's Hospital
Houston, TX, USA

Rebecca Scherzer
Pediatrics
Nationwide Children's Hospital/The Ohio State University College of Medicine
Columbus, OH, USA

Jocelyn Schiller
Pediatrics
University of Michigan–Ann Arbor
Ann Arbor, MI, USA

ISBN 978-3-031-59872-2 ISBN 978-3-031-59873-9 (eBook)
https://doi.org/10.1007/978-3-031-59873-9

This Springer imprint is published by the registered company Springer Nature Switzerland AG
The registered company address is: Gewerbestrasse 11, 6330 Cham, Switzerland

Preface

Dear Students,

Welcome to Pediatrics—be ready to be challenged and to have fun! We hope this book will help you be successful on your pediatric rotations. You will most likely work in inpatient and outpatient pediatric settings to gain exposure and experience in both routine well child care and the management of acute and chronic medical problems. You will begin to appreciate the importance of longitudinal relationships and observe the dynamic process unique to the pediatric patient and their family. This book covers the fundamental knowledge and skills required for pediatric care, including the physical, emotional, and social development of children, and the diagnosis and management of common pediatric conditions. The book also focuses on interprofessional communication, breaking bad news, and strategies to improve your own learning. Lastly, we have emphasized a patient-centered approach, highlighting the importance of building strong relationships and providing high-quality care that is appropriate for each child's unique needs.

This book is designed to serve as a reference during your pediatric rotations including the core clerkship, sub-internship, and electives. The book is organized into sections that cover the major areas of pediatric medicine, including newborn care, common inpatient and outpatient infectious disease considerations, common procedures, and approach to well child care. Sections include practical examples to illustrate key concepts and help you apply knowledge to real-world scenarios. You can read the entire book over the course of the rotation cover to cover. Or you can refer to chapters and focus your reading based on patients you see in your rotation. The chapters are short with high-yield information. There are only a few references per chapter so you can focus on the most useful references.

Whether you hope to enter the field of pediatrics or have chosen a career path that does not include the care of children, the information and skills you learn in pediatrics courses will help you become a better physician, and the knowledge you gain may help you be a better sibling, parent, aunt, uncle, or grandparent! Friends and family may ask you for medical advice, even if the concern is not in your area of specialty. But having completed pediatrics courses, you will feel some comfort in providing initial guidance to friends and family who approach you with their concerns.

We wish you the best of luck as you navigate through your pediatric courses and become more confident in your knowledge and skills.

Columbus, OH, USA — Nancy Liao
Columbus, OH, USA — John Mahan
Houston, TX, USA — Sanghamitra Misra
Columbus, OH, USA — Rebecca Scherzer
Ann Arbor, MI, USA — Jocelyn Schiller

Contents

Chapter 1
The Power of Play

Marial Biard and Sara Reynolds

Introduction

Working with children in medical settings is one of the most challenging and most rewarding experiences for healthcare providers. The basis for successful outcomes is built on the provider establishing a respectful and trusting relationship with the child and their caregivers. Developing good rapport leads to improved clinical outcomes, patient satisfaction, and compliance with treatment. Relationships with pediatric patients differ significantly from those in adult care, as clinicians are working to develop the trust of both the patient and their adult caregiver simultaneously. This chapter will help demystify how to communicate and establish rapport with children, highlight the importance of verbal and nonverbal communication, and provide helpful tips and tricks to incorporate play into bedside interactions.

Establishing Rapport

Rapport involves effective communication and portrayal of an understanding of another's feelings and ideas. It is important to engage pediatric patients with verbal and nonverbal communication through a psychosocial-based service lens. The steps below specifically address establishing rapport quickly and efficiently in high-stress environments.

M. Biard (✉) · S. Reynolds
Texas Children's Hospital, Houston, TX, USA
e-mail: mabiard@texaschildrens.org

N. Liao et al. (eds.), *Pediatric Rotations*,
https://doi.org/10.1007/978-3-031-59873-9_1

Equip Yourself for Success Prior to Meeting the Patient

Preparing prior to entering the room sets you up to establish immediate rapport. While some information might not be readily available in the chart, knowing ahead of time what pertinent information is needed from the patient and their caregiver(s) eases the flow of communication so that interactions can evolve from transactional to relational.

Things to have prepared before you enter a room:

1. **Basic information**—The patient's name, or preferred name, pronouns, caregivers, and reason for your visit. Once you have made an introduction, you can confirm the patient's preferred name by asking "What name do you prefer to be called" or "Hi, are you Jordan? Is that the name you'd like me to call you?"
2. **Developmental knowledge and awareness**—Review child development and consider what a neurotypically developing child might be doing or interested in (school, sports, music, popular movies, etc.).
3. **Ask permission to enter the room**—This area is their home away from home, and it is important to be respectful of that space by knocking on the door and asking for permission to enter by saying "May I come in?"

Introductions

A positive introduction is crucial in the trajectory of your partnership with each patient and family you serve. Initial greetings help set the tone for an empathetic and supportive relationship. Upon entering, it is customary practice to introduce yourself by name and role (medical student, nurse practitioner, etc.), state the reason for your visit, and identify the key players in the room (i.e., family members, caregivers, etc.). Involve the child in the discussions; this might look like asking questions such as "Are you Sally? Is that what you would like for me to call you?" Asking the child directly about who is with them during the visit gives the child an opportunity to be part of the conversation and help identify the person/persons accompanying them just as we do not assume a child wishes to be called by their given name, we also cannot assume the person in the room with the patient is their parent. If the accompanying adult does not indicate their relationship, it is important to ask what their role is in the patient's life and medical care.

Scenario #1 Physician Meeting a Patient and Caregivers for the First Time

Knock on door, wait for response

Physician: "*Hello I am Dr. Kris, I'm here to talk to you about how you have been feeling lately. May I come in and speak to you?*"

Patient: "*Sure, come in.*"

Physician: "*Thank you, is Sally the name you like to go by?*"

Patient: "*Yes, thank you for asking.*"

Physician: "*Great. Sally, tell me who is here with you today?*"

Patient: "*That's my mom and that's my grandma.*"

After establishing the names and roles of everyone in the room, you can transition into the reason for your visit.

"I Spy." Finding Commonalities and Shared Experiences

There is a strong correlation between positive physician–patient interactions and patient satisfaction scores. Taking time during the visit to genuinely interact and develop rapport with your patient and their caregivers allows for a "mutually beneficial partnership" that is the cornerstone of family-centered care. A quick way to establish a rapport with your patient is to find information throughout the room that you can identify and share as a common interest. Having a solid understanding of child development and the interests of a typically developing child allows you to have a general idea of what your patient might be interested in. Asking questions creates a dialogue and foundation for information gathering.

Establishing trust in a clinical relationship involves the medical provider demonstrating empathetic care, competence, and integrity. Once an element of commonality has been established by sharing information or attempting to make a unique connection between you, the patient, and the caregiver, the groundwork for trust has been put in place. As in the examples above, your connection point does not have to be an extended conversation; just a short touchpoint indicating to the patient and caregivers you are interested in them as individuals and not solely a medical issue that needs to be addressed.

Examples include:

- "*I like your Astros jersey. I really like Altuve. Who is your favorite player?*"
- "*Those are cool Legos. What is your favorite thing to build with them? Can you show me what you are making today?*"
- "*Those are great headphones, what music are you listening to? Who is your favorite artist right now?*"

Body Language and Nonverbal Cues

Our nonverbal gestalt is the compilation of body movements, posture, and facial expression coming together to convey one message. The use of body language helps convey your character and provides insight into how you conduct yourself, both are essential in establishing the foundation of rapport.

Facial expression is a nonverbal communication tool that typically suggests what emotions people are experiencing. In this context, facial masking is the minimalization of facial expression to decrease interpretation of what someone may be thinking. It is a skill that develops as we age, therefore, children have a more transparent presentation of what they are experiencing. By paying attention to facial cues of the patient and caregivers, you are attempting to look through a window into how they perceive the interaction. It is important to remember that the window goes both ways, which requires you to be thoughtful of your own facial expressions. If a question from a caregiver leads to you clarifying previous statements, be conscious of how you may physically express emotions on your face.

Body language and gesturing are the other valuable tools in nonverbal communication. Part of the impact your physical behavior has on patients and families can be explained by the concept of empathy, or the ability to share in another person's emotions or feelings. When someone speaks, the listener often tends to mirror the speaker's attitudes. This places great importance on being conscious of body language during patient interactions. If you appear relaxed and confident, your patients can also feel relaxed and confident. In turn, body language can discretely convince patients and families that you are sincere and trustworthy; therefore, helping patients and families pay attention to what you say and evaluate it on its own merits.

Gesturing is a very prominent piece of body language often utilized to emphasize aspects of speech. To make sure your gestures are appropriate make sure you are using movements that align with your message. Appropriate gesturing will serve as a powerful instrument for convincing your patients and families of your sincerity, earnestness, and enthusiasm. See Table 1.1 for suggestions to improve nonverbal communication.

Table 1.1 Nonverbal Communication Tools

Nonverbal communication	Information to share	Examples and application
Body positioning	The angle and plane your body is in and/or facing during an interaction	• Turn to face the child and caregiver • Remain closer to the door until introductions are made and rapport is established • While remaining comfortable strive to lower your body until you and the patient are eye-to-eye • Sit in a chair or couch at bedside • Ask if you can sit at the foot of their bed

Nonverbal communication	Information to share	Examples and application
Body language	These are the movements, and shape your body takes during an interaction	• Hands in neutral position (relaxed at your side, in your pockets, or holding papers/materials) • Gestures that are calming and/or align with your speech • Minimal fidgeting
Eye contact	The duration of time spent looking directly into someone's eyes	• Eye contact's significance varies across cultures and is something to be aware of prior to entering a room • In many western cultures, when speaking it is important to look at your co-conversationalist 50% of the time • When listening this number increases to 70%. This communicates a sincerity in your attention and openness
Gestalt	These are the principles of nonverbal communication when they are all combined	• Confident stance • Fluid gesture • Appropriate eye contact • Open/child friendly body language • Enthusiasm

Verbal Communication

The act of verbal communication is using words to convey a message. Though considered easy, verbal communication is frequently where communication breakdowns occur. Things can get "lost in translation" when medical team members attempt to succinctly deliver vital information while translating that information from advanced medical terminology to laymen's terms. This is especially true for children who require a more direct and condensed form of communication to easily understand the message within the words. Using a combination of the nonverbal communications tools you have learned with the following verbal tips will serve you well in being an effective communicator. See Table 1.2 for suggestions on how to improve verbal communication.

Once these elements of verbal and nonverbal communication are combined, you should feel a positive shift in the increase of engagement and an ease in your interaction with patients and families. This means a positive rapport has been established, and from this foundation, relaxation and an element of play are welcomed and easily incorporated.

Table 1.2 Verbal Communication Tools

Verbal Communication	Description	Example
Developmental level	This refers to the academic or cognitive level for the conversation for everyone involved to understand the message being communicated. U.S. population has an average reading level of seventh to eighth grade education. When verbally conversing, it is suggested to speak at a sixth grade reading level as it helps critical information, such as medication instructions, be understood.	• Adhering to a sixth grade reading level for most adults who are not familiar with a medical setting is a good place to start. From there, you can use deductive reasoning to tailor the cognitive level of future conversations • Clear wording that can be understood by most developmental ages • Use concrete examples; short simple phrasing works best to avoid confusion
Prosody	The patterns of stress, rhythm, and intonation in a language	• Prosody is what keeps humans from sounding like robots. This is where we put emphasis on certain words or syllables in a phrase to communicate intent
Dynamic level	This is the variation in loudness when someone is speaking	• If you enter a bright room with windows open and the patient is engaged in preferred activity (TV, games, etc.) your voice can be louder and more cheerful • Masks are now highly present in clinical practice; this can create for muffled or unclear speech. Make sure to project through your mask
Tone/inflection	The tone or pitch of voice is used to convey a more precise meaning for our words and provides insight into how we are feeling	• Assess the status of the room and allow your voice to match • If you walk into a dark room, windows drawn, with minimal auditory stimulation, this means your voice should be quiet and soft

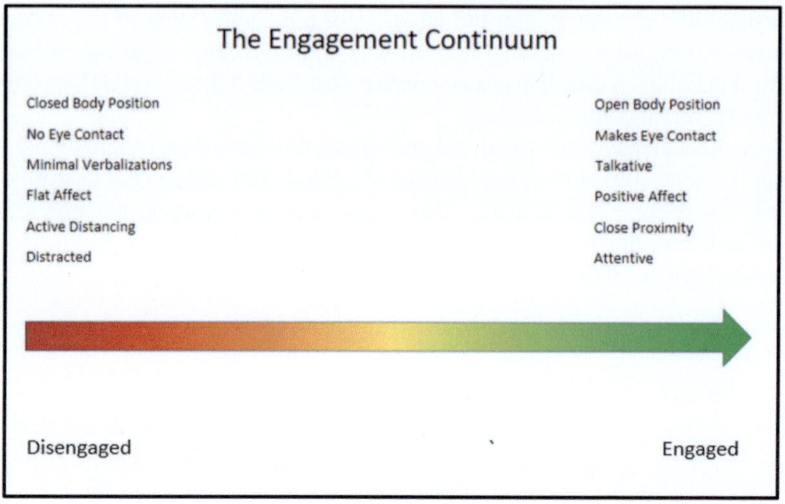

Incorporating Play into Your Practice: Why Play?

Play has been described as the "work" of children; it is how children make sense of their world, develop social skills, learn new concepts, and conquer fears. Play is especially critical in healthcare settings, where the unknown and illness often heighten the child's fear and anxiety. Although you may have a limited time frame for interacting with a patient and caregiver, you can still use a playful demeanor to support patients and families. Engaging the child in this way allows them to have some control throughout the visit and may help reduce fears related to seeing a doctor through active participation. Play can also be utilized to help patients understand unfamiliar language, clarify misconceptions, or decrease anxiety surrounding a minor procedure. Being intentionally playful with your patient population can have a positive effect on both you and your patient/caregiver.

Decreasing Anxiety

The following example describes utilizing a child's comfort item (i.e., stuffed animal) to address the fear of getting a shot and play out a potentially threatening interaction to help the patient better understand and cope with the medical environment.

Scenario #2 Using Medical Play to Assist with Medicine Administration

Physician: "*Hi Diego, I'm Dr. Brandon. I see you brought your teddy bear. What is their name?*

Patient: "*His name is Pickles. Are you going to give me a shot?*"

Physician: "*Today I want to make sure that you are growing and are healthy. I am going to listen to you with my stethoscope and we might need to give you medicine in your arm. Let us check out Pickles first. Can you show me how we should listen to their heart with a stethoscope?*"

Scenario #3 Explaining Medical Terminology in a Playful Manner

Patient: "*Why do I need to have a CAT scan? I'm not a cat*"

Physician: "*Are you sure? Let's hear your best meow.*"

Patient: "*Meow. I'm still not a cat though.*"

Physician: "*You're right. We don't scan cats here. A CAT scan takes pictures of the inside of your body so we can see what is happening in there.*"

Redirection

Distraction, redirection, and alternate engagement all reference a common technique utilized by psychosocial support staff to focus the patient's attention away from stimuli that is producing fear or anxiety. Redirection provides a way to cope with pain, fear, and anxiety often experienced during situations where patients need motivation and additional support to display compliance in their medical treatment. Redirection commonly looks like finding a source of stimuli such as music or a game to focus patients' attention on rather than the ongoing procedure.

Scenario #4 Different Ways to Introduce Redirection Prior to Removing Stitches

Physician: "*How about you and Dad look through this book and try to find all the balloons on each page while I remove your stitches?*"

Physician: "*Do you have a favorite movie? What is the best part of that movie? Let's watch that part while I remove your stitches.*"

Physician: "*How many times do you think we can sing ABC's while I remove your stitches? I bet we can't get to five! Who do you think will sing the loudest?*"

Incorporating something familiar/favored into a patient's attention field will help distract them and allow them to focus on something they enjoy over something that brings pain/anxiety.

Relaxation

Another way to address anxiety in an efficient manner is to remind patients and families of the importance of relaxation. While this can be a challenging task to execute in acute medical settings, relaxation is important in helping relieve stress and tension from the body. There are succinct ways to help incorporate relaxation into practice through play. Several methods rely on preexisting physiological constructs within our body system. One such method used in relaxation is deep breathing. Deep breathing slows the sympathetic nervous system and helps down-regulate our stress centers. Child life professionals often use bubbles and windmills to provide a concrete visual of the child's breathing so they can understand what deep breathing looks like. If these resources are available to you, incorporate them as you see fit. However, all you truly need is a sense of imagination and playfulness to provide a moment of relaxation and calming.

Scenario #5 Using Imagination and Play to Incorporate Relaxation into an Examination

(Patient age < 6) Physician: "*Wow look! A magic butterfly has landed on my hand! What do you say we try three big breaths to send it flying across the room. Ready? Deep breath in... go!*"

Patient and Physician both exhale deeply pretending to send the butterfly flying across the room/treatment area.

Physician: "*That was great. Two more big breaths!*" etc.

Scenario #6 Incorporating Deep Breathing for Relaxation into Examination

Physician: "*Let's take a few deep breaths together before we start. Oh! Let's make this a game. We can see who can breathe out the longest. Ready? Big breath in... now slowly blow out.*"

By using familiar concepts such as butterflies and incorporating a game-like mentality into relaxation exercises, everyone can continue with the visit in a calmer, more relaxed state.

Caregiver's Presence

A strong tool to utilize when decreasing anxiety in children is the caregiver or other person accompanying the patient. Often, children base their emotions and perceptions on how the people they know, love, and trust are responding to any given situation. Here are some helpful examples of ways to utilize the caregiver as a positive tool for anxiety management:

1. **Learn and utilize the caregiver's name**—This communicates effort and openness on your behalf. It also shows closeness to the caregiver which translates as closeness to the child.
2. **Listen to the caregiver for procedural tips and tricks regarding their child**—Ask a caregiver if they have advice for how to make medical care (i.e., exam, procedure, etc.) go easier. They are experts on their child and will know how lights, placement, sounds, etc. will work best for their child and by extension, everyone involved in the process.

3. **Allow for comfortable positioning**—Is the reason for your visit still achievable if the patient is in their mother's lap? Can they be holding grandma's hand? Helping facilitate closeness to their caregivers allows the patient to feel safe and secure. This frequently helps the procedure or examination go much more smoothly.

Another way to promote a relaxed environment is to make sure the caregiver's anxiety is being addressed. Keeping caregivers informed and utilizing them as the expert on their child are important to calm and focus the caregiver. To enhance the child's care and continue to support the caregiver remember that in every interaction you are serving as a role model and helping establish a foundation for treatment that will carry over into the child's home and daily living.

Play to Help Meet Goals

As Mary Poppins once said. "In every job that must be done, there is an element of fun. You find the fun and snap! The job's a game..." While you cannot pull out a spoon full of sugar, you can incorporate fun into your plan of care for patients/caregivers. To achieve successful clinical outcomes, you need buy-in from the patient and their caregiver in implementing strategies to help them succeed. By setting goals and providing positive feedback, you are able to produce intrinsic motivation, self-determination, and desired adherence.

- **Setting goals**—These can be part of your initial rapport building and introduction. When stating the goal for the visit and subsequent treatment plan, everyone is familiar and more prepared to work together as a team. Goals should be short, easy to understand, and a collaborative effort between the physician and the patient/caregiver. Taking the time to explain and increase understanding of what is happening within the patients' medical treatment helps align them to the overarching goal of your visit.
- **Providing positive reinforcement**—This provides the patient and caregiver with a sense of accomplishment and allows their reward center to activate. Praising specific behaviors encourages continued behaviors while also validating coping strategies. Be brief and specific when providing encouragement and praising desired behaviors. Additionally, praise the child for completing the task, even if they cry. Crying is a coping strategy! Having small rewards, such as stickers or other small prizes may also help a child to feel a sense of accomplishment and have tangible reminders of success.
- **Child Friendly Language**—Using child-friendly language when educating a patient on a new diagnosis or sharing information pertinent to their medical treatment can sometimes seem daunting; however, imagination and creativity are strong allies to this task. They take information that is difficult to process and weave it into a metaphor which is easier for children to comprehend. First gather

baseline information in/around the patient's understanding of what is happening to them. Asking them to tell you in their own words why they are meeting with you provides valuable insight and may offer language you can use to help them understand.

Scenario #7 Meeting with a 10-Year-Old Who Has Been Newly Diagnosed with Leukemia: Dialogue

Physician: "*Morning, J, I'm Doctor N. Can you tell me why you are here today?*"

Patient: "*My mom said I have cancer.*"

Physician: "*Ok, do you know what cancer is?*"

Patient: "*Not really. I just know mom says it's attacking my body and making me sick which is why I feel so tired.*"

Physician: "*You and mom are both right. I am here to help you learn about what cancer is and to tell you how we plan to help heal your body.*"

By establishing what the patient understands about their visit or illness, you are better able to develop a plan of care or provide education tailored to their personal comprehension. Here is where creativity comes into the process; you could use the child's language of "attack" to create a castle metaphor or use the feeling tiredness to create a metaphor where the body is a factory, and the bone marrow machine is currently broken. Do not be afraid to use online resources for assistance in getting creative. Modeling can also include showing informational videos made specifically to help educate children in language they can understand.

Scenario #8 14-Year-Old Patient Who Is Not Being Compliant with Their Diabetes Regimen

Your patient is 14 years old and struggling to manage their diabetes.

When you arrive, introduce yourself and instead of immediately stating the goal or intent of your visit, begin by asking open-ended questions about barriers to their care. Letting them be the narrator of their own story helps them to feel more independent and to increase their decision-making role.

The patient indicates they cannot remember to take medication on time and forgets to bring supplies to school. Acknowledge their statements and converse with them using open-ended questions to help facilitate problem solving. Asking a patient about their daily routine such as "Talk me through your morning. How do you wake up for school?" helps provide insight into available technology/support for them. If they use their phone, you can continue by asking what their favorite apps are and if they have considered downloading an app or using a reminder setting to help.

Having information about apps or different ways other patients set reminders to check their blood sugar provides a peer model of success while still providing them with the choice over which platform they utilize. Incorporating personal examples increase relatability and show that you are listening and problem solving *with* the patient instead of *for* the patient.

Continuing the conversation in this ebb-and-flow rhythm will help create motivation on the patient's behalf and support continued problem solving between you and the patient, such as "What are the reasons you are having a tough time carrying supplies to school? Do you have a backpack? Are fanny packs cool or lame?" These answers will provide you with more choices to present the patient for problem solving. "How about trialing taking a purse, fanny pack, or small pencil case with your supplies inside to school the next few days?" This back-and-forth problem-solving style is a wonderful way to incorporate positive reinforcement in a developmentally appropriate way. "A pencil case is a great idea! Very incognito & perfect size to keep everything together and easy to access. Love it!"

Recap

Play is especially critical in healthcare settings to help and engage pediatric patients. While medical providers do not always have the capacity to play in clinical settings, it is possible to incorporate playfulness into medical practice. Moments like the ones described in this chapter may seem trivial but can have a lasting impact on the foundation you create as a caregiver to a family unit.

Further Reading

Abendroth K, Whited J. Motivation, rapport, and resilience: three pillars of adolescent therapy to shift the focus to adulthood. Perspect ASHA Spec Interest Groups. 2021;6:1–9.

Apker J, Shank S, Baker M, Hatten K, VanSweden S. Observing and identifying hospitalist best communication practices in patient interactions. Hosp Top. 2019;97(4):156–64.

Bayer ND, Taylor A, Atabek Z, Santolaya J, Bamat TW, Washington N. Should we call you mom and dad? Caregiver preferences and pediatric physician and nurse manner in greetings. Hosp Pediatr. 2019;9(12):989–92. Epub 2019 Nov 12

Mărginean CO, Meliţ LE, Chinceşan M, Mureşan S, Georgescu AM, Suciu N, Pop A, Azamfirei L. Communication skills in pediatrics—the relationship between pediatrician and child. Medicine. 2017;96(43):e8399.

Toussaint L, Nguyen QA, Roettger C, Dixon K, Offenbächer M, Kohls N, Hirsch J, Sirois F. Effectiveness of progressive muscle relaxation, deep breathing, and guided imagery in promoting psychological and physiological states of relaxation. Evid Based Complement Alternat Med. 2021;2021:5924040.

Chapter 2
Taking a Pediatric History

Ashley Shamansky and Rena Kasick

History of Present Illness (HPI)

The pediatric interview varies depending on the age and cognitive abilities of the child. Caretakers are often present during the encounter and may be the primary historian; however, it is best to avoid assumptions and clarify who is with the child during the interview. You may consider addressing the child first, "Who did you bring with you today?" or asking the adult directly "Tell me, how are you related to the patient?" You may learn that your patient has two mothers or fathers, is taken care of by other family members, or is in foster care. Children as young as preschool age may be able to start providing you with accurate and reliable information [1]. A school-aged child can often provide initial accounts of the problem they are seeing you for with others offering supplemental history. When you evaluate a preteen or teenage patient, part of the interview may be conducted one-on-one without the parent/guardian in the room.

Getting on the patient's eye level helps build rapport. You can start by asking about a toy, a cartoon character on their clothing, or their favorite hobby. As you begin taking the history, use the patient and parent's expectations to set the agenda.

During history taking, consider the setting. Are you seeing the patient in an outpatient pediatric office for a health maintenance visit, an urgent care for a sick visit, the hospital for a new admission? The setting helps direct the history and the types of questions you ask.

A. Shamansky (✉)
Department of Pediatrics, Geisinger Commonwealth School of Medicine, Danville, PA, USA
e-mail: alshamansky1@geisinger.edu

R. Kasick
Department of Pediatrics, Nationwide Children's Hospital/The Ohio State University College of Medicine, Columbus, OH, USA
e-mail: rena.kasick@nationwidechildrens.org

N. Liao et al. (eds.), *Pediatric Rotations*,
https://doi.org/10.1007/978-3-031-59873-9_2

Even in a health maintenance visit, you want to determine if the patient and/or parent have any questions or concerns. As you collect the HPI, you want to determine the chief complaint (CC) and begin exploring it. There are several mnemonics to aid you in obtaining this information including, but not limited to OLD CARTS, CODIERS, PQRSTU. As the general principles in characterizing a chief complaint do not change from children to adults, it is recommended that you review your history taking materials or texts.

Onset
Location
Duration
Character
Alleviating/Aggravating
Radiation
Timing
Severity

Birth History

The birth history of a patient should be obtained when the child is less than 2 years of age or in settings where it may be relevant to the child's presenting problem (i.e., a patient in neurodevelopmental clinic presenting for developmental delay). Components of the birth history can be further divided into prenatal, natal, and postnatal history.

- Questions that may be asked in the prenatal history include maternal and paternal age, abnormal anatomy scans or prenatal testing, exposures during pregnancy (medications, illicit drugs, alcohol, tobacco, infections), and prenatal care (history of gestational diabetes, hypertension, antiphospholipid syndrome).
- Natal period questions include mode of delivery, interventions utilized (forceps or vacuum), fetal presentation, duration of labor, complications during labor (maternal bleeding, failure to progress, abnormal fetal tracing), maternal fever, labor duration, length of rupture of membranes, amniotic fluid color, and gestation (pre-term, term, post-dates).
- Postnatal questions include resuscitation measures used (if any), APGARS, nursery or neonatal intensive care unit (NICU) complications (hypoglycemia, jaundice, neonatal abstinence syndrome, congenital anomalies, birth injuries), medications/vaccinations given (vitamin K, erythromycin ointment, hepatitis B vaccine), feeding method (breast or bottle), and when the infant first passed meconium.

Developmental History

The thoroughness and content of the developmental history are dependent on age and CC. During certain visits, it may be appropriate to ask if the child's development is on track. Other times you may want to explore each developmental domain and when the developmental milestone occurred. Example questions include: "How has your child's development been? What new things are he/she/they doing? Has he/she/they ever stopped doing something they previously were able to do?" If there is delay, ask if it is progressive or non-progressive. In school-aged children, assessment of development may be important to determine if the patient is above, at, or below grade level, if they have specific plans developed such as a 504 or Individualized Education Plan (IEP), and what those plans procure for the child with regard to additional classroom support. Validated screening tools, such as the Ages and Stages Questionnaire (ASQ) or Modified Checklist for Autism in Toddlers (M-CHAT), can be used to assist in the acquisition of this information.

Past Medical History

It is important to understand a child's past medical history as it may impact how you manage the CC. During a health maintenance visit, it is necessary to review their medical conditions, severity of the condition, age of diagnosis, and understand how the chronic medical problem(s) impacts daily life.

- Medical diagnoses, past or present, including accidents, injuries, and ingestions with date of diagnosis for each condition. For chronic conditions, include the name/location of the current subspecialist(s), if any.
- Past hospitalizations, including dates, hospital name, diagnosis.
- Past surgeries, including the date, hospital name, and the name of the surgeon or where the surgery happened.
- Current medications, including dose, route, and frequency. Be sure to include all over the counter medications and homeopathic preparations. Children often take medication in liquid formulations, and caregivers may report a dosage in milliliters (mL). It is important to convert the dose from mL's to milligrams (mg) or milligrams per kilogram (mg/kg).
  Example: 10 kg child taking ibuprofen reported as taking 5 mL
  Ibuprofen concentration: 100 mg/5 mL
  Dose is 100 mg
- Allergies, both drug and environmental, including the reaction type, triggers, and severity of reaction.
- Verify immunization status and need for catch-up/annual vaccinations. The most up-to-date vaccination schedules and guidance can be found on the Center for Disease Control and Prevention website. If not up-to-date, be as specific as possible about the reason(s) why. Remember to ask specifically about certain vac-

cines like influenza and SARS-CoV2 that fall outside of the routine childhood schedule.

During a well child visit, pediatricians also assess the child's and caregivers' understanding of their medical problem(s) and provide appropriate anticipatory guidance. In the emergency room or hospital setting, a focused past medical history is prudent.

Feeding History

A detailed feeding history is particularly important for infants and any child who receives tube feeds. Document the type of formula (including kcal/oz) as well as any additives (thickening agents, protein powder, etc.), frequency, volume, and mode of intake. For breastfed infants, describe the frequency and duration of feeds, and whether there have been any concerns about latch, milk transfer, or maternal supply. You should also note the age at which solid foods were introduced and the types and amounts of current solid food intake. If there are any formulas or foods that are poorly tolerated, you should note that here as well.

Surgical History

A surgical history includes the operation or procedure, indication, laterality, date, and/or age of the child at the time of operation and postoperative complications, if any. A recent surgery may heighten the index of suspicion for postoperative complications. For example, in a child who presents with severe abdominal pain, an abdominal surgery may increase consideration for possible postoperative complications, such as infection, adhesions, or ileus.

Family History

There are special considerations for family history in the pediatric population. A complete family history includes medical conditions and age at diagnosis of family members within three generations including biological siblings, parents, and grandparents. Inquiring about consanguinity (ask "Are the parents of the patient related in any way?"), chromosomal abnormalities, pattern of growth, and other congenital diseases may be pertinent. For example, a family history of congenital heart disease may be significant in a newborn who is having oxygen desaturations in the nursery.

Social History

Understanding their home and school circumstances may reveal psychosocial factors that impact the care you provide. There is no particular order in which to obtain this history and many questions may overlap. For the younger child, you should cover home environment, education, eating, activities, and safety. Consider using more open-ended questions to obtain the social history, especially with sensitive topics where it may be best to allow the patient the freedom to engage in the encounter and share personal information.

The social history includes information about who lives in the home with the child (or homes—don't forget to ask about other homes where children spend a significant amount of time) including the ages of other children. You should also ask about who else cares for the child during the day (daycare, nanny, relative, etc.). Other appropriate information may include:

- Exposure to second-hand smoke, lead (include the year the dwelling was built), other toxins
- Primary water source (city water, well water, bottled water, etc.)
- History of food insecurity, homelessness, insurance status
- Occupation of parent(s) or primary caretaker(s)
- Presence of pets in the home
- Sleeping arrangements (particularly for infants)
- Smoke detectors and carbon monoxide detectors in the home
- Firearms in the home

The preteen and teenage years are a time of exploration and are quite formative. Due to the sensitive and confidential nature of some topics, it is recommended to ask the parent to step outside the room during this part of the interview. Normalizing this interaction empowers the patient in the care of their own physical and mental health and helps to strengthen the physician–patient relationship. You should provide a statement of confidentiality and convey circumstances in which confidentiality is breached, such as when the shared information will harm or compromise the safety of the patient or those around them.

It is important to ask about illicit substances as well as tobacco and alcohol. Define what substance(s), route(s) of delivery, frequency of use, and environment(s) where each substance is used. Asking about sexuality is also part of the social history. Most clinicians will start having these discussions around the age of 11 or 12. Topics to be covered will vary by age and presenting complaint. Some questions to consider:

- Gender identity
- Sexual orientation
- Age at first sexual encounter
- Types of sexual activity and number of partners
- Pregnancy and sexually transmitted infection (STI) prevention
- History of STI testing and treatment
- History of forced or coerced sexual activity

The adolescent social history can be outlined with the HEEADSSS mnemonic which stands for home, education, eating, activities/employment, drugs, sex, suicidality, and safety [2]. Table 2.1 outlines the mnemonic with examples of questions and tips for collecting this information.

As noted with other portions of the pediatric history, completing every aspect of the social history noted above is exhaustive. Use your setting as well as the patient's CC to help focus the social history.

Table 2.1 HEEADSSS assessment [2]

	Challenges/pitfalls	Suggested questions
Home	Do not assume that children have a typical nuclear family or that children live at only one home	"Where do you live?" "Who lives at home with you?" "Do you feel safe at home?" "Who can you talk to when you're upset?"
Education	You can begin your interview with these questions, as they may be easier to answer	"What grade are you in?" "How are your grades? Have there been changes in how you are doing in school?" "What do you like (not like) about school?" "What is your favorite class?" "What are your future plans or goals?"
Eating and exercise	Inquiring about self-esteem and body-image is important	"Tell me about your diet?" "Are you happy with your weight?" "Have you ever restricted your diet or vomited to lose weight?" "Do you exercise? What do you do for exercise? How frequently?"
Activity/ employment	This category is another category that is easy to break the ice with when talking to an adolescent. It allows the adolescent to talk about what they enjoy	"Tell me what you do in a typical day?" "Tell me about your friends?" "What do you do for fun?" "Do you have a job? Did you work over the summer?" "Do you participate in any clubs or sports at school?"
Drugs	Adolescent years are a time of self-exploration. It is important to ask these questions using nonjudgmental language. If the adolescent is using substances, you can also use motivational interviewing to determine whether they want to stop	"Do any of your friends use drugs (like marijuana or take pain pills), tobacco products, or drink alcohol?" "Have you ever used recreational drugs, tobacco products (including e-cigarettes and vaping), or drink alcohol?" "Do you use prescription drugs that we not prescribed by a doctor for you?" "Have you ever felt pressured to try these things?" "Where do you get the money for them?" "Are you interested in trying to cut down or stop?"

Table 2.1 (continued)

	Challenges/pitfalls	Suggested questions
Sexuality	Sexual history taking may be uncomfortable for the patient. Normalizing the interview using nonjudgmental language is helpful. "I ask these sensitive questions to all of my teenagers so I can help understand and better take care of you" remember, it is best to not assume the answer your patient may provide you. Sexual activity can include oral, vaginal or anal intercourse. You may need to make this clear to the patient	"What gender do you identify as?" "What pronouns would you prefer me to use with you?" "Are you in or have you ever been in a relationship with anyone?" "Many people your age are starting to explore sexual activity. Sexual activity can include oral, vaginal, or anal intercourse. Have you ever been sexually active?" "What contraception or protection have you considered or used?" "Have you ever felt pressured into sexual activity?" "Have you ever had an infection that you got because of sexual activity?"
Suicidality	Caretakers may have apprehension about the child's psychological health and instead raise concerns for behavioral changes they notice If your suicidality screen is positive, it is important to raise your concern immediately to your attending physician so immediate care can be provided to ensure the patient's safety	"Tell me about your mood lately…" "How do you feel right now?" "Have you ever been so sad you have thought about hurting yourself?" "Have you ever tried hurting yourself?"
Safety	It is important to screen for general safety as well as gun safety	"Are there any guns or weapons in the home?" "Where and how are they stored?" "Do you feel safe at home/work/school?" "Is there a time or place (or person) where you feel unsafe?"
Social media	It is important to screen for behaviors that might put children at risk for human trafficking and child pornography	"Which social media platforms do you use?" "Do you ever share your personal details on social media?" "Have you ever felt bullied online?"

Review of Systems

Depending on the environment in which you are seeing your pediatric patient, your review of systems may be focused on areas related to the chief complaint. For example, in the emergency department, if you are seeing a child for an asthma exacerbation, you may focus on asking questions regarding HEENT, cardiovascular, and respiratory systems. However, during a health maintenance visit, you may perform a more comprehensive 10–14 point review of systems that is age appropriate. Refer to Table 2.2, for example, review of systems questions.

Table 2.2 Pediatric review of systems

	Newborn to 12 months	12 months to 3 years	3–12 years	>13 years	Clinical relevance
General	Fussy, irritable, lethargy		X	X	A neonate with fevers and irritability may suggest possible meningitis and would typically require lumbar puncture to obtain cerebrospinal fluid for diagnostic testing
	Fever, weight loss/gain, change in activity, fatigue				
HEENT	Changes in vision, esotropia/exotropia, frequent colds, otitis media, congestion, nosebleeds, sore throat, hearing problems (newborn screening), ear pain, ear drainage, teething, noisy breathing/snoring				Delayed tooth eruption beyond 10 months old may point to prematurity, underlying genetic abnormalities, developmental (endocrine) disorders, or nutritional deficiencies
Cardiovascular	Sweating, color change with feeding	X	X	X	Toddlers or older children with tetralogy of Fallot may instinctively squat when they are short of breath in efforts to increase blood flow to the lungs
	X	Squatting		X	
	X	X	Tachycardia, exercise intolerance, palpitations, syncope with activity, chest pain with activity		
Respiratory	Cough, wheezing, shortness of breath, stridor, cyanosis, retractions, nasal flaring, hemoptysis				Frequent nighttime cough or wheezing in a child may indicate poor asthma control
Gastro-intestinal	Vomiting (bloody/bilious), diarrhea, constipation, hematemesis, hematochezia, melena, jaundice				Profuse, persistent vomiting in a child at any age should increase consideration for structural causes of obstruction such as malrotation/volvulus
	X	X	Nausea, abdominal pain		
Genito-urinary	Hematuria, edema (periorbital, sacral)				Nocturnal enuresis in a child older than 5–7 years of age should include evaluation for stressors, trauma, constipation, bladder or kidney disease, and rarely neurological disease in an otherwise normal child
	X	Dysuria, frequency, urgency, enuresis (nocturnal/diurnal), discharge			
	X	X	X	Sexual activity, LMP, sexual activity, STI exposure, details of menarche	

Table 2.2 (continued)

	Newborn to 12 months	12 months to 3 years	3–12 years	>13 years	Clinical relevance
Endocrine	Growth pattern				A neonate who is diagnosed with failure to thrive, tracking below the third percentile for weight, may be due to inadequate caloric intake, malabsorption, or increased energy expenditures
	X	Polyuria/polydipsia			
	X	X	Heat/cold intolerance		
Musculo-skeletal	Trauma, scoliosis				A teen with knee pain who participates in running/jumping sports may have patellofemoral syndrome, Osgood-Schlatter, or iliotibial band friction and is diagnosed by physical exam
	X	Myalgias, arthralgias, limp, weakness			
Neurologic	Change in alertness, fussiness, seizure activity, developmental delay or regression, trauma, loss of consciousness, changes in tone/weakness				A child who begins to lose previously acquired milestones should raise concern for autism, Rett syndrome, and other neurodegenerative diseases
	X	Tics			
	X	X	Headache		
Hematologic	Easy bruising, bleeding, lumps (neck/axilla/groin)				Bruising behind the ears, trunk, or buttocks in a non-ambulatory should raise concern for non-accidental trauma
Skin	Rashes, hair problems, hives				A diaper dermatitis that is brightly erythematous with satellite lesions is characteristic of a candida infection
Psychiatry	X		Mood changes, anxiety, insomnia, changes in appetite, ability to focus/concentration, changes in energy level, suicidal ideation		A child who has a positive screen for suicidality should be assessed for intent and access to lethal means and immediately referred to psychiatric services and/or emergency department to ensure safety

Special Considerations

The Nonverbal Child

Some pediatric patients have complex medical problems and are nonverbal. Often the parent/guardian provides the history in these cases. For example, depending on the environment, nursing reports or objective data from monitors provide additional information. If you are seeing a nonverbal child, consider how you may interact with them. It is recommended to ask the patient/guardian about their baseline communication methods and for guidance on how to interact with them. Always greet the patient directly and tell them what parts of the exam you will conduct, just as you would with neurotypical patients. Ask "How does your child typically share their needs with you?" or "How do they let you know if they are happy or if something is wrong?" and "What kind of things does are they able to do?" or "What kind of things do they like to do?" If you are fortunate to have continuity with these patients, you may learn that there are certain "likes" that will bring about a smile and other nonverbal cues that may clue you into pain or discomfort.

References

1. Mendelsohn JS, Quinn MT, McNahh WL. Interview strategies commonly used by pediatricians. Arch Pediatr Adolesc Med. 1999;153(2):154–7. https://doi.org/10.1001/archped.153.2.154.
2. Goldenring JM, Rosen DS. HEEADSSS 3.0: the psychosocial interview for adolescents updated for a new century fueled by media. Contemp Pediatr. 2014:16–28.

Chapter 3
Age-Based Strategies for Physical Exams

Amanda Padilla and D'Juanna White-Satcher

Background

The performance of the physical exam goes much smoother when the patient is comfortable with the examiner. Many young patients may have stranger anxiety, and since examining a child involves invading their personal space, a child may resist being examined. As children get older, they may associate doctor's offices with painful experiences like getting shots and thus may have some fear and anxiety associated with doctors and exam tables. The best way to overcome this is to develop rapport with the patient as soon as you enter the room. For children old enough to communicate, you should incorporate them in the history portion of the exam as much as possible.

For younger and less cooperative children, the order of exam should be adjusted, with the least invasive exams occurring first and the most invasive last. Typically, the heart and lung exam should be attempted first, and the ear and oropharynx exams last. Physical restraint should not be routinely used to examine patients.

As you perform the exam, you should explain to the patient what you are about to do. You should make sure you are "telling" the patient not "asking" their permission to do portions of the exam. You can allow them to make some choices but not choose whether to be examined. For example, "I'm about to examine your ears, do you want me to check the right ear or the left ear first?" not "Can I check your ears?"

A. Padilla (✉) · D. White-Satcher
Division of Academic General Pediatrics, Department of Pediatrics, Baylor College of Medicine, Houston, TX, USA
e-mail: ap24@bcm.edu; satcher@bcm.edu

N. Liao et al. (eds.), *Pediatric Rotations*,
https://doi.org/10.1007/978-3-031-59873-9_3

Considerations for the Physical Exam of the Newborn/Early Infant

- Before touching an infant, make some commentary based on your observations about the baby or caregiver/baby connection. Comments such as—"What a sweet baby!" or "Oh, he looks just like you!" or "She can't take her eyes off of you" can be made.
- Explain to the infant's caregiver(s) everything you are doing and why.
- Examine as much as possible in the caregiver's arms. The caregiver's lap can be used as an exam table for abdominal and hip examinations.
- Heart and lung exams should be completed first, as this is the least invasive portion of exam.
- When examining the red reflex, it is best if the infant opens their eyes spontaneously. Darkening of the room or putting the infant in a vertical position often makes them open their eyes.
- Ear and oral exams should be saved for last as they can be performed even if the baby is crying.

Considerations for the Physical Exam of the Older Infant/Toddler

- During the history portion of the encounter, try to interact periodically with the patient, playing "peek-a-boo" type games.
- Consider using small stethoscope toys, especially those with lights or noise makers as distractors. These should be disinfected between patients.
- Utilize the caregiver's lap for the exam.
- As the child outgrows the caregiver's lap, an exam table can be made using the laps of the caregiver and examiner. The examiner should sit knee-to-knee with the caregiver—the child's head and upper body will remain on the caregiver with legs resting on examiner.
- Alternatively, the caregiver can sit on the exam table with the child in their lap, and as the child outgrows the lap, the child's lower body and legs will rest on exam table.
- If the child is walking around playing, the examiner can stoop down to their level to engage. Part of the exam can be done in this manner if the patient is cooperative.
- Parts of the exam can be demonstrated on stuffed animals, siblings, or caregivers to encourage the patient to cooperate.
- Save the oral exam for last. If the patient is crying or screaming with the ear exam, you can pivot your strategy and quickly examine the oropharynx.
- If you need to use a tongue depressor to examine the oropharynx, make sure the patient is well-restrained by the caregiver so they are not injured.

Considerations for the Physical Exam of Pre-school/School-Aged Children

- Explain what you will be doing in advance using age-appropriate language.
- For some children in this age range, it still helps to demonstrate the exam on a toy, sibling, or caregiver first.
- The patient may choose whether to be examined on the caregiver's lap or exam table.
- To help a child feel comfortable sitting on the exam table, you can bring in some crayons and allow the child to sit on the table and draw on the exam paper.
- In more cooperative patients, standard "head-to-toe" order of exam can typically be utilized. However, if the child is less cooperative, proceed as you would in younger children by performing least invasive exam portions first.
- If you have difficulty examining the oropharynx, use a tongue depressor as a last resort. You can demonstrate panting like a puppy and ask the patient to mimic. Doing this improves visualization of the posterior pharynx.
- For lung auscultation, if patient is not taking big breaths upon instruction:
  - Tear off a strip of exam paper and hold it about 1 ft away from the patient and ask patient to blow the paper away.
  - Use light on otoscope or pen light and ask the child to try to blow the light out-as the child takes a deep breath, you turn off the light.
- To assess abdominal tenderness, after listening for bowel sounds, use the stethoscope to apply slight pressure to the abdomen as you watch the child's face for signs of discomfort such as grimacing or crying. If a child is ticklish, you may pause the exam for a moment, distract the child, and try again.

Considerations for the Physical Exam of Tween/Teens

- Standard "head-to-toe" order of exam can be utilized.
- Incorporating the tween/teen in the history-taking portion of the encounter will help them feel more comfortable with you.
- Be sensitive to the fact that some tween/teens may be self-conscious about physical changes in their bodies and may be uncomfortable sitting in a gown for an extended period of time. They may also be uncomfortable changing clothes in front of their caretaker and siblings. If possible, you should take the history with the tween/teen in street clothes and then ask if they would prefer their caretaker/siblings to leave while they change into the gown.
- Take advantage of the exam time to discuss puberty and self-hygiene.

Focusing on the Pediatric Ear Exam

Examining the ear of a child is one of the more challenging parts of the physical exam especially because it is performed best when the child is stationary. For infants, this exam can be performed successfully in a caregiver's arms. The head of the infant should be held up against the caregiver's chest wall by the caregiver. You can then stabilize the head against the chest wall.

For most children, the ear exam is not difficult to perform. There are many toddlers who will sit on an exam table or the caregiver's lap without moving as their ears are examined. Incorporate play into the exam. Ask the child if you will find dinosaurs in their ears or whistle as you exam and say "I'm looking for birds." Some children, however, cannot hold still independently and will require some caregiver assistance/restraint. All ear exams should be attempted first without restraint. Prior to attempting the exam, explain what you are about to do, and that the child needs to hold still. If the child cannot hold still independently, then mild restraint may be needed to ensure that a successful ear exam is possible. School-age children should not be restrained for an ear exam unless the exam is critical to the visit.

Approach to the Ear Exam If Caregiver Assistance/Restraint Is Needed

- The body should be stabilized as movement can make the ear exam challenging and injury can occur.
- Examining in the caregiver's arms vs. exam table depends on the cooperativity of the patient, the size of child in comparison to caregiver, and the caregiver's ability/willingness to help restrain a child in their arms.
- In-arms approach:
  - The child's back should rest against the front of the caregiver's chest and their head should be turned and able to rest fully on the caregiver's chest.
  - The examiner stabilizes the head, and the caregiver stabilizes the child's body and hands with their arms. The caregiver may need to cross their legs over the child's legs to prevent movement/kicking.
- Exam table approach
  - The child's back should be against the exam table, and head should be turned.
  - The examiner stabilizes the head, and the caregiver stabilizes the body by holding their shoulders flat against the table while gently lying on their child. Some caregivers are unable to do this, and another care team member may be needed.

Genital and Breast Exam

- A chaperone must be present for genitourinary and breast exams.
- Caregivers should be present for all pre-pubertal patients.
- Explain in age-appropriate language exactly what is going to be done and why.
- Discussing "private areas," inappropriate touching, and why physicians do this exam in the presence of caregiver is appropriate.
- If patient is uncooperative/resistant, this exam should be deferred (and documented as such)

Examining the Child with Developmental/Intellectual Disabilities or Limited Verbal Communication

Examining a child with developmental disabilities or limited verbal communication may add complexity to the medical assessment. As with examining all patients, it is important to consider specific needs and limitations the child may have, to be flexible during the clinical encounter, and to provide the appropriate amount of time to adequately and appropriately assess the patient. Following are some helpful strategies and tips for examining children with cognitive or communication impairment.

Starting the medical encounter:

- Approach the child and family and introduce yourself by name and credentials prior to touching the patient. Even if the patient has severe cognitive impairments that limit communication, always speak with them as if they can hear and understand you.
- Sometimes it can be helpful to ask the family how their child communicates with them. This allows you to better understand how they may communicate with you during a physical exam. This may include gestures, signing, eye gaze, moaning or vocalizing, or physical touch. Children with disabilities may have better receptive language skills than expressive language skills.
- Ask caregivers about any difficulties that could arise during the exam. Often, caregivers can provide suggestions for how to accomplish more difficult parts of the exam such as the best way to examine the patient's mouth or ears.
- Allow time for the patient to get used to your presence before examining them. Be sensitive to sensory issues they may have like not liking their head being touched or being sensitive to loud noises. Some patients will calm to the sound of their favorite song or by seeing or holding a beloved toy or comfort object.

Examining the patient:

- Talk to your patient throughout the exam and prepare them for the next part of the physical exam.
- Allow your patient to remain in a comfortable position and clothed for as long as possible. A child who has spasticity or uses a wheelchair may become uncom-

fortable on an exam table for the duration of a visit. Though there may be limitations to how the exam takes place, most patients will need to be moved from their wheelchair to examine their back and genitourinary areas.

- Be flexible with the exam. Sometimes a patient will become overwhelmed and require a break. When able, use play or distraction to help facilitate the exam.
- Don't be afraid to ask for help. Transferring patient from the wheelchair to table may require two people. Some patients will need to be restrained by more people than just their caregiver for critical portions of the exam. Always try to use the least restrictive restraint that is needed and clarify with your clinical instructor prior to restraining a patient.
- Some children with disabilities have medical technology dependence. These may include a tracheostomy and ventilator, gastrostomy tube, and mobility aids like braces. When in doubt, ask the caregiver or your clinical instructor the best way to examine a patient with these devices.
  - Tracheostomy ties should not be removed during routine care, and the tracheostomy should not be manipulated unless under supervision.
  - Gastrostomy tubes can be touched and turned gently, but be careful to keep tubes away from the patient's hands as they may pull the tube out. Gastrojejunostomy tubes should not be manipulated.

Pain Assessment in Pediatric Patients

Assessing pain can be challenging in pediatric patients due to variability in child development and pain presentation. Pain expression looks different in infants compared with school-age children or adolescents and can be particularly challenging in the child with developmental or intellectual disabilities. There are a variety of validated pain scales that can be used to help assess pain and discomfort and can be incorporated into the physical exam during a pain assessment (Table 3.1). It is important to use the correct pain scale for the clinical scenario and to frequently reassess the patient after procedures and/or interventions. Some pain scales are validated for postoperative pain, others assess sedation or procedural pain, and most pain scales are validated for specific age groups.

In general, pain often presents with physical signs, some of which are visible during examination. Pain can lead to changes in vital signs including tachycardia, hypertension, and tachypnea. It can also be visible as changes in facial expression or grimace, increased crying or withdrawn or tired appearance, writhing and constant movement, or guarding and staying very still. The reason for the pain and developmental age affect and influence pain behaviors. For example, a young toddler may hit their head or pull their hair if they are having a headache, while an adolescent might retreat to a dark room and be very quiet or withdrawn when

Table 3.1 Examples of validated pain scales for pediatric patients

Pain scale	Method of assessment	Population
Neonatal Pain Agitation and Sedation Scale (N-PASS)	Observational scale of pain behaviors, five categories with five-point scale (−2 to +2). Sedation is categorized with negative numbers and pain with positive numbers	Neonates, sedated neonates, postoperative patients
Crying, Requires Oxygen, Increased Vital Signs, Expression, and Sleeplessness (CRIES)	Observational scale of pain behaviors, five categories with three-point scale	Neonatal, postoperative patients
Faces, Legs, Activity, Cry, Consolability Scale (FLACC)	Observational scale of pain behaviors, five categories with three-point scale	Validated in young children, used in 0–18 years, postoperative patients
Revised Faces, Legs, Activity, Cry, Consolability Scale (R-FLACC)	Observational scale of pain behaviors based on FLACC with added patient-centered pain behaviors, tailored for the child with cognitive impairment or oral communication difficulties	Nonverbal children or children with cognitive impairments

experiencing similar pain. A child with appendicitis will avoid rapid movements and show guarding during an abdominal exam, while a child with gastroenteritis may writhe in pain intermittently.

For all patients, assessing pain requires integration of the physical exam with a thorough pain history. Children are often able to start using some basic pain language like "hurt" or "ouch" at two years old but often struggle to localize pain or relay information about the timing of pain until they are approximately 7 years old. Children as young as 3 years of age can use the Faces Pain Scale-Revised, Wong-Baker FACES scale, or Oucher scales, which have greater reliability as the patient ages. These scales use facial depictions of pain either with cartoon drawings of faces or photographs of children in progressive levels of distress accompanied by a numerical scale. Children ages 7 years and above can use numerical pain scales to indicate the severity of their pain, with pain expression becoming more advanced as language skills and cognitive development improve.

Pain expression can look different in children with cognitive impairment and developmental disabilities. The most reliable indicators of pain for a child with cognitive impairment are their individual pain behaviors and knowledge of the patient's baseline. For some children, this can include changes in tone, tremors or abnormal movements, head banging or breath holding, screaming, and other verbal outbursts. Discussions with caregivers who know the child's baseline communication patterns are therefore necessary in evaluating pain for the child. For children with developmental disabilities, consider using a measurement method consistent with their developmental level or a scale developed for these patients specifically.

Further Readings

Krechel SW, Bildner J. CRIES: a new neonatal postoperative pain measurement score. Initial testing of validity and reliability. Paediatr Anaesth. 1995;5(1):53–61. https://doi.org/10.1111/j.1460-9592.1995.tb00242.x.

Merkel SI, Voepel-Lewis T, Shayevitz JR, Malviya S. The FLACC: a behavioral scale for scoring postoperative pain in young children. Pediatr Nurs. 1997;23(3):293–7.

Tsze DS, von Baeyer CL, Bulloch B, Dayan PS. Validation of self-report pain scales in children. Pediatrics. 2013;132(4):e971–9. https://doi.org/10.1542/peds.2013-1509. Epub 2013 Sep 2.

Chapter 4
Challenging Conversations in Pediatrics

Melanie C. Marsh

Introduction

Learning effective communication skills is vital for having productive and appropriate daily interactions with patients, their caretakers, and other professionals in our healthcare team. Medical professionals, particularly medical students, may feel ill-equipped to handle certain patient's scenarios, especially when sharing potentially life altering news. Difficult discussions in the field of pediatrics pose unique challenges, different from those in adult medicine. We must navigate family dynamics while delivering meaningful, age-appropriate messages to children and their caregivers. We may have limited experience in these conversations as they fortunately happen less frequently in pediatrics. What may be an everyday occurrence to one family could be considered life altering or difficult to another, thus further emphasizing the importance of meeting the family where they are. This chapter will review some strategies to build confidence in these types of discussions.

What patients and caretakers want:

- Uninterrupted face-to-face communication
- Clear and honest communication
- Information given in understandable terms
- Emotional support
- Time to ask questions

M. C. Marsh (✉)
Hospital Pediatrics, Advocate Children's Hospital, Park Ridge, IL, USA
e-mail: Melanie.Marsh@aah.org

N. Liao et al. (eds.), *Pediatric Rotations*,
https://doi.org/10.1007/978-3-031-59873-9_4

Specific Patient Scenarios

Breaking Bad News/Sharing Life Altering News

It is normal to feel just as nervous or anxious about these meetings as your families. Preparing and planning in advance can be highly instrumental for success. All essential team members should consider having a planning meeting separate from the family first. Depending on the age of the child, it may be helpful to have two separate meetings: one first with the caregiver (where the focus is specially to plan what should be shared with the child) and one with the caregiver and child. Assigning a non-parent family member or friend to document/take notes during the meeting can be helpful to relieve this burden from parents. See Table 4.1 for the modified SPIKES protocol for delivering bad news.

Table 4.1 An approach to breaking bad news (SPIKES)—modified for pediatrics

Important components	Successes	Pitfalls
Setting	• Make sure everyone who needs to be there is present (this includes medical team members and pertinent family members) • Determine if child is going to participate in the meeting • Make sure there is comfortable seating for everyone involved and that everyone is seated at eye level • If needed, ensure that in-person interpreters are secured in advance • All team members should introduce themselves and their role	• Having too many people in the room or multiple people talking at once • Distractions/pagers going off • People entering and leaving the room during the meeting • Having young children, including siblings present at time of discussion
Perception	• First ask what the family already knows; often the family is aware of the diagnosis or the news before it is shared • Expand upon this foundation	• Assuming that all family members are on the same page or have the same educational background
Involvement	• Set an agenda at the beginning • Acknowledge and include any cultural, racial, and religious beliefs (this can affect how information is shared) • Pause often and ensure the family has ample time/opportunity for questions	• Paternalistic, medical provider-driven discussion (what you may think is the most important part of the talk may be what the parent cares about least)

Table 4.1 (continued)

Important components	Successes	Pitfalls
Knowledge	• Limit information to several key points • Check often for family's understanding • Plan for follow-up meetings to discuss in depth detail • Use visuals and diagrams when pertinent • Acknowledge uncertainty	• Use of medical jargon, fast pacing • One-way conversations • Overly positive or negative conversation (balance hope and realism)
Emotion, empathy	• Acknowledge emotions and feelings in the room (use expressions like I understand how this could be a surprise) • Empathize with the family; It is ok to wish for something different for the family (i.e., I wish I had different news for you) • Validate the emotional responses and explore with follow-up questioning	• Saying things like "I know how you must feel" • Including personal stories (this is not a time for you to share about your family members or friends)
Strategy, summary, and self-reflection	• Reflect back to the family what was said, use teach back method • Ensure the family has had enough time to process the shared information (it will likely take multiple discussions before most of what was said is heard) • Establish a timeline for further discussions and next steps • Provide information about support services (social work, spiritual care)	• Continuing a path where emotions are explored but no plan is set in place • Allowing personal and professional boundaries to cross

Adapted from Baile WF, Buckman R, Lenzi R, Glober G, Beale EA, Kudelka AP. SPIKES-A six-step protocol for delivering bad news: application to the patient with cancer. Oncologist. 2000;5(4):302–11. doi: 10.1634/theoncologist.5-4-302. PMID: 10964998

De-escalating Upset Families

Caregivers, parents, and family members may feel angry for a variety of reasons. Sometimes it may seem more reasonable or justified than other times, but all portrayed emotions require thoughtful communication to maintain a respectful and strong medical provider-family alliance. Table 4.2 outlines one standardized method for approaching these situations:

Table 4.2 How to use "Take the HEAT" practically

Elements	Best practices and tips
Hear the family out (introduction, initiation of conversation, listening, and nonverbal skills)	• Introduce self, use patient name, sit down • Acknowledge there is a concern and actively solicit information • Stay fully attentive without distraction/disengaged behavior • Allow patients to completely discuss concerns, provide verbal and nonverbal acknowledgment that you are listening
Empathize (further explore and validate emotion or parent/patient experience; acknowledge emotional state of patient/parent)	• Interpret implicit or unstated message behind patient/parent emotion and offer sympathetic statements • Ask open-ended questions and offer validating or normalizing statements through open dialogue
Apologize	• State "I'm sorry" and respond to patient emotion (e.g. "I am sorry that you are upset") • Apologize for any errors, if appropriate
Take action (verbal commitment to next steps)	• Discuss specific action steps to be personally taken and indicated when/how follow up with the family will occur • Provide a summative statement, gain agreement to the plan from family, ask if family has additional questions/needs

Adapted from Delacruz N, Reed S, Splinter A, et al. Take the HEAT: A pilot study on improving communication with angry families. Patient Educ Couns. 2017;100(6):1235–1239. doi:10.1016/j.pec.2016.12.012

Tricky Topics-Gun Safety, Vaccine Hesitancy, Child Abuse Concerns

Gun Safety

Gun safety can be an emotionally loaded and polarizing topic for many families. The conversation should be incorporated into anticipatory guidance for age-appropriate safety, to avoid making it seem that it is a conversation about personal preferences. It is not against the law to discuss and counsel on firearm safety.

Why Guns Are a Risk

– Most adolescent suicides occur in the home, and guns may be in the home (often owned by the parent)
– Most acts are impulsive (with time to action <5 min)

- There is high fatality with firearm-associated suicide attempts, more than any other means
- Many school-age children know where the firearm is kept in the house, even if parents think they do not

Safety Steps

- The first recommendation is to remove the gun(s) from the home
- If families plan to keep the gun(s), they should be (1) unloaded, (2) locked in a safe, and (3) stored separately from ammunition

How to Make Counseling Relevant to Milestones

At a minimum, counseling should be incorporated into well child checks. And more often for families at high risk, including those with history of domestic violence, emotion/mental/physical bullying, prior mental health concerns, and/or known history of drug or alcohol abuse.

Birth: This can be a time of significant change for families. New parents might be open to changes for the safety of their child. Incorporating this type of discussion from the beginning will make the counseling seem less intrusive later and appear as just a part of a routine visit.

Toddler: Children are starting to explore and often do not understand the concept of "no" or do have lasting memory about dangerous items. Similar to opening cabinets with cleaning solutions or medicines, children will look and find things that seem interesting but may in fact be lethal.

Preschool: These children are more curious, looking for cause and effect, and are likely to play at other's homes. However, they continue to lack judgment about consequences. They may also not share with parents or know how to tell parents if there is something unsafe in their environment. Encourage families to ask questions of other parents. It can be normalizing by framing it about their child.

Child: School-age children may not be supervised as often. They may also have seen gun-related violence in videos or the media. They may try "play enacting" things they have seen.

Adolescent: Children in this age group are more likely to be risk-takers and can be pressured by peers. They may also display impulsive behaviors and experiment with alcohol and drugs, which disinhibit behaviors even further.

Vaccine Hesitancy

Vaccine hesitancy is a complicated medical and social issue. Many factors contribute to this (Table 4.3), and there are no easy or quick solutions. A critical first step is for the medical team to create strong rapport with families because it can help to make vaccine counseling more effective. The American Academy of Pediatrics (AAP) partnered with the FrameWorks Institute to recommend the following evidence-based talking points:

- Talk about the benefits of vaccination for the common good
- Talk about improving vaccine access as a preventive public health measure
- Focus on how vaccines are beneficial to the child's long-term health and well-being
- Use computer or smartphone updates metaphor to explain how the immune system improves its performance through vaccination
- Use a literacy metaphor to explain how the immune system learns how to respond to viruses through vaccination

Additional steps to take when talking about vaccines:

If no concerns for vaccine hesitancy:

1. Present the vaccinations as "due" as part of routine healthcare and disease prevention
   (a) For example, say, "The flue vaccine is due today"
2. Ask for clarifying questions or concerns

Table 4.3 Contributors to vaccine hesitancy

Caregiver factors	Medical provider factors	Combined factors
Concerns for vaccine safety (i.e., development of autism, painful to the child, vaccine additives, vaccines causing illness such as influenza, etc.)	Insufficient time to provide dedicated, thoughtful counseling	Poor rapport
Uncertainty regarding the necessity of vaccines (i.e., diseases being prevented are not serious such as chicken pox, not all vaccines are needed such as HPV in a child who is not sexually active, flu vaccines are sometimes not fully effective so why give?)	Little to no reimbursement for nurse-only visits and nursing counseling	Dissemination of false information (via social media, community or religious leaders, etc.)
Lack of vaccine knowledge	Lack of deep understanding of caregiver barriers and fears	
Mistrust (i.e., pharmaceutical companies, medical professionals, or the government)	Discomfort and limited experience in providing vaccine counseling	

If suspected concerns for vaccine hesitancy:

1. Budget additional time to understand the root cause. Ask about their questions and concerns.
2. Acknowledge their concerns
   (a) For example, say, "It makes sense to me, after you explained it, why you would be concerned."
3. Seek permission to correct misconceptions. Examples:
   (a) "Would it be ok for me to explain a little further how vaccines are developed/tested?"
   (b) "Would it be ok for me to explain a little more about why the flu vaccines cannot give someone the flu?"
4. Explain what clinical trials are and review the safety of vaccines but be open about what is known about immunizations and what is not known.
5. Review reasons for vaccination and risks of not immunizing in a nonconfrontational way
   (a) Use stories or anecdotes, share if you have a personal experience with taking care of a child with vaccine-preventable illness
6. Reiterate importance of the current recommended schedule. Alternative vaccine schedules have not been evaluated for better safety or efficacy.
7. Present the vaccinations as required for routine healthcare and disease prevention

For more resources to help tackle these discussions, visit the AAP website. https://www.aap.org/en/patient-care/immunizations/communicating-with-families-and-promoting-vaccine-confidence/.

Child Abuse Concerns

Those who care for children are in a unique and vital position to identify and prevent child abuse. It is never an easy or pleasant conversation but one that needs to happen even when suspicion is low. It is important to remind parents that your job is not to uncover what happened or potential perpetrators of the abuse but rather to identify injuries and imminent harm. If you focus on the medical management and not the social situation, these cases can be less daunting. Of course, your job also includes contacting the appropriate personnel to complete the social/safety investigation. Leaving this role to persons specifically trained in child abuse is better for you and for the child. It is common to make the mistake of launching into the social aspect of the incident, but this carries the risk of potentially confusing the child further and compromising later formal forensic interviews. Table 4.4 outlines several issues that may arise in these scenarios and strategies on how to approach them.

Table 4.4 Sample strategies to consider during discussions involving possible child abuse [1]

Challenges	Proposed strategies
Once child maltreatment is broached, the parent seems to "shut down"	• Despite the possibility of child abuse, remember that a parent may him/herself be the victim of violence and discrimination, and "shutting down" may be a learned response to the judgments of others, to fear, to anxiety, or to worry—as well as the possibility of non-cooperative guilt. • Establish rapport and ensure confidentiality but clarify: "Everything we discuss today is confidential unless I feel that you or someone else is at risk. If that is a concern, then we will discuss things together"
It may be challenging to provide respect and kindness to a parent who may have hurt a child or been complicit in them getting hurt	• You may experience "moral distress" when dealing with families suspected of abuse, since it is natural to be protective of the child; yet as should be the case for all critically ill children, appropriate support for the parents should be offered, including a bereavement counselor, chaplain, or other persons identified by the parents as providing important psychological and spiritual support. • Acknowledging and naming this possibility of conflict is an important first step; recognizing that a "defensive parent" is also reacting to a high-stress situation; compassion, understanding, and nonjudgmental must be intentional
I am not familiar with my ethical or legal obligations in balancing limits to parent autonomy vs the duty to protect the child	• The pediatric ethical assumption of a "best interest standard" complicates matters, since a parent has wide latitude in deciding what is in their child's interest. However, physical, sexual, emotional, or psychological abuse of any kind is never in the best interest of the child. Hence, you have a moral/ethical obligation to act when suspected child abuse occurs. • Avoiding confrontation with the family may be a foregone conclusion and is NOT a reason not to report. On the other hand, "confrontation" may also be managed in a compassionate, empathetic way using the HEAT principles
What can I do to establish rapport quickly?	• Families will feel supported and put their trust in you if you take time to establish rapport. Trying to build trust with the family, however difficult in cases of child abuse, is critical to an optimal outcome. • Nonverbal communication is just as important as verbal communication. • Take the time to sit down and look everyone in the eye. • In suspected child abuse, some forms of communication (e.g., smiling) may not be appropriate, but the ability to communicate concern—verbally and nonverbally—is essential. • Suspected child abuse cases are just as serious as definitive child abuse and will require a similar commitment of resources

Addressing Students' Feelings

The health and happiness of our patients and their families are of utmost importance. But, also important is the long-term mental health and professional sustainability for our healthcare colleagues. It is easy to believe that difficult situations and conversations get better with time. However, just because we have been doing something for a long time doesn't necessarily mean that we are better at it. In fact, dealing with these types of situations repeatedly without practicing these skills or debriefing after challenging events can lead to burn out. Burn out can negatively affect patient care in many ways including poor communication, medical errors, and negligence. It is essential that we not only protect patients as the first victim but also health care workers as potential *second victims*.

Second Victim Syndrome/Phenomenon

The concept was first described in 2000 by Dr. Albert W Wu in his article on medical error. The second victim syndrome/phenomenon occurs in response to a traumatic event involving a patient that causes distress and unrest to the healthcare provider who feels responsible for the outcome. There are several stages of this process (Fig. 4.1).

If we don't focus on supporting each other and creating a culture of acceptance and empathy, many of us will never reach the final stage in a positive way. It is especially important that we support each other during our medical education as trainees can be particularly susceptible to second victim syndrome, which can affect confidence and professional identity. See Table 4.5 for steps to support a second victim.

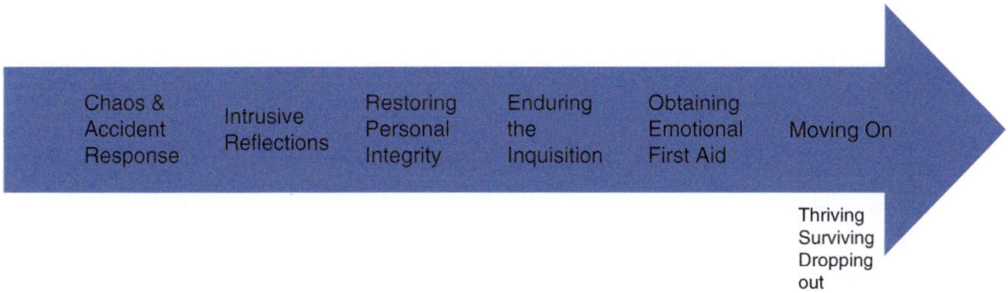

Fig. 4.1 Stages of second victim recovery trajectory. (Adapted from Scott SD, Hirschinger LE, Cox KR, McCoig M, Brandt J, Hall LW. The natural history of recovery for the healthcare provider "second victim" after adverse patient events. Quality and Safety in Health Care. 2009;18(5):325–30. doi:10.1136/qshc.2009.032870)

Table 4.5 Providing peer support to a second victim

Recognition	Second victims may demonstrate: • Deviation from normal behavior • Emotional overreactions to stimuli • Decreased morale (low energy, little enthusiasm, cynical, decreased communication, etc.) • Difficulty in concentration and confusion • Lower job efficiency • Avoidance of friends, colleagues, classmates
Understanding and compassion	Create a safe environment for discussion based on understanding and compassion and in which the assumption is that the intentions of the provider were good. Do not admonish or punished the person for their errors. Recognize human fallibility
Supportive care	Engage in active listening • Clarification—Giving or requesting more information for better understanding. • Paraphrasing—Rephrasing back what you just heard. • Reflection • Summarization—Summarizing the conversation, recapping major points of interest Do say • Are you OK? • What do you need? • How are you feeling? • I know you didn't intend to cause harm. I know it's so hard to tell a patient about that diagnosis. I know it's so hard to care for a patient whose family is angry. Do NOT say • Everything will be OK • Don't worry about it
Referral	If you feel more support is needed, offer opportunities to employer assistance programs or similar counseling opportunities in the setting of psychological stress

Adapted from Pratt S, Kenney L, Scott SD, Wu AW. How to develop a second victim support program: a toolkit for health care organizations. Jt Comm J Qual Patient Saf. 2012 May;38(5):235–40, 193. doi: 10.1016/s1553-7250(12)38030-6. PMID: 22649864 and Merandi J, Liao N, Lewe D, Morvay S, Stewart B, Catt C, Scott SD. Deployment of a Second Victim Peer Support Program: A Replication Study. Pediatr Qual Saf. 2017 Jun 21;2(4):e031. doi: 10.1097/pq9.0000000000000031. PMID: 30229168; PMCID: PMC6132481

Building Resilience

It is sometimes unclear what makes one person more resilient than the next in challenging scenarios. But just like any other skill, the most important piece of resiliency is continued practice. There are often workshops or courses offered at medical schools that focus on adaptations in the face of stress specific to a career in medicine. Take advantage of these resources before traumatic or challenging situations occur. They can help us feel more prepared when we encounter something challenging. Most importantly, focus on self-care; re-engage in things that provide enjoyment, pursue hobbies, cultivate social connections, spend time outdoors, and make sure sleep and physical needs are being met. And finally, we should be kinder to ourselves.

Reference

1. Melanie C Marsh, Suzanne M Reed, John D Mahan, Lydia Schneider, Ashley K Fernandes, Nancy Liao, Isaac Spears, Stephanie Lauden. Advanced Multimodal Communication Curriculum for Pediatric Residents. J Med Educ Curric Dev. 2021;8:23821205211035239. https://doi.org/10.1177/23821205211035239. eCollection 2021 Jan-Dec.

Further Reading

Alelwani SM, Ahmed YA. Medical training for communication of bad news: a literature review. J Educ Health Promot. 2014;3:51. https://doi.org/10.4103/2277-9531.134737.

Christian CW, et al. The evaluation of suspected child physical abuse. Pediatrics. 2015;135(5):e1337–54. https://doi.org/10.1542/peds.2015-0356.

Edwards KM, Hackell JM, THE COMMITTEE ON INFECTIOUS DISEASES TCOPAAM. Countering vaccine hesitancy. Pediatrics. 2016;138(3):e20162146. https://doi.org/10.1542/peds.2016-2146.

Wolfe AD, Frierdich SA, Wish J, Kilgore-Carlin J, Plotkin JA, Hoover-Regan M. Sharing life-altering information: development of pediatric hospital guidelines and team training. J Palliat Med. 2014;17(9):1011–8. https://doi.org/10.1089/jpm.2013.0620.

Chapter 5
Presenting Patients

Mohammed Najjar

Background

Oral case presentation in clinical settings is the most important and most frequently used method of communication among the members of patient care team. The goal of oral case presentation is to pass along relevant patient information (history, physical examination, laboratory results, and the presenter's understanding of the case) in an organized and efficient way for a specific audience to develop similar clinical understanding of patient's medical problem and reach similar diagnostic conclusion in order to develop shared management plan.

Oral case presentations play an important and unique role in medical education. It allows the presenter (learner) to plan questions and actions before the patient interview, to synthesize the information for the oral presentation, and to learn from the feedback. The preceptor will have a chance to identify areas for growth knowledge and suggest points for improvement.

Presenting Patients

General guidelines for oral presentations

- Brief yet succinct to maintain listener's attention. Should be 3–10 min, depending on the type of presentation.
- Emphasis on the "history of present illness" and the "assessment and plan"

M. Najjar (✉)
Division of Hospital Medicine, Department of Pediatrics, Nationwide Children's Hospital/
The Ohio State University College of Medicine, Columbus, OH, USA
e-mail: Mohammed.Najjar@nationwidechildrens.org

N. Liao et al. (eds.), *Pediatric Rotations*,
https://doi.org/10.1007/978-3-031-59873-9_5

- Presented from memory and presenter should keep eye contact with listeners during presentation. May refer to notes intermittently.
- Differs from written case presentation. Only mention relevant and pertinent facts that are expected to help listeners understand the current problem(s) and reach similar conclusions.

New Admission to Inpatient Service

Purpose: Organize the presenter; present enough information for listener(s) to understand the chief complaint and build a differential diagnosis and management plan; allow the presenter to explain the medical reasoning that led to the assessment and management plan; give the instructor/preceptor a chance to assess the presenter, offer input, and provide feedback.

Basic structure:

- Chief complaint
- History of present illness
- Relevant information from family, social, and past medical history
- Physical examination
- Laboratory and imaging
- Assessment and plan

Chief complaint: contains four elements, presented in one sentence:

- Patient's age and sex
- Patient's active and ongoing medical problems (three to four most relevant and mentioned by name only)
- Patient's reason for presentation/admission
- Duration of symptoms
- No surprises should appear in the history of present illness after the chief complaint sentence

Chief Complaint
John is a 7-year-old male with history of well controlled mild intermittent asthma presented with 3 days of congestion, cough, and increase work of breathing.

History of present illness (HPI) is the essential part of the oral presentation and the source of approximately 90% of the correct diagnosis.

Components:

- All "positive" statements (i.e., what occurred) precedes "negative" elements (i.e., what was absent).

– “Positive” statements are presented in chronological order with attention to details.
– If the current problem is related to the patient’s past medical history, the HPI begins with one to two sentences to summarize this problem using (date of diagnosis, how was the diagnosis made, current symptoms and treatment, complications, and objective measures of the chronic problem available (e.g., Hemoglobin A1C for diabetes, most recent surgical revision for ventriculoperitoneal shunt).
– “Negative” statements include three main categories of findings that are important to mention: (1) constitutional elements, (2) signs and symptoms relevant to the system of chief complaint, i.e., if patient has dysuria, mention no discoloration of urine, no flak pain, etc. (3) important risk factors, such as prenatal exposure, second-hand smoke exposure, etc. Ask yourself: “What could my patient have been exposed to cause this presentation?”
– Brief description of medical care, prior relevant lab results and medical management if the patient had been seen previously for the same problem in primary care, urgent care, or the emergency department, or had been transferred from another hospital, etc.

Chief Complaint	<u>Example of a presentation on a patient newly admitted to the hospital.</u> John is a 7 year old male with history of well controlled mild intermittent asthma presented with 3 days of congestion, cough and increase work of breathing.
Relevant Past Medical History (PMH)	John has a history of mild intermittent asthma, first diagnosed when he was 3 year old. His asthma has been well controlled with PRN Albuterol inhaler with spacer and last admission for asthma exacerbation was more than one year ago. No PICU admissions.
Current problem “Positive” elements, pay attention to chronology and details.	Patient started to have congestion, runny nose, and dry cough 3 days prior to presentation. Albuterol as needed was helping during the first 2 days, however over the last 24 hours it wasn’t. His mother noticed increased work of breathing and exercise intolerance, so she brought him to the Emergency Department (ED).
“Negative” elements: constitutional complaints, other elements relevant to targeted system, and important risk factors.	There is no history of fever, weight loss, diaphoresis, edema or decreased oral intake. No history of sputum production, hemoptysis, chest pain, or cyanosis. His mother denied recent significant exposure to allergens like dogs, cats, or pollens. Of note, his brother recently had an upper respiratory infection (URI).
Prior evaluation	In ED: John was found to have moderate increase work of breathing and tight chest. He received a dose of systemic steroid, dual inhalation therapy (Albuterol and Ipratropium) X3 with minimal improvement so IV line was inserted and a dose of parenteral Magnesium sulfate was given. Patient improved. He was then admitted to the inpatient service for further management.

Past Medical and Surgical History, Family History, Social History, and medications: Present only relevant information from family, social and past medical history: brief summary of other PMH elements including growth and developmental milestones, medications, relevant family and social histories. You should obtain this information in detail but only present what is most relevant.

Presentation of Past Medical and Surgical History, Family History, Social History, and Medications

He has a history of eczema and allergic rhinitis. He is on Zyrtec 10 mg once daily, hydrocortisone 1% cream PRN and lotion. There is no family history of asthma.

Physical Examination (PE): Start with a short statement to summarize vital signs, then mention all abnormal findings on PE. Among normal findings, only mention pertinent negative findings.

Presentation of the PE

On PE, Patient is a febrile, has tachypnea respiratory rate of 35–40 bpm, tachycardia with heart rate 140–150 bpm, normal blood pressure, and saturation above 94% on room. He has mild intercostal and subcostal retractions, generalized expiratory wheezing with mild decreased air entry over lung bases. No nasal flaring, no cyanosis, no crackles, and no rhonchi. His capillary refills <2 s. Ear nose and throat exam is normal except for clear rhinorrhea and nasal congestion. Cardiovascular examination is within normal limits except for the tachycardia.

Laboratory testing and imaging: Include all abnormal laboratory and imaging findings. Compare the results with previous testing if available. Among normal laboratory tests and imaging, mention only pertinent negatives and present the results as they appear in traditional order (Electrolytes: Sodium/Potassium/Chloride/Co2/BUN/Cr/Glucose). Provide your interpretation of the findings.

Presentation of the Labs and Imaging

No laboratory testing was performed in the ED. CXR shows bilateral streaky consolidations involving lower lobes. Most probably atelectasis in this clinical setting.

Assessment and plan: This is one of the most important components of the oral presentation. Begin your assessment with a "positive" statement that includes age, gender, and relevant past medical history; Then move to mentioning only significant symptoms, signs, PE, laboratory, and imaging; Then present the differential diagnosis.

- List three to five differential diagnosis starting with the most to the least probable. Mention why certain diagnosis is likely or less likely according to your medical reasoning.
- If the patient has more than one problem or diagnosis, list each problem separately and have a differential diagnosis for each.
- Discuss the management plan, your justification for these decisions, and possible anticipated side effects.

If you are presenting a patient after a night call, add one to two sentences to update the team about what happened and what treatment you gave overnight.

Presentation of an Assessment and Plan
John is a 7-year-old male, known to have well-controlled mild intermittent asthma, presented with 3 days of congestion, cough, and increased work of breathing. PE is significant for no hypoxia, moderate respiratory distress, wheezing, and mildly decreased air entry in both lung bases. Presentation is most likely due to status asthmaticus triggered by viral infection with bilateral lung atelectasis, confirmed by CXR. This is not likely to be foreign body aspiration or vocal cord dysfunction. In the ED, he received albuterol and ipratropium nebulizer treatments, systemic steroids, and then magnesium sulfate due to poor clinical response of initial asthma exacerbation treatment. He was then admitted to the floor in stable condition.

Overnight he was continued on the asthma pathway with Q2 hour albuterol treatments and systemic steroids. He has stable saturations on room air, and his vital signs are within normal limits except for mild tachycardia.

Daily Presentation in Inpatient Service

Purpose: Inform listener(s) of events from the past 24 h; focused discussion about the assessment and update the management plan; allow presenter to explain medical reasoning behind decisions.

Structure: Start with an opening one liner to remind listener(s) of the patient name, age, chief complaint, working diagnosis, reason for hospitalization, and duration of hospitalization.

You can then use the Subjective, Objective, Assessment and Plan (SOAP) structure to present your facts.

- Subjective (S): Highlight changes in clinical status as communicated by patient or family members.
- Objective (O): Present objective data collected from chart review and your encounter with the patient. Vital signs (ranges); intake and output, key PE find-

ings (highlight changes over the last 24 h), and updates in labs and imaging with you interpretation of data.

- Assessment (A): You can present assessment as detailed in the H&P section.
- Plan (P): Present your plan by problem or by organ system(s). Choose as many organ systems as you see fit for your patient's condition. Early on during practice, it is preferable to go through the main categories in your head to make sure you are not missing any relevant areas. The broad organ system categories include: neurological; psychiatric; cardiovascular; pulmonary; gastrointestinal; renal/genitourinary; hematologic/oncologic; endocrine/metabolic; infectious; tubes/lines/drains. Include any recommendations from consultants. Always include discharge criteria and plan to set clear expectations and improve communication.

Notes

Consider using system-based presentation of the plan for complicated patients with many problems during the current hospitalization. Consider using problem-based presentations for patients with more simple presentations.

SOAP structure can be used for oral presentation and for note writing.

Family-Centered Rounds

Family-centered care was recommended by the Institute of Medicine as an essential component to improve patient safety, communication, and quality of care. Family-Centered Round (FCR) has become a corner-stone for family centered care in inpatient pediatrics services in the United States and Canada. It is defined as multidisciplinary bedside rounds whereby both the patient and family are able to participate in medical decision-making. This multidisciplinary team includes the physician and the bedside nurse and can include a case manager, social worker, pharmacist, dietitian, respiratory therapist, physical therapist, occupational therapist, discharge planner, consulting physicians, and learners. The size of the team is usually determined by the patient's needs, case complexity, and the availability of resources in the institution.

Components of FCR are described by Muething, et al.

- *On admission*: A staff member describes the process of FCR to the family. The family decides how rounds are conducted: at bedside, family joins the team outside of the patient's room or family chooses not to participate in rounds and only receives an update by the responsible physician or nurse after rounds.
- *On rounds*: the intern or medical student responsible for the patient:
- Enter the room first to wake the family and reconfirm their interest in joining rounds.
- Introduces the team, explains the process and goals of FCR, welcomes family involvement and their right to interrupt to correct a mistake in the history or to clarify medical terminology.

- Presents the case using simple language. Eye contact is made with the team and family members. The family is included in discussing management plan and discharge goals.
- To increase efficiency: team members are assigned roles and could complete certain tasks during rounds. This includes placing orders, discharge summaries, prescriptions, and home care plans. Additionally, the presence of nurses and other relevant staff member like pharmacists, dietitians, and discharge planners should improve communication and efficiency in decision-making process.
- The supervising physician (attending physician, fellow or senior resident) oversees the process. They may correct professionalism and communication difficulties. The supervising physician can model appropriate behaviors and pick opportunities for bedside teaching. The patient's family must be informed and agree upon this process.

Notes
You can use oral presentation skills detailed above for family-centered rounds but make sure to use clear and simplified language for patients and families to understand.

Outpatient Oral Presentation

There are four common types of visits for pediatrics outpatient clinics:

- New outpatient visits
- Well child checks
- Follow-up patient visits
- Patients presenting for an acute problem

Oral presentations for each type of visit have a unique purpose. Use the general principles detailed above to present each category in a precise way and emphasize the components that are most important for the type of visit. As with other types of presentations, outpatient oral presentations help to organize the student thought processes and give the preceptor a chance to assess the presentation, offer input, and provide feedback.

General Structure:

- Reason for the visit: to establish care, address specific patient's concerns (acute illness, medication referral, referrals, etc.), assess growth and development, etc.
- Relevant acute or subacute history
- Review of systems
- Past medical, surgical, family, and social histories
- Growth and diet
- Developmental milestones
- Medications and allergies

- Sexual history, if appropriate
- Smoking, alcohol or other drug use
- Vital signs and physical examination
- Relevant labs and imaging
- Assessment and plan

New Outpatient Visit

Purpose: Review patient's past and current history and address new concerns; identify health problems that need further evaluation and/or treatment.

Well Child Check

Purpose: Review patient's past and current history; focus on developmental milestones growth and diet; review and catch up on vaccinations; practice anticipatory guidance and preventative medicine; review of medications.

Follow-Up Patient's Visits

Purpose: Review relevant interval heath care events; identify new health care problems and address them; review of medications and make appropriate changes.

Patients Presenting for an Acute Problem to the Primary Care Physician (PCP)

Purpose: Identify, risk factors in patient's history that could have led to the acute visit; give presenter a chance to practice reasoning and generate appropriate assessment and plan.

Special Considerations when Presenting Pediatric Patient

Intake and Output

Reporting intake and output is important on daily presentations for pediatric inpatients. Details of this report are usually discussed with bedside nurse and nurse assistants before or during rounds. The intake specifies all what goes in patient's body over a period, usually 24 h (enteral feeding, parenteral nutrition/IV hydration, IV flushes, etc.). The output represents that which comes out of the body (urine output, emesis, output from drains, liquid stools, etc.)

The purpose is to assess nutritional status of a patient (volume of formula feeding of an infant, time of breast feeding, volume of enteral tube feeding, food intake and frequency to enable caloric counts) and hydration status (enteral and parenteral fluid intake, volume of fluids with IV medications, frequency of vomiting, frequency and consistency of stooling, volume of surgical wound drain, etc.). Additional information can be determined according to patient's situation (for example patients with chest tube and pleural effusion: volume, amount, color, and consistency of drained pleural fluids are important to determine management plan; patients with diabetes insipidus: volume of each void and its relation to the timing of deamino D-arginine vasopressin (DDAVP) dose is important to adjusting the medication).

Growth and Weight Gain in Infants and Children

The mean weight of a full term newborn is 3.25 kg (+/− 0.9 kg). Infants could lose 6–10% of birth weight during the first 5–7 days of life secondary to normal diuresis of excess fluid after birth. They regain birth weight around day 10 of life. Infants then are expected to gain 30 g (+/− 15 g) every day for the first 3 months of their lives. They usually triple their birth weight by 1 year of age.

It is important to interpret anthropometrics (height, weight, head circumference, and calculated Body Mass Index (BMI)) according to age at least once during every inpatient and outpatient pediatric visit. Growth should be evaluated over time by plotting these values on growth charts. The Center for Disease Control and Prevention (CDC) recommends that health care providers in the United States use the World Health Organization (WHO) growth charts to monitor growth for infants up to 24 months of age, then use the CDC growth charts for children age 2 years and older. You can download WHO and CDC growth charts from the CDC website. https://www.cdc.gov/growthcharts/.

Using Z-Scores

Z-scores represent standard deviations (SD) from the mean for height/length, weight, head circumference, weight for length/height, and BMI. They are values used by the WHO to define normal range of growth and provide cut offs for overweight status, obesity, or malnutrition. Data for z-scores were collected from healthy breastfed infants and young children from diverse countries. The use of these scores is recommended for infant and toddlers younger than 2 years of age. They can be accessed on: https://www.who.int/tools/child-growth-standards/standards. CDC uses percentiles on growth charts. Results of both systems correlate but don't correspond exactly.

- Z-score −2 to +2: anthropometrics are within normal limits (within 2 SD from the mean)
- Z-score < −2: the parameter is more than 2 SD below the mean, z-score (−2 to −2.9) correlates with moderate malnutrition
- Z-score < −3: the parameter is more than 3 SD below the mean, z-score < −3 correlates with severe malnutrition
- Z-score > +2: the parameter is more than 2 SD above the mean

Caloric Requirements for Infants and Children

Energy requirement for a child is the amount of food energy needed to support growth and development. There are different tools we can use to calculate Estimated Energy Requirements (EER) for children in different age groups but generally, we can use median weight and height to estimate. See Table 5.1 for EER based on sex and weight.

To calculate the amount of breast milk and/or formula infants need, determine EER as detailed above and calculate the total volume needed according to the caloric concentration of the type of food the infant is ingesting. Breast milk, regular powder, or premixed formulas has 19–20 kcal/oz. Premature infant formula and fortified infant formulas contain variable caloric content per fluid ounce but are typically above 22 kcal/oz.

Vital Signs

Report vitals as a spot measure for outpatients and as a range over the last 24 h for inpatients.

Temperature: when body temperature is reported, make sure to report the value of the measurement in Celsius or Fahrenheit, site of measurement (forehead, axilla, ear, oral or anal), range of temperature values, frequency of fevers, maximum temperature, and trend.

Table 5.1 EER for healthy boys and girls of median weight and height (weight and height at 50th percentile for age)

Age	Boys EER (kcal/kg/day)	Girls EER (kcal/kg/day)
0–2 months	107	104
3 months	95	95
4–35 months	82	82

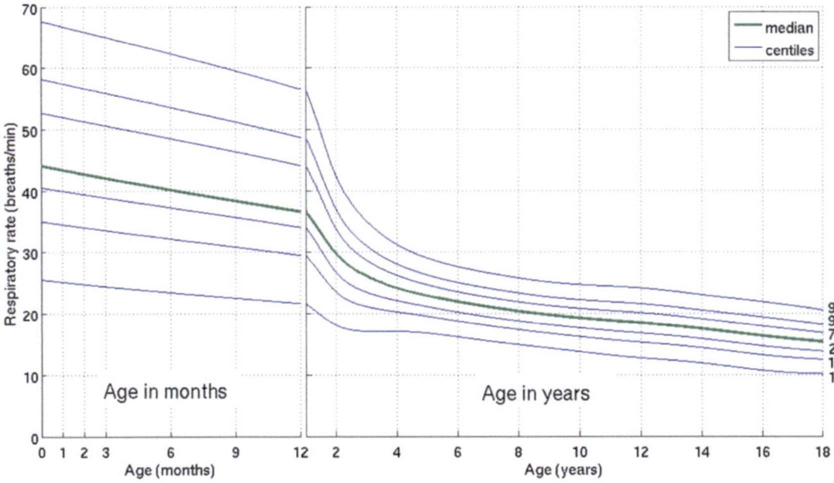

Fig. 5.1 Normal respiratory rate by age. (Reprinted with permission from Fleming S, Thompson M, Stevens R, Heneghan C, Plüddemann A, Maconochie I, Tarassenko L, Mant D. Normal ranges of heart rate and respiratory rate in children from birth to 18 years of age: a systematic review of observational studies. Lancet. 2011 Mar 19)

Respiratory Rate (RR): Interpret RR according to age (Fig. 5.1), child's activity level, and amount of respiratory support, if any.

Heart Rate (HR): Interpret HR according to age (Fig. 5.2), child's activity, temperature (may be additionally elevated with fever, and level of comfort.

Blood Pressure (BP): Blood pressure is interpreted based on a child's sex, age, and height percentile. You also need to consider a child's activity level, site of measurement (BP is normally higher in the lower extremities—a common site of measurement for infants), and level of comfort (elevated if crying or in pain).

Before reporting an abnormal value, make sure that the measurement was done while the patient was in a comfortable position and not fussy, using an oscillometer device and an appropriate cuff size on the right arm. If the BP is still abnormal, repeat the measurement using auscultation then average the results. See Table 5.2 for BP parameters by age. Complete charts of normal values can be found in the recommended additional resource, Flynn, et al. 2017. Hypotension is generally defined as <5 percentile for sex, age, and height. You can also use the Pediatric Advanced Life Support (PALS) formula systolic BP < 70 + 2 (age in years) to define hypotension for ages 1–10. See Table 5.3 for BP categories and stages of hypertension by age.

Application Exercises

1. Calculate the estimated energy requirement and feeding schedule for 3 month-old previously healthy, breast feeding boy who weighs 6.5 kg.

   A. Using Table 5.1, a 3-month old male infant requires 95 kcal/kg/day. 95 kcal/kg/day × 6.5 kg = 617.5 kg/day, therefore the EER is 617.5 kcal/day.

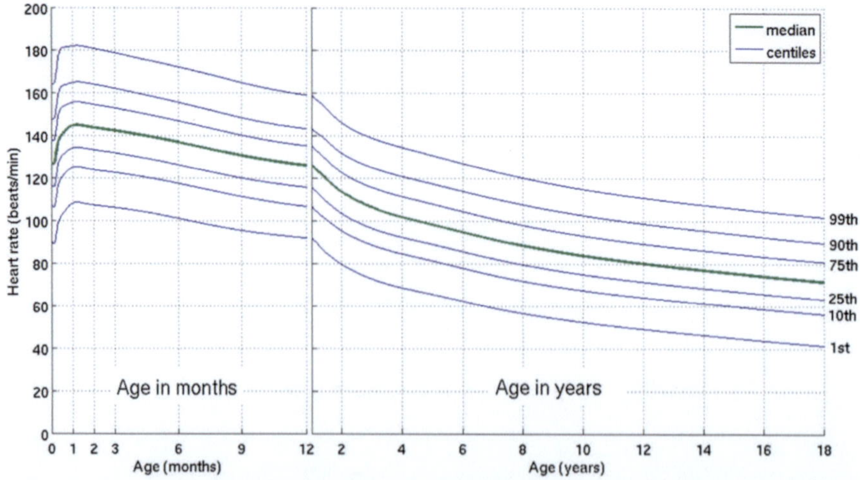

Fig. 5.2 Normal heart rate by age. (Reprinted with permission from Fleming S, Thompson M, Stevens R, Heneghan C, Plüddemann A, Maconochie I, Tarassenko L, Mant D. Normal ranges of heart rate and respiratory rate in children from birth to 18 years of age: a systematic review of observational studies. Lancet. 2011 Mar 19)

Table 5.2 BP parameters by age

Age	5th percentile[a]	50th percentile[a]	90th percentile[a]	9fifth percentile[a]
Toddler (1–2 years)	85–87/41–44	86–89/42–46	88–91/44/48	88–91/44–49
Preschooler (3–5 years)	88–91/47–52	90–94/49–54	92–96/51–56	93–96/51–56
School-aged (6–9 years)	93–96/54–57	95–99/56–60	97–101/58–62	98–101/59–62
Preteen (10–12 years)	97–102/59–61	100–105/61–62	102–108/62–64	103–109/63–64
Adolescent (13–15 years)	104–107/62–63	108–111/64–65	110–112/65–67	111–112/66–68

[a] Based on Flynn, et al. 2017, reflects averaged values for male and female sex and 50th percentile for height

Table 5.3 BP categories and stages of hypertension by age

Age	Normal BP	Elevated BP	Stage 1 HTN	Stage 2 HTN
1–13 years	<90th percentile	≥90th percentile to <95th percentile or 120/80 mmHg to <95th percentile (whichever is lower)	≥95th percentile to <95th percentile + 12 mmHg or 130/80 to 139/89 mmHg (whichever is lower)	≥95th percentile +12 mmHg or ≥140/90 mmHg (whichever is lower)
≥13 years	<120/<80 mmHg	120/<80 to 129/<80 mmHg	130/80 to 139/89 mmHg	≥140/90 mmHg

Adapted from Flynn, et al. 2017

B. Breast milk is estimated to be 20 kcal/30 mL (1 oz). 617.5 kg/day ÷ 20 kcal/30 mL = 926 mL of breast milk per day. 926 mL × 30 mL/oz = 30.9 oz. A 3-month-old typically feeds six to eight times a day. If he eats 8 times a day, schedule = 115 mL or 3.9 oz. breast milk every 3 h.

2. Calculate the estimated energy requirement and feeding schedule for a 6 month old, previously healthy girl who weighs 8 kg and drinks regular formula.

   A. Using Table 5.1, a 6-month-old female infant requires 82 kcal/kg/day. 82 kcal/kg/day × 8 kg = 656 kcal/day therefore the EER is 656 Kcal/day.
   B. Regular formula has 20 kcal/30 mL (1 oz). 656 kcal/day ÷ 20 kcal/30 mL = 984 mL of formula per day. 984 mL × 30 mL/oz = 32.8 oz. A typical 6 month old will drink formula four to five times a day. That equates to 164 ml or ~5.5 oz five times a day.

Further Reading

Flynn JT, Kaelber DC, Baker-Smith CM, Blowey D, Carroll AE, Daniels SR, de Ferranti SD, Dionne JM, Falkner B, Flinn SK, Gidding SS, Goodwin C, Leu MG, Powers ME, Rea C, Samuels J, Simasek M, Thaker VV, Urbina EM, SUBCOMMITTEE ON SCREENING AND MANAGEMENT OF HIGH BLOOD PRESSURE IN CHILDREN. Clinical practice guideline for screening and management of high blood pressure in children and adolescents. Pediatrics. 2017;140(3):e20171904. https://doi.org/10.1542/peds.2017-1904. Epub 2017 Aug 21. Erratum in: Pediatrics. 2017 Nov 30; Erratum in: Pediatrics. 2018 Sep;142(3).

Kleinman RE, Greer FR. Pediatric nutrition. 7th ed. American Academy of Pediatrics; 2014.

Muething SE, Kotagal UR, Schoettker PJ, Gonzalez del Rey J, DeWitt TG. Family-centered bedside rounds: a new approach to patient care and teaching. Pediatrics. 2007;119(4):829–32.

Chapter 6
Note Writing

Vignesh Doraiswamy and Claire Sevov

Note Writing

Clinical notes serve a variety of purposes in modern medical care. Documentation records the care provided, communicates the plan of care to the entire care team, and supports the level of service billed by the attending physician. Clinical documentation may also be cited as evidence in a court of law. Therefore, it is important to approach note writing with careful consideration, particularly when you're learning this skill for the first time. Before diving into specific types of documentation, Table 6.1 details three basic rules to avoid the pitfalls of documentation in the electronic medical record (EMR).

Finally, the Twenty-First Century Cures Act requires most documentation to be immediately available to patients and caregivers so you should always consider them as part of your audience. Keep your language factual and non-judgmental and consider how some commonly used words may be misinterpreted by a non-medical audience. Phrases such as "the patient complains of abdominal pain" may sound perfectly neutral to someone with medical training but could easily be misconstrued by a patient.

V. Doraiswamy (✉) · C. Sevov
Department of Pediatrics and Department of Internal Medicine, Nationwide Children's Hospital/The Ohio State University College of Medicine, Columbus, OH, USA
e-mail: vignesh.doraiswamy@osumc.edu; claire.sevov@osumc.edu

N. Liao et al. (eds.), *Pediatric Rotations*,
https://doi.org/10.1007/978-3-031-59873-9_6

Table 6.1 Pitfalls of documenting in the electronic medical record (EMR)

Be careful with auto-populated fields	The EMR can pull in information from different parts of the chart with templates and "smart phrases." These tools increase efficiency but can crowd your note with unhelpful or inaccurate information. For example, if using an automated function to pull in the family history, it's still up to you to independently verify and update the information. Another example is using an automated function to pull in all radiographic studies for a patient who has been admitted for 5 weeks
Use copy/paste functions cautiously	Copying and pasting a progress note from day to day has become a routine time-saving practice in most health systems. You MUST ensure that all sections of the note are updated appropriately to reflect the changing clinical situation. For example, a patient who was extubated 24 h prior should not still have "endotracheal tube in place" documented in the physical exam
Leave out "-day" words	Because you will likely use the copy/paste function at some point, it's best to avoid the use of words like "today," "yesterday," "Tuesday," etc. If you forget to change one of these words, your note will be incorrect the next day. We suggest using actual dates to avoid this pitfall

Problem-Based vs. Systems-Based Plans

The Assessment and Plan could be considered the most important section of any note and will be discussed in detail below. The two primary ways to organize the plan are referred to as "problem-based" or "systems-based" formats. Pediatricians in both the inpatient and outpatient settings usually prefer problem-based plans. This is organized by naming each of the patient's problems followed by the plan of action to address that specific problem. A more detailed discussion of how to create a problem list with examples can be found later in this chapter. By convention, problems should be prioritized in order of severity or importance with the primary problem addressed first. A systems-based plan, organized by organ system, is often preferred in a critical care setting. Table 6.2 provides a general overview of where patient care issues fit in a systems-based plan. We suggest that even when using a systems-based approach to the plan, the best practice is to name each problem you are addressing within that system (see Table 6.3).

For instance, a toddler with a history of hereditary nephropathy admitted to the hospital for pyelonephritis and sepsis might have the following problem and systems-based plans:

Table 6.2 Example of system-based categorization of patient problems

Cardiovascular	Shock Arrhythmias Cardiac dysfunction Abnormal blood pressure
Respiratory	Respiratory failure Asthma/bronchiolitis/cystic fibrosis/etc
Neurologic	Pain Need for sedation secondary to primary problem (such as sedation for intubation) Encephalopathy/delirium Seizures Neurological injuries Increased intracranial pressure
Infectious disease	Active infections (suspected or proven)
Gastrointestinal	Diet, enteral feeding, parenteral nutrition Tubes (naso/orogastric or jejunal, percutaneous tubes, rectal tubes) Stool frequency and character (diarrhea or constipation), bowel regimen Gastrointestinal (GI) bleeding Surgical issues involving the GI tract (ostomies, bowel trauma) Hepatic/pancreatic pathology such as elevated liver enzymes, cholecystitis, cirrhosis, and pancreatitis Other gastrointestinal disorders Need for stress ulcer prophylaxis (if not mentioned elsewhere)
Renal/ genitourinary	Fluid balance issues (e.g., overload, diuresis, risk for dehydration due to inadequate intake) Oliguria or anuria Electrolytes imbalances (Note: Some providers like to make a separate "FEN" category that lumps together fluids, electrolytes, and nutrition.) Acid-base issues, such as metabolic acidosis Other renal and genitourinary pathology such as hematuria, renal calculi, obstruction, and kidney injury (acute or chronic)
Hematologic	Cell line dyscrasias (e.g., anemia, thrombocytosis, thrombocytopenia, leukopenia) Coagulopathies (e.g., disseminated intravascular coagulation, thrombotic thrombocytopenic purpura, idiopathic thrombocytopenia) Bleeding issues and transfusion thresholds Thrombosis, including venous thromboembolism risk and prophylaxis
Endocrine	Glucose control, insulin needs Thyroid derangements, adrenal insufficiency, other hormonal imbalances

Table 6.3 Example of problem vs. system-based plan

Problem-based plan	System-based plan
1. Sepsis 2. E. coli pyelonephritis 3. Acute on chronic renal dysfunction 4. Chronic hypertension	Cardiovascular: 1. Sepsis 2. Chronic hypertension Infectious disease: 1. E. coli pyelonephritis Renal: 1. Acute kidney injury 2. Chronic kidney disease

History and Physical Exam Note

The History and Physical Exam (H&P) note documents the events leading up to the patient's hospitalization, their medical history, their physical exam, the physician's clinical reasoning about the underlying medical issues that led to hospitalization, and the initial diagnostic and therapeutic plan of care.

Components of an H&P include the following:

Reason for Admission: Also referred to as the "Chief Complaint," the patient's primary reason for admission should be clearly documented at the beginning of your note. Usually this is a single word or phrase such as "shortness of breath." Context will be provided in the next History of Present Illness. Note: Some clinicians will use the patient's exact words in quotations, but it's not always appropriate to do so.

History of Present Illness (HPI): This is where we tell the patient's story, usually as a chronological account of the events leading up to hospitalization. It begins with a sentence introducing the patient's age, relevant comorbidities, and the reason for admission. This is followed by a summary of the events leading up to admission. Depending on the time course of the illness, this summary could span a few days or a few years. The HPI should also include any relevant medical history, family/social history or risk factors, and pertinent positive and negative review of systems related to the Chief Complaint. In pediatrics, we often have many different storytellers (caregivers +/− patient) so it's always important to record who is providing each part of the history. For patients admitted through the Emergency Department (ED), a short paragraph at the end of the HPI is usually dedicated to describing the initial findings and management in the ED. For patients initially managed at an outside institution, you should document the name and location of the medical facility rather than refer to it as an "outside hospital" as this will assist with obtaining records in the future.

A complete history also includes a past medical history, developmental history, family history, and social history. Please see Chap. 2 for detailed discussion on relevant questions for these portions of the history.

Review of Systems: Refer to Chap. 2 for a more extensive discussion of the pediatric Review of Systems. This is usually presented in a list organized by system. You may wish to highlight pertinent positives and negatives with bold text or underlining. If you're unable to obtain a Review of Systems (e.g., because of a patient's mental status or refusal to answer your questions), you should state that rather than leaving this blank.

Physical Exam: See Chap. 3 for advice on age-based strategies to obtain a comprehensive Physical Exam. For documentation purposes, the Physical Exam is usually broken down into some variation of the following categories:

- Vital signs
- General appearance
- Head, Ears, Eyes, Nose, and Throat (HEENT)
- Neck

- Cardiovascular
- Respiratory
- Abdomen
- Genitourinary
- Back
- Extremities
- Neurologic
- Skin
- Psych/mental status

The Physical Exam is very vulnerable to copy/paste errors. It is important to update your physical exam daily and not include exam maneuvers that you did not actually perform that day (e.g. "tympanic membranes without effusion or erythema" should NOT be in the note unless you actually looked with an otoscope on that calendar day). Also be wary of including unfamiliar abbreviations to avoid documenting something that you didn't observe.

Clinical Data: This section includes any new labs, cultures, pathology, imaging, or procedure findings. It may also include prior findings (e.g., an echocardiogram from 6 months ago) that are relevant to the current medical management. You do NOT need to include all imaging findings or labs from the entire hospital stay, only what is relevant to current clinical care. You should state that you reviewed the clinical data and summarize the findings. Comment specifically if you personally review any radiology studies and if you discussed with a radiologist.

Assessment: The assessment should not be a restating of the opening line of the HPI. Instead, it should be a brief synthesis of your findings from the History, Physical Exam, and Clinical Data. Many learners use the IDEA framework below to help formulate the assessment [1] (Table 6.4).

The formulation of relevant differential diagnoses is often challenging for students. You may be tempted to add in diagnoses just to increase the number of items on your list, or you may rely on someone else's documentation. It can also be frustrating to be told to "work on expanding (or refining) your differentials" without much guidance. The CARD framework is one helpful way for you to approach building a differential diagnosis (Table 6.5).

Plan: The plan should be an organized outline of the diagnostic and therapeutic interventions you are providing for the patient. The first and the most important step in organizing your plan is to determine how to categorize the patient's problems.

Table 6.4 The IDEA framework for formulating an assessment

Interpretive summary	Includes a very brief synthesis of the relevant medical history and presenting symptoms/clinical findings
Differential diagnosis	Clearly state the one diagnosis you believe is most likely based on the available information
Explanation	Explain why you think that is the most likely diagnosis
Alternative diagnoses	List the alternative diagnoses you are considering and why you think they are more or less likely based on clinical information

Table 6.5 The CARD framework for generating a differential diagnosis

Common causes of the problem	Common diagnoses are just that—common
Atypical presentations of common diagnoses	Atypical presentations of common diagnoses are generally more likely than rare diagnoses
Rare diagnoses	These are the "zebras" that you learn about in medical school. You are unlikely to encounter them but if you never think of them you will miss them
Don't miss diagnoses	These are life-threatening diagnoses that must be considered and ruled out

Problem Type	Simple Problems List	Processed Problem List
Symptoms	Cough Fever ↓wet diapers	1. Acute Hypoxic Respiratory Failure secondary to RSV Bronchiolitis Cough Fever Tachypnea Tachycardia Hypoxia Leukocytosis Positive RSV CXR findings
Exam	Tachypnea Tachycardia Sunken fontanelle Dry mucous membranes Hypoxia	
Labs	Leukocytosis ↑BUN and Creatinine Positive RSV	2. Severe Dehydration with Acute Kidney Injury ↓wet diapers Sunken fontanelle Dry mucous membranes ↑BUN and Cr
Imaging	CXR with patchy opacities	

Fig. 6.1 Example of how to generate a simple problem list and then synthesize into a processed problem list

What you name as the problem should be as specific as possible without creating premature closure. For patients with multiple problems, you should prioritize your problem list by acuity and urgency. Sometimes it can be difficult to know exactly how to lump or split different pathology when creating a problem list. A good first step is to write a detailed list of the patients' problems (including all symptoms and abnormal vitals, exam findings, labs, microbiology, pathology, and imaging findings). From this list you will need to determine what findings can be grouped together under a single problem (see Fig. 6.1).

If a patient has multiple active problems, it can be helpful to give each problem its own focused assessment including your prioritized differential (see the IDEA framework above). Once your problem list is established, you should create a bulleted list of action items for each problem including (1) diagnostic plans, (2) therapeutic plans, (3) monitoring, (4) consultative plan, and (5) follow-up plans. You may not have a bullet point in each of these categories for every problem but thinking about it in a systematic way can prevent you from forgetting important aspects of the patient's care.

For the RSV bronchiolitis patient, the plan might look like:

Acute Hypoxemic Respiratory Failure Secondary to RSV Bronchiolitis

- Obtain influenza swab to rule out concurrent infection
- Provide supplemental oxygen as needed to keep SpO2 > 90%
- Monitor on continuous pulse oximetry while on supplemental O2
- Consult ICU if work of breathing increases
- Will need primary care follow-up at discharge

Inpatient Daily Progress Notes

The inpatient Daily Progress Note is a follow-up note, written daily after admission, and serves as an update on the patient's condition, the medical team's impressions, and the plan of care. This information is utilized by many different people involved in the patient's care including nurses, therapists (e.g., physical therapy), medical and surgical consultants, social workers, discharge planners, billing and coding professionals, and insurance companies. Once again, patients and their families may also view these notes. The four components of a Daily Progress Note are the subjective, objective, assessment, and plan. There are two common formats referred to as "SOAP" and "APSO," depending on whether you place the assessment and plan at the end of the note or the beginning of the note.

Subjective/Interval Events: The subjective refers to what the patient, parent, nurse, etc. tell you about how the patient is doing, as well as any concerns (e.g., "patient's mother is worried that the albuterol inhaler is not as effective as the nebulized treatments"). This should include at least a two-point review of pertinent systems. Interval events include any major changes to the clinical status or plan such as new fevers, escalating respiratory support, canceled procedures, etc. These updates should be brief since you will discuss all new clinical data and your clinical reasoning in other sections of the note.

Objective: There are only a few minor differences in the necessary information for the objective section in a daily progress note as compared to the H&P. You may choose to include laboratory or imaging results that are not necessarily new on that calendar day if they remain an important part of your medical decision making (e.g., blood culture sensitivities or MRI findings on presentation). You should not include older results that are irrelevant to the current plan of care (e.g., an abdominal radiograph to confirm placement of a nasogastric tube that has since been removed).

Assessment: The assessment in the daily progress notes should be a brief summary of how the patient presented, what the working diagnosis is, and how the patient is responding to treatment. This does not need to change every single day but should not be static from admission to discharge.

For example, on the fifth day of a hospitalization:

- WRONG: "Taylor is a 9-year-old child with developmental delay who presented with fever, cough, and left lower lobe infiltrate on chest X-ray concerning for pneumonia."
- RIGHT: "Taylor is a 9-year-old child with developmental delay who initially presented with fever and cough, found to have complicated left lower lobe pneumonia with parapneumonic effusion, now improving on IV antibiotics status post chest tube placement."

Plan: As the patient's hospitalization progresses, you may need to change the problems that were initially listed in the H&P. For instance, "Fever of Unknown Origin" may become "Kawasaki Disease" as more clinical information becomes available. The problem list should be dynamic, with problems ordered to reflect the current issues being addressed. For prolonged hospitalizations, some clinicians will keep a list of "Resolved Problems" at the bottom of the Plan. The daily progress note should also include a final section titled "Disposition" where you discuss the approximate timeframe for expected discharge and what needs to happen before that time.

For example:

Disposition: Plan to discharge home with home health care services, likely in the next 72 h, pending final culture results, transition to oral antibiotic regimen, and removal of chest tube.

Discharge Summaries

The discharge summary is the final provider-generated note of a patient's hospital stay and is meant to be a summary of the hospitalization. In addition to all the previously mentioned stakeholders who view your inpatient notes, the discharge summary is a communication with all future care providers, including inpatient skilled nursing, rehabilitation or long-term care facilities, home health care nurses, the primary pediatrician, outpatient consultants, and emergency or inpatient physicians caring for the patient during future admissions.

There is some disagreement about the best way to write a discharge summary. Some people prefer to write a narrative summary including why the patient was admitted, what occurred during the admission, and what needs to be followed up on. This can work well for generally healthy patients with one main problem addressed during the admission. For more complex patients, it's generally advisable to use a problem-based summary to ensure that important information about management of secondary problems is not missed and any subspecialists seeing the patient in follow-up can easily find the most relevant information within the note. You will not go wrong with a brief narrative overview of the hospitalization followed by a

Table 6.6 Do's and don'ts for the discharge summary

Do include
• The primary diagnosis for hospitalization • Description of treatment received including any ongoing treatment at discharge (e.g., completing an antibiotic course) • Follow-up care needs (labs, appointments, clinical findings to monitor, etc.) • Important lab/imaging results (culture sensitivities, special labs, echocardiograms, cross-sectional imaging, etc.) • Immunizations received while inpatient • Pending results • Any other new chronic diagnoses (and new treatments) • Discharge medication list (needs to be correct!!)
Don't include
• The admission HPI word-for-word • Every lab or imaging result from the entire hospital stay • Minute details about day-to-day events in the hospital (e.g., "patient weaned from 2L supplemental O2 to 1L at 5 pm on hospital day 2 but then increased to 1.5L at 7 pm and back to 1L at 2 am the next morning") • Abbreviations or test names that are not universally understood (for example, your hospital system's name for a viral respiratory panel may be specific to your institution) • Pejorative language about the patient or patient's caregivers • Accusatory or judgmental language about care received from other providers

problem-based summary of important findings, medication changes, and follow-up needs. We do not find a systems-based approach particularly useful for the discharge summary. Refer to Table 6.6 for some general tips on what always needs to be included whichever format you choose.

Outpatient Notes

All outpatient pediatric visits and documentation are one of two types: a well-child visit or an acute visit. Though the principles of documentation for both of these visit types are generally the same as inpatient notes, outpatient notes tend to be shorter and more focused on either the developmental assessment of the child or the acute visit issue.

Well-Child Visit: The well-child visit is an opportunity to complete a comprehensive assessment of the child and their developmental environment. It allows us to identify and investigate abnormalities and find opportunities to promote optimal growth and development.

There are four main components of a preventative well-child visit, all of which should be performed and documented accurately:

- Detailed age-appropriate developmental and behavioral assessment
- Thorough and detailed physical exam (refer to "Physical Exam" above) including review of growth parameters

- Age-appropriate screening tests (e.g., lead, hemoglobin, Autism screens), procedures (such as vaccinations), and referrals (such as eye or dental)
- Anticipatory guidance

A fair portion of time during a well-child visit may include discussion of age-appropriate anticipatory guidance for the child's parents/caregivers, but it is often acceptable to document which anticipatory guidance topics were discussed without needing a detailed discussion of each bit of guidance. Please see Chap. 37 for specifics on the approach to well-child visits including discussion of preventative care, anticipatory guidance, and developmental milestones.

Most practice locations will have age-specific templates for every well-child visit from the newborn to 18-year-old visits that you can use to help organize your note. The CDC's developmental milestones are also an excellent reference [2].

Acute Visit: A "sick" or "acute" visit is a common occurrence in pediatric clinics. These visits usually address one or two acute issues and are much shorter in duration. This requires a thorough but efficient approach. If the child returns to the clinic, urgent care, or is admitted to the hospital for the same issue, the documentation of their initial presentation to care is very important.

Like inpatient notes, acute visit notes can also be in SOAP or APSO format depending on preference. The subjective, objective, assessment and plan sections generally contain the same information as for inpatient notes (see "Daily Progress Notes" section of this chapter) with some modifications described below.

Reason for Visit and Subjective: A short summary that describes the patient and their pertinent medical history as well as reason for their visit should be documented at the beginning of your note. This is where you will document what you obtain from the patient/caregivers. This should also include a focused and pertinent review of systems.

Objective: Just as you did in your inpatient notes, be sure to document vital signs, weight and growth parameters as well as your focused physical exam findings. While you may not have as much diagnostic data, it will be important to document whatever point-of-care testing you perform in the clinic (rapid strep, rapid RSV/Flu, spirometry results, etc.).

Assessment: In the assessment section of an acute visit note, you should offer an interpretive summary of what led to the patient's presentation and what you think is going on (including what else is on the differential).

Plan: The plan should list your diagnostic, therapeutic, and/or consultative plan for the patient. In addition, a very important part of the plan (or this can be a separate section at the end) should include the child's acute visit anticipatory guidance. This documents your discussion with the child/caregiver regarding expected time frame for improvement or resolution of symptoms as well as what signs and symptoms would warrant return to clinic or seeking emergency care. You should clearly state whether specific follow-up is recommended in a given time frame or only on an as needed basis.

References

1. Baker EA, Ledford CH, Fogg L, Way DP, Park YS. The IDEA assessment tool: assessing the reporting, diagnostic reasoning, and decision-making skills demonstrated in medical students' hospital admission notes. Teach Learn Med. 2015;27(2):163–73.
2. Centers for Disease Control and Prevention. CDC's developmental milestones. 2022. https://www.cdc.gov/ncbddd/actearly/milestones/index.html. Accessed 29 Mar 2022.

Chapter 7
Consults and Handoffs

Nancy Liao and Kristen Lewis

Requesting Expert Consultation

Preparation

Expert consultation can add significant value to patient care. When requesting a consult, first consider what you need from the consultant. Only request a consult if you require:

- Assistance with a diagnosis based on clinical finding/symptoms/laboratory and radiology data
- Assistance with determining a diagnostic or therapeutic management plan
- Procedural intervention
- Engagement in a patient's close follow-up plan.

Requesting consultation to simply have a team "on board" without a goal from their input is much less likely to add value. If you are uncertain of the specific reason for requesting a consult, consider asking your team, "Can you help me understand what question we have for the consultant?" or "Can you explain what we hope the consultant will add to the patient's care?" These are non-threatening ways to promote your understanding and advocate for appropriate consultation.

N. Liao
Pediatrics, Nationwide Children's Hospital/The Ohio State University College of Medicine, Columbus, OH, USA
e-mail: nancy.liao@nationwidechildrens.org

K. Lewis (✉)
Department of Pediatrics and Department of Internal Medicine, Nationwide Children's Hospital/The Ohio State University College of Medicine, Columbus, OH, USA
e-mail: kristen.lewis@osumc.edu

N. Liao et al. (eds.), *Pediatric Rotations*,
https://doi.org/10.1007/978-3-031-59873-9_7

Prepare what you plan to say when you contact the consultant. Think through each of the items in the following CONSULT mnemonic (Table 7.1). A high-quality consult request is clear, concise, and in most cases will take less than 1 min to complete.

Table 7.1 CONSULT mnemonic for requesting a consult [1]

	Information to share	Example
Contact the consultant, courteously	– Your name, training level, and team – Verify you have contacted the correct person for a consult request	"Hi, I'm xx, the sub-intern on the hospital pediatrics team. Are you the person covering ENT consults?"
Orient	– Patient name, location, and MRN	"I would like to request a consult on patient xx in room xx. I can provide you the MRN if helpful"
Narrow question	– Ask a focused question that specifically states the primary issue and what you hope the consultant can contribute to the patient's care	"The patient is being admitted with a peritonsillar abscess which I believe requires I&D. I would like you to evaluate her for the procedure"
Story	– Patient's age, (if relevant) birth history, and sex – Include **pertinent** HPI and hospital course – Include **pertinent** exam findings and testing results – Share your team's assessment – If you have a diagnostic question, have a differential in mind, and share the work-up you have already conducted – If you have a therapeutic question, have an anticipated management plan in mind – Amount of information is appropriate for the complexity of the case	"xx is a 3 year old previously healthy female who presented with fever and sore throat. Significant tonsillar asymmetry on exam led to a CT being obtained which h revealed a 1 × 1.5 cm abscess in her left tonsil. She is currently NPO, receiving IV fluids and IV antibiotic therapy with ampicillin/sulbactam"
Urgency	– Today? Tomorrow? Urgently now? – Specifically state this information – Be ready to provide justification for your stated urgency	– "I believe it would be best for you to see her today to definitively treat the abscess"

Table 7.1 (continued)

	Information to share	Example
Later	– Make a follow-up plan of how to be contacted – If provided with preliminary recommendations, use closed-loop communication and repeat the information back to make sure you have understood correctly	– "Can you please call me with your recommendations at number xx after you have seen the patient?"
Thank you	– Always be polite and courteous throughout	– "Thank you for your assistance. Our team appreciates it!"

Additional Tips:

- Have patient information readily available when you contact the consultant. Sit in front of a computer if using electronic health record. This will allow you to look up unanticipated data that the consultant requests.
- If your schedule allows, consider asking the consultant to contact you when they are going to see the patient. You will benefit from more in-depth learning, and the patient will benefit from highly coordinated care.
- When possible, ask to observe procedures or diagnostic testing that consultants perform or recommend. This will also promote deeper understanding.
- If you do not fully understand the reasoning behind a consultant's recommendations, ask for clarification. This is yet another opportunity to promote your learning and will allow you to more effectively and confidently discuss the plan of care with your patients.

Pitfalls:

- Lack of a specific question—This can result in unnecessary requests for consults or completed consults that do not fully address your patient's and team's concerns.
- Overly verbose presentation—This can lead to frustration and is disrespectful of your consultant's time. Focus on the information your consultant requires to answer your key question.
- Lack of closed-loop communication—This can lead to confusion regarding the specific question for the consultant or confusion regarding the consultant's recommendations.
  - When planning to request a consult, state to your team your key question for the consultant, and confirm you are correct.
  - When the consultant provides you with recommendations, repeat back their recommendations and ask clarifying questions as necessary.

Special Situations

Curbside Consults

A curbside consult occurs when an expert provides patient care recommendations without completing a full, independent evaluation of the patient. While this practice is historically common and convenient, it places patients at risk. Recommendations from curbside consults can unknowingly be based upon inaccurate or incomplete information, and hence result in different recommendations than those obtained through formal consultation. Students generally should not be performing curbside consults.

The Reluctant Consultant

Consultants are called upon to balance competing professional demands on a daily basis. From tending to their own patients' care needs and managing the workload of consults, to performing procedures, consultants often have long and busy days in the hospital. While rude or unprofessional behavior is not acceptable, do your best to foster collegial collaboration between your team and the consultant. If this should happen, discuss with your senior resident or attending. Succinct, pertinent patient information, clear consultation questions, and knowing your patient well will help in this endeavor. Keep high-quality patient care as your top priority, and advocate for this on behalf of your patient whenever necessary.

Patient Handoffs

Patient handoffs occur at numerous junctures during the care of hospitalized patients. Handoffs occur when patients change care locations within the hospital (for example between the emergency department and the medical unit), when care providers change shifts (for example between the day team and the night team), when patients are discharged from the hospital, and more. A clear transfer of professional responsibility for patients' care defines these handoff time points. Unfortunately, handoffs expose patients to risk, with errors in communication contributing to adverse events. These communication errors may be a part of either written handoffs, verbal handoffs, or both.

Consider the following I-PASS mnemonic (Table 7.2) as a scaffold for conducting a written or verbal handoff of hospitalized patients. I-PASS was developed in the pediatric setting, and when used consistently has been shown to reduce patient harm. Not all institutions use the I-PASS mnemonic, though most do adopt a common handoff format with which you should familiarize yourself. These handoff tools often share common features with I-PASS.

Table 7.2 I-PASS mnemonic to handoff a patient [2]

	Information to share	Example
Illness severity	– Identify the patient's clinical stability and trajectory. – Consider stable, "watcher," unstable	"This patient is a watcher"
Patient summary	– Provide summary statement, "one liner"	"xx is a 4 month old male with no significant history admitted with acute viral bronchiolitis with associated hypoxia"
	– Events leading up to admission. Keep this concise	"His symptoms began with an upper respiratory infection 3 days ago, but when he developed increased work of breathing last evening, he was brought to the emergency department"
	– Hospital course. Keep this brief and relevant	"We have placed him on 0.5 L NC and been suctioning him prior to feeds. This afternoon he did have an episode of significantly increased retractions and tachypnea, but with additional suctioning, these both improved. We have continued to allow him to take PO and have not started IV fluids"
	– Ongoing assessment and plan. What do you think is going on?	"xx remains at risk for worsening respiratory distress"
Action list	Identify a to do list	"Please monitor respiratory rate and night round to assess work of breathing"
Situation awareness/ contingency planning	Give a plan	"If called with increased work of breathing or tachypnea with respiratory rate > 60, please go to see the patient. Consider nasal suctioning if it has not already been done. If increased work of breathing or tachypnea continue despite nasal suctioning, consider starting O2 via high flow nasal cannula." "If respiratory rate is consistently above 60 despite suction and oxygen, please make him NPO and start IV fluids"
Synthesis by receiver	Ensure receiver summarizes what was heard, asks questions, restates key action/to do items	"Ok, xx is a 4 month old with viral bronchiolitis. He is on 0.5 L O2 and requiring nasal suctioning. I will plan to round on him this evening. If he has increased work of breathing, will trial nasal suction, then consider high flow nasal cannula and make him NPO. Does he have an IV in place?"

Additional Tips:

- Consider organizing your sign out such that the patients at highest risk for instability are prioritized, both in order of presentation and in the amount of time you spend on them. This increases the attention paid by the recipient on these patients
- Incorporate "to-do-lists" and "if-then" communication into handoffs

- Conduct verbal handoffs in a distraction free zone
- Ensure closed-loop communication between participants

Pitfalls:

- Vague language
  - Provide clear and concrete information as much as possible. For example, instead of "if the nurse calls with hyperglycemia, give insulin." Say, "The patient's correction factor is to give 1 unit of short acting insulin (Humalog) for blood glucoses every 50 points above 150."
- Disorganized or omitted information
  - Following a standardized framework for every handoff (such as I-PASS) can help prevent disorganization and omissions of pertinent information.
- Irrelevant details
  - The attention span of the person receiving the handoff will wane. Keep the information that you provide focused and relevant.
- Inaccurate or outdated information
  - Hospitalized patients' statuses change on a daily basis. Accurate information one day may be outdated and inaccurate the next. Be sure to update the written information you provide daily.

References

1. Podolsky A, Stern DT, Peccoralo L. The courteous consult: a CONSULT card and training to improve resident consults. J Grad Med Educ. 2015;7(1):113–7. https://doi.org/10.4300/JGME-D-14-00207.1.
2. Starmer AJ, Spector ND, Srivastava R, et al. I-PASS, a mnemonic to standardize verbal handoffs. Pediatrics. 2012;129(2):201–4. https://doi.org/10.1542/peds.2011-2966.

Chapter 8
Interprofessional Communication

Margaret Redmond and Rakhi Gupta Basuray

Professionalism, Collaboration, and Communication

Professionalism is a conceptual understanding, a manifestation of a profession's moral and ethical principles toward whom it serves. Medicine has one of the oldest examples of a professionalism standard, the Hippocratic oath. As you may have observed, modern, Western medicine is increasingly delivered in a team-based approach and draws from professional standards within nursing, social work, pharmacy, and other collaborating professions. Patients can receive better healthcare when delivered by a coordinated team of providers.

Communicating effectively within these teams is critical to assure safe, quality care and is a key component of professionalism. In other chapters of this book, structured forms of interprofessional communication are reviewed such as how to present patients, write notes, and hand off a patient. However, much communication within and around a medical team is less structured and can have common pitfalls. When concerns arise, consider the following communication competencies outlined by the Interprofessional Education Collaborative (IPEC), a national collaboration between 15 health professions, working toward improving population health by improving team-based care (Table 8.1). As patient advocates with shared common goals, being mindful of others' expertise can facilitate improved outcomes.

M. Redmond (✉)
Division of Allergy and Immunology, Department of Pediatrics, The Ohio State University/Nationwide Children's Hospital, Columbus, OH, USA
e-mail: margaret.redmond@nationwidechildrens.org

R. Gupta Basuray
Division of Hospital Pediatrics, Department of Pediatrics, The Ohio State University/Nationwide Children's Hospital, Columbus, OH, USA
e-mail: rakhi.guptabasuray@nationwidechildrens.org

N. Liao et al. (eds.), *Pediatric Rotations*,
https://doi.org/10.1007/978-3-031-59873-9_8

Table 8.1 IPEC communication sub-competencies (Adapted)

1	Utilize communication tools and techniques to facilitate interactions and discussions
2	Implement universally understandable terminology
3	Express oneself with clarity, respectfully and confidently
4	Actively listen and encourage others
5	Seek, respond, and provide instructive feedback in a timely and sensitive manner
6	Use respectful language during difficult, conflicting, or crucial conversations
7	Recognize individual experiences and positions as assets
8	Promote the importance of teamwork

Adapted from Interprofessional Education Collaborative [3]

Vignette #1

You are rounding in the newborn nursery. Your patient was born to first-time parents eager to get home. The family recently immigrated to the area and needs social support services to ensure a safe transport home and appropriate sleep environment for the baby. You are informed that the mother has been discharged from the hospital, but you do not feel the baby is currently ready for discharge. You are conflicted about separating mom and baby.

Considerations for Vignette #1:

- *Work with your interprofessional team members to gather additional information regarding support options for the family.*
- *Explain your hesitation about discharging the baby.*
- *Solicit historically utilized resolutions in similar situations.*
- *This will take extra time and could impact workflow efficiency. By maintaining patient safety as your anchor, further collaboration with social services and throughput considerations may improve outcomes for your patient's entire family.*

Context is key for approaching communication in a professional manner. Though most of the research looking at interprofessional communication is centered in a Western concept, standards in other parts of the world have commonalities such as altruism, honesty, accountability, and respect. Differences in expectations or preferred modes of address, however, can be present.

Vignette #2

Your team has recently added a nursing team member who trained in a different healthcare system. Your team is very focused on collaboration and members working independently within their scope. However, the recently added team member is relying on you to manage patient care activities that you believe are within their scope of care.

Considerations for Vignette #2:

- *Lead with curiosity.*
- *Ask questions about roles within the health care system in which they were trained.*

It is possible that the previous health care model was more authoritarian or that patient care activities were allocated between team members in a different way. Once that understanding has been reached, you can discuss expectations to reduce the opportunity for miscommunication.

The Healthcare System's Contribution to Communication Complexities

It is important to remember that errors in health care are best addressed when systems, not individuals, are analyzed. Errors can be divided into two categories: those immediately detectable and due, in part, to lapse in memory or negligence, and those inherently present within a system, though only revealed when triggered. Errors stemming from communication align with the latter. Improving interprofessional communication requires understanding of system deficiencies and complexities. A historic tradition of hierarchy, tendency toward individualism, dilution of accountability, and heterogeneity within and between professionals are a few elements. Compounding this is the frequent, transient nature of team members, often rotating between various settings and roles. Competing objectives such as providing sound patient care alongside the objective of efficiency can result in frustration as you juggle too much on your own. You may personally and professionally align with competing morals and ethics, such as supporting the rights of an adolescent which may be in conflict with preferences of a custodial caregiver. Variation in expectation adds another layer of complexity and exists between units or departments. Normal behaviors in a pediatric emergency department may not be normal in a pediatric psychiatry unit. Lastly, rules, either explicit or implicit, may fluctuate. The preferred organization of a patient presentation between attendings is a ripe example and can make it difficult for you to anticipate and plan. Successful communication requires sensitivity and accommodation of these complexities in our ever-changing health care system.

Groupthink

Being part of a team has endless benefits but must be balanced against challenges that can manifest from communication that occurs within the group. One such concept is groupthink. In short, this is the emergence of consensus without each person critically analyzing variables and potential outcomes. Though intentions may be well-meaning, to be supportive and unified, or externally driven by pressures created by systems and administration, creativity and individual instincts can become silenced and lead to harbored ill-feelings, conflict, and suboptimal patient care. Awareness of this phenomenon, in addition to employing counterbalancing measures, such as explicitly stating team goals during discussion and intentionally seeking and exploring alternative perspectives and solutions can enhance interprofessional communication.

Vignette #3

You are sitting in a team meeting to discuss next steps for a complex patient involving several subspecialists and surgeons. The patient has had chronic, debilitating abdominal pain. Medications are not adequately managing the symptoms which are limiting the patient's ability to participate in rehab, counseling, and the practice of mindfulness. The family is anxious to resolve the symptoms with surgery. The surgical team can operate on the patient this week if appropriate. You wonder if medical child abuse could be in the differential diagnosis having recently attended a didactic on this topic.

Considerations for Vignette #3:

- *What is the best way to voice your concern?*
- *Is there harm from raising this suspicion?*
- *Could harm manifest if your suspicion is not voiced?*

Offer your concern in a non-accusatory manner as part of a discussion on shared patient goals. Doing so has the potential to further ensure patient safety.

Modes of Interprofessional Communication

The primary goal of all interprofessional communication is to share knowledge about the patient in a timely and respectful manner. As technology advances, the ways health care teams communicate have become more varied. In general, there are two primary forms of communication: verbal and written. Verbal communication can be in person or via phone. Written communication can be via e-mail, electronic medical records, secure chat functions, text message, or social media. There are many modes for communication, and managing them all in a timely fashion is a challenge.

Vignette #4

You are on call for a group of patients admitted to the hospital and are simultaneously receiving notifications from various team members via *page, calls on your communication badge* (i.e., *Vocera™), and messages by secure chat—all while another team member stops by the work room to ask a question. How do you prioritize communication?*

Considerations for Vignette #4:

A common pitfall is to prioritize the first page received. However, this can cause more urgent needs to become overlooked. It is also tempting to communicate in an abrupt manner when pulled in many directions. Remember to take one communication at a time. When responding, if the initial task is not urgent, let the team member know you will address it as soon as you are able and proceed to assess the next communication. If the first task is urgent and may take some time to complete, do not be afraid to seek help from other members of your medical team in resolving the other communications. Keep track of uncompleted tasks so when you are able, you can address them.

Another common pitfall with multiple communication modalities is redundancy. This can negatively impact patients in several ways. One is when important information is overlooked by a team member believing they have already addressed information through a previous similar communication. This risk can be mitigated with **closed loop communication**, the acknowledgment of communication and confirmation of understanding between team members.

Vignette #5

You are sent a secure chat message by a nurse. She notifies you that your patient needs a change to the dietary status prior to planned procedure the following day. You change the order. A few minutes later you receive a page from the nurse that the dietary order needs to be changed. You believe this page was sent at the same time as the secure chat message and ignore the page. It is later revealed the dietary order was incorrectly modified and your patient's procedure was delayed.

Considerations for Vignette #5:

Even though there are many demands on your time, it is important to close every loop. Responding to the second secure chat stating you placed the order and confirming it was correct may have prevented the error. Even if a page feels redundant, call and close the loop. These extra steps will take time but will help reduce miscommunication and potential patient harm.

Interprofessional communication extends beyond the work setting. Social media is used to educate patients or other health care professionals on a variety of topics. Social media can also be used to advocate for legislation or societal awareness surrounding health and the system of health care. A common pitfall is to not lead with respect for patients or other professionals in these relaxed settings. Because social media can feel like a private setting, it can easily become a venue for sharing inappropriate information that cannot be erased or recalled. This may violate professionalism standards, institutional policies, and privacy laws if patient information is discussed.

Navigating Interprofessional Communication

Research has shown that most medical professionalism is learned by watching behaviors of senior healthcare professionals. You are beginning your journey in interprofessional communication and have the opportunity to think critically about the behaviors you see on your teams. Consider if specific behaviors are those you wish to perpetuate. All members of the team influence the team culture from the first day they arrive and are regarded by patients as representatives of healthcare. Effective interprofessional communication can help build life-long relationships between disciplines and can result in creative solutions to patient care. These relationships take time and require work to develop.

We will next review three communication skills to maximize your interprofessional communication.

1. **Understanding of roles**: Sometimes deficiencies in communication occur because of a misunderstanding of roles. Ask members of your team how they would describe their role. This can be a useful exercise in listening as well.
2. **Attribution of ideas**: When discussing patient care, take a proactive approach in acknowledging the source of an idea and use your voice to amplify that idea if you think it is valuable for optimal patient care.
3. **Making amends**: All of us are going to make mistakes. It is critical to address errors and make amends when possible.

Vignette #6
A group of nursing students are joining rounds for the day. One of your peers remarks that rounds are too crowded and that maybe the nursing students should not be included. Your attending does not overhear this remark, but it is clear the nursing students did, as well as one of the interns on the team. After rounds, you notice the intern take your fellow medical student aside for a private conversation.

Considerations for Vignette #6
Carve out time to talk with the nursing students. Ask questions about what they learned from rounds. Each health care team member provides necessary aspects of patient care and understanding the nursing students' goals and take-away from rounds can impact the way you participate on rounds. Each participant on rounds can thereby learn to complement each other and ultimately deliver optimized patient care. Getting to know about nursing students' training and what they value about their future career in health care is a way to start building bridges now.

Vignette #7
During rounds, the pharmacist is making dosing recommendations. You believe that the consulting specialist recommended a different medication. You are feeling stressed as rounds are running long and many patients still need to be seen. You interrupt the pharmacist and tell them they are recommending the wrong

medication and push past their recommendations. Following rounds, you are reviewing the consult note and realize that the pharmacist was correct.

Considerations for Vignette #7:

After discussing your error with your attending and team, apologize to the pharmacist and acknowledge your error.

Conclusion

Current Western healthcare models rely on large teams of diverse professionals to deliver high quality care to patients. Respectful and effective communication is paramount to promote patient safety, reduce avoidable errors, and facilitate excellent patient outcomes. Healthcare systems, however, harbor communication pitfalls. Through open lines of communication, a clear understanding of professional roles and goals, and encouragement of participation, these pitfalls may be averted. Mindful and active development of interprofessional communication skills can help you become an effective and reliable leader of your healthcare team.

Bibliography

1. Fallat ME, Glover J, American Academy of Pediatrics, Committee on Bioethics. Professionalism in pediatrics. Pediatrics. 2007;120(4):e1123–33. https://doi.org/10.1542/peds.2007-2230.
2. American Board of Pediatrics. Education and Training Committee. Teaching, promoting, and assessing professionalism across the continuum: a medical educator's guide. https://www.abp.org/professionalism-guide. Accessed 27 Mar 2022.
3. Interprofessional Education Collaborative. Core competencies for interprofessional collaborative practice: 2016 update. Washington, DC: Interprofessional Education Collaborative; 2016.
4. Al-Rumayyan A, Van Mook W, Magzoub ME, Al-Eraky MM, Ferwana M, Khan MA, Dolmans D. Medical professionalism frameworks across non-western cultures: a narrative overview. Med Teach. 2017;39(sup1):S8–S14.
5. Varpio L, Hall P, Lingard L, Schryer CF. Interprofessional communication and medical error: a reframing of research questions and approaches. Acad Med. 2008;83(10 Suppl):S76–81. https://doi.org/10.1097/ACM.0b013e318183e67b.

Chapter 9
How to Promote Your Learning

Scott Carney

Pre-rotation Activities

Enhancing individual learning during pediatric rotations requires students to navigate a variety of different situations, educators, and experiences which can be accomplished through advanced preparation, expectation setting, and reflection throughout the rotation. Understanding the schedule allows for learners to identify where and when structured learning will happen or be provided, when they will be expected to create self-study opportunities, and when they will be able to create mental respite and self-care to "reload" for the remainder of the rotation. Identifying and reviewing what resources will be provided during the rotation allow for the individual learner to know the responsibilities they will have, and the clinical and educational experiences planned during the clerkship to enhance the student's learning. Each rotation provides differing amounts of study materials, lecture materials, test/preparation questions, procedural opportunities, and mentorship opportunities. Knowing at the onset of the rotation what will and will not be provided allows for the learner to seek out those opportunities that are offered and can enhance their learning. Table 9.1 reviews how to prepare for a rotation.

S. Carney (✉)
Division of General and Hospital Pediatrics, Department of Pediatrics, Prisma Health – Columbia/University of South Carolina School of Medicine, Columbia, SC, USA
e-mail: Scott.Carney@prismahealth.org

N. Liao et al. (eds.), *Pediatric Rotations*,
https://doi.org/10.1007/978-3-031-59873-9_9

Table 9.1 Pre-rotation preparation

Advanced preparation	Prior to the rotation, acquaint oneself with the overall organization, expectations, and resources available during the rotation	1. Review given rotation materials distributed by the course 2. Identify learning resources-books, institutional policies, clinical guidelines, hand books, etc. (senior medical students and house staff are a great resource for this)
Understanding the flow	Ask questions on the first day of the rotation with the attending and/or team	1. Where/when to arrive? 2. When do rounds start? When does the first patient arrive in clinic? 3. Are patients self-assigned or distributed? 4. What are call/shift responsibilities? 5. Where/when does formal teaching occur? 6. When does the day conclude?

Table 9.2 Expectation setting

Setting self-expectations	Prior to the rotation engage in reflection to identify key goals and learning objectives	1. What skills am I focusing on? 2. What do I want out of this rotation? 3. Where are my areas for improvement?
Understanding general expectations	On the first day of the rotation with the attending and/or team	1. What are expectations for patient presentations? 2. How many patients am I expected to see? 3. What are expectations for notes? 4. What are expectations for student-driven conversations with families and patients?
Negotiating shared goals	On the first few days of the rotation with the attending and/or team	1. Explicitly share your goals for the rotation and what you want to improve 2. Come to agreement on when feedback will be given

Setting Expectations

Starting with what one's self-expectations are during the rotation sets the stage for future success. While understandable that not everyone has an interest in pediatrics, the clerkship years provide an opportunity to view ones preferred field of medicine through a new lens. For example, a student that may see their future in orthopedics can focus on pediatric orthopedic issues to not only enhance their learning but also stay engaged during the rotation. Even those that see themselves carrying for the other end of the age spectrum in geriatric medicine can learn from pediatrics by focusing on parallel areas such as delirium management, learning about effective communication with families, etc. By developing personal expectations for the rotation and aligning them with the expectations of the clerkship, the learner stays engaged, ignites passion, and sees purpose in what they are doing through the clerkship. Table 9.2 suggests some key questions to guide expectation setting.

Mid-rotation

By the middle of the rotation, learners should take the opportunity to promote and evaluate their learning and request feedback for improvement from the clinical team members. Availability and comfort in providing feedback often vary between faculty members, residents, and clerkship directors but by learning to seek out direct feedback each student gains valuable skills that will translate across other rotations and last through the remainder of their professional career. Some of these areas are easier to assess than others (e.g., medical knowledge) and helping evaluators by asking specific questions regarding performance may lead to improved feedback. Table 9.3 outlines key questions to ask.

Table 9.3 Questions to ask during feedback session

Clinical performance (History and physical exam skills, diagnostic and therapeutic decision-making)	• How should I improve taking a social history in an adolescent? • What parts of my exam skills am I now comfortable in performing and which have I not become adept at or struggle with? • Are there ages of patients I struggle to examine confidently or have not yet seen regularly? • Do I organize my history and exams into a logical comprehensive fashion? • Are my assessment and plans cohesive? Do I routinely leave portions of assessments or plans out? • Am I moving forward on the RIME model of medical education (Reporter—Interpreter—Manager—Educator) to at least interpreting interactions?
Medical knowledge	• What are my knowledge gaps in general related to/what do I struggle with? (Pathophysiology? Anatomy? Pharmacology? Eetc.) • What pediatric specific conditions have I learned about and mastered at this point? • What is the best way for me to reinforce knowledge obtained and build upon it? (Question banks, patient interactions, discussion, focused reading, etc.)
Documentation	• Have I had the opportunity to practice documentation of a variety of sources? (Inpatient admission H&P; outpatient clinic note; daily progress note; discharge summary) • What are my areas for improvement related to daily documentation?
Communication skills	• How do you think my interaction with patient X went? • How are my interactions with members of the health care team? • How can I improve my presentations during rounds, am I using effective patient centered language? • Do I find the appropriate balance of professionalism and putting families/patients at ease during visits?

In addition to self-reflection during the mid-portion of the rotation, students should recognize what learning opportunities lie ahead and evaluate requirements that still must be completed. To help in planning for the end of the rotation and any testing which may occur, students can create a plan for completion of required rotational elements and a study schedule. This will aid students avoiding the need to finish up tasks in the final days and which can create undue stress or pose a risk of potentially failing to complete requirements due to elements out of their control (e.g., faculty member on vacation).

End of Rotation/Post Rotation

The culmination of the clinical experience provides students with the opportunity to reflect on the rotation, their own self-efficacy toward learning, pitfalls, improvements, and things worth considering for future rotations or self-learning moving forward. This is not done in a vacuum as a variety of avenues are available to aid in assessment. Similar to the mid-rotation, the end of the rotation should be a time of self-reflection as well as eliciting feedback of the learner to improve clinical skills and enhance medical knowledge. Asking questions of oneself and soliciting feedback from a variety of different individuals such as pediatric residents, faculty members, and the clerkship director can provide ongoing areas for improvement as well as areas in which the student is already succeeding. Table 9.4 reviews end of rotation questions.

Table 9.4 End of rotation reflection

Overall rotational evaluation	• What went well? • What did I enjoy that I didn't think I would? • What did I not enjoy that I thought I would? • What could have gone better? • What did I learn that I can apply to other areas? • How did I grow?
Areas I succeeded in	• What was an area I performed well in clinically during the rotation? • What was an area I demonstrated good medical knowledge? • What was a meaningful patient experience I was a part of?
Areas I can continue to grow in	• What opportunities should I have taken more advantage of? • What was a communication skill, clinical skill, or piece of medical knowledge I still need to work on? • Did I seek out feedback to improve?
Ways to continue to build upon successes and improve shortcomings	• How did I support my learning during this rotation? • What resources did I find particularly effective/ineffective?

Framing the feedback provided in a more general sense provides a chance for students to apply it to future practice and rotations exclusive of the pediatric experience. It may seem that getting feedback in the newborn nursery will be of little use to someone planning to go into dermatology but learning how to describe and discuss benign rashes with a worried individual may prove useful in the future.

For some, the end of the rotation provides an opportunity for ongoing mentorship and assistance with future needs as well. If a student has enjoyed their experience, had a meaningful interaction with residents or faculty members or potentially envisions pediatrics in their future, the end of the rotation provides a time to acknowledge those thoughts/feelings and to act upon them. Creating lasting connections and asking about ongoing mentorship and potential opportunities whether with faculty or residents can build bridges for future relationships that will benefit students in many meaningful ways. Alerting faculty to potential future needs (letters of recommendation) if applicable can benefit students in long term.

The Clinical Setting

Each clerkship and organization will have varying expectations regarding the "how to" of the clinical aspect of the pediatric clerkship but the following should serve as a guide to "Surviving Pediatrics." Getting the most out of the clinical aspects of the rotation regardless of location, however, involves three key elements: patient ownership, seeing oneself as a part of the healthcare team, and ongoing investment and engagement in learning whenever possible. We will focus on two areas of the rotation that students will find themselves in, the inpatient setting and general outpatient clinic.

Inpatient Rotations

Rounding in the pediatric inpatient environment is often fast paced and can seem overwhelming with frequent patient turnover, high volumes of admissions, medical complexity, and at times competing demands from families, staff, or faculty. Understanding how to orient to the daily flow can aid students in success in managing the seemingly chaotic atmosphere. As with any rotation, understanding setting and team expectations through effective orientation and question asking at the onset is at its core the foundation for success.

Pre-rounding

The purpose of pre-rounding is to gather necessary information for formal rounds and informed discussions with patients, families, and staff prior to team-based rounds. Pre-rounding can serve as an opportunity for learners to practice patient and family specific communication, create therapeutic alliance, and bolster nuanced physical exam skills, while also allowing for students to learn how to confront and address uncertainty both within themselves as well as for families. See Table 9.5 for a pre-rounding checklist. It is appropriate to defer to the collective team at times when learners are unsure.

Table 9.5 Pre-rounding checklist

Task	Roles	Student actions
Patient handoff	• Typically led by house staff • Learners should actively engage in note taking • Students may be encouraged or discouraged from asking questions	Learn of events which transpired, new updates, or key pieces of information shared which may not have made it into the medical record
Information gathering from the electronic medical record (EMR)	• Learners should create a step-by-step routine • Record information for later presentations either electronically or by written record for later discussion (safeguard any written documents to protect personal health information of patients) • Perform pediatric specific calculations (see Chap. 5)	Review: 1. All notes (nursing/staff, resident, specialist, etc.) created since the last time the student reviewed the EMR 2. Newly obtained labs or radiographic studies and those that are pending/still to be obtained 3. Intake and output for the past 24 h 4. Current medication list including as needed medications and the frequency of those medications 5. Vital signs and **trends** over the past 24 h or since admission 6. Note milligram per kilogram dosing of certain medications, urinary output as represented by milliliter per kilogram per hour, and nutritional intake as kilocalories per kilogram per day for infants
Visiting patients/families	• Create active discussion with families and when possible, patients • Meet with house staff to discuss developments in pre-rounding	7. Inquire about overnight events/events since they were last seen 8. Update any known developments 9. Ask about specific questions/needs that need to be addressed on rounds 10. Perform guided/specific physical exam

Rounds

Formal rounding during inpatient rotations typically follows pre-rounding. At its core rounding in pediatrics is a team-based approach involving multiple layers of support and expertise with the family and patient at the center of it all. Table 9.6 describes the roles and responsibilities of inpatient team members. The components of the rounding team will vary but at times may include a faculty member, pediatric or non-pediatric residents rotating on inpatient services, pediatric nursing staff, pharmacists, allied health providers (PT, OT, ST), nutritionists, and respiratory therapists, the role of each is loosely defined in the following table. The standard for pediatric inpatient rounding since 2012 has involved family centered rounds [1]. Chapter 5 details presentations on family centered rounds. During rounds when not presenting a patient, students should remain engaged and advance their learning from peers. Rounds are an opportunity to observe others' presentations, participate in patient discussions and bedside teaching be it from peers, residents, faculty, or staff.

Table 9.6 Roles and responsibilities of the inpatient team

Faculty	Responsible for oversight of rounds, teaching, alteration to plans when necessary/clarification
Resident	Primary care provider for patients/families. Primary communicator/liaison between families and team. Input orders. Generate formal plans of care and care coordination
Nursing staff	Primary bedside care provider. Patient advocate. Educator of daily care
Pharmacist	Oversight of medications, dosing, adjustments. Aid in conversion of IV to oral medications. Aid in medication calendar and med teaching
Allied health professional (Physical therapy, occupational therapy, speech therapy)	Aid in improvement of functions of daily living. Assessments for functionality for patients
Nutritionist	Provide nutritional assessments. Goals for caloric needs. Options for optimal nutritional development
Respiratory therapist	Oversee respiratory needs of patients. Provide respiratory medications and teaching to families and patients
Social worker	Provide assessment of social barriers to care and resources for families both within and external to hospital setting. Link to community resources

Table 9.7 Post-rounds to-do list

1. Aid in contacting consultants, other team members not present on rounds and discussing needs/updates
2. Follow up on labs or imaging ordered during rounds that may have occurred which will impact care. Obtain any outside medical records discussed during rounds
3. Write daily progress notes on patients seen
4. Check in or re-examine patients
5. Create self-reflection and evaluation on lessons learned, areas to improve, and what went well during rounding with team

Post-rounds

The post-rounding time should be a period to aid in completion of work with the team via communication with internal or external care providers as well as a reflective and preparatory time for students. Table 9.7 provides an ordered task list.

Outpatient Rotations

Students rotating in the outpatient pediatric setting are provided with many learning experiences in a variety of settings. A structured/well-planned approach to those experiences can optimize the clinical rotation.

The Daily Flow

The daily workflow from clinic to clinic may vary but students should prepare in a systematic way, including pre-clinical activities when possible and post-clinical activities to reinforce learning. Keys to succeeding in the daily flow of outpatient clinic are outlined in Table 9.8 below.

Table 9.8 Outpatient clinic daily workflow

Pre-clinic activities	1. Identify patients and families which they may be seeing that day 2. Chart review of the patient(s) to learn about prior visits and plans for the upcoming visit • Pay particular attention to prior physical exam findings, diagnostic workup, vital signs (including growth parameters), medication lists, and other providers who may have seen the patient 3. Discuss with team (faculty/residents) known learning opportunities that may transpire during clinic day
During clinic activities/ pitfalls	4. See patients in a timely manner upon arrival to prevent disruption to clinical flow 5. Focus on obtaining facts/exam skills pertinent to the reason for visit as well as learning pertinent exams vs comprehensive exams and when each is relevant 6. Prepare to defer when appropriate to residents/faculty when families attempt to address multiple areas during the visit 7. Focus on creating succinct presentation skills as opposed to full history and physical exams when appropriate • Presentations should focus on a full history of present illness (HPI); pertinent updates to past medical, social, or family history; key physical exam findings; and finally diagnostic and therapeutic plans
Post clinic activities	8. Completion of daily visit notes 9. Reflection on areas of improvement/success during clinic visits and feedback from team on ways to improve 10. Discussion of clinical questions unanswered from clinic day along with plan for self-study

Conclusion

Pediatric rotations provide ample opportunity for students to hone their clinical skills and enhance their medical knowledge for use not only in the field of pediatrics but as clinicians in general. Through preparation, investment, and engagement students can build on life-long learning skills which will translate into real-world practice throughout their careers.

Reference

1. COMMITTEE ON HOSPITAL CARE and INSTITUTE FOR PATIENT- AND FAMILY-CENTERED CARE. Patient- and family-centered care and the pediatrician's role. Pediatrics. 2012;129(2):394–404. https://doi.org/10.1542/peds.2011-3084. Epub 2012 Jan 30.

Chapter 10
Abdominal Pain

Andrew Shieh and Emily L. Jacobson

Background

Abdominal pain is pain that occurs between the thorax and pelvis and can be acute, recurrent, or chronic. It is one of the most common chief complaints in children, accounting for 9% of primary care visits and 5–10% of emergency department visits. Although most children who present with abdominal pain will have a self-limiting condition, the presence of pain may be a sign of a serious surgical or medical emergency. Evaluation of abdominal pain requires a detailed history, complete physical exam, and consideration for laboratory investigation and imaging studies. Making a timely diagnosis among the diverse etiologies is often challenging, and an incorrect diagnosis can be devastating or cause a patient to undergo unnecessary diagnostic tests. The disposition of patients with acute abdominal pain relies on interpreting the available information to make a diagnosis and providing thorough anticipatory guidance to patients.

A. Shieh (✉)
Department of Emergency Medicine, University of Michigan Medical School, Ann Arbor, MI, USA
e-mail: shandrew@med.umich.edu

E. L. Jacobson
Department of Pediatrics, Department of Internal Medicine, University of Michigan Medical School, Ann Arbor, MI, USA
e-mail: jacobsoe@med.umich.edu

N. Liao et al. (eds.), *Pediatric Rotations*,
https://doi.org/10.1007/978-3-031-59873-9_10

Pathophysiology

The type of pain associated with a particular condition may change as the disease progresses. Pain is transmitted through different afferent nerve fibers and can be triggered by three different pathways: visceral, somatic, and referred. Localization can be confounded by the type of fibers involved in the abdomen. Visceral nerve fibers are found in the intestinal mucosa, mesentery, and muscles of the abdominal wall. They respond to stretch, such as when bowel is distended, and perceive pain that is usually gradual in onset and long duration. The pain sensed is dull and diffuse because the nerves are not well myelinated, have fewer nerve endings, enter the spinal cord at multiple levels, and are bilaterally innervated. Generally, visceral pain in the lower esophagus, stomach, and duodenum is perceived in the epigastric region. Visceral pain in the small intestine is felt in the umbilical region, and colonic visceral pain is felt in the lower quadrants. Autonomic nerves are involved with visceral nerve fibers, and many patients may experience nausea, vomiting, diaphoresis, and anxiety.

Somatic nerve fibers are located in the skin, muscle, and parietal peritoneum. They transmit pain due to inflammation, stretching, and tearing. These nerves are myelinated and travel within spinal nerves that transmit to specific dorsal root ganglia. As a result, the pain tends to be more focal, sudden in onset, and sharp in quality. Irritation of the parietal peritoneum, regardless of etiology, often leads to pain that worsens with movement and minimal palpation. The pain of appendicitis, with sharp pain localized to the right lower quadrant, is an example of somatic pain.

Pain in the abdomen may also be referred to or from other parts of the body. The pain is typically felt in the dermatome region that corresponds to visceral nerve input to the spinal cord. For example, children with pneumonia may have referred pain in the abdomen.

History

Obtaining a history is the most important step to considering a diagnosis. In pediatrics, an important piece of history is often the age of the patient, as certain diagnoses become more or less likely depending on age. Young children are often not able to localize their pain. Caregiver report of associated symptoms is often vital in making the correct diagnosis. Similar to any chief concern of pain, it is important to consider onset, duration, periodicity, location, migration, characterization, severity, and precipitating and alleviating factors for pain. Given the breadth of possible diagnoses, it is also important to obtain a full review of symptoms, prior medical history, and family history. Past medical history remains important as special populations of patients are at risk for less common but severe conditions. For example, patients with sickle cell disease are at risk for splenic sequestration. One must also consider different diagnoses in the adolescent and/or sexually active child; it is important to take a confidential history in this age group. Finally, the social history can provide key clues to the etiology as well as the impact symptoms are having on the patient's life and function. A complete history may not always be provided by the patient or caregiver, and thus, clinicians must sometimes ask specific questions to gather information. Based on the differential diagnosis, one may also need to ask clarifying questions specifically related to conditions of consideration. For example, if ingestion is possible, one would want to ask about medications in the house, or if diabetic ketoacidosis (DKA) is felt to be likely, it is prudent to ask about polyuria or polydipsia. Finally, it is important to note any red flag symptoms such as bilious emesis, bloody diarrhea, nocturnal pain, unintentional weight loss, or delayed puberty. Below are the other common questions to ask to help narrow the differential diagnosis and acutely manage the patient presenting with abdominal pain:

- *Is fever present?*—Consider infectious causes of abdominal pain such as gastroenteritis, appendicitis, pharyngitis, urinary tract infection, and pneumonia
- *Does the patient have vomiting or diarrhea?*—Fluid losses, electrolyte abnormalities, and physical exam findings of poor perfusion should be addressed immediately
- *Is the pain worse with movement or is there involuntary guarding or rebound tenderness?*—Peritoneal irritation can suggest acute surgical issues (appendicitis, trauma, perforation)
- *Is there involuntary weight loss?*—May suggest inflammatory bowel disease (IBD), celiac disease, or malignancy. Eating disorders should also be considered
- *Is bilious emesis present?*—Malrotation/volvulus and necrotizing enterocolitis should be considered in neonates as well as intussusception in those with colicky pain
- *Are pale, acholic stools and/or jaundice present?*—Consider biliary or hepatic disease
- *Are other symptoms present?*—Associated symptoms such as sore throat, rash, or joint pain may suggest referred pain or other systemic process
- *Is the pain chronic with previous negative work-up and imaging?*—Consider functional abdominal pain if there are no alarming findings
- *Is there a family history of abdominal pain or autoimmune conditions?*—Consider celiac disease, IBD, vasculitis, and diabetes mellitus

Physical Examination

Acute abdominal pain can be caused by benign etiologies or serious conditions that require surgery. Unfortunately, no physical exam findings are absolute, but a combination of overall appearance and red flag findings may suggest serious illness. In particular, pay close attention to lethargy, hemodynamic instability, dehydration, and peritoneal signs such as rebound or guarding as they often signal conditions warranting urgent evaluation and management. Attention should be given to performing a complete physical exam in all initial assessments:

- Vital signs
- Growth charts and plotting growth parameters
- General: assess for appearance, activity, alertness, obvious discomfort
- Examine the chest, lungs, back, flank

- Abdomen: inspect, auscultate, palpate, percuss. Look for distension or signs of peritoneal irritation (rebound tenderness, guarding, avoidance of motion)
  - Examination maneuvers specific for appendicitis: McBurney's sign (tender to palpation at two-third the distance from umbilicus to right anterior superior iliac spine), Rovsing's sign (palpation in left lower quadrant increases pain in right lower quadrant), obturator sign (pain with internal rotation of hip with right knee flexed), Psoas sign (pain with right thigh extension with patient lying on left side)
  - Palpable masses: May be benign (e.g., fecal burden in left lower quadrant) or worrisome (e.g., pyloric stenosis, tumors such as neuroblastoma or Wilms tumor)
- Genital: urethral orifice, vaginal orifice, scrotal exam, rectal exam, bimanual exam in all sexually active adolescent females with dysuria or vaginal discharge (evaluate for cervical motion, uterine, or adnexal tenderness), speculum exam (indicated when adolescent female has persistent symptomatic vaginal discharge, bleeding, or high suspicion for foreign body)
  - Ensure chaperone is present for all sensitive exams
  - Advise patient and obtain informed consent prior to performing exam
  - For infants and preadolescent children, a caregiver should remain close to the child
  - Genitourinary exam should be conducted in the knee-to-chest or frog-legged position for girls
  - Boys should be examined in the standing position with feet spread shoulder width for the genitourinary exam
  - Rectal exam should be conducted in the lateral decubitus position for both sexes
  - The genitourinary and rectal exams should be performed as the last part of the physical exam
- Hips: range of motion (flexion of hips may provoke peritoneal irritation)
- Neurological: gait, difficulty with walking or jumping
- Integumentary: skin turgor, capillary refill as indication of hydration status and perfusion

It is important to observe patients with serial exams given the evolution of the physical exam may help with diagnosis and is important for acute patient management.

Laboratory Assessment

Laboratory assessment for children presenting with abdominal pain is variable depending on symptoms, age and sex of patient, acuity of presentation, and differential diagnosis. Any test ordered should have a reason for being ordered, and no test result alone can make a diagnosis. For example, a complete blood cell count

(CBC) with differential and C-reactive protein (CRP) can confirm a provider's suspicions for an inflammatory process but alone cannot diagnose appendicitis. Adolescent females should undergo a pregnancy test regardless of whether they use contraception or have not yet experienced menarche. Additional work-up can be considered based on location of pain and symptoms (Table 10.1).

Table 10.1 Diagnostic assessment based on history and physical examination

Symptom	Diagnostic evaluation	Rationale and tips
Unexplained fever, weight loss	CBC, CRP, ESR	Basic screening for inflammatory state
	Blood glucose, urinary ketones, venous blood gas, beta-hydroxybutyrate	Assess for diabetes mellitus and DKA
	Cortisol (random or morning)	Screen for adrenal insufficiency
	Metabolic panel	Screen for adrenal insufficiency, electrolyte derangements
Diarrhea	Stool studies (PCR based, ova and parasite, *Clostridium difficile toxin)*	Evaluate for infectious cause if diagnosis will change management
	Fecal calprotectin	Screening test for IBD
Bilious emesis	Two view abdominal X-rays (upright and flat views)	Evaluate for air-fluid levels suggesting obstruction or ileus
	Upper GI series	X-ray imaging to evaluate for malrotation, volvulus
Urinary symptoms (dysuria, urgency, frequency, hematuria)	Urinalysis with urine culture	Evaluate for UTI, glomerulonephritis, nephrotic syndrome
	Renal ultrasound	Assess for pyelonephritis, renal abscess, nephrolithiasis
Right upper quadrant or epigastric pain	Metabolic panel	Evaluate for elevated liver enzymes or cholestatic pattern
	Lipase	Assess for pancreatitis
	Helicobacter pylori testing	Consideration when assessing dyspepsia
	Right upper quadrant ultrasound	Evaluate for biliary tree anatomy or obstruction
Urethral discharge, lower abdominal pain, testicular pain	Vaginal swab, urine, urethral swab (NAAT)	Evaluate for C*hlamydia trachomatis, Neisseria gonorrhoeae*, PID
	Urine or serum β-hCG	Evaluate for pregnancy
	STD blood tests (RPR, HIV, hepatitis B surface antigen)	All sexually active adolescents should be tested for HIV at least yearly
	Ultrasound (pelvic or testicular)	Assess for ovarian or testicular torsion

Abbreviations: *β-hCG* beta-human chorionic gonadotropin; *CBC* complete blood count; *CRP* C-reactive protein; *DKA* diabetic ketoacidosis; *ESR* erythrocyte sedimentation rate; *GI* gastrointestinal; *HIV* human immunodeficiency virus; *IBD* inflammatory bowel disease; *NAAT* nucleic acid amplification test; *PCR* polymerase chain reaction; *PID* pelvic inflammatory disease; *RPR* rapid plasma reagin; *STD* sexually transmitted diseases; *UTI* urinary tract infection

Imaging

Diagnostic imaging should be guided by the differential diagnosis after obtaining a thorough history and performing a complete physical exam. Similar to laboratory evaluation, not all children presenting with abdominal pain require diagnostic imaging. For example, the diagnosis of constipation can often be made based on history and physical exam alone. Imaging is vital in certain scenarios, though, such as in traumatic injury and when there is concern for acute surgical pathology.

Traumatic Abdominal Injuries

Abdominal injury may result from penetrating or blunt trauma, and children with severe blunt trauma may present with only mild abdominal pain. The most common mechanisms of blunt injury include falls and motor vehicle collisions, while penetrating injuries are commonly caused by gunshot and stab wounds. Lacerations of the spleen and liver are the most common traumatic intra-abdominal injuries because these organs lie outside the rib cage. After performing a physical exam to identify possible significant intra-abdominal injury (e.g., liver laceration, splenic hematoma or rupture, colonic perforation), a focused assessment with sonography using bedside ultrasound may be used to quickly evaluate for free fluid or hemoperitoneum. However, given that some patients with severe solid organ injury have minimal intra-abdominal fluid, ultrasound should not be the only diagnostic test performed to exclude intra-abdominal injury after trauma. Hemodynamically stable patients should undergo emergent computed tomography (CT) scan. Advanced imaging should be obtained only in patients who are hemodynamically stable, while unstable patients with abdominal trauma should undergo emergent evaluation by a surgeon.

Surgical Pathology or Prior Abdominal Surgery

In neonates and young infants, an abdominal radiograph should be obtained to assess for pneumatosis consistent with necrotizing enterocolitis. In patients with prior abdominal surgery presenting with acute pain and other symptoms concerning for obstruction (vomiting, significant distension, inability to pass gas or stool, hypoactive bowel sounds), abdominal radiography, including upright and flat views, should be obtained. Ultrasonography is helpful to assess the need for urgent surgical intervention in diagnoses such as non-reducible intussusception, incarcerated hernia, testicular or ovarian torsion. Ultrasonography is also useful in the diagnosis of cholecystitis or ruptured ovarian cyst. In older children, an ultrasound should be obtained if acute appendicitis is suspected, but the diagnosis cannot be excluded if the appendix is not visualized. A CT scan may be required due to its excellent sensitivity and specificity for appendicitis and other surgical emergencies, but should only be obtained after risks of radiation are discussed. A CT scan should be obtained to evaluate for a ruptured tumor, ruptured ectopic pregnancy, or perforated viscus with diffuse peritonitis. Magnetic resonance imaging (MRI) has excellent diagnostic reliability as well without radiation exposure.

Colicky Pain

Patients with episodic colicky pain (intermittent acute abdominal pain) should undergo evaluation for intussusception with ultrasonography, even if there is no history of bloody stools. Inguinal hernias may become incarcerated during viral illness or crying and require urgent evaluation with ultrasonography. Ultrasonography of the liver, gallbladder, and kidneys is useful in older children if other symptoms such as jaundice, urinary symptoms, flank pain, and vomiting are present. Ultrasonography has poor sensitivity to identify small renal calculi, so patients may require a helical CT scan for detection of calculi.

Palpable Masses

Children with severe constipation may present with a palpable mass in left lower quadrant of the abdomen, and stool burden may be evaluated with a radiograph if there is suspicion for obstruction or an alternative diagnosis is being considered. Ultrasound should be ordered to evaluate for intussusception if a sausage-shaped mass is palpated in the right mid-abdomen. Evaluation for possible intra-abdominal mass may require a CT scan and eventual MRI.

Abnormal Uterine Bleeding

Transabdominal or transvaginal pelvic ultrasonography can be used to evaluate structural abnormalities of the vagina, uterus, and ovaries. Relevant findings may include vaginal or cervical outlet obstruction, ovarian cysts and masses, ovarian follicles, or complications of pregnancy.

Differential Diagnosis

The differential diagnosis for children presenting with abdominal pain is broad and can be overwhelming. One needs to consider both common diagnoses for age along with life-threatening diagnoses that cannot be missed. It can be helpful to have a

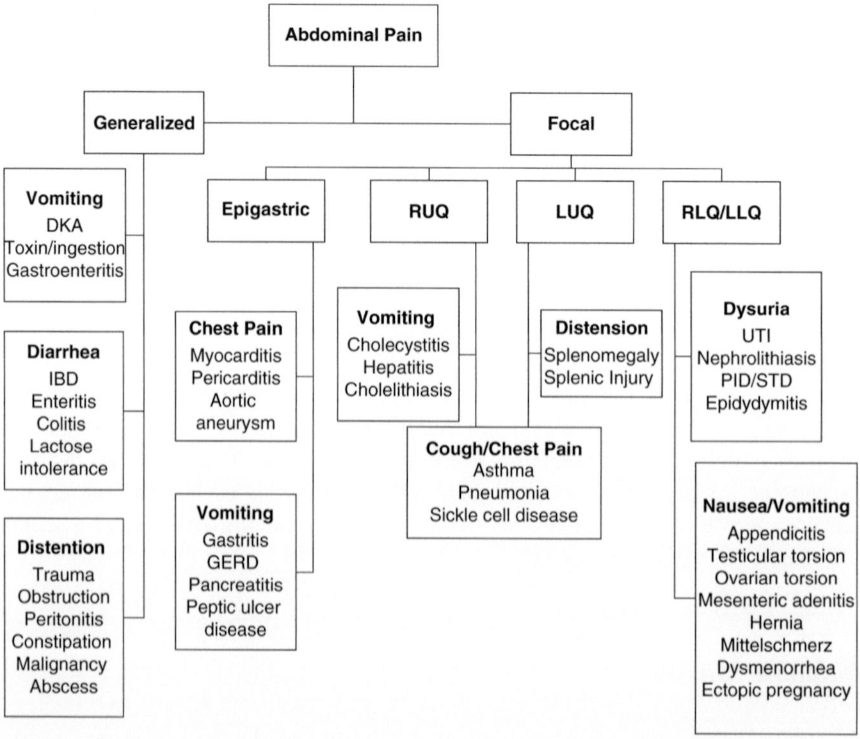

Fig. 10.1 General approach to pediatric abdominal pain. Abbreviations: *DKA* diabetic ketoacidosis; *GERD* gastroesophageal reflux disease; *IBD* inflammatory bowel disease; *LLQ* left lower quadrant; *LUQ* left upper quadrant; *PID* pelvic inflammatory disease; *RLQ* right lower quadrant; *RUQ* right upper quadrant; *STD* sexually transmitted diseases; *UTI* urinary tract infection

systemic approach for thinking through possible diagnoses. Potential systematic approaches to group diagnoses include by location of pain, system involvement (i.e., endocrine, renal), or associated symptoms (i.e., diarrhea, urinary symptoms) (Fig. 10.1). Below are different systemic approaches to diagnose the etiology of a child's abdominal pain along with highlights of common and/or life-threatening conditions.

Causes of Acute Abdominal Pain <5 Years Old

The table below highlights a systems-based approach to diagnose abdominal pain in children under 5 years old (Table 10.2). While a dedicated review of all causes of abdominal pain in children under 5 years old is out of the scope of this book, it is important to highlight a few conditions in this population.

Table 10.2 Causes of acute abdominal pain in children <5 years old

System	Acuity	Condition	Notes
Gastrointestinal	Life threatening	Necrotizing enterocolitis	Premature infants or infants with congenital heart disease. Often associated with bloody stool
		Intussusception	Paroxysmal pain, bloody stool, vomiting
		Malrotation with volvulus	Severe pain, vomiting, obstruction, bloody stools
		Appendicitis	Migration of pain from periumbilical region to RLQ
		Incarcerated hernia	Manually reduce if no systemic signs of toxicity
		Obstruction	Higher risk with previous surgery, often associated with emesis
	Common	Constipation	Peak occurrence in toddler to pre-school aged children
		Protein sensitivity (milk, gluten), FPIES	Can be associated with vomiting, diarrhea, bloody stools. Dietary history is important
		GERD	Complications include failure to thrive in infants with treatment dependent on growth. Can exacerbate underlying respiratory issues in older kids
		Mesenteric adenitis	Diagnosis of exclusion, main differential diagnosis is appendicitis
Infectious		Gastroenteritis	Viral, bacterial, or parasitic
		UTI/pyelonephritis	Common cause for fever in this age group
		Pneumonia	Common in underlying respiratory disease, immunosuppression, neuromuscular disease
		Hepatitis	Associated with jaundice, change in stools
		Viral illness	May be associated with respiratory symptoms or rash
Endocrine		Diabetic ketoacidosis	May be first presentation of type 1 diabetes mellitus
Rheumatologic		Henoch-Schönlein purpura	Associated with palpable purpura in dependent areas, joint pain, and hematuria
Renal		Hemolytic uremic syndrome	Triad of acute microangiopathic hemolytic anemia, thrombocytopenia, oliguric renal failure

(continued)

Table 10.2 (continued)

System	Acuity	Condition	Notes
Hematological/oncologic		Malignancy (neuroblastoma, hepatoblastoma, Wilms tumor)	Assess for lung metastases or mediastinal tumor (neuroblastoma)
Other		Trauma (accidental or child abuse)	Spleen and liver are most prone to injury
		Ingestion	Consider lead, medications in the home, foreign body ingestion

Abbreviations: *FPIES* food protein-induced enterocolitis syndrome; *GERD* gastroesophageal reflux disease; *RLQ* right lower quadrant; *UTI* urinary tract infection

Necrotizing Enterocolitis (NEC)

NEC manifests by ischemic necrosis of the intestinal mucosa and is one of the most common emergencies during the newborn period. The most important risk factor is prematurity, but other factors include cyanotic heart disease, growth restriction, birth asphyxia, gastroschisis, sepsis, history of exchange transfusion, antenatal cocaine abuse, and premature rupture of membranes. Patients present with feeding intolerance and occult or grossly bloody stools. Systemic signs may include shock, temperature instability, respiratory failure, and apnea. Physical exam findings include distention, tenderness, and absent bowel sounds. Abdominal radiograph reveals dilated loops of bowel and air-fluid levels; pneumatosis intestinalis (gas in the wall of the intestines) may be subtle, but is pathognomonic of NEC. Initial stabilization is directed toward abdominal decompression, fluid resuscitation, and parenteral antibiotics. Most patients require bowel rest for at least 10 days followed by slowly increased enteral feedings based on clinical condition. Surgery is indicated for perforation, pneumoperitoneum, or cellulitis of the abdominal wall.

Intussusception

Intussusception is the telescoping or invagination of one part of the intestine into an adjacent part of intestine, most commonly ileocolic. It tends to present in children between 3 months and 3 years old. Symptoms and signs include acute colicky abdominal pain, emesis, altered mental status, and a palpable mass on exam. Stools may be a mixture of blood and mucous, appearing as "currant jelly", but this a late finding and only occurs in a minority of patients. Given the risk for bowel ischemia and perforation, prompt diagnosis and management are vital. Diagnosis is usually confirmed by ultrasound demonstrating a "doughnut" or "target sign" of bowel.

Treatment for ileocolic intussusception involves intravenous hydration, surgical consultation, and reduction (typically first-line management is to use a pneumatic enema). Compared to ileocolic, small bowel-small bowel intussusception typically spontaneously reduces.

Malrotation/Volvulus

Malrotation is due to abnormal in utero development and results in the abnormal location and fixation of the intestines. This can lead to development of volvulus, or twisting of the intestines, and subsequent bowel obstruction and ischemia. Volvulus most commonly presents in young infants with bilious emesis and abdominal distension. Abdominal radiograph can help rule out other causes of obstruction. This is typically followed by an upper gastrointestinal series to confirm malrotation and volvulus. If confirmed, urgent surgical consultation is necessary.

Henoch-Schönlein Purpura (HSP)

Henoch-Schönlein Purpura is the most common systemic vasculitis in children characterized by palpable purpura, arthralgias, colicky abdominal pain, and renal involvement. There is often a preceding upper respiratory viral illness or streptococcal infection. The painless purpura and edema are predominantly gravity dependent areas (e.g., legs, buttocks, scrotum). Bloody stools may be also present. Initial laboratory tests should include urinalysis to evaluate for hematuria or proteinuria. CBC may reveal leukocytosis, but normal hemoglobin and platelet count. Abdominal ultrasound should be considered to screen for intussusception. The condition is usually well managed with non-steroidal anti-inflammatory drugs or acetaminophen and usually spontaneously resolves within 8 weeks. Corticosteroids may be indicated in patients with severe abdominal pain but does not shorten the overall clinical course. Patients require follow-up with their primary physician for routine urinalysis and blood pressure monitoring for at least 6 months to screen for development of kidney disease.

Constipation

Constipation is one of the more common causes of abdominal pain in toddlers and pre-school aged children. It can be associated with a child withholding stool to prevent painful defecation triggered by changes in toilet training routine, stress, diet, and starting school. While symptoms vary by age group, it typically presents with hard, infrequent, and difficult movements to pass stool. Functional constipation is most common, but it is important to consider red flag components of history and symptoms to rule out other conditions associated with constipation. For example, passage of meconium in a neonate after 48 h should raise suspicion for Hirschsprung disease or cystic fibrosis. Significant vomiting with constipation should lead to further evaluation to exclude bowel obstruction. The treatment of functional constipation varies based on the age of the patient, but should involve adequate initial disimpaction, behavioral treatment, and medication management.

Causes of Acute Abdominal Pain >5 Years Old

The differential diagnosis for young children compared to older children has some similarities and differences. For example, gastroenteritis and urinary tract infections can occur in both age groups and present with similar symptoms. Other conditions such as streptococcus pharyngitis or inflammatory bowel disease are more common in the older age group. Older children may also be able to participate more in providing a history and cooperate with the physical exam. Because of this, a pain-localization systematic approach to the differential diagnosis may be beneficial (Table 10.3). Below is expanded information on selective causes of abdominal pain in this age group.

Table 10.3 Causes of acute abdominal pain >5 years old

	Life threatening	Common	Less common
Generalized	IBD/megacolon Peritonitis Obstruction (prior abdominal surgery) DKA Toxin/ingestion	Acute gastroenteritis Colitis Constipation Viral syndrome Trauma Functional abdominal pain Lactose intolerance	IBD Malignancy Intra-abdominal abscess
Epigastric	Peptic ulcer disease (with perforation) Aortic aneurysm	Gastritis GERD	Pancreatitis Myocarditis Pericarditis
RUQ	Cholecystitis Acute fulminant hepatitis	Pneumonia Asthma	Cholelithiasis
RLQ	Appendicitis Testicular torsion Ovarian torsion Ectopic pregnancy	UTI Mesenteric adenitis Dysmenorrhea Mittelschmerz	PID Epididymitis Nephrolithiasis Hernia
LUQ		Pneumonia Sickle cell disease	Splenomegaly
LLQ	Testicular torsion Ovarian torsion Ectopic pregnancy	Urinary tract infection Dysmenorrhea Mittelschmerz	PID Epididymitis Nephrolithiasis Hernia

Abbreviations: *DKA* diabetic ketoacidosis; *GERD* gastroesophageal reflux disease; *IBD* inflammatory bowel disease; *PID* pelvic inflammatory disease; *UTI* urinary tract infection

Appendicitis

Acute appendicitis is the most common abdominal condition in children requiring surgery. Risk factors for perforation of the appendix and other complications include age below 4 years old and prolonged duration of symptoms beyond 36 h. The abdominal pain typically presents as vague, colicky periumbilical pain that migrates to the right lower quadrant within 12 h after onset of pain. Ultrasonography is widely accepted as the first-line imaging modality for diagnosis. If ultrasound is equivocal, advanced imaging is required to reliably exclude appendicitis. Once the diagnosis is confirmed, antibiotics should be given preoperatively to reduce risk of abscess formation. The choice of when or if patients receive an appendectomy is variable based on a variety of factors.

Gastroesophageal Reflux Disease

Gastroesophageal reflux is a normal physiologic process occurring in healthy infants and older children. Gastroesophageal reflux disease results when clinical symptoms result from reflux due to delayed gastric emptying or decreased neural protective reflexes of digestive tract. Infants younger than 6 months of age with reflux may present with frequent spitting up of small amounts of breastmilk or formula, feeding discomfort or intolerance, or back arching with feeds. A thorough diet history and reassuring physical exam are adequate to make the diagnosis of uncomplicated reflux. Adolescents usually present with recurrent abdominal pain, regurgitation, or heartburn symptoms. For infants who are feeding well and gaining appropriate weight, treatment with an H2 blocker or proton pump inhibitor is often not indicated and instead, efforts should be directed toward parental education. Formula changes usually do not significantly improve symptoms, but if protein allergy is suspected, a short trial of a hydrolyzed formula may be beneficial.

Functional Abdominal Pain

Functional abdominal pain is the most common cause of recurrent pediatric abdominal pain. The Rome IV criteria in 2016 defines functional abdominal pain as episodic pain that does not occur solely during physiologic events (e.g., menses, eating), cannot be attributed to an organic medical condition after appropriate evaluation, and occurs four or more times per month for greater than 2 months. It occurs in approximately 0.3–8% of children with higher prevalence in girls, children of ages 4–6 years old, and early adolescents. This condition includes nausea and vomiting disorders (cyclic vomiting syndrome, rumination syndrome, aerophagia), abdominal migraine, functional dyspepsia, and irritable bowel syndrome. Laboratory studies are often not necessary for functional abdominal pain unless testing is indicated when alarming symptoms or physical exam findings suggest nonfunctional disorder. Treatment for functional abdominal pain should be approached from a psychosocial perspective and may include a combination of psychotherapy, diet, pharmacology, and alternative medicine. Cognitive-behavioral therapy with mind-body techniques focused on stress management, and anxiety can result in significant short-term improvement in pain.

Management

Treatment for abdominal pain depends on the condition. All children who are seriously ill or injured should be stabilized in the emergency department immediately. Severe cardiorespiratory disease and shock may present with abdominal pain, and careful attention should be paid to airway, breathing, and circulation to prevent further clinical deterioration. Seriously ill children or those who require immediate surgical evaluation for traumatic injury, appendicitis, intussusception, or incarcerated hernia should be prioritized. Once patients are stabilized, efforts should be directed toward further diagnosis and symptom plus condition management. Patients should not be discharged from the hospital until the patient is able to tolerate oral intake without significant recurrence of pain. The prognosis depends on the cause of abdominal pain.

Conditions Requiring Immediate Surgical Consultation

- Volvulus (gastric, midgut, sigmoid)
- Closed loop or high-grade bowel obstruction
- Incarcerated hernia
- Non-reducible intussusception
- Malrotation with volvulus
- Acute appendicitis
- Diffuse peritonitis
- Ruptured tumor
- Testicular torsion
- Ovarian torsion
- Ectopic pregnancy

Conditions with Initial Medical Management

- Constipation
- Pancreatitis

- Cholecystitis
- Partial small bowel obstruction
- Renal calculi
- Intestinal adhesions without bowel compromise
- Inflammatory bowel disease
- Abdominal abscess
- Ovarian cyst
- Oncological diseases
- Toxic megacolon or typhlitis

Conditions with Medical Management

- Gastroenteritis
- Urinary tract infection
- Hepatitis
- Pelvic inflammatory disease
- Pneumonia
- Ileus
- Diabetic ketoacidosis
- Peptic ulcer disease
- Henoch-Schönlein Purpura
- Hemolytic uremic syndrome
- Intoxication
- Dysmenorrhea
- Functional abdominal pain

Anticipatory Guidance

Children should return to the emergency department or be hospitalized when a surgical or medical emergency is suspected. Patients who are unable to tolerate enteral nutrition or maintain hydration at home should be evaluated. Patients and families should monitor for signs of dehydration such as decreased urine output, lack of tears, dizziness, and fatigue. Patients should be advised to seek medical guidance and evaluation if pain migrates, worsens in severity, and becomes characteristically associated with other symptoms including weight loss, persistent diarrhea or vomiting, or does not improve. Further anticipatory guidance is tailored to the specific diagnosis and known complications of such conditions. If there is ongoing involuntary weight loss, deceleration of linear growth, persistent vomiting or diarrhea, or persistent pain, expert consultation should be sought.

Application Exercises

1. A 9-year-old boy presents to the emergency department with periumbilical abdominal pain that began last night and is now worsening. The pain is severe and constant. The patient now has non-bloody, non-bilious vomiting prior to presentation. Physical exam reveals a temperature of 38.5 °C. Abdominal exam reveals abdominal tenderness in the right lower quadrant with rebound tenderness. The patient also has guarding in other regions of his abdomen with palpation. What imaging modality would you order first?

   A. Computed tomography
   B. Magnetic resonance imaging
   C. Ultrasonography
   D. Upper gastrointestinal X-ray series

   Answer C: The first-line diagnostic study to evaluate for appendicitis is ultrasonography. However, sensitivity and specificity can vary depending on patient anatomy, body habitus, age, and operator-experience. CT and MRI have higher sensitivity and specificity for diagnosis. However, CT exposes the patient to radiation and MRI may not be readily available at all pediatric centers. Upper gastrointestinal X-ray series would be useful in the diagnosis of malrotation in patients who are hemodynamically stable unless volvulus (presents with bilious emesis) is present.

2. A 2-year-old boy presents with intermittent abdominal pain that began approximately 10 h ago. In between the episodes, the boy has no distress and is very active. He has attempted to drink, but experiences vomiting due to pain. He has no diarrhea. Physical exam reveals no fever. You witness an episode of pain in which the boy holds his abdomen and screams in pain. Under which circumstance would surgical intervention be indicated as the initial management for this boy?

   A. Currant jelly stools
   B. Recurrence of symptoms 1 h after a reduction attempt
   C. Failure of ibuprofen to alleviate the pain
   D. Hypotension and tachycardia are present

   Answer D: The classic triad of intussusception is intermittent colicky abdominal pain, "currant jelly" stools, and vomiting. It is the most common abdominal emergency in children between ages 6 months and 36 months. There are a variety of nonsurgical techniques to reduce an intussusception including different types of enemas and methods of visualization. Successful reduction is achieved over 80% of the time. If the initial reduction is only partially successful and the patient remains hemodynamically stable, another attempt can be tried. However, hemodynamically unstable patients should have surgery immediately.

3. A 13-year-old obese boy presents to the emergency department with 2 days of vomiting and severe abdominal pain. The pain is constant and radiates toward his back. He has no diarrhea. Physical exam reveals a temperature of 38.1 °C with heart rate of 110 beats per minute. He is comfortable in bed without vomit-

ing. Abdominal exam reveals epigastric abdominal tenderness. There is no right upper quadrant tenderness. His laboratory studies reveal a lipase level that is over four times the normal limit. How would this boy be best managed?

A. Start broad spectrum parenteral antibiotics
B. Restrict intravenous fluids to half maintenance rate
C. Treat pain with frequent morphine doses
D. Place a nasogastric tube to continuous suction and allow him to have nothing by mouth for 1 week

Answer C: Pancreatitis is characterized by two of the following three features: abdominal pain, elevated pancreatic enzymes at least three times the upper limit of normal, and radiologic evidence of pancreatic inflammation. Up to 25% of cases are idiopathic. Management of pancreatitis is supportive and requires aggressive fluid resuscitation, usually with fluids at one-and-a-half times to two times maintenance rate. Pain should be managed with non-steroidal anti-inflammatory drugs and narcotics. For severe systemic illness or necrosis of the pancreatitis, broad spectrum antibiotics should be used. Nasogastric decompression should be used if the patient is actively vomiting. Early nutrition is usually appropriate when pain is improved.

4. A 4-week-old boy presents to the emergency department with abdominal distension and bilious vomiting that began 6 h earlier. He has had three episodes of vomiting and is unable to feed formula. There is no blood in the stool. On abdominal exam, the boy is in acute pain. His vital signs are normal except for mild tachycardia. His abdomen is distended without rigidity, tympanitic to percussion, and diffusely tender. Which imaging study should be ordered next?

A. Radiograph of abdomen
B. Ultrasonography of abdomen
C. Upper gastrointestinal series
D. Computed tomography of abdomen

Answer C: An upper gastrointestinal series is the best test to diagnose malrotation and will reveal abnormal position of the third and fourth portion of the duodenum in malrotation and the "corkscrew" sign when midgut volvulus is present. To exclude malrotation, the duodenum should be retroperitoneal on lateral radiographs and the ligament of Treitz should cross midline to the left of the spine. An abdominal radiograph cannot exclude the possibility of malrotation. Given potential for volvulus and obstruction, malrotation is a true surgical emergency.

Further Reading

Baker RD. Acute abdominal pain. Pediatr Rev. 2018;39(3):130–9.
Hyman PE. Chronic and recurrent abdominal pain. Pediatr Rev. 2016;37(9):377–90.

Shah SS, Zaoutis LB, Catallozzi M, Frank G. Gastroenterology. In: The Philadelphia guide: inpatient pediatrics. 2nd ed. McGraw Hill Education; 2016. p. 132–54.
Thapar N, Benninga MA, Crowell MD, Lorenzo CD, Mack I, Nurko S, Saps M, Shulman RJ, Szajewska H, van Tilburg MAL, Enck P. Paediatric functional abdominal pain disorders. Nat Rev. Dis Primers. 2020;6(89):1–23.

Chapter 11
Acid–Base and Electrolyte Disorders

Ashley Rawson, Andrew Schwaderer, and Myda Khalid

Background

Common pediatric ailments such as viral gastroenteritis, respiratory infections, and type 1 diabetes often present with electrolyte and/or acid/base derangements. The objective of this chapter is to focus on some of these metabolic derangements often encountered in the pediatric clinic, emergency room, and hospital setting: metabolic acidosis, metabolic alkalosis, respiratory acidosis, respiratory alkalosis, hyponatremia, and hypernatremia. A basic understanding of these abnormalities will allow for more prompt diagnosis and management of several pediatric illnesses.

Pathophysiology

Acid/base balance is tightly controlled by multiple processes including intracellular and extracellular buffering agents, elimination or retention of carbon dioxide (CO_2) via respiration, and acid excretion or bicarbonate retention by the kidney tubules.

A. Rawson (✉)
Division of Pediatric Nephrology, Department of Pediatrics, Our Lady of the Lake Children's Hospital, Baton Rouge, LA, USA
e-mail: ashley.rawson@fmolhs.org

A. Schwaderer · M. Khalid
Division of Pediatric Nephrology, Department of Pediatrics, Riley Hospital for Children/Indiana University, Indianapolis, IN, USA
e-mail: schwadea@iu.edu; khalidm@iu.edu

N. Liao et al. (eds.), *Pediatric Rotations*,
https://doi.org/10.1007/978-3-031-59873-9_11

Metabolic Acidosis and Respiratory Acidosis

Metabolic acidosis is indicated by a low blood pH < 7.35 and serum bicarbonate (HCO_3) < 22 mmol/L. In contrast, a respiratory acidosis is indicated by an increase in the arterial partial pressure of carbon dioxide (pCO_2) > 45 mmHg with a low blood pH < 7.35. Metabolic acidosis is the result of one or a combination of these mechanisms: increased acid production, increased acid intake, decreased renal acid excretion, or increased bicarbonate loss from the gastrointestinal tract or the kidney. Metabolic acidosis can also result as a compensatory mechanism in the setting of respiratory alkalosis, a process that occurs over days. Conversely, respiratory compensation in the setting of metabolic acidosis occurs rapidly within 12–24 h. Respiratory acidosis is the result of one or a combination of these mechanisms: increased CO_2 production, hypoventilation, abnormalities in respiratory drive, anatomic chest wall abnormalities, or abnormal respiratory musculature.

Metabolic Alkalosis and Respiratory Alkalosis

Metabolic alkalosis is indicated by an increased blood pH > 7.45 and serum bicarbonate (HCO_3) >29 mmol/L. A metabolic alkalosis is generated by loss of acid from extracellular fluid, addition of bicarbonate via intake or decreased excretion, or volume contraction. The alkalosis is sustained by a low serum chloride and/or potassium. Like metabolic acidosis, metabolic alkalosis can also result as a compensatory mechanism in the setting of respiratory acidosis. Respiratory alkalosis results in an arterial pH > 7.45 and is secondary to a reduction in the arterial partial pressure of carbon dioxide (pCO_2) < 35 mmHg. Often this is from hyperventilation that may be secondary to pain and anxiety.

Hypernatremia

Hypernatremia is defined as a serum sodium >145 mEq/L and is typically due to excess salt or inadequate water, the latter being more common. Osmolality is tightly controlled in the body, and unexpected movements in water across cell membranes can result in swelling or shrinking of cells, the most important being in the brain.

Hyponatremia

Hyponatremia is defined as a serum sodium <135 mEq/L. Hyponatremia can occur in the setting of volume depletion, euvolemia, and hypervolemia. In the setting of volume depletion as is often seen with gastroenteritis, the patient loses water through vomiting and diarrhea and the losses are replaced by a hypotonic solution (too much water, such as diluted baby formula). This results in a decrease in circulating volume which stimulates antidiuretic hormone (ADH) promoting reabsorption of water by the kidney tubules. Hyponatremia in euvolemic or hypervolemic states can be due to the inappropriate release of ADH or edematous states resulting in too much water, respectively. Neurologic sequelae like seizures and altered mental status are caused by rapid fluids shifts across neuronal cell membranes causing brain edema and usually occur with serum sodium levels ≤120 mEq/L.

History

Each component of the history is vital to determining the underlying cause of acid, base, and sodium disorders. Listening to patients and their families provides a wealth of information often allowing diagnosis and management to target the correct pathology.

Hydration Status

Intake and output are important for evaluation of sodium balance and acid/base derangements. Patients with vomiting and diarrhea may be dehydrated and therefore hyper or hyponatremic. He/she/they may have hydrated with a hypotonic solution that resulted in a low serum sodium. Consider the patient's ability to control their intake and output as well. Infants who are formula fed or breastfed are unable to control their hydration status. How is mother's milk supply? Is the patient a formula fed infant? How is the family preparing the infant's formula? Incorrect formula mixing is a common etiology of sodium derangements in infants. Patients who are significantly developmentally delayed may not experience a brain signal telling them to drink and patients who are g-tube dependent may be unable to control their own hydration status. Ask if these patients have been tolerating their feeds and what their feeding regimen is.

Urine output and stool output will also give you an idea of hydration status. A patient with good urine output is unlikely to be dehydrated unless a renal concentrating defect is present, for example, diabetes insipidus which we will discuss below. High stool output or excessive vomiting is also likely to result in electrolyte abnormalities and dehydration.

Ingestions

Multiple ingestions and exposures can result in acid/base derangements. Consider the patient's environment: Are any medications or household cleaners stored in the home within the patients reach? In older patients, it is important to take a good history of mental health disorders or current stressors to evaluate for risk of intentional ingestions.

Growth and Development

Changes in acid/base balance also alter a child's ability to grow and develop normally. Ask the family about developmental milestones expected for that patient's age and evaluate their growth chart.

Physical Exam

Vitals

Vital signs offer critical clues to acid/base disorders and derangements in sodium. Patients with acid/base disorders may have unusual breathing patterns. An example of this is Kussmaul breathing that is seen in diabetic ketoacidosis. These patients have labored, rapid breathing and you may also note a fruity smell to their breath from the increased ketones in their blood. Many patients with metabolic acidosis will have rapid breathing to expel more CO_2 (respiratory compensation). The opposite may be seen in patients with metabolic alkalosis.

Heart rate is also very important. Tachycardia is seen in dehydration prior to low blood pressure. However, consider the presentation of the patient as fever can result in tachycardia as well. An elevated blood pressure could indicate a fluid overloaded status. In patients with severe sodium derangements that have resulted in neurological findings, you may note bradycardia and irregular respirations as well.

Weight

Weight is important when trying to determine a child's fluid status. If possible, obtain the weight of a child prior to their acute illnesses. Consider reviewing records from the patient's primary care physician to obtain a recent weight. Decreases in weight can indicate dehydration, and increases may indicate fluid overload. You should also examine the child's growth chart.

See Table 11.1 for considerations in the physician exam.

Table 11.1 Physical exam findings to consider

System	Considerations	Reasoning
Vitals and general	Shorter or smaller than expected Lethargic Blood pressure and volume status	Chronic acid/base disorders often result in poor growth. Severe acid/base and sodium derangements can present as lethargy. Patients with hypertension and volume overload may have a hypokalemic metabolic acidosis
Head	Microcephalic Sunken fontanelle	Microcephaly can indicate a neurological deficit or developmental delay. May not have a thirst signal. Sunken fontanelle occurs in dehydration
EENT	Sunken eyes and dark circles, dry mucous membranes, no tear production	Are indicators of dehydration and decreased circulating volume
Cardiovascular	Peripheral edema	Is associated with conditions resulting in hypotonic hypervolemic hyponatremia like nephrotic syndrome and heart failure
Respiratory	Rapid respiratory rates Irregular respirations	Can occur with respiratory compensation for a metabolic acidosis May indicate increased intracranial pressure
Abdominal	Abdominal hardware present	Stool losses through an ostomy can be associated with a metabolic acidosis
Skin	Doughy skin turgor	Can be associated with hypernatremia
Neurological	Seizure activity, increased tone, brisk reflexes, and nuchal rigidity	May indicate severe hyper or hyponatremia

Laboratory Assessment/Imaging

Assessment of patients with acid/base disorders can be challenging if the patient has developed respiratory or metabolic compensation. However, we will present a step-by-step process that will help you interpret the findings.

If you suspect an acid/base disorder in a patient, the first step is to determine the blood pH by obtaining an arterial, venous, or capillary blood gas. The pH will tell you if patient is acidemic ($pH < 7.35$) or alkalemic ($pH > 7.45$). With the blood gas, take note of both the pCO_2 and bicarbonate. The next step is obtaining an electrolyte panel that includes bicarbonate, sodium, chloride, and potassium. Your electrolyte panel bicarbonate should correspond closely with the bicarbonate seen on the blood gas (small differences may result due to the different instruments used to analyze blood gas versus chemistry samples).

If the patient is acidemic, the next step is determining if it is primarily a respiratory acidosis or a metabolic acidosis. In general, respiratory acidosis patients will have elevated pCO_2 and metabolic acidosis patients will have low serum bicarbonate. Should the patient have a low serum bicarbonate and a metabolic acidosis is suspected, the next step is determining the anion gap to classify the acidosis as a normal or high anion gap acidosis. The anion gap is calculated using the equation below:

$$AG = [Na] - [Cl] - [HCO_3]$$

A normal anion gap is between 8 and 14 mEq/L. A high anion gap indicates circulating organic acids in the blood (differential is noted below). In the setting of a high anion gap, additional labs to consider are toxicology screening, microscopic urinalysis, salicylate level, serum lactate, serum osmolality, and beta-hydroxybutyrate. In the setting of a normal anion gap, obtain urinary electrolytes to assess for renal tubular acidosis (Fig. 11.1).

Metabolic alkalosis is less common and is divided into conditions that are chloride responsive or non-responsive. Urinary chloride differentiates between these two types. A low urine chloride <10 mEq/L is seen in chloride responsive conditions. A normal to high urine chloride >10 mEq/L occurs in chloride non-responsive conditions.

Physical exam and thorough history are crucial in diagnosing respiratory acidosis and alkalosis. The respiratory rate and anatomy of the chest wall should be evaluated. Imaging studies such as a chest X-ray or computed tomography (CT) of the chest may give clues to the underlying cause of respiratory disorders.

Keep in mind that alterations in pCO_2 and bicarbonate could also be due to a compensatory process. The pH of the body is determined by the ratio of dissolved CO_2 (carbonic acid) and bicarbonate. When more dissolved CO_2 is present, the pH will be lower and vice versa. When there is an increase in dissolved CO_2 from a pathologic process, the body will increase the bicarbonate to stabilize the ratio thereby compensating for the pathologic change. For example, the kidneys will hold on to more bicarbonate when an asthmatic is trapping CO_2 in the lungs. Respiratory

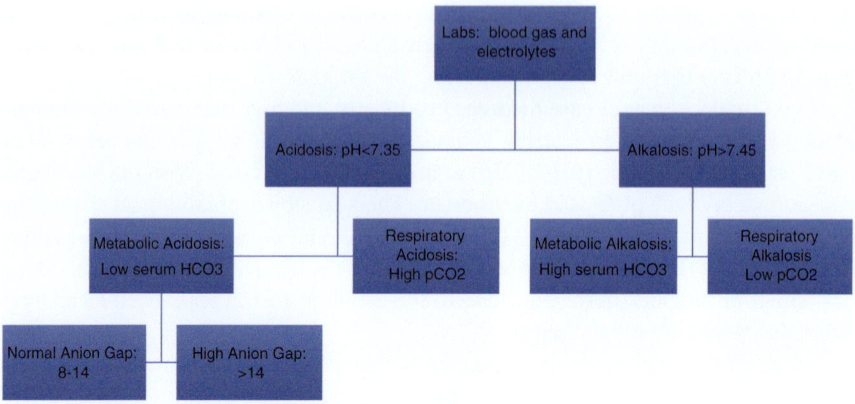

Fig. 11.1 Laboratory assessment in the setting of acid/base disorders

compensation for metabolic processes results in a change in the pattern of breathing to expel or retain CO_2. This process is rapid beginning within 30 min and complete by 24 h. Metabolic compensation for respiratory processes on the other hand takes 3–5 days to complete although some buffering can occur within minutes (acute compensation). The kidneys will increase hydrogen ion secretion and retain more bicarbonate in the setting of acidosis and decrease hydrogen ion secretion in the setting of alkalosis. Easily accessible calculators exist to calculate the expected compensation result using formulas such as Winter's Formula.

If you notice the pCO_2 or serum bicarbonate are not where you would expect them to be due to compensation, then you may be dealing with partial compensation or a mixed acid/base disorder (with multiple independent abnormalities).

Hypernatremia and Hyponatremia

An electrolyte panel, serum osmolality level, urine osmolality level, and urine sodium are typically the four most important laboratory assessments needed to discover the etiology for sodium disorders. Under normal conditions, when serum sodium is low, urine sodium should also be low, and if serum osmolality is low, the urine osmolality should also be low and vice versa. Aberrations in this pattern will guide you toward your diagnosis. It is also important to remember that the concentration and volume of urine analyzed will alter urine sodium levels. When investigating patients with low sodium levels, rule out factors affecting the serum sodium assay such as hyperlipidemia as seen in children with nephrotic syndrome. This is an example of spurious or false hyponatremia. Elevated triglyceride levels make serum sodium appear spuriously low. You can calculate the corrected sodium using the equation below:

$$\text{Decrease in sodium}\left(\text{mEq}/\text{L}\right) = \text{Triglycerides}\left(\text{mg}/\text{dL}\right) \times 0.002$$

Factitious hyponatremia occurs in children with hyperglycemia. Elevated glucose results in an increase in serum osmolality and tonicity causing water to shift from the intracellular space to the extracellular space decreasing the serum sodium concentration. You can calculate the corrected sodium in this situation using the equation below:

$$\text{Corrected sodium}\left(\text{mEq}/\text{L}\right) = \text{Measured sodium}\left(\text{mEq}/\text{L}\right) + \left[0.024 \times \left(\text{Serum glucose}\left(\text{mg}/\text{dL}\right) - 100\right)\right]$$

Key Differential Diagnosis

Metabolic Acidosis: High Anion Gap Acidosis (HAGMA)

Multiple mnemonic devices exist to represent causes of HAGMA; however, GOLDMARK seems to be the most frequently used at this time. Table 11.2 lists diagnoses suspected in the setting of HAGMA. Remember that a high anion gap means that an unmeasured anion is present in the blood and is what all of these diagnoses have in common.

Diabetic Ketoacidosis (DKA)

DKA is a very important cause of HAGMA in pediatrics. Patients with type I diabetes are especially at risk of DKA, in fact DKA is often how a child with type I diabetes presents. In these patients, due to the lack of insulin, metabolism of fatty acids results in an increase in ketoacids (beta-hydroxybutyrate being one), a higher hydrogen ion concentration and ensuing metabolic acidosis. Remember that compensation for metabolic acidosis takes only minutes, so these patients will exhibit Kussmaul respirations, which are rapid and labored, to decrease the pCO_2 and increase the blood pH. These patients can rapidly become dehydrated given an osmotic diuresis from elevated serum glucose, and emesis.

Ingestions

Ingestions are another important cause of HAGMA. Ethylene glycol (anti-freeze), for example, is important to consider. It is a common household item and has a sweet taste that is enticing to toddlers. In the body, ethylene glycol is metabolized to glycolic acid which results in a high anion gap. Oxalate is also produced as

Table 11.2 Causes of HAGMA

G	Glycols—ethylene glycol (anti-freeze, de-icing solutions, inks, hydraulic brake fluid) and propylene glycol (anti-freeze, e-cigarette liquid)
O	Oxoproline—pyroglutamic acid (toxic metabolite from acetaminophen ingestion)
L	Lactate—standard lactate from lactic acidosis (inborn errors of metabolism, poor tissue perfusion, iron overdose, mitochondrial disorders, crush injuries)
D	D-lactate—exogenous lactic acid produced by gut bacteria (often seen in short gut syndrome patients)
M	Methanol—includes alcohols in general, results in production of formate and formic acid
A	Aspirin—salicylic acid
R	Renal failure—uremic acidosis
K	Ketones—diabetic ketoacidosis, isoniazid, starvation ketosis

ethylene glycol is further metabolized. A key finding in these patients is the presence of oxalate crystals in the urine that are visualized via urine microscopy.

Ethylene glycol, methanol, and paraldehyde also produce an osmolar gap that can further hint toward the diagnosis. The osmolar gap is a difference between measured and calculated serum osmolality. Salicylates and NSAIDs are other common household staples whose overdose can result in HAGMA. Salicylate toxicity can be more difficult to diagnose as the immediate ingestion also results in stimulation of the respiratory center causing a respiratory alkalosis.

Metabolic Acidosis: Normal Anion Gap Metabolic Acidosis (NAGMA)

The etiology of NAGMA is much less varied than those seen above. In Table 11.3, a useful mnemonic for typical causes of NAGMA (USEDCARP) is presented. By far the most common cause in children is diarrhea. Diarrhea results in loss of potassium and bicarbonate in the stool. In renal tubular acidosis (RTA), proximal tubular RTA or type II RTA results from an inability to reabsorb bicarbonate. The proximal tubule resorbs many ions and small proteins so a hint toward this diagnosis may be a loss of additional ions in the urine. These patients may have glucosuria, phosphaturia, and proteinuria. Broad proximal tubular dysfunction is also called Fanconi's syndrome. These patients are still able to acidify their urine and will often have lower urinary pH on a urinalysis. Distal RTA or type I RTA results from an inability to acidify urine. Additional H+ ions in the urine are excreted in the form of ammonium which has a net positive charge. It is often complexed with chloride which has a negative net charge. If there is an inability to acidify urine, less ammonium is being released and complexed with chloride. Urinary ammonium is not typically measured in the lab, but urinary sodium, potassium, and chloride are easily measured. When acidification of the urine is happening appropriately, the urine net charge (as calculated by the sum of urine sodium and urine potassium minus the urine chloride) should be net negative because urine ammonium (positive charge) is not measured. If urine ammonium is not being produced readily, the urine net charge may appear positive. Other rare causes of normal anion gap acidosis are outlined in Table 11.3.

Table 11.3 Causes of normal anion gap acidosis

U	Ureteral diversions—ureterosigmoidostomy, ureteroenterostomy
S	Small bowel diversions, Sulfamylon
E	Extra chloride—normal saline administration, magnesium chloride
D	**Diarrhea, Diarrhea, Diarrhea**—by far most common causes of NAGMA
C	Carbonic anhydrase inhibitors, cholestyramine
A	hypoAldosteronism, hyperAlimentation, adrenal insufficiency
R	Renal tubular acidosis
P	Pancreatic fistula

Table 11.4 Causes of metabolic alkalosis

Chloride responsive: metabolic alkalosis with urinary chloride <10 mEq/L	Chloride non-responsive: metabolic alkalosis with urinary chloride >10 mEq/L
Vomiting: pyloric stenosis, cyclic vomiting syndrome, and bulimia	Renal: Bartter's and Gitelman's syndromes
Laxative abuse	Adrenal: Hyperaldosteronism and Cushing's syndrome
Nasogastric suction	Exogenous steroids
Diuretics (thiazides and loops)	Alkali ingestion
Cystic fibrosis	Refeeding syndrome

Metabolic Alkalosis

As mentioned above, metabolic alkalosis is less common; the differential is less varied and, as presented in Table 11.4, can be classified as chloride responsive or non-responsive. Chloride responsive conditions include persistent vomiting as seen in pyloric stenosis, bulimia, and cyclic vomiting syndrome. Affected patients lose hydrogen ions, electrolytes such as potassium, and volume. They can be hypokalemic due to aldosterone secretion in response to volume depletion. Hypokalemia is also due to increased cellular exchange of hydrogen ions and potassium (hydrogen ions coming out of the cell in exchange for potassium ions coming into the cell). Diuretics cause alkalosis in a similar fashion. Pyloric stenosis is an important cause to consider in infants with projectile vomiting. Chloride non-responsive conditions are even more unusual. The underlying cause is often excess mineralocorticoid activity. These patients are volume expanded, hypertensive, and hypokalemic. An exception to this rule is patients with Bartter's and Gitelman's syndromes. These syndromes are the result of abnormalities in the channels in the thick ascending limb of the loop of Henle and the distal convoluted tubule. Channel abnormalities lead to excessive urine chloride wasting.

Respiratory Acidosis and Alkalosis

Respiratory acidosis results from increased CO_2 in the blood by many different mechanisms. One mechanism is suppression of the CNS respiratory drive. This could be the result of CNS infections, trauma, toxins (opioids), or a postictal state. Other possible CNS causes are Guillain-Barre, myasthenia gravis, or botulinum toxin which depresses the movement of the respiratory musculature resulting in CO_2 retention. Bronchiolitis, asthma, pneumonia, cystic fibrosis, and bronchopulmonary dysplasia are common causes of respiratory acidosis in pediatrics.

Conditions in which there is decreased oxygen delivery to tissues result in an increased respiratory rate and cause respiratory alkalosis. Some examples include anemia, high altitude, and hypotension. Other more common causes of increased respiratory rate are anxiety, stress, pain, and hyperthermia. Lastly, pulmonary disorders that cause inflammation and irritation in lung tissues may decrease arterial oxygen partial pressure. The body may attempt to compensate by increasing minute ventilation and breathing off more CO_2. Examples include pulmonary edema, airway obstruction, and interstitial lung disease.

Hypernatremia

It is helpful to think of the cause of hypernatremia as either water loss or excessive salt intake. For instance, infants who are breastfed are at risk for hypernatremia in the first 1–3 weeks after birth. These infants may develop severe dehydration due to inadequate transfer of breast milk (water loss) to the infant, leading to water loss as fluid intake does not keep up with normal insensible and urine losses. This can happen when the mother has either low production of breast milk or the physiologic decrease in human milk concentration does not occur. Another example of water loss or loss of more fluid relative to electrolytes includes overly diluted urine like in the setting of central or nephrogenic diabetes insipidus. In diabetes insipidus, the body is not releasing antidiuretic hormone (ADH) or not responding appropriately to ADH. Children with renal diseases such as dysplasia can have limited ability to concentrate urine adequately and be unable to drink enough to keep up with high urine volumes. Loss of fluid through the skin through burns or sweat and gastrointestinal losses through profuse watery diarrhea or vomiting in the setting of gastroenteritis often result in hypernatremia. Keep in mind that children with neurological deficits and developmental delay are at higher risk of hypernatremic episodes due to inability to regulate fluid with oral fluid intake. Excessive salt intake causing hypernatremia is often iatrogenic. The administration of high volumes of normal saline is the most common iatrogenic cause. There have also been reports of salt poisoning in child abuse cases that could cause hypernatremia.

Hyponatremia

It is helpful to categorize causes of hyponatremia by tonicity and volume. A combination of labs that help you to determine tonicity, osmolality, and volume will lead you to the correct differential diagnosis. Children with low sodium and low tonicity or osmolality should have low urine osmolality. In the setting of low serum sodium and low serum osmolality, high urine osmolality of greater than 100 mosm/kg indicates inability to excrete excess free water. This is usually the case in children with syndrome of inappropriate antidiuretic hormone (SIADH) or renal failure. Children who are edematous and appear fluid overloaded likely have increased total body water but the effective circulating volume may be low. For this reason, the body releases ADH resulting in water retention and dilution of the serum sodium. This is

Table 11.5 Categories of hyponatremia

Hyponatremia type	Description	Key lab and exam considerations
Hypertonic	Increased osmoles (for example from hyperglycemia, or infusion of mannitol or intravenous immunoglobulin in the serum cause a shift in) relatively hypotonic	High serum glucose, high measured serum osmolality
Isotonic	Measurement of sodium results in a lower level because an increased lipid/protein component dilutes out the physiologically relevant aqueous sodium component	High serum triglycerides
Hypotonic		
Hypovolemic	Isotonic losses replaced by relative free water (e.g., excessively diluted baby formula) Cerebral salt wasting	Low urine sodium High urine sodium
Euvolemic	Syndrome of inappropriate secretion of antidiuretic hormone (SIADH)	High urine sodium and osmolality
Hypervolemic	Edematous state (e.g., nephrotic syndrome, congestive heart failure, cirrhosis, capillary leak)	Low serum albumin, edema, high urine protein, abnormal liver function tests and/or decreased cardiac function on echocardiogram

seen in patients with cirrhosis, heart failure, nephrotic syndrome, and other conditions where serum proteins are low (e.g. malnutrition, liver disease, protein losing enteropathy, extensive burns). Lastly, a child may be producing dilute urine as you would expect in the presence of low sodium. In this case, the patient may be losing salt in the urine and will have an elevated urine sodium such as in cerebral salt wasting. The patient may be taking in large amounts of hypotonic fluid like in the case of psychogenic polydipsia. See Table 11.5 for more information and key lab and exam findings for hyponatremia.

Management

Metabolic Acidosis

Management of metabolic acidosis is directed toward the underlying cause. For instance, DKA requires volume repletion and insulin administration. Treatment of lactic acidosis secondary to decreased perfusion can involve volume administration or pressors to improve oxygen delivery. Some ingestions may have specific antidotes that can be administered such as fomepizole in methanol ingestions and others may require urinary alkalinization (salicylates) to promote loss in the urine or dialysis to clear the toxin and its derived metabolites directly (ethylene glycol). In patients with NAGMA, the management is again determined by the cause. Patients with diarrhea causing only mild acidosis may simply require hydration. Patients with more severe bicarbonate losses from diarrhea or renal tubular acidosis may require sodium bicarbonate replacement. It is important to approach bicarbonate repletion slowly as significant side effects of too rapid correction or excessive treatment are possible such as hypocalcemia, hypernatremia, hyperosmolality, and/or overcorrection leading to alkalosis. Bicarbonate should be infused slowly, and labs should be checked frequently to monitor the response to treatment. Once the acute episode of acidosis has resolved, some patients like those with RTA will require chronic oral bicarbonate supplementation.

Metabolic Alkalosis

Management again targets the underlying cause. Anti-emetics are used to decrease vomiting, and surgery is required to correct pyloric stenosis. Consider a reduction in diuretic doses, if diuretics are being used. Pairing thiazide and loop diuretics with potassium sparing diuretics may also be helpful. In patients at risk of refeeding syndrome, start feeds at low rates and volumes and work up slowly.

Respiratory Acidosis and Alkalosis

Management of respiratory disorders is discussed in other chapters of this textbook.

Hypernatremia

Hypernatremia is often accompanied by fluid loss as discussed above; therefore, treatment of hypernatremia usually requires fluid and salt repletion. If a patient is severely volume depleted, then replacing volume with an isotonic solution takes precedent over sodium correction. However, it is important to only give enough fluid to stabilize the patient and improve tissue perfusion. Rapid correction in hypernatremia could result in cerebral edema if fluid resuscitation is overzealous. The next step is to calculate the patient's free water deficit using the equation below.

$$\text{Free water deficit}(\text{L}) = 0.7 \times \text{wt}(\text{kg})[\text{current sodium} / \text{desired sodium}]$$

The free water deficit should be replaced at a rate calculated to decrease the serum sodium no faster than 0.6 mEq/L/h or 15 mEq/L/day. If the sodium is decreasing faster than 0.6 mEq/L/h, either decrease the rate of IV fluid or increase the concentration of sodium in the IV fluids. Frequent lab monitoring is critical, and the sodium should be checked every 1–4 h.

Hyponatremia

Treatment of hyponatremia differs slightly depending on the duration of low sodium. Children with acute hyponatremia (low sodium for less than 48 h) are more likely to tolerate more rapid correction but are also more likely to have neurological symptoms such as seizures. If neurological symptoms are present, then it is important to raise the sodium more quickly, consider administering 3% hypertonic saline. In mild to moderate acute hyponatremia, hypertonic saline is usually unnecessary, and treatment is determined by the underlying cause. Gastrointestinal illness may require fluid and salt repletion with normal saline. SIADH on the other hand is often treated by fluid restriction and sometimes oral sodium supplementation. Patients with chronic hyponatremia are at higher risks of cerebral side effects if too rapid correction occurs. It is still appropriate to consider the use of 3% hypertonic saline if the patient is experiencing neurological sequelae. The aim is to raise the sodium a few mEq/L to stop neurological symptoms but not to fully correct the serum sodium. Assuming total body water is 50% of weight, 1 mL/kg of 3% hypertonic saline will raise the sodium about 1 mEq/L. The infusion rate should raise the sodium by 1 mEq/L/h until symptoms improve. For chronic hyponatremia that is mild to moderate, one should calculate the sodium deficit using the equation below.

$$\text{Na deficit} = \left[\text{normal Na} - \text{serum Na}\right] \times \text{body weight}\left(\text{kg}\right) \times 0.6$$

The goal of treatment should be to raise the serum sodium by no more than 8 mEq/L/day.

Frequent lab monitoring is critical. Too rapid correction can result in osmotic demyelination.

Anticipatory Guidance

Acid/Base Disorders

While anticipatory guidance will be different for each diagnosis, some general reminders for parents are listed below:

1. Keep all medications in a cabinet that is out of reach of children. Consider adding a lock to the cabinet as your child ages.
2. Keep all cleaning supplies and car fluids in a locked cabinet.
3. Should you suspect that your child has ingested a medication, cleaning fluid, or car fluid take your child to the ER or call 911.
4. Take note of older children's mental status and look for signs of depression: increased/decreased sleepiness, easily angers, trouble concentrating, isolation, and no longer getting joy from joyful activities.

5. Talk to your pediatrician about your child's growth and be willing to do blood work if there are any concerns.
6. Know and be comfortable telling physicians about your child's past medical history and surgical procedures.
7. Take notice of changes in urination, stooling, intake, and output.

Hyponatremia/Hypernatremia

1. If your child is on a feeding or fluid regimen, make sure that you can tell medical employees the details of that regimen.
2. Never dilute baby formula beyond the recommended mixture. Always follow the mixing instructions provided unless instructed otherwise by a physician.
3. Take notice of changes in urination, stooling, intake, and output.
4. Encourage your child to take multiple water breaks while participating in outdoor and indoor sports.
5. Use an oral electrolyte solution to rehydrate your child in the case of vomiting.
6. If your child in unable to tolerate oral intake, take the child to the ER.

Application Exercises

You are seeing a 5-year-old male child in the emergency room. His mother reports that he has been losing weight over the last 4 weeks. She has also noticed him urinating frequently and drinking more water than usual. Over the last few hours, he has had multiple episodes of vomiting. His mother encouraged him to take small sips of Pedialyte, but he has not tolerated any oral intake. After you take a thorough history and perform a physical exam, you order labs including a complete metabolic panel (CMP), venous blood gas, serum osmolality, complete blood count, and urinalysis. His CMP is remarkable for sodium of 132 mmol/L, potassium of 4.5 mmol/L, chloride of 102 mmol/L, bicarb of 10 mmol/L, BUN of 54 mg/dL, Cr of 0.92 mg/dL, and glucose of 400 mg/dL. His urinalysis reveals 3+ glucose and 2+ ketones. His blood gas shows a pH of 7.02, pCO_2 of 20 mmHg, and bicarb of 11 mEq/L. CBC is unremarkable. Serum osmolality is 306 mOsm/kg. You believe the most likely diagnosis for this patient is DKA in new onset type 1 diabetes mellitus.

1. What physical exam findings would you expect to see in this patient?
2. Why is this patient's sodium decreased?
3. Identify the acid/base disorder seen in this patient?
4. Why is this patient's CO_2 decreased?

Answers

1. What physical exam findings would you expect to see in this patient?

   A. Physical exam findings that you might expect to find in a patient with diabetic ketoacidosis

      (i) Kussmaul respirations—deep and rapid respirations
      (ii) Fruity smelling breath
      (iii) Signs of dehydration—sunken eyes, tachycardia, possibly hypotension, poor skin turgor, dry mucous membranes
      (iv) Neurological manifestations—lethargy, drowsiness, and obtundation

2. Why is this patient's sodium decreased?

   A. Glucose is mainly restricted to the extracellular fluid. When the concentration of glucose increases, the osmotic gradient across the cellular wall is increased. This osmotic force drives water across the cellular wall to the extracellular space. The extra water dilutes the sodium concentration in the extracellular fluid.

3. Identify the acid/base disorder seen in this patient?

   A. First note the pH on this patient's blood gas. The pH is lower than 7.35 meaning the patient is acidotic.
   B. The next step is determining whether this is a respiratory or metabolic acidosis. In respiratory acidosis, the CO_2 is increased which is not the case in this patient. In metabolic acidosis, the bicarb is decreased which is the case in this patient.
   C. Now that you have determined that the patient has a metabolic acidosis, you should calculate the anion gap.

$$AG = [Na] - [Cl] - [HCO_3]$$

$$132\,mmol/L - 102\,mmol/L - 10\,mmol/L = 20\,mmol/L$$

   The anion gap is elevated, so this patient has HAGMA which is consistent with DKA presentation.

4. Why is this patient's CO_2 decreased?

   A. The patient's CO_2 is decreased due to acute respiratory compensation for metabolic acidosis. CO_2 is decreased by about 1.2 mmHg for every 1 mEq/L decrease in the serum bicarb.

Further Reading

Jain A. Body fluid composition. Pediatr Rev. 2015;36:141–52.
Reid-Adam J. Hyponatremia. Pediatr Rev. 2013;34:417–9.
Schwaderer AL, Schwartz GJ. Back to basics. Pediatr Rev. 2004;25:350–7.
Schwaderer AL, Schwartz GJ. Treating hypernatremic dehydration. Pediatr Rev. 2005;26:148–50.
Wolfsdorf JI, Glaser N, Agus M, Fritsch M, Hanas R, Rewers A, Sperling MA, Codner E. ISPAD clinical practice consensus guidelines 2018: diabetic ketoacidosis and the hyperglycemic hyperosmolar state. Pediatr Diabetes. 2018;19:155–77.

Chapter 12
Asthma and Status Asthmaticus, Allergies, and Eczema

Deepa Patadia, Lily C. Pien, and Kara McNamara

Asthma and Status Asthmaticus

Background/Pathophysiology

The 2021 Global Initiative for Asthma *Global Strategy for Asthma Management and Prevention* offers the following definition of asthma: "Asthma is a heterogeneous disease, usually characterized by chronic airway inflammation. It is defined by the history of respiratory symptoms such as wheeze, shortness of breath, chest tightness and cough that vary over time and in intensity, together with variable

D. Patadia (✉)
Department of Allergy and Clinical Immunology, Respiratory Institute, Cleveland Clinic, Cleveland, OH, USA

Ohio University Heritage College of Osteopathic Medicine, Cleveland, OH, USA
e-mail: PATADID@ccf.org

L. C. Pien
Department of Allergy and Clinical Immunology, Respiratory Institute, Cleveland Clinic, Cleveland, OH, USA

Cleveland Clinic Lerner College of Medicine of Case Western Reserve University, Cleveland, OH, USA

Office of Educator and Scholar Development (OESD), Center of Educational Resources, Education Institute, Cleveland Clinic, Cleveland, OH, USA
e-mail: PIENL@ccf.org

K. McNamara
Pediatric Allergy and Immunology, Cleveland Clinic, Cleveland, OH, USA

Cleveland Clinic Lerner College of Medicine of Case Western Reserve University, Cleveland, OH, USA
e-mail: mcnamak@ccf.org

N. Liao et al. (eds.), *Pediatric Rotations*,
https://doi.org/10.1007/978-3-031-59873-9_12

expiratory airflow limitation." Asthma involves persistent inflammation of the airways, with airway smooth muscle hyperplasia, mucous plugging, and thickening of the airway walls. Asthma phenotypes have been described and can be useful in guiding therapy in some severe asthma cases. Examples of asthma phenotypes include allergic, exercise-induced, aspirin-sensitive, neutrophilic, and occupational asthma. Allergic asthma is the most common type of childhood asthma.

In the United States, 12.7% of children younger than 18 years have been diagnosed with asthma at some time. Childhood asthma is more prevalent in males than females; this reverses by adulthood. When compared to White children, the prevalence of asthma is higher in children of American Indian or Alaska Native descent, in Black children, and in Puerto Rican children. The racial and ethnic disparities in asthma prevalence are driven by many complex factors, including social, structural, biological, and behavioral components.

Recurrent wheezing and cough are common in young children, often associated with viral respiratory infections. However, not all of these children will develop asthma. The Modified Asthma Predictive Index and the Pediatric Asthma Risk Score are tools that can help determine risk of asthma development in young children with recurrent wheezing. They use criteria including parental history of asthma and the patient's atopic comorbidities to predict risk of future asthma development in these children. Asthma activity can vary over time, with many children improving with age. However, severe asthma tends to persist into adulthood. There is no cure for asthma, but it is usually a manageable chronic disease with proper diagnosis and treatment.

History

Taking a history is an important part of the evaluation and management of asthma. Table 12.1 outlines key questions to ask patients.

Physical Examination

When well, the physical exam of a patient with asthma can be normal. During periods of asthma activity, abnormal physical findings may be present. Table 12.2 provides key assessments to conduct in the physical exam for a patient with asthma.

Laboratory Assessment/Imaging

Pulmonary function testing is helpful in documenting airflow obstruction in children 5 years and older. The typical finding of asthma is expiratory airflow obstruction, or reduced ratio of air exhaled in the first second to total air exhaled on

Table 12.1 Relevant components of the asthma history

Features of asthma symptoms
What symptoms are occurring? (i.e., cough, wheezing, dyspnea)
What triggers the symptoms? (i.e., exercise, allergen exposures, viral illnesses, cold air, laughter)
What relieves the symptoms? (i.e., rest, SABA[a], avoidance of triggers)
What comorbidities are present that may contribute to asthma symptoms? (i.e., allergic rhinitis, gastroesophageal reflux, inducible laryngeal obstruction, obesity)
Symptom timing and frequency
How often do symptoms occur during the daytime and at nighttime?
Are symptoms constant or intermittent?
How many asthma exacerbations have occurred in the past year?
Symptom severity
Has the patient needed to seek acute care in the clinic or emergency department?
Has the patient ever been admitted to the hospital for asthma symptoms?
Has admission to the intensive care unit or intubation ever been necessary?
Asthma treatments
How often have systemic corticosteroids been necessary to treat asthma symptoms?
What controller medications does the patient use and how often are medications missed?
What is the frequency of SABA[a] use for symptoms?
Is the patient experiencing side effects or adverse effects of the asthma medications?

[a] *SABA* short-acting beta-agonist. These are medications that are used as needed for quick-relief of asthma symptoms. Examples include albuterol and levalbuterol

Table 12.2 Pertinent physical exam findings in asthma

System	Key points
Vital signs	Include blood pressure, heart rate, respiratory rate, temperature, and pulse oximetry. Important in recognizing degree of illness in an acute visit
General	Observe nutritional and developmental status—abnormalities may suggest an alternate diagnosis Observe work of breathing—respiratory rate and effort, head bobbing, nasal flaring, grunting, retractions
HEENT	Look for signs of allergic rhinitis or upper respiratory tract infection as a trigger Presence of nasal polyps suggests an alternate diagnosis, such as cystic fibrosis
Cardiac	Abnormal findings suggest an alternate diagnosis, such as congenital heart defect
Respiratory	Auscultate for wheezing, reduced breath sounds, prolonged expiratory phase of respiration Wheezing may be absent in severe exacerbations if there is reduced airflow Re-examination after treatment with short-acting beta-agonist in the office can be useful in acute visits
Skin	Look for signs of atopic dermatitis

spirometry (reduced FEV1/FVC), with reversibility after bronchodilator administration. Spirometry can appear normal in patients with asthma that is not active at the time of the test; therefore, normal spirometry does not rule out asthma. Fractional excretion of nitric oxide (FeNO) measurements are useful in children 5 years and older for asthma diagnosis and monitoring, but are not recommended to be used in isolation. FeNO is a measure of asthma-related inflammation in the lungs. Peak expiratory flow measurements can also be useful in documenting asthma activity.

Allergen mitigation strategies are recommended for patients with symptoms related to allergen exposure by history or based on allergy testing. Referral to an allergist should be considered in the management of patients with asthma.

Laboratory evaluation, including peripheral eosinophil count and total IgE can be helpful in identifying asthma phenotypes and may impact management of patients with severe asthma who are candidates for biologic therapy. Imaging studies generally are not necessary in diagnosing asthma. Chest imaging may be used to exclude other diagnoses, such as pneumonia or foreign body aspiration.

Key Differential Diagnosis

Table 12.3 outlines a key differential diagnosis for asthma and provides some distinguishing features on physical examination.

Management

The GINA guidelines divide asthma control into two domains: symptom control and future risk of adverse outcomes. Symptom control is assessed based on frequency of daytime and nighttime symptoms, frequency of short-acting beta-agonist (SABA) use, and activity limitation. Asthma control should be assessed at every visit. Poor symptom control is associated with increased risk of exacerbations. In pediatric patients, it is important to ask about missed school days due to asthma, ability to participate in activities such as sports, and impact of asthma on their life. The Asthma Control Test or Asthma Control Questionnaire are helpful tools in assessing symptom control. Future risk of adverse outcomes is based on history of one or more exacerbations per year, low FEV1, peripheral eosinophilia, smoking, poor inhaler technique, nonadherence, and socioeconomic issues.

Table 12.3 Key differential diagnosis in asthma

Diagnosis	Distinguishing features
Foreign body aspiration	Young child with sudden onset of symptoms and access to a small object
Cystic fibrosis	Presence of nasal polyps, sinus disease, failure to thrive, and associated GI manifestations
Bronchopulmonary dysplasia	History of prematurity
Structural abnormalities (e.g., vascular rings)	May present as stridor
Congenital heart disease	Abnormal cardiac exam
Infection	Presence of fever, abnormal chest X-ray, crackles on physical exam
Inducible laryngeal obstruction	Inspiratory stridor

The NAEPP guidelines discuss asthma severity and control. Both are divided into two domains: impairment and risk. Impairment is the frequency and intensity of symptoms and the impact on function. Risk is the likelihood of asthma exacerbation or loss of lung function over time.

When managing asthma, the goal is to control symptoms and reduce future risk of adverse outcomes (exacerbations, medication side effects, persistent airflow limitation). Asthma control is assessed, adjustments are made to the asthma therapies, and response to therapy is reviewed frequently. Therapies are stepped up if asthma remains uncontrolled and stepped down when good control is achieved, to determine the minimum effective dose of medication. The choice of asthma treatment depends on patient's age and asthma severity.

Traditionally, asthma treatments were divided into "controller" therapies (such as inhaled corticosteroids and long-acting beta-agonists) which were taken on a scheduled basis, and "on-demand" therapies (such as short-acting beta-agonists) that were used to treat asthma symptoms when they occurred. Controller medications were adjusted according to the classification of asthma activity (mild, moderate, or severe persistent), based on frequency and severity of symptoms. More recently, some traditional "controller" therapies have been found to be useful when used on-demand or for short periods of time in certain patient populations. The most recent asthma treatment guidance includes this approach. Examples include recommendations for short courses of daily inhaled corticosteroid (ICS) and on-demand short-acting beta-agonist (SABA) with respiratory infections in children under age 4, as needed use of ICS and SABA concomitantly in patients age 12 and above with mild persistent asthma, and use of daily and on-demand ICS-formoterol for treatment of patients 4 years and old with moderate persistent asthma. Table 12.4 reviews asthma medications, their mechanisms of action, and how they should be used. The reader is recommended to review the GINA guidelines and the NAEPP guidelines for detailed information on medication management.

Asthma exacerbations are episodes of acutely worsening symptoms or lung function and represent a change from the patient's usual state. Appropriate chronic treatment of asthma to reduce the risk of exacerbations, as well as recognition and treatment of exacerbations are important components in the management of asthma. Mild exacerbations can be managed in the outpatient clinic setting. Severe exacerbations require treatment in the emergency department.

A patient is considered to be in status asthmaticus if they do not respond to initial bronchodilator therapies. Severe asthma exacerbations can result in hypoxia, respiratory failure, and even death; therefore, appropriate treatment of exacerbations is very important. The patient should be assessed by history and physical, with special attention to the vital signs and work of breathing. The assessment can also assist in identifying any alternative diagnoses. Treatment of an acute exacerbation includes oxygen therapy to maintain appropriate oxygen saturations, inhaled SABA and ipratropium, and systemic corticosteroids (oral preferred). IV magnesium may be considered in patients who fail to respond to initial therapy. The patient should be reassessed frequently and the decision on whether hospitalization is needed should depend on clinical response. Severe asthma exacerbations can require admission to the intensive care unit, with need for intubation and mechanical ventilation. Frequent

Table 12.4 Medications used in asthma management

Medication	Mechanism of action	Use in asthma
Short-acting beta-agonist (SABA) (e.g., albuterol, levalbuterol)	Activates beta-2 receptors, resulting in bronchodilation; effect is rapid, but of a short duration	On-demand medication for relief of acute asthma symptoms
Inhaled corticosteroid (ICS)	Anti-inflammatory effect; reduces airway hyperresponsiveness	Controller therapy traditionally; now used on demand along with SABA in some situations
Long-acting beta-agonist (LABA)	Activates beta-2 receptors, resulting in bronchodilation; effect is for a long duration	Always used in combination with ICS in treatment of asthma. ICS/LABA is used as controller therapies. ICS/formoterol may be used for on-demand treatment in some cases
Leukotriene antagonist (e.g., montelukast, zafirlukast)	Block cysteinyl leukotriene-induced bronchospasm	Controller therapy
Inhaled anticholinergics	Competitive inhibitors of muscarinic receptors; promote bronchodilation	Add-on controller therapy
Biologics (e.g., omalizumab, dupilumab, mepolizumab, benralizumab, reslizumab, tezepelumab)	Block asthma-related inflammation by targeting particular inflammatory molecules or receptors (e.g., IgE, IL-5, IL-4, IL-13, or TSLP)	Add-on controller therapy
Systemic corticosteroids	Anti-inflammatory effect	Management of acute exacerbations

treatments with bronchodilators and close monitoring of respiratory status are needed for patients admitted for asthma exacerbations or status asthmaticus.

Anticipatory Guidance

1. There is no cure for asthma, but it can be very effectively managed
2. Asthma activity varies over time, and health care providers may adjust asthma medications accordingly
3. Not all young children who wheeze go on to have asthma

Allergic Rhinitis

Background

Allergic rhinitis (AR) is a common, chronic, and inflammatory hypersensitivity disorder within the nose with a prevalence of up to 40% of children. Eye symptoms, known as allergic conjunctivitis, are seen in up to 60% of patients with AR. While AR is not a life-threatening disorder, due to its enduring nature, it impacts the quality of life of affected children and has social and economic effects. Associated diseases include rhinosinusitis, asthma, otitis media, and sleep disorders. AR can be classified by its severity (mild, moderate, severe), frequency (intermittent, persistent), and allergic exposures (seasonal, perennial) to assist with diagnosis, treatment, and management.

Pathophysiology

AR is an immunologic, inflammatory disorder that is mediated by specific IgE antibody produced against selected airborne allergens such as cat, dog, dust mites, molds, and pollens. When there is reintroduction of a specific allergen, the allergen will bind and cross-link to IgE antibodies bound to allergic cells (mast cells in the nose, circulating basophils). Allergic cells are then activated and de-granulate, releasing mast cell inflammatory mediators, such as histamine, leukotrienes, prostaglandins, tryptase, bradykinin, and platelet-activating factor. Histamine causes the well-known symptoms of itching, sneezing, and nasal drainage, known as the early phase response. A late-phase response, characterized by congestion and inflammation, is mediated by leukotrienes, prostaglandins, and inflammatory cells, such as eosinophils, basophils, and T cells that infiltrate nasal mucosa.

Clinical History

Seasonal AR is less common in children who are younger than the age of 2. Common clinical symptoms include sneezing, sometimes paroxysmal, itching of the nose, eyes, palate and ears, nasal congestion, and nasal drainage, posteriorly or anteriorly. Onset of these symptoms is quickly seen after allergen exposure and can persist even after the allergen is no longer present due to the late-phase response. Children may not explicitly complain of itching but can be seen rubbing and scratching the nose and eyes. Nasal congestion can manifest as mouth breathing, snoring, decrease sense of smell and, if chronic, with dental misalignment/malocclusions. Nasal drainage is usually clear to whitish; other signs of drainage may present as habitual sniffling, snorting, coughing, and throat clearing. Allergic conjunctivitis symptoms include bilateral itching, redness/hyperemia, watering with discharge, and swelling of the conjunctiva and eyelids. Systemic symptoms reported occasionally are drowsiness, fatigue, and headaches. Fever is not common, and if present, warrants further consideration of chest, sinus, or ear infections.

The identification of triggers when possible is a key in the clinical history of AR. Asking the time of year when symptoms are present helps determine seasonal or perennial AR. If being outdoors elicits symptoms, pollen allergy is likely. If exposures to cats or dogs consistently are associated with sneezing and itching, animal allergy should be suspected. Dust mite exposure can be more difficult to pinpoint; however, AR due to this allergen occurs indoor and can be year-round.

Table 12.5 Responsible airborne allergens and time of year with allergic symptoms

Responsible airborne allergen	Time of year symptoms present (variation with specific geographic region)
Tree pollen (e.g., as birch, maple, oak)	Spring
Grass pollen (e.g., timothy, orchard, Bermuda)	Late spring and early summer
Weed pollen (e.g., ragweed)	Late summer through fall
Mold (e.g., Alternaria, Cladosporium)	Can be year-round, late summer, and fall
Indoor allergens (e.g., cat, dog, mice, dust mites, cockroach)	Year-round, may be worse during the winter

Dust mite allergens can be found in carpets, pillows and mattresses, curtains, and stuffed animals. Table 12.5 outlines the times of the year when different airborne allergens are present in the environment.

Physical Examination

Areas to carefully examine are the nose and the mouth. Eyes, ears, and lungs should also be included in the examination to look for signs of associated disorders. A nasal crease across the bridge of the nose can be seen and is caused by the persistent upward rubbing of the nose to relieve itching and drainage (known as the "allergic salute"). Nasal mucosa of the inferior and middle turbinates can be swollen and pale in color, with clear to whitish nasal discharge draining anteriorly or posteriorly. Cobblestoning (irritated and inflamed lymphoid tissue that appears as pebble-like bumps) in the posterior pharynx can be present. Other oral signs are mouth breathing, a high-arched palate (sometimes termed a "gothic palate"), and misalignment of dental structures.

Swelling and redness of the eyelids can be seen due to chronic scratching in efforts to relieve itching. Allergic shiners, or bluish discoloration of the lower eyelids, related to swollen veins or venous stasis in the periorbital tissue, and lower eyelid creases, known as Dennie-Morgan lines have also been noted in AR patients. Allergic conjunctivitis occurs when the conjunctiva is affected and inflamed by airborne allergens. Stringy discharge from the eyes also indicates involvement. Examination of the ears is helpful as some children have Eustachian tube dysfunction and will develop otitis media with effusion. Lungs should be examined for wheezing and decreased breath sounds as allergic asthma can be seen or develop in children with AR.

Laboratory Assessment/Imaging

As allergen-specific IgE is responsible for the symptoms of AR, the workup involves testing for IgE. Allergen-specific IgE can be identified in two ways: in vivo skin prick testing (SPT) and in vitro specific IgE (sIgE). SPT offers several advantages over sIgE as results are immediate, visible to the patient and family members, and has higher sensitivity. Younger children may be less intimidated by SPT as compared to a needle stick used for sIgE testing. Barriers to SPT are the need to stop oral antihistamines for 5 days prior to testing, skin disorders (atopic dermatitis/eczema, hives, dermatographism) that are not controlled, and uncontrolled asthma. Selection of specific airborne allergens is based upon the clinical history, possible triggers, and the age of the child. As allergen-specific IgE only indicates sensitization, there must be correlation of the results of the SPT to the patient's clinical history, meaning that the patient with specific IgE sensitization should have symptoms with the specific allergen exposure.

Key Differential Diagnosis

Table 12.6 lists key differential diagnosis of rhinitis and conjunctivitis and provides some distinguishing features on physical examination.

Table 12.6 Key differential diagnosis of rhinitis and conjunctivitis

	Distinguishing features
Differential for allergic rhinitis	
Infection (viral, bacterial)	Purulent discharge; can be recurrent; shorter duration of symptoms if viral infection; can be seen with immunodeficiency disorder; absent to minimal itching
Vasomotor irritant rhinitis	Triggers are strong smells such as perfumes, cigarette smoke, and changes in temperature; negative skin tests
Foreign body	Foul-smelling discharge; young child
Obstruction	Can be related to adenoidal or nasal turbinate hypertrophy; foreign body; nasal septal deviation; may be unilateral congestion/obstruction; trisomy 21; congenital abnormality such as choanal atresia; encephalocele, meningocele; nasal polyps seen with cystic fibrosis; tumors
Rhinitis medicamentosa	Dependence on over-the-counter topical decongestants
Differential for allergic conjunctivitis	
Infection	Viral infection can bilateral or unilateral and associated with other viral upper respiratory symptoms Bacterial infection with symptoms of purulent drainage, bilateral or unilateral
Nasal lacrimal duct obstruction	More typically unilateral symptoms, onset early birth or early infancy, lack of itching

Management

There are three major management components of AR: allergen avoidance measures, medications, and immune modulation.

Allergen Avoidance Measures

Once specific allergic triggers have been identified, complete elimination of the trigger would be ideal. Practically speaking, complete avoidance of triggers is difficult to implement, may be expensive, and sometimes upsetting to patient and family. Effective avoidance measures usually require a multipronged approach (Table 12.7).

Complete avoidance is often challenging as there can be exposures to allergens at other relatives' and friends' homes. Avoidance measures can be expensive and may not be financially affordable for all families. The difficulty of avoiding allergenic triggers leads to the use of medications (Table 12.8).

Immune Modulation

Immune modulation for AR is the only management that can alter/modify the allergic response. Current forms are subcutaneous injections, commonly known as allergy shots, and sublingual immunotherapy, known as SLIT, which is available in the US in tablet form. Indications for immune modulation are severe symptoms, inadequate symptoms control with avoidance and medications, and adverse effects to medications.

Table 12.7 Responsible allergic triggers and strategies to decrease exposure

Responsible allergic trigger	Strategies to decrease allergen exposure
Animals (e.g., cat, dog, other pets)	– Removal from home – Washing animals regularly
Dust mites	– Allergenic protective covers on the bed – Removal of carpeting in bedroom, and elsewhere in home – Removal of drapes and curtains, stuffed toy animals – Weekly washing of bed linens in hot water
Outdoor allergens	– Use of air-conditioning – Wearing mask outdoors – Staying indoors during high pollen count days

Table 12.8 Commonly prescribed medications for allergic rhinitis

	Indications	Dosing	Other issues
Oral medications			
– Antihistamines over-the-counter, such as cetirizine, fexofenadine, loratadine, levocetirizine	Predominant drainage, itching, sneezing; many approved for age >2 y/o; check individual medication for age <2 y/o	Use preventively and daily; all approved for daily use; check individual medication for specific dosing	Avoid older first-generation antihistamines due to increased side effects; cetirizine can cause some drowsiness
– Leukotriene receptor antagonist medication, such as montelukast (prescription needed)	If symptoms not controlled with nasal spray, or antihistamines; less effective	Use preventively and daily; check individual medication for specific dosing	Also used in the treatment of asthma; has a black box warning about possible neuropsychiatric effects
Intranasal sprays			
– Corticosteroid spray over-the-counter, such as fluticasone/Flonase, budesonide/Rhinocort AQ, mometasone/Nasonex, triamcinolone/Nasacort	First-line treatment of choice, useful in relieving the predominant symptom of nasal congestion; several approved for age >2 y/o; check individual medication for age <2 y/o; also beneficial for vasomotor irritant rhinitis	Most approved for 1–2 sprays per nostril daily use; check individual medication for specific dosing	Proper technique for use should be provided; avoid spraying septum to prevent septal irritation; low systemic bioavailability decreases the concerns about systemic side effects
– Antihistamine nasal spray such as azelastine/Astelin (prescription needed)	Quick onset of action	>5 y/o, dose ranges from 1 to 2 sprays twice a day depending upon patient's age	Can taste bitter; can be used in combination with intranasal steroid spray

Anticipatory Guidance

1. AR is a chronic disease.
2. Avoidance measures can be helpful, but medications may be needed for more control of symptoms. Medications can be used year-round or when seasonally needed. Most are available over-the-counter; however, instructions provided by the health care provider can assist in adherence and benefit.
3. Further evaluation by an allergist can involve skin testing to identify specific allergic triggers and consideration of immune modulation.

Eczema

Background and Pathophysiology

Eczema, or atopic dermatitis, is a common chronic skin condition which affects up to 20% of children. It is associated with atopy and can be a first step of the "atopic march" and precede the development of other atopic diseases including food allergy, allergic rhinitis, and asthma. Eczema is due to a defect of the skin barrier. When the skin barrier is dysfunctional, this leads to trans-epidermal water loss and allows external factors such as irritants and allergens to cross the damaged barrier. This in turn leads to dry skin as well as inflammation and increased risk for allergic diseases such as food allergy.

This condition is multifactorial, and some genetic factors have been identified. One example is a loss of function mutation in filaggrin (FLG) which can be identified in many patients with early onset eczema. The immune system plays a role, and immune dysregulation is present in eczema with a predominantly type 2 inflammation present in the skin. Cytokines such as IL-4, IL-13, and IL-31 are involved as well as thymic stromal lymphopoietin (TSLP). IgE-mediated allergies, such as food or environmental allergies, can exacerbate eczema but are not typically the sole etiology of eczema. Irritation to the skin by external factors can exacerbate eczema, including frequent scratching. For this reason, eczema is sometimes called "the itch that rashes" since the scratching can lead to increased inflammation which in turn increases the itch in a vicious cycle.

The microbiome of the skin is altered in patients with eczema. Studies have shown reduced diversity in the bacterial species in individuals with eczema and an increase in *Staphylococcus aureus*, in both active eczema lesions and non-lesional skin. This alteration in the microbiome can increase risk for secondary infection and can impact local cytokine production.

History

Similar to other rashes, a critical first step of the history includes focusing on the description of the rash. Important questions include: What does the rash look like? Where is the rash located? How long does the rash last during a flare? Is the rash itchy? What treatments have been attempted and have those treatments been effective? Eczema tends to present at a young age, with the majority of cases beginning within the first year of life. The severity tends to wax and wane, but many children will have gradual improvement over time.

In addition to asking questions to help confirm a diagnosis of eczema, questions regarding the impact on quality of life can assist in developing a treatment plan. Consider questions such as: Does the eczema and itching disrupt the child's sleep? Is the child able to focus in school?

Table 12.9 Distribution of eczema by age

Infants and young children (<2 years)	Older children and adolescents
Most commonly involves cheeks and extensor surfaces Sometimes diffuse Often spares diaper region	Most commonly involves flexural surfaces, especially antecubital fossae and popliteal fossae Can involve wrists, ankles, behind the ears

Physical Examination

The major focus of the physical exam for eczema is examination of the skin. The distribution of eczema varies by age (Table 12.9).

Examination of the skin reveals erythematous papules and plaques. Erythema can appear more violaceous or can be more difficult to appreciate in darker pigmented children. The skin can also appear very dry (xerosis). With chronic inflammation, some children will develop lichenification (thickening of the skin) or pigment changes (either hyper- or hypo-pigmentation). There might be visible excoriation, cracking or fissuring of the skin. Palmar hyperlinearity can be noted, particularly in individuals with filaggrin mutations. Between flares, children with eczema can have normal appearing skin.

Laboratory Assessment/Imaging

Eczema is a clinical diagnosis. Laboratory testing is not commonly utilized in the diagnosis of eczema; however, certain laboratory findings can be identified. Patients with eczema frequently have elevated serum IgE levels. Skin biopsy is not used for diagnosis, but may occasionally be obtained to rule out other diagnoses. Histology can show epidermal changes such as spongiosis, acanthosis, and hyperkeratosis.

Key Differential Diagnosis

The differential diagnosis for eczema includes other pruritic rashes such as contact dermatitis (either irritant or allergic), seborrheic dermatitis, and psoriasis (Table 12.10). There are primary immunodeficiency diseases associated with an eczematous rash, such as Hyper-IgE syndrome or Wiskott-Aldrich syndrome. When there is new onset of eczematous appearing rash in older children and adults, cutaneous T cell lymphoma should be considered.

Table 12.10 Differential diagnosis of eczema

Differential diagnosis	Key distinguishing features
Contact dermatitis	Distribution dependent on trigger
Seborrheic dermatitis	Less pruritus, often greasy appearing rather than dry, flaky, most commonly involves scalp and face
Psoriasis	More commonly involves diaper region, scaling
Immunodeficiency	Additional clinical features which could include recurrent infections, dysmorphic features, failure to thrive, family history of immunodeficiency
Cutaneous T cell lymphoma	Older age of onset

Management

The management of eczema can be divided into two main categories. One which involves daily skin care to aid in maintaining the integrity of the skin barrier and measures to help prevent flares. The other involves therapies directed at decreasing inflammation.

Daily skin care emphasizes aggressive moisturizing multiple times a day, daily bathing, and avoidance of irritants. The frequency of bathing is controversial; large, well-controlled studies are lacking, but most experts now recommend daily bathing followed by immediate application of emollient or moisturizer. Thick creams or emollients are preferred over lotions. Gentle products are recommended for children with eczema since there is increased risk for developing contact dermatitis to various triggers such as fragrance or preservatives which can be found in soap or emollient/moisturizers.

Aeroallergens such as animal dander, dust mites, or pollen can exacerbate eczema and, if allergy testing indicates sensitization, avoidance measures can be used. The understanding of the relationship between food allergy and eczema has grown and changed significantly in the recent past. Although food triggers are occasionally noted in patients with severe eczema, there are a variety of reasons that food allergy testing and/or elimination diets for eczema are not routinely recommended by allergists. This includes the poor positive predictive value of allergy skin testing to foods without appropriate clinical history and the possible increased risk of future IgE mediated/anaphylactic allergy to foods with avoidance diets. With growing knowledge of food allergy over the last several decades, it is now recognized that early exposure and regular exposure to specific allergenic foods promote tolerance. Conversely, delaying introduction or eliminating specific foods from the diet can promote allergic sensitization.

Although the skin care regimen can help reduce frequency and severity of flares, most children will also need at least intermittent use of pharmacologic therapies to address inflammation (Table 12.11). There are a large number of pharmacologic treatment options for eczema which are summarized in the table below.

Table 12.11 Pharmacologic treatments for eczema

Category of medication	Examples	Route of administration
Topical corticosteroids	Hydrocortisone, triamcinolone, desonide, fluticasone	Topical
Calcineurin inhibitors	Tacrolimus, pimecrolimus	Topical
Phosphodiesterase 5 inhibitor	Crisaborole	Topical
Monoclonal antibodies		
Anti-IL-4αR (which inhibits IL-4 and IL-13 signaling)	Dupilumab	Subcutaneous injection
Anti-IL-13	Tralokinumab	Subcutaneous injection
Jak kinase inhibitors	Ruxolitinib, abrocitinib, upadacitinib	Topical or oral
Systemic immunosuppressants	Cyclosporine, methotrexate	Oral
Phototherapy		

Topical corticosteroids (TCS) remain the mainstay of therapy for mild to moderate eczema for a variety of reasons including topical application, low cost, and wide availability. Side effects can occur with long-term use, thus lower potency steroids are utilized when feasible, particularly for sensitive areas such as the face and groin. In addition, topical steroids are utilized during acute flares and then either tapered or held when the skin is clear. For more severe eczema, a rapidly growing number of biologic therapies are now available and are often preferred over the less targeted oral immunosuppressants. Some biologics, such as dupilumab, have favorable side effect profiles, but the high cost and route of administration (subcutaneous injection) can sometimes preclude wider use.

Several other adjunctive therapies are available. Oral antihistamines can help provide itch relief. Controlled clinical studies have not shown any significant improvement in eczema with the use of oral second-generation antihistamines but first-generation antihistamines (diphenhydramine, hydroxyzine) can provide benefit primarily due to sedative effect and thus decreased nighttime pruritus.

A non-pharmacologic treatment option is wet wraps. This involves application of wet dressings, often in the form of wet socks and/or wet cotton pajamas overnight, to maximize hydration of the skin and reduce itch. Dilute bleach baths are sometimes used to decrease *S. aureus* colonization although evidence from well-controlled studies is lacking.

Anticipatory Guidance

1. Eczema is a waxing and waning chronic condition for which there is no cure, and managing symptoms can be difficult. It requires hard work to follow a rigorous daily skin care regimen and adherence to medication regimens.

2. The etiology of eczema is multifactorial. Typically no single specific cause can be found.
3. The relationship between eczema and allergies is complex. It is unlikely that avoiding something like a specific food will resolve the eczema entirely. Allergy testing can sometimes have a role, but this should be carefully considered with a physician. Broad food allergy testing is not recommended and should be avoided.

Application Exercise

1. A 6-month-old female infant presents to the pediatric office for a rash. Mom reports that the rash started about 2 months ago and tends to come and go. The rash is red and located on the cheeks, the extensor surface of the elbows, and the abdomen. Her skin is also very dry. Mom has been applying petroleum jelly daily to the skin and rash but she feels like it doesn't help very much. She has also tried using over-the-counter hydrocortisone which helped briefly. The infant is breast fed, although mom occasionally supplements with a milk-based formula. She is growing well and is overall a happy baby. However she is not currently sleeping very well and seems to be scratching during the night. Which treatment option would be the most appropriate next step?

   A. Instruct mom to eliminate milk from her diet and switch to an extensively hydrolyzed formula for supplementation.
   B. Prescribe cetirizine as needed in the evening to help control the itch.
   C. Prescribe hydrocortisone 2.5% ointment to use as needed up to twice a day on the rash.
   D. Instruct mom on using the petroleum jelly more frequently.

   Answer C: Prescribe hydrocortisone 2.5% ointment to use as needed up to twice a day on the rash. The description of the rash is consistent with eczema. In this case, the infant is suffering from eczema flares that have not been adequately controlled with the use of an emollient plus very low potency, over-the-counter topical steroid. A stronger treatment is needed to control the inflammation, and the hydrocortisone 2.5% ointment is the best option. The role of foods in eczema is complex, but empiric elimination diets are no longer routinely recommended for a variety of reasons, thus A is incorrect. Oral antihistamines, like the cetirizine in option B, are sometimes used as adjuncts but second-generation antihistamines do not have strong evidence for benefit in eczema. Finally, while using the petroleum jelly or other emollient more frequently may offer some utility, given the lesions that are currently reported, this is unlikely to be sufficient alone and anti-inflammatory treatment is also needed.

Further Reading

Bousquet J, Schünemann HJ, Togias A, Bachert C, Erhola M, Hellings PW, et al., Allergic Rhinitis and Its Impact on Asthma Working Group. Next-generation Allergic Rhinitis and Its Impact on Asthma (ARIA) guidelines for allergic rhinitis based on Grading of Recommendations Assessment, Development and Evaluation (GRADE) and real-world evidence. J Allergy Clin Immunol. 2020;145(1):70–80.

Cloutier MM, Baptist AP, Blake KV, et al. 2020 Focused updates to the asthma management guidelines. A report from the National Asthma Education and Prevention Program (NAEPP) coordinating Committee Expert Panel Working Group. J Allergy Clin Immunol. 2020;146(6):1217.

Dykewicz MS, Wallace DV, Amrol DJ, Baroody FM, Bernstein JA, Craig TJ, et al. Rhinitis 2020: a practice parameter update. J Allergy Clin Immunol. 2020;146(4):721–67.

Fishbein AB, Silverberg JI, Wilson EJ, et al. Update on atopic dermatitis: diagnosis, severity assessment and treatment selection. J Allergy Clin Immunol Pract. 2020;8(1):91–101.

Global Initiative for Asthma (GINA). Global strategy for asthma management and prevention. 2021. Available from: www.ginasthma.org.

Langan SM, Irvine AD, Weidinger S. Atopic dermatitis. Lancet. 2020;396(10247):345–60.

Chapter 13
Bronchiolitis

Nora Biary and Pooja Desai

Background/Pathophysiology

Bronchiolitis is a clinical syndrome of respiratory distress commonly triggered by a viral infection of the lower airways in children below 24 months of age. It is the most common cause of hospitalization for children below 12 months of age, primarily in the fall and winter months. Although bronchiolitis can be caused by a number of viral pathogens, the most common virus responsible is respiratory syncytial virus (RSV). Viral bronchiolitis is contagious and can be spread through contaminated surfaces or via inhaled infectious droplets. Once in the nasal epithelium, the virus causes symptoms of upper respiratory infections (URI). In some patients, the infection spreads to the bronchioles (lower respiratory tract). This leads to inflammation of the lining of the bronchioles, which leads to edema and necrosis of the epithelial lining as well as mucous production. This in turn leads to narrowing of the bronchioles and obstruction which is responsible for the clinical presentation of bronchiolitis.

Typically, children have a viral prodrome with upper respiratory symptoms (e.g., rhinorrhea, cough), followed by lower respiratory symptoms which may include tachypnea, wheezing, crackles or rales, and increased work of breathing (e.g., use of accessory muscles, nasal flaring, and/or grunting). Lower respiratory symptoms generally develop by around day 2–3 of illness, peak on days 3–5, and then resolve within a week, though the cough may linger for several weeks. The acute course may be prolonged depending on age at diagnosis, severity of illness, and other comorbidities or associated high risk conditions.

Clinical severity of bronchiolitis can vary, from those who can be observed outpatient to those who require mechanical ventilation in the intensive care unit (ICU).

N. Biary · P. Desai (✉)
Department of Pediatrics, University of Michigan Medical School, Ann Arbor, MI, USA
e-mail: pjdesai@med.umich.edu

N. Liao et al. (eds.), *Pediatric Rotations*,
https://doi.org/10.1007/978-3-031-59873-9_13

It is typically difficult to predict how severe a patient's course of illness will be. However, children with hemodynamically significant congenital heart disease, immunodeficiency, neuromuscular weakness, chronic lung disease, prematurity and complex medical conditions are at risk of more severe disease, potentially requiring closer observation, longer hospitalizations and more interventions.

Most cases of bronchiolitis last around a week, with symptoms usually at their worst midway through. Patients who are at risk of more severe disease or those who required invasive ventilation may have a longer course of illness. In the majority of cases, children with bronchiolitis are expected to have a full recovery.

History

The medical history is an important piece of the initial evaluation for children with bronchiolitis. Asking caregivers about symptom onset and trajectory can help characterize the severity of illness and development of possible complications. Fever pattern can help gauge day of illness as well. Inquiring about respiratory symptoms such as cough, congestion, rhinorrhea, as well as breathing concerns—specifically if caregivers have noticed any labored or noisy breathing is important. Children with bronchiolitis may wheeze as a part of their presentation, therefore some symptoms can overlap with reactive airway disease. It may be helpful to learn whether the child has wheezed or responded to beta agonists in the past and if there is a family history of asthma. Additionally, respiratory symptoms can make feeding more challenging in the setting of nasal congestion; therefore, taking an accurate feeding history as well noting the number and quality of wet diapers can help discern the degree of dehydration, if present. Finally, providers should inquire about potential sick contacts such as sick family members or daycare exposures.

Physical Exam

The physical exam findings of bronchiolitis are largely related to respiratory status (see Table 13.1). Additional signs of illness are related to hydration status. On auscultation, there might be a prolonged expiratory phase and shifting coarse or fine crackles/rales indicative of mucus in small airways. Hypoxemia (oxygen saturation <95%) is commonly detected on pulse oximetry.

Table 13.1 Physical examination findings in bronchiolitis

Vital sign abnormalities to watch for	• Fever (temperature >100.4 °F) • Tachycardia • Elevated systolic blood pressure • Tachypnea initially, though bradypnea can present if a children in respiratory failure
Respiratory symptoms	Upper respiratory symptoms—viral prodrome • Nasal congestion • Rhinorrhea Lower respiratory symptoms • Cough • Expiratory wheeze • Increased work of breathing – Retractions (intercostal, subcostal, suprasternal) – Nasal flaring – Head bobbing—use of neck muscles to help breathing – "Belly" or abdominal breathing—use of abdominal muscles to assist in pulling the diaphragm down to help breathing – Grunting
Signs of dehydration (in typical order of presentation)	Dry mucous membranes Decreased skin turgor Tachycardia Prolonged capillary refill Sunken anterior fontanelle

Workup

Bronchiolitis is a clinical diagnosis. See Table 13.2 for key differential diagnosis. Chest radiographs and laboratory studies are not indicated as a part of routine workup and evaluation as they are not necessary to make the diagnosis of bronchiolitis alone. However, if there are concerns for a secondary bacterial infection (e.g., pneumonia manifested by high fever or acute respiratory deterioration, or sepsis manifested by hypotension/shock), complications (e.g., consolidation or abnormal breath sounds suggesting pneumonia or pneumothorax), or if there is uncertainty about the diagnosis, then further studies may be useful in evaluation. Testing for specific viruses in children with bronchiolitis is typically conducted if the result will alter management (e.g., discontinuing palivizumab prophylaxis, antibiotic management, anti-influenza therapy, isolation or quarantine for severe acute respiratory syndrome coronavirus 2 (SARS-CoV-2), or cohorting of hospitalized patients or caregivers).

Key Differential Diagnoses

Table 13.2 Differential diagnosis of bronchiolitis

RAD/asthma	• Similar presentation to bronchiolitis, has prolonged expiratory phase/wheezing due to narrowing of bronchioles • Bronchiolitis is a disease in patients aged <2 years, while RAD/asthma is not limited by age • Family history of asthma or personal history of atopic disease increases likelihood of RAD/asthma diagnosis
Bacterial pneumonia	• Like bronchiolitis, presents with fevers and respiratory distress • Presents with higher grade fevers and focal exam findings without wheeze • Prodrome of viral URI symptoms, such as rhinorrhea is not always present
Foreign body aspiration	• Usually presents with sudden onset wheeze and cough with no preceding URI symptoms, including no rhinorrhea • Exam with diminished breath sounds and expiratory wheezing usually on the right side
Congenital airway obstructive lesion/vascular rings	• Wheezing is usually caused by external tracheal compression • Unlike bronchiolitis, patients present with a recurrent wheeze with associated stridor
Gastroesophageal reflux disease	• Usually chronic symptoms • Symptoms include wheezing, emesis, failure to thrive

RAD reactive airway disease, *URI* upper respiratory infection

Management

The management of bronchiolitis is supportive and consists of observation of work of breathing, fever management, and gentle, frequent suctioning of the external nares. Maintaining hydration is important given the risk of insensible losses caused by tachypnea, secretions, fevers and decreased oral intake. In an outpatient setting, caregivers should continue to provide fluids and monitor urine output. In the hospital setting, children may require intravenous fluids as a bolus or maintenance rate fluids. While feeding by mouth is comforting to the sick child, it is important to recognize that patients with significant respiratory distress are at risk of aspiration. Children with significant respiratory distress should have nothing by mouth (NPO) to prevent aspiration, and in anticipation of the possibility of decompensation that leads to intubation. Indications for admission for bronchiolitis include significant work of breathing and tachypnea with risk of decompensation, hypoxemia, and dehydration. Younger infants may present with apnea which would also be an indication for admission.

Children with hypoxemia may receive supplemental oxygen via nasal cannula or face mask if they are hypoxemic. Those with moderate to significant work of breathing may be started on high flow nasal cannula (HFNC) which delivers heated and humidified oxygen to improve gas exchange and decrease the work of breathing. Decreasing work of breathing is essential as respiratory failure can have severe and potentially fatal consequences, including risk of shock from dehydration and even cardiac arrest. Other modes of respiratory support such as continuous positive airway pressure (CPAP) or mechanical ventilation can be provided in the intensive care unit. Respiratory support is titrated to the needs of the patient. As the child's respiratory status improves, respiratory support can be weaned.

The use of inhaled bronchodilators (albuterol) is not recommended in otherwise healthy patients, as studies have shown no significant benefit. Steroids, antivirals, antibiotics, inhaled anticholinergics (ipratropium) and deep nasopharyngeal suctioning are also not recommended. The patient is deemed stable for discharge once they are able to maintain normal oxygen saturations on room air, are breathing comfortably, and are able to maintain hydration on their own.

Anticipatory Guidance

When infants and children are diagnosed with bronchiolitis, it is important to educate caregivers and give appropriate anticipatory guidance, especially since this illness often worsens a few days into the course before improving. Generally counseling involves discussing symptoms, home management, and instructions about when to seek medical care.

Management at home for bronchiolitis is supportive, focused mainly on maintaining hydration and clearing secretions. Hydration with liquids is more important than eating solids when children are acutely ill. For infants and children with bronchiolitis, feeding may be disrupted due to nasal congestion, therefore watching for wet diapers as a metric for hydration is important. A general rule is a minimum of about 3–4 wet diapers per day, with no longer than 6–8 h between diapers. A cool mist humidifier can help with nasal congestion while children are sleeping. Caregivers should perform gentle nasal suctioning with saline drops as needed, to help loosen secretions. Acetaminophen or ibuprofen (ibuprofen only if older than 6 months) can be used as needed to relieve fever/discomfort. Over the counter, cough suppressants and cold medications are not recommended. Honey should be avoided for children below 12 months of age due to the risk of botulism; however, it can be given to toddlers over 12 months of age for cough relief. Avoiding smoking and exposure to secondhand smoke is important, as inhaled smoke can irritate lungs further. And finally, frequent hand washing is important to prevent further spread of infection to other family members and caregivers.

Guidance regarding seeking medical care should address and caregiver comfort with their child's clinical status. Signs of worsening illness include faster breathing than usual or labored breathing. Labored breathing refers to accessory muscle use (e.g., belly breathing, subcostal retractions, intercostal retractions, or tracheal tugging), and grunting noises at the end of expiration. Other signs of worsening illness include inability to feed or stay hydrated because of breathing concerns (which can also be noticed by a decrease in wet diaper frequency to less than 3 per day), persistent fever for 5 or more days, or even a new fever in a child who was otherwise clinically improving. Worsening fussiness, sleepiness, or refusal to feed/persistent vomiting in setting of respiratory symptoms are also reasons to seek medical care. Finally, if the caregiver is worried about the child's clinical status, they should be encouraged to discuss with their pediatrician. If there is any concern for life-threatening emergency such as florid respiratory distress or lethargy, the caregiver should be instructed to call 911 for emergency support.

Follow up for children with bronchiolitis is largely based on clinical course. If a child was hospitalized, follow up with their primary care physician (PCP) in clinic/office is advised within 1–3 days after discharge. If not hospitalized, children may still require intermittent visits to the PCP for respiratory checks during the acute period of illness. Those who do not improve significantly by day 7 should also have close follow up with their PCP, who will then help guide further care. It is important to remember that the cough can persist for a few weeks.

Application Exercises

1. A 7-month-old previously healthy boy is brought to the emergency department by his parents for increased work of breathing. They report that he's been breathing fast and heavy since he woke up this morning. He's had a runny nose and has been sneezing for the past 2 days. He attends daycare, where several children have been sick. His father reports having childhood asthma, and there is a family history of atopy. On exam, you note a respiratory rate of 65 breaths/min, head bobbing, subcostal retractions, and diffuse wheezes. Which of the following is the most appropriate next step?

   A. Trial a dose of albuterol
   B. Start antiviral
   C. Start High Flow Nasal Cannula (HFNC)
   D. Continued observation

   Answer C: Given the prodrome of URI symptoms, history of recent sick contacts, and current clinical presentation, this patient likely has viral bronchiolitis. The treatment is supportive. HFNC can help ease work of breathing. Although patients with bronchiolitis can wheeze, beta agonists are not indicated for the management of bronchiolitis. At this time, this patient's history and exam are more consistent with bronchiolitis than community acquired pneumonia; therefore, antibiotics are not indicated. Given that this patient is tachypneic and having respiratory distress, continued observation is not the best option.

2. A 4-month-old previously healthy girl is brought to her pediatrician's office by her mother for 4 days of cough, rhinorrhea, and nasal congestion. Today her mother noticed she was breathing a little faster. She is nursing for shorter amounts of time, but more frequently, and wet diapers are normal. She has not been sleeping well and wakes frequently due to nasal congestion. On exam, vitals are temp 37 °C, HR 120, RR 40, SpO_2 98%; there are some intermittent

intercostal retractions, coarse breath sounds, occasional wheeze, flat anterior fontanelle, and good capillary refill. The mom is asking what should be done next.

A. Refer the patient to the emergency department for evaluation and admission for respiratory and hydration support
B. Reassurance and supportive care with clear anticipatory guidance and close primary care physician follow-up
C. Obtain chest X-ray
D. Obtain respiratory swab to determine pathogen

Answer B: The child in this vignette has bronchiolitis given the prodrome of URI symptoms followed by signs of lower respiratory tract involvement. Given she has normal urine output, is well hydrated on exam, and only intermittent retractions, she can be monitored at home with clear guidance about when to present to emergency care if needed, along with scheduled PCP follow-up. Reassurance about the natural trajectory of bronchiolitis can help comfort caregivers as well. Given her stability, referral to the ED is not necessary at this time. Beta agonists are not indicated in the management of bronchiolitis. Her exam is not consistent with a focal lung infection; therefore, antibiotics would not be indicated.

Further Reading

Kronman MP, Crowell CS, Vora SB. Bronchiolitis. In: Marcdante KJ, Kliegman RM, Schuh AM, editors. Nelson essentials of pediatrics. Philadelphia, PA: Elsevier; 2023.
Ralston SL, Lieberthal AS, Meissner HC, Alverson BK, Baley JE, Gadomski AM, et al., American Academy of Pediatrics. Clinical practice guideline: the diagnosis, management, and prevention of bronchiolitis. Pediatrics. 2014;134(5):e1474–502. Erratum in: Pediatrics. 2015;136(4):782.
Silver AH, Nazif JM. Bronchiolitis. Pediatr Rev. 2019;40(11):568–76.

Chapter 14
Burns and Wounds

Clifton Lee and Ashlie Tseng

Wounds

History

As with many diagnoses, the history and physical exam are extremely important in the assessment of wounds. When taking a history, interviewers should obtain mechanism of injury, past medical history, developmental milestones, nutritional status, current medications, allergies, and immunization status, particularly tetanus. These histories will help elucidate if there are factors that may impact wound healing.

Physical Exam

Pay close attention to vital signs and identify issues that need to be addressed urgently or emergently. For example, hypovolemia from bleeding can lead to tachycardia and hypotension. Infectious concerns can manifest with tachycardia, tachypnea, fever, and blood pressure changes (hypotension or widened pulse pressure). Look for bleeding or evidence of further injury that requires additional management such as musculoskeletal injury including fractures, tendon injury, and neurovascular damage. Assess for evidence of infection or the presence of foreign bodies.

C. Lee (✉) · A. Tseng
Department of Pediatrics, Children's Hospital of Richmond at VCU, Virginia Commonwealth University School of Medicine, Richmond, VA, USA
e-mail: clifton.lee@vcuhealth.org; ashlie.tseng@vcuhealth.org

N. Liao et al. (eds.), *Pediatric Rotations*,
https://doi.org/10.1007/978-3-031-59873-9_14

Laboratory Assessment/Imaging

Routine laboratory assessment and imaging are not indicated. Certain considerations may warrant further workup based on the history and physical exam. Laboratory evaluation including complete blood count, coagulation studies, and type & cross may be obtained if there is continued bleeding or severe blood loss. Consider imaging to look for retained foreign bodies. Radiographs can identify retained metal while ultrasound studies can better evaluate for other types of foreign bodies.

Differential Diagnosis

Wounds can have traumatic and nontraumatic etiologies. Accidental injuries are the most common cause of wounds but nonaccidental trauma should always be on the differential. Nontraumatic etiologies include child abuse, infections, pressure injury, or dermatologic diseases.

Management

Patients should have an initial triage and assessment and be medically stabilized as necessary. Once that has been assured, the next step is to properly irrigate the wound. Typically, sterile saline is used but there is evidence that tap water is not associated with a higher risk for infection. More important than fluid choice is achieving higher pressure during irrigation, such as with a syringe. Antiseptics are not commonly used given the lack of clear benefit in reducing infection rates and the risk of harm with some solutions. Necrotic or devitalized tissue needs debridement to ensure adequate wound healing.

The next consideration in management is wound closure. There are three types: primary, secondary, and delayed (Table 14.1).

A topical anesthetic such as lidocaine, epinephrine, and tetracaine can be used for pain control/analgesia. When suturing or stapling in the ED setting, injected lidocaine is used. Peripheral nerve blocks are less common but are used for more extensive repairs.

Table 14.2 outlines some situations when consultation with specialists may be necessary.

Fortunately, most patients can be managed without admission to the hospital, though hospitalization can be considered in patients concerns for sepsis, failure of outpatient management, or complicating injuries requiring further intervention. Optimal healing requires a moist environment; however, the wound cannot be so wet that edges of the wound become macerated.

Table 14.1 Types of wound closure

Types of wound closure	Description	Considerations
Primary	Repair at the time of presentation by using surgical tapes, tissue adhesives, sutures, or staples	No concerns for infection Low concern for wound dehiscence (low tension on incision line, little tissue loss) Cosmetic concerns in the face Benefits: minimal scarring, faster wound healing
Secondary	No closure, allowing the wound the heal naturally	Wounds presenting later for care, typically >8 h Any concern for infection in conjunction with appropriate infectious treatment, or in situations of gross contamination Wounds that cannot be closed without tension
Delayed	Intentional delay of primary wound closure	May be considered with contaminated wounds after treatment of infection Includes skin grafts or flaps

Table 14.2 Specialty consults

Specialty	Indications
Plastic surgery	Concerning for disfigurement Wounds involving the vermilion border
Pediatric or plastic surgery	Wounds that require debridement or skin grafting
Neurosurgery	Penetrating injury to the skull
Orthopedic surgery	Concern of damage to adjacent bones
Child abuse specialists and social work	Concern for nonaccidental trauma
Psychology	If significant traumatic injuries or nonaccidental trauma
Physical and occupational therapy	Injuries that cross joints Wounds that cause limitations to activities
Nutritionist	Poor underlying nutrition Concern for deficiencies such as vitamin C or zinc Extensive wounds that require high protein diet to promote healing

Complications and Other Considerations

Routine prophylaxis with antibiotics is not required. Certain patient and wound factors may make infectious complications more likely. Patient factors include nutritional deficits or immunocompromised status. Types of injury such as bites, puncture wounds, or late presentation for care are examples of wound-specific factors. When there is concern for infection, the antibiotic regimen should be tailored to the

Table 14.3 Indications for tetanus vaccination and TIG

	Wound type	
Vaccine status	Clean	Dirty
Unvaccinated	Complete primary series	Complete primary series Administer tetanus immune globulin (TIG)
Vaccinated	Last vaccine: <10 years: None >10 years: Tetanus vaccine booster	Last vaccine: <5 years: None >5 years: Tetanus vaccine booster

possible exposures. Coverage for methicillin resistant *Staphylococcus aureus* should be considered, and antibiotic choice should be based on local resistance patterns. Amoxicillin clavulanate is commonly used for human and animal bites and provides coverage of aerobic bacteria and anaerobic oral flora. Treat for 3–5 days for prophylaxis and 5–14 days for infection.

Wounds at high risk for tetanus include puncture wounds, wounds contaminated with dirt, soil, saliva, or feces, and those with devitalize tissue (such as burns, crush injuries, frostbite). As mentioned above, tetanus immunization status is important to establish. See Table 14.3 for guidance on tetanus vaccination and use of tetanus immune globulin (TIG). Refer to the United States' Center for Disease Control website for the most up-to-date information on tetanus vaccines. Rabies should be considered in certain types of animal bites (bats, raccoons, skunks, foxes), and the rabies vaccine and/or immunoglobulin may be administered, and the public health department should be notified.

Burns

Background

Injuries are a leading cause of death among children in the United States of which 0.7% are caused by fires or burns. Although approximately 90% of pediatric burn injuries happen at home, adolescents are more likely to be burned outside the home. The type of burn injury is related to the age and the developmental stage of the child. Toddlers and preschool children are more likely to sustain scald, intra-oral, and electrical burns, while flame and chemical burns are more likely in older children. Boys are more likely than girls to be burned. Death is very rare in children with scald burns; however, mortality significantly increases with cases of nonaccidental trauma. Larger total body surface area (TBSA) burns tend to be related to flame-related exposure. Long-term outcomes are favorable for children with access to multi-specialty burn centers.

Pathophysiology

Burn wounds trigger local and systemic changes which increase in intensity with the size and depth of the wound. The local response to a burn injury includes microvascular vasoconstriction and thrombosis in peripheral unburned tissue. The systemic response to a burn injury results from a complex array of changes including neurohormonal changes, fluid loss, hypoproteinemia, and hypotension. In children with large burns, a systemic response can manifest as high fevers and multi-organ dysfunction. During the first 1–2 days after a burn injury, a hypodynamic state with decreased cardiac output and metabolic rate is commonly seen. In addition to these physiologic changes, there are several unique anatomic and physiologic concerns for children with burn injuries. Airway protection with endotracheal intubation is necessary in children with smoke inhalation due to airway edema.

Younger infants may require a higher volume of fluid per unit body weight than older children due to less mature renal concentrating abilities. Children have higher metabolic needs than adults; thus, early nutritional support is beneficial. Finally, children have a relatively large body surface area which makes them more susceptible to hypothermia.

History

Careful and detailed histories should be obtained from all caretakers as well as the child if possible. Ask about the surrounding circumstances, the type of burn, and how the patient sustained the injury. The mechanism of injury should fit with the age and developmental stage of the child. If not, be concerned for nonaccidental trauma. Inconsistencies in the history or a delay in seeking medical assessment may also raise suspicion.

Burns sustained in an enclosed fire will be associated with smoke inhalation. Contact burns that occur with a hot surface such as glass-front fireplaces, oven doors, and irons are common with younger children. Most electrical burn injuries occur when children put objects in the outlets or bite on the cords. The most common chemical agents that cause burn injury include oven cleaners, aerosols, drain cleaners, bleach, and hair dye. Exposure in adolescent patients can be related to a suicide attempt.

Physical Exam

A comprehensive physical examination including a detailed documentation of the injuries should be noted and photographed. Begin with a primary survey. The assessment of the airway is of highest priority. This is followed by breathing (adequacy of ventilatory effort), circulation (blood pressure and evaluation for shock), disability (neurologic stability), and exposure (assessment of injuries). This is followed by the secondary survey which facilitates cataloging all injures and minimizing delayed care of injuries missed by the initial examination. The secondary survey includes a review of the injury mechanism and a careful head-to-toe examination. The initial evaluation of the burn injury includes an accurate determination of the wound size and depth. Assess for any injuries or burn patterns may be indicative of nonaccidental trauma. Burns range from superficial (epidermis only), partial thickness (involving part or most of dermis), and full thickness (involving the dermis and subcutaneous structures). This assessment is important for initial management as well as the establishment of likely timeline for healing. Estimate the total body surface area (TBSA) of a burn using the Lund and Browder burn chart (Fig. 14.1). An alternate rule is that the patient's palm and fingers represent 1% of the body surface.

Laboratory Assessment/Imaging

Initial laboratory and imaging evaluations largely depend on the type of burn injury and the need for initial fluid resuscitation. Electrolytes, glucose, and kidney function should be obtained as well as a liver function test. A complete blood count, coagulation panel, and a type and cross may also be needed if concomitant hemorrhagic shock is suspected. Initial imaging studies are determined by the history and a careful physical examination. If a nonaccidental trauma is suspected, additional studies are needed such as a skeletal survey and a non-contrasted head CT (computed tomography).

Management

The overarching goals of burn management are to maximize perfusion and oxygenation to the affected tissues to promote healing and to minimize wound infection. The fundamentals of burn resuscitation are managing the airway, accurately calculating the TBSA, hemodynamic stabilization, evaluating for additional trauma, adequate pain management, and appropriate disposition. Any burn with greater than 10% TBSA requires IV fluid management. The Parkland formula is commonly used to calculate fluid requirements. 4 mL × body weight (kg) × TBSA = total fluids in the first 24 h. The first half should be given within 8 h, followed by the second half over the next 16 h. Children may need analgesic and anxiolytic medications during the initial wound evaluation and debridement (Table 14.4).

Tetanus considerations are also important in burn care. If nonaccidental trauma is suspected, appropriate consultations with Social Work and a Child Abuse Specialist should be obtained. There may be institutional variation with the criteria

Lund and Browder Charts for area of body burnt

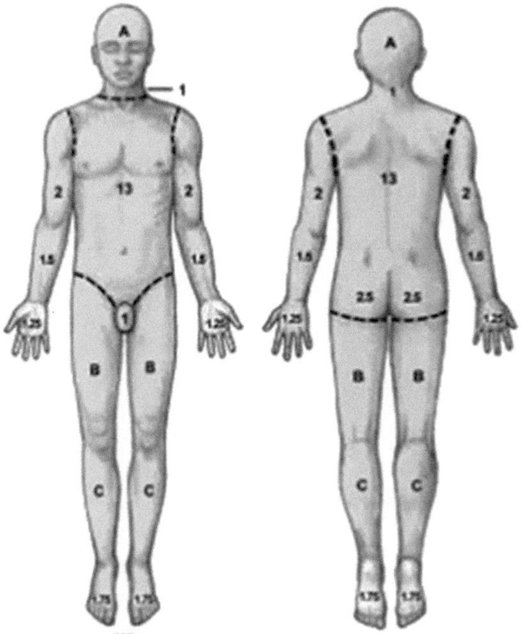

Burnt area	%
Head	
Neck	
Trunk (front)	
Trunk (back	
Arm (right)	
Arm (left)	
Hand (right)	
Hand (left)	
Buttock (right)	
Buttock (left)	
Genitals	
Leg (right)	
Leg (left)	
Feet (right)	
Feet (left)	
Total burn area	

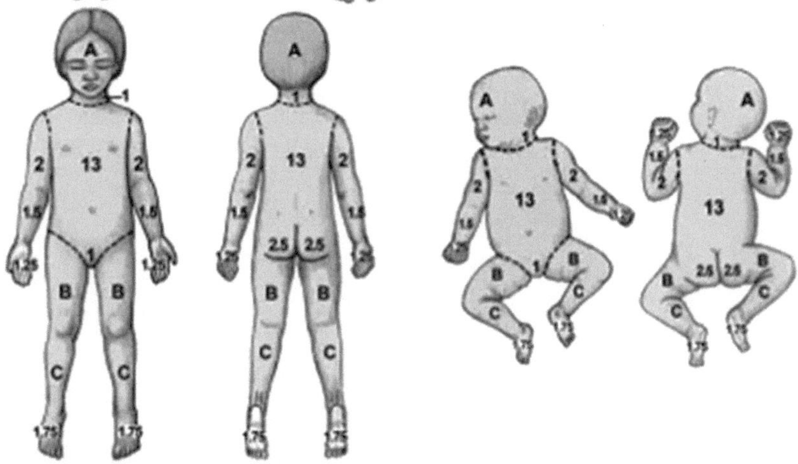

Age (years)	Under 1	2–4	5–9	10–14	15	Adult
A — ½ of head	9½	8½	6½	5½	4½	3½
B — ½ of one thigh	2¾	3¼	4	4½	4½	4¾
C — ½ of one leg	2½	2½	2¾	3	3¼	3

Fig. 14.1 Lund and Browder chart (from the American Burn Association)

Table 14.4 Burn depth classification and documentation with prognosis to aid in patient education (from Strobel and Fey, *Emerg Med Clin N Am*, 2018)

Classification	Depth	Examination description	Healing time	Risk for scar	Pain control	Wound care
Superficial (first degree)[a]	Epidermis	• Erythematous • No blister • Painful	4–5 days	None	• Ibuprofen • Acetaminophen	• Aloe vera • Emollient moisturizers
Superficial partial-thickness (second degree)	Epidermis and dermis	• Pink, moist, blanching with intact capillary refill • Blister • Painful when blister deroofed and open to air	7–10 days	• Minimal • Dark-skinned individuals may lose melanin and be hypopigmented during healing	• Narcotic 30 min before dressing change	• Soap and water twice daily dressing change with bacitracin or petroleum jelly and non-adherent gauze • Commercial long-term dressings Mepilex Ag (Molnlycke, Norcross, GA, USA) or Aquacel Ag (ConvaTec, Princeton, NJ, USA) • Silver sulfadiazine has fallen out of favor because it has more adverse effects (i.e. sulfa allergy, kernicterus in neonates, anemia G-6-PD) without proof of superiority

Classification	Depth	Examination description	Healing time	Risk for scar	Pain control	Wound care
Deep partial-thickness (second degree) and indeterminate-thickness	Deeper dermis	• Erythematous or yellow, nonblanching • Dry to waxy • Blister easily unroofs • Possibly not painful if nerve fibers involved • Presence of hair follicles • Capillary burst with red punctum of bleeding at times	2–3 weeks	Probable	• Narcotics 30 min before dressing changes • Acetaminophen • Ibuprofen	• Acticoat (Smith & Nephew, Canada) • Surgical consultation for early excision and grafting of indeterminate-thickness and full-thickness burns decreases infection, cost, and mortality rates • Physical therapy and occupational therapy
Full-thickness (third degree)	Dermis	• White, waxy, and leathery • Lack hair follicles • Insensate	Weeks	Definite	–	Surgical consultation for early excision and grafting
Fourth degree	Subcutaneous tissues into the fascia, muscle, tendon, bone	• Deep structures visualized	Months	Definite	• Narcotics • Ibuprofen • Acetaminophen	Surgical consultation

used to determine patient transfer to a specialty burn center; however, in general, a transfer should be considered for burns: >5% TBSA; involving the face, hands, feet, perineum, or joints; circumferential burns; burn associated with another injury or inhalation injury; suspected nonaccidental trauma; electrical burns or chemical burns.

Anticipatory Guidance for Wounds

Education should be provided to patients and caregivers about monitoring for signs of infection. Pain control can generally be accomplished with a combination of acetaminophen and ibuprofen. As wounds and burns heal, they may become pruritic. Diphenhydramine, hydroxyzine, or cetirizine can be used for itching. The healing wound should be moisturized regularly with petroleum jelly to promote healing. Finally, the scar should be protected from sun exposure with sunscreen (sun protection factor 25 or greater) to improve cosmetic appearance. For patients with burns, prevention strategies should be discussed. For example, hot irons, hair curling irons, and hot beverages should be placed out of reach of young children. Outlets should be covered, and electrical cords should be inspected for loose wires. Smoke detectors should be inspected regularly. Families should have a home fire evacuation plan.

Application Exercises

1. You are seeing a 15-year-old patient who presents to the emergency room due to an injury to her foot. She was helping her parents build a fence and stepped on a nail that pierced through her sandal. On examination, you see a small puncture wound at the base of her heel and soil under her toenails. Immunization records show that she completed her five dose DTaP series appropriately and the last dose was at 4 years of age. What is the next appropriate step in management?

   A. No need for any tetanus toxoid vaccination or tetanus immunoglobulin
   B. Administer TIG immediately but there is no need for tetanus toxoid vaccination
   C. Administer tetanus toxoid vaccination but there is no need for TIG currently
   D. Administer both tetanus toxoid vaccination and TIG during this encounter

   Answer C: The patient requires a tetanus-containing vaccine given that it has been more than 5 years since her last dose but does not require tetanus immunoglobulin. This patient is not immunocompromised and does not require TIG since she has completed primary vaccination. Tetanus in an immunocompetent patient following primary vaccination is extremely rare.
2. A 4-year-old boy is evaluated in the Pediatric Emergency Department due to a burn injury sustained from a house fire. Per EMS report, there was considerable smoke exposure prior to extrication from the house. Vital signs are as follows: temperature is 37 °C, pulse is 120 beats/min, respiratory rate is 38 breaths/min,

and blood pressure is 96/55 mmHg. On physical examination, he is drooling. There is presence of soot on his nostrils. On auscultation, faint inspiratory stridor is heard. Approximately, 10% TBSA is affected with combination of partial and full thickness burns.

What is the most appropriate management?

A. IV fluid resuscitation with lactated Ringers bolus (20 mL/kg)
B. Apply non-occlusive dressing over the burns
C. Pain management with IV morphine
D. Immediate endotracheal intubation
E. Careful examination and documentation of the burn injuries

Rationale: Answer D: Immediate endotracheal intubation. The airway should be secured if the patient exhibits any of the following: hoarseness, stridor, drooling, respiratory distress, or altered mental status. Presence of soot on the nostrils indicates inhalation injury. In children, due to a smaller airway diameter, even a small amount of edema can cause exponential airway narrowing. Thus, the airway must be secured.

Further Reading

Black KD, Cico SJ, Caglar D. Wound management. Pediatr Rev. 2015;36(5):207–15.
Navanadan N, Renna-Rodriguz M, DiStefano MC. Pearls in pediatric wound management. Clin Pediatr Emerg Med. 2017;18(1):53–61.
Sheridan RL. Burn care for children. Pediatr Rev. 2018;39(6):273–86.
Strobel AM, Fey R. Emergency care of pediatric burns. Emerg Med Clin N Am. 2018;36(2):441–58.
Suman A, Owen J. Update on the management of burns in paediatrics. 2019. BJA Educ. 2020;20(3):103–10.

Chapter 15
Common Procedures

Meghan McClure and Krista Preisberga

Introduction

Minor medical procedures are frequently performed in pediatric patients in the emergency departments (EDs), acute care floors, and designated procedural areas. The skills required to perform common procedures can be learned throughout medical school with the help and supervision of experienced physicians. It is important for you to understand the indications, potential complications, as well as the procedural steps for each of the following common pediatric procedures.

Obtaining Consent

All procedures, however minor, require written or verbal consent prior to initiation of the procedure. The consent process includes discussion of the following elements: (1) purpose and indications of the procedure, (2) benefits of the procedure to the patient, and (3) known risks involved with the procedures and measures taken to minimize those risks. An official hospital form should be signed by the patient (if over 18), parent/guardian, person obtaining consent, and a witness. Only truly emergent, life-saving, procedures may be performed with implied (not documented) consent if a parent/guardian is unavailable to provide consent.

M. McClure (✉) · K. Preisberga
Division of Pediatric Hospital Medicine, Department of Pediatrics, Baylor College of Medicine, Houston, TX, USA
e-mail: meghan.mcclure@bcm.edu; preisber@bcm.edu

N. Liao et al. (eds.), *Pediatric Rotations*,
https://doi.org/10.1007/978-3-031-59873-9_15

Pre-procedural Diet Guidelines

Specific guidelines may vary between institutions; however, the American Society of Anesthesiologists practice guidelines state that for healthy patients of any age undergoing a sedated non-emergent procedure, fasting recommendations are 8 hours for a heavy meal containing fried or fatty foods, 6 hours for a light meal, formula, or non-human milk, and 2 hours for clear liquids (water, fruit juices without pulp, tea, black coffee, etc.). Breastmilk processing time falls between clear liquids and formula with a recommended fasting time of 4 hours. Some procedures or imaging studies may require specific NPO (nil per os) timelines; for example, gastric emptying studies or upper GI fluoroscopic evaluations, and fasting recommendations should be discussed with performing provider at time of ordering.

Procedures

Peripheral and Central Venous Access

Venipuncture is used for obtaining blood for diagnostic purposes or placement of intravenous catheters for therapeutic administration of fluids and medications. When obtaining blood for sampling without a need for catheter placement, the butterfly needle is used most frequently followed by hypodermic needle. Both range in size from 14 gauge (largest diameter) to 27 gauge (smallest diameter). If catheter placement is needed, the IV needle is sheathed in the catheter that remains in the vein as the needle is retracted. Complications from peripheral IV placement include bleeding, phlebitis, cellulitis or other site infections, and pre-syncope/syncope.

Supplies Needed

1. Non-sterile gloves
2. Butterfly needle/needle + vacuum container
3. Blood collection tubes
4. Alcohol swabs
5. Non-sterile gauze
6. Bandages

Venipuncture in Antecubital Fossa Procedure

1. Wash your hands. You should wear non-sterile gloves for this procedure.
2. Apply tourniquet 3–4 in. above expected puncture site and ask patient to make a fist to help visualize an accessible vein.
3. Clean skin with alcohol swab starting from the expected puncture site and moving in circular fashion outwards to cover an area of at least 4 cm diameter.
4. Allow skin to air dry completely for 30 seconds.

5. Hold patient's arm below expected puncture site firmly to draw the skin taut and anchor vein. Once you visualize the vein you want to use, insert the needle bevel-up in the same direction that vein is running, holding needle at 15° angle with arm.
6. When you see blood return ("flash"), firmly attach collection tubes.
7. When you have inserted the last collection tube and only need ~1 cc more of blood, release the tourniquet.
8. Remove needle from patient's arm, lock the needle immediately, and press down on the puncture site with gauze. Place sterile bandage.

Central venous catheters (CVC) are large bore catheters that terminate in the super vena cava or inferior vena cava and ensure reliable venous access with rapid delivery of medication. There are four types of CVCs: non-tunneled, tunneled, Peripherally Inserted Central Catheter (PICC), and port-a-cath. Placement of CVCs requires additional dedicated training and is beyond the scope of this book. The PICC line is most often encountered by students when request is made for removal. The PICC line terminates in the SVC as with other central lines but has its insertion point peripherally. Potential complications related to PICC removal include air embolism, site infection, or bleeding.

Supplies Needed

1. Non-sterile gloves
2. Suture removal kit
3. Sterile 2 × 2 gauze
4. Alcohol swab
5. Sterile dressing (gauze + Tegaderm bandage)

Removal of PICC Line Procedure

1. Explain the procedure to the patient.
2. Wash your hands. You should wear non-sterile gloves for this procedure.
3. Place patient supine with arm abducted, place a pad under the patient's arm that has the PICC line, and remove the dressing carefully from insertion site.
4. Remove PICC from stabilization device (this may require cutting 1–2 sutures).
5. Cleanse exit site with alcohol swab and allow to air dry × 30 s.
6. Ask patient to hold breath at end of expiration.
7. Hold sterile 2 × 2 gauze directly to exit site with non-dominant hand. With dominant hand, slowly remove catheter using gentle, even pressure.
8. Apply firm pressure to exit site with gauze dressing until hemostasis is achieved and apply sterile dressing to site.
9. Measure PICC line to compare with insertion record. Inspect for intact tip. If evidence of break or incorrect catheter length, order a chest and/or extremity radiograph to confirm retained fragment and discuss with interventional radiology for endovascular retrieval.

Enteral Feeding Tubes

Maximizing nutrition is of utmost importance in pediatrics, and feeding by mouth is always preferred over enteral administration of nutrition; however, enteral feeds may be necessary based on a patient's diagnosis/condition. If a patient is expected to resume nutrition per os in less than 6 months, a short-term solution is placement of a nasogastric (NG) or nasojejunal (NJ) feeding tube. If timing of impaired oral nutrition is expected to last 6 months or longer, placement of a more secure enteral tube is preferred. In these instances, a gastrostomy (direct connection from viscera to skin) may be created allowing for direct skin to stomach access.

Indications for initiation of enteral tube feeds are when a patient is unable to safely consume the nutrition due to neuromuscular deficit, anatomic abnormalities of the oropharynx, aspiration risk, unwillingness to consume a specified caloric requirement due to food aversion, or anorexia. Contraindications to enteral feeding include gastrointestinal obstruction, perforation, or ischemia.

Nasogastric tube placement can be performed at bedside by any trained provider. Nasojejunal tube generally requires placement with image guidance to ensure tip of the tube rests in the jejunum. Any post-pyloric tubes are more technically challenging to place, and many are weighted at the tip to prevent malposition. Thus, bedside placement of NJ tubes is not routinely performed.

Supplies Needed

1. Non-sterile gloves
2. Appropriate diameter NG tube (see below guidelines)
3. Lubricant jelly
4. Adhesive tape cut 4–5 in., ripped vertically along half of length
5. 1% lidocaine spray (optional)
6. 10 mL syringe
7. Emesis bucket

NG Tube Placement Procedure

1. Determine the correct diameter size of tubing needed. General guidelines are as follows:

    (a) 10 French for infants up to 2 years
    (b) 12 French for 2–5 years
    (c) 14 French 6–11 years
    (d) 16 French for older than 12 years of age

2. Measure the length of tubing using the tube in a straight line from bridge of the nose to the tragus and then straight line from tragus to xiphoid process (see Fig. 15.1). This will be the cm mark at the nares when successfully inserted.
3. Obtain verbal consent and explain the procedure to the child with age-appropriate language. This is generally best accomplished with the help of child life specialists.

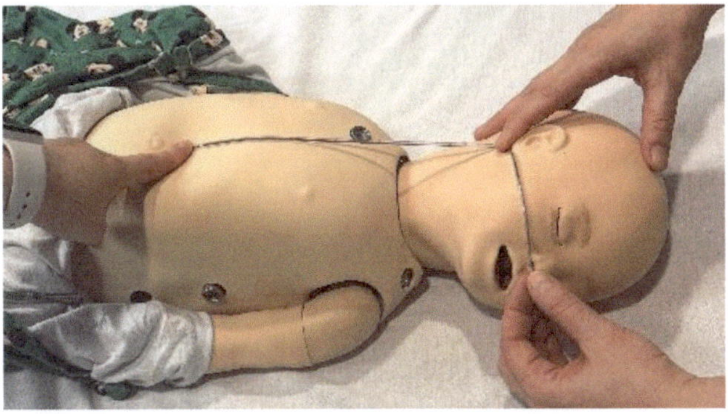

Fig. 15.1 Proper measurement of nasogastric tube length prior to placement

Clinical pearl: You can spray 1% lidocaine to the chosen naris and posterior oropharynx before tube placement to anesthetize the area and minimize discomfort.

4. Wash your hands. You should wear non-sterile gloves for this procedure.
5. Place lubricant jelly over the distal tip of the tubing.
6. With the patient sitting up, insert the tube into the chosen naris and advance gently down the posterior nasopharynx applying gentle pressure. Point the tube posteriorly and then down to stay below the nasal turbinate. You will feel mild resistance. However, if you feel strong resistance, do not force the tube. Ask an attending for help.

   Clinical pearl: Ask the child to swallow while the tube is passing the lower oropharynx to help guide it into the esophagus. This will also help with the gag reflex.
7. Once you reach the marker measured previously, use 10 mL syringe to aspirate the stomach contents for a pH check to determine placement. A pH < 6 would be expected for gastric contents.
8. Secure the tube in place with adhesive tape to minimize movement. Wrap the tails of the tape in opposite directions around the tube.
9. Additional step of confirming placement with X-ray can be performed prior to initiating enteral feeds.

Long-term use of NG or NJ tubes can lead to frequent displacement, nasopharyngeal infections, tissue irritation, and potential for perforation into the esophagus. One permanent feeding tube option is balloon gastrostomy tube (shown in Fig. 15.2). The most common problem associated with balloon G-tubes is accidental removal of the tube from the stoma either from a leak in the balloon or traction on the tube itself. G-tubes can be easily replaced at bedside. G-tube placement with a smaller size tube can result in gastric content leaking from stoma site and skin irritation. These can be avoided by ensuring that the correct size G-tube is provided.

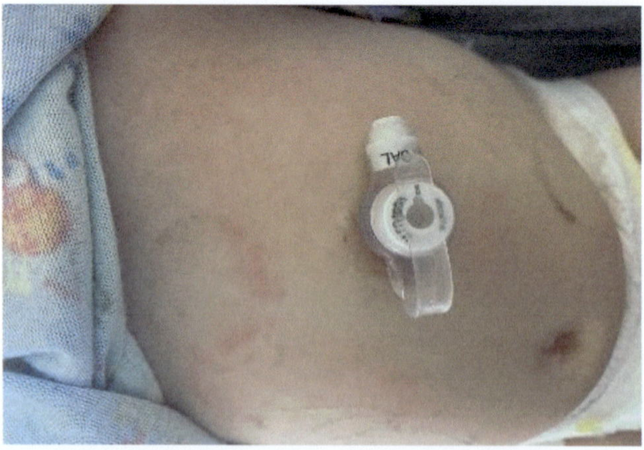

Fig. 15.2 Mickey G button in place. Note port labeled BAL for balloon inflation. Capped feeding port in center

Supplies Needed

1. Non-sterile gloves
2. G-tube kit- proper size and type (Mic-key, AMT, Cor-Pak)
3. Water-soluble lubricant
4. 5 mL syringe filled with water

Balloon G-Tube Replacement Procedure

1. You must first remove the old tube if still present. Wash hands and put on non-sterile gloves.
2. Attach a 5 mL syringe to port labeled "BAL" and slowly pull back on plunger until all the water from the balloon is removed. This will deflate the balloon so you can gently remove G-tube from stoma site.
3. Once stoma is open, clean the area with sterile saline and 4 × 4 gauze, lubricate new G-tube with petroleum jelly, and insert the new G-tube into the stoma site using a slight twisting motion back-and-forth until the port nears skin. Attach a 5 mL syringe and instill 3 mL of water into balloon (can add up to 5 mL of water if tube is not secure to skin). Excess amount of force can result in creation of false tract and tissue damage. If unable to replace the tube using gentle pressure, surgery should be contacted for evaluation. One size smaller tube or a urinary Foley catheter of equivalent diameter can be used to keep the stoma from closing any further.
4. Check placement by using two of the three following techniques: (a) Pull back gently on GT to make sure it is abutting against the wall of the stomach. (b) Attach syringe to feeding port and pull back stomach contents. Contents can be simply reinjected through feeding port after confirmation. (c) Inject water into feeding port to ensure no resistance to flow.

Lumbar Puncture

Lumbar punctures (LP) are common procedures done in the pediatric ED, acute care floors, and neonatal care units. They are most commonly indicated in diagnostic evaluation of cerebrospinal fluid (CSF) for autoimmune processes or infection, particularly in the neonatal period. They can also be used to obtain measurement of CSF opening pressure in cases of severe headache (concerning for intracranial hypertension or pseudotumor cerebri) or in the administration of chemotherapy agents for oncologic patients.

Absolute contraindication to performing an LP would include skin infection directly over the site, lumbar vertebral abscess, epidural abscess, or any focal infection that could lead to dissemination of infection to the CNS with needle introduction. If there is concern for increased intracranial pressure as evidence by papilledema, abnormal level of consciousness, seizure, or focal neurologic exam, the patient requires head imaging prior to attempting this procedure to avoid risk for herniation. Additionally, presence of a known anatomic abnormality such as Chiari malformation would require consultation with a neurosurgeon prior to proceeding with LP.

Relative contraindications would include coagulation abnormalities and platelet dysfunction. Patients with scoliosis or with a larger body habitus can present a challenge and might require image- or ultrasound-guided LP by an interventional radiologist.

Supplies Needed

1. Personal protection—sterile gloves, gown, facemask, eye protection
2. Oral sucrose and topical lidocaine for neonates
3. Lumbar puncture tray (see Fig. 15.3a)
4. One additional spinal needle (see Fig. 15.3b)
5. Biohazard bag for transport of specimen
6. Specimen labels with correct patient name and identification

Lumbar Puncture Procedure

1. If using topical lidocaine cream for infants, place over the intended puncture site at least 30 min prior to the procedure. Cover with a non-absorbent dressing.
2. Call a time-out to identify the correct patient, identify all team members, and name the procedure being performed, marking the date and time of the start of the procedure.
3. Remove the tray from the plastic wrapping and place on a sturdy surface near your patient.
4. Position child (see Fig. 15.4a):

   (a) Lateral decubitus position with neck flexed and knees to chest. Care should be taken to allow the spine to be as straight as possible as bending at the hip will create a curvature making it more challenging to enter the correct space.

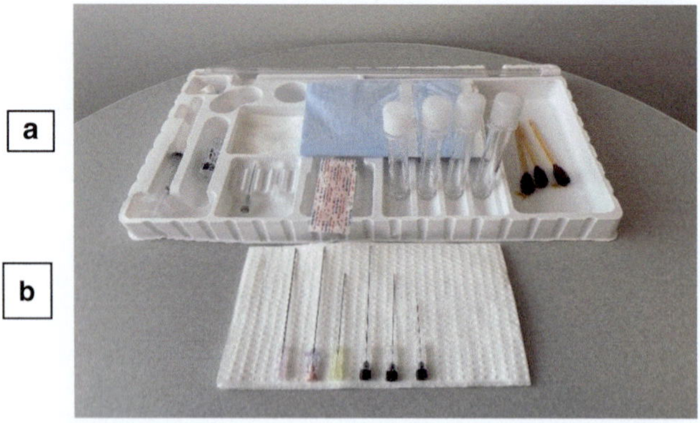

Fig. 15.3 (a) Standard LP tray contents: betadine cleanser packet with three swabs, four 10 mL collection tubes (labeled 1–4), lidocaine without epinephrine 1%, 3 mL syringe with one 20- and 25-gauge needle, 22-gauge spinal needle with stylet in pediatric tray or 20-gauge spinal needle with stylet in adult tray, Sterile drapes, 4 × 4 sterile gauze and adhesive bandage. Adult tray contains additional supplies: monometer, extension, 4 way stopcock. (b) Choosing the length of the 22-gauge needle is dependent on size of the child. Generally, 1.5 cm is used for children less than 1 year of age, 2.5 cm in children less than 5 years of age. Additionally, for large adult size patients, an 18-gauge spinal needle could be used

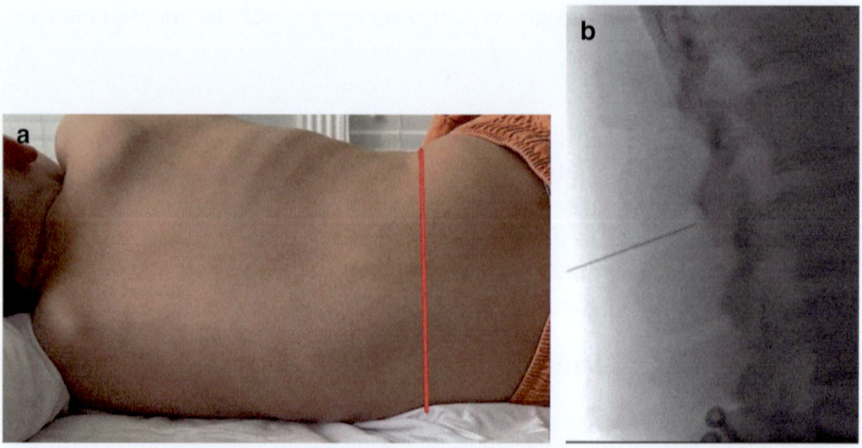

Fig. 15.4 (a, left) Proper lateral decubitus positioning for LP with identified L4/L5 level. (b, right) Sagittal view of intravertebral space and proper angle of LP needle

(b) Sitting, tucked position can be utilized in awake patients. Having a good holder for infant positioning is essential as they tend to move throughout the process.

5. Identify the L3–L4 interspace by palpating bilateral iliac crests and imaging a straight line between the two crests. The spinous process can be visually seen on thin body habitus and smaller children.
6. You should then gown and put on sterile gloves. Open the tray taking care to only touch the paper in which the tray is wrapped. Place specimen tubes upright for easy collection.
7. Sterilize the anticipated puncture site with antiseptic solution, start at the proposed site and work outward in a circular manner. Repeat two more times with the provided swabs taking care to remain sterile.
8. Drape area with sterile drapes, leaving proposed site exposed.
9. Check child's position to ensure correct spine flexion, maximizing intralaminar space.
10. If patient is deeply sedated or anesthetized, the use of local lidocaine is likely not needed. In awake patients, infiltration of dermis and subcutaneous tissue with lidocaine is usually required to avoid significant pain with this procedure. The lidocaine infusion can be painful on its own with many patients reporting a strong burning sensation on injection.

    Clinical pearl: Using buffered lidocaine can significantly reduce the pain of infusion; however, this preparation has to be obtained from pharmacy in advance.
11. Infusion of lidocaine is done slowly with small aliquots of 0.25 mL at a time as the needle is advanced further into the deeper tissue. Allow 5 min for full numbing to take effect.
12. Using a 20- or 22-gauge spinal needle and stylet, puncture skin in the L4–L5 interspace aiming toward umbilicus. The bevel of the needle should face upward if the patient is in lateral decubitus position or sideways if sitting up. This will ensure the bevel separates the nerve fibers and should be parallel to the cauda equina.
13. Advance needle until there is a decrease in resistance. This might not always happen, thus removing the stylet to see if CSF flows should be done as the needle is advanced past 4 cm. If one encounters resistance, the needle can be slightly withdrawn, and angle adjusted and advanced.

    Clinical pearl: In young children, the spinous process is more horizontal and thus having the needle angle only slightly cephalad should be sufficient. In older children, the spinous process becomes progressively angled downwards, thus requiring more cephalad entry (see Fig. 15.4b).
14. If measuring opening pressure, patient must be in lateral decubitus position. The patient can slowly adjust position. Ensure the legs are straight prior to measurement. Remove stylet, connect the stopcock and the manometer to spinal needle and measure opening pressure prior to specimen collection.

    Clinical pearl: Normal opening pressure is less than 25 cm H_2O. Value above 28 mm H_2O is considered elevated in children.

15. Allow CSF to drip into collecting tubes—generally 1–2 mL of CSF can be collected per tube. If LP was performed for treatment of increased intracranial pressure, more fluid can be removed and closing pressure can measured again prior to removing the needle.
16. When CSF collection complete, replace stylet and withdraw needle. Use the sterile gauze to apply gentle pressure to the puncture site and cover it with adhesive bandage.
17. Clean antiseptic solution off with damp warm towel to prevent skin irritation.
18. Ensure the specimen tubes are labeled. Generally, Tube 1 is sent for cell count, Tube 2 for glucose and protein, Tube 3 for gram stain and culture, Tube 4 for additional studies.

Potential Complications After LP

1. Most common complication of LP is headache. The persistent leak of CSF can result in decreased pressure. This type of headache is relieved by laying down and returns upon sitting or standing. Persistent headache can necessitate a need for a "blood patch" to stop the ongoing CSF leak and is normally done by anesthesiology providers.
2. Local pain at the needle entry site is usually mild soreness.
3. Localized infection near the puncture site can result from poor sterile technique. Once the spinal needle has punctured the skin, readjustment of the angle should be done without completely removing the needle. You should never remove and re-puncture the skin with the same needle.
4. Bleeding along the needle tract is generally rare in patients with normal coagulation profile. Holding anticoagulation for 24 h prior to this procedure to avoid formation of hematomas is routinely recommended.
5. In oncology patients with bone marrow suppression, it is recommended that platelets are above 50K prior to performing a LP.
6. Herniation of cerebellar tonsils is an extremely rare complication that occurs in patients with intracranial masses or abnormal anatomy such as Chiari malformation.

Laceration Repair

Laceration repairs are primarily done in the ED setting and are indicated for the primary closure of a wound and to restore perfusion to injured tissue. Contraindications to performing a laceration repair would include wounds required to heal by secondary intention (e.g., animal bites) or wounds that are grossly contaminated and may cause severe infection if closed immediately. Complex repairs by specialists such as plastic surgery or orthopedics may be required for lesions on the face or hands, particularly when crossing the vermillion border of the lips or crossing over joint spaces. Complications of the procedure can include wound infection, dehiscence, or retained foreign body.

Supplies Needed

1. Personal protection: sterile gloves, face/eye shield, surgical cap
2. Sterile drapes
3. Laceration repair kit, including needle holder, tooth forceps, scissors
4. Anesthetic options:
   (a) Topical: LET (lidocaine, epinephrine, tetracaine) or EMLA (lidocaine, prilocaine)
   (b) Injections: 1% lidocaine with/without epinephrine for local anesthesia (load in a 10 mL syringe, 25 gauge needle)
5. Antiseptic skin prep solution: chlorhexidine or povidone-iodine solution
6. Sterile NS in 60 mL syringe with splash guard or NS spray bottle for irrigation
7. Towels and bowl
8. Suture (see Table 15.1)

Laceration Repair Procedure

1. Position patient and expose area to adequate lighting on flattened surface.
2. Clean area around wound in an outward circular fashion with antiseptic solution.
3. Anesthetize wound either by placement of topical anesthetic covered by an occlusive bandage for 15–20 min prior to procedure or by injecting anesthetic in the plane between dermis and subcutaneous tissue by injecting in a fan-like distribution around the wound and surrounding area.
   Clinical pearl: When injecting, pull back with slight traction so that you make sure to avoid blood vessels.
4. Wearing eye protection and non-sterile gloves, use a 60 mL syringe with splash guard or NS spray bottle and irrigate the wound (100 mL of NS/cm of laceration).
5. Drape area and explore wound with forceps for foreign body, tendon, nerve, or vessel injury while carefully removing devitalized tissue.

Table 15.1 Selection of Appropriate Suture

Location	Suture type	Removal time
Scalp	4-0 or 5-0 nylon	5–7 days
Face	6-0 nylon	4–6 days
Neck	5-0 nylon	4–6 days
Trunk	4-0 vicryl	7–10 days
Extremities/ buttocks	4-0 or 5-0 vicryl	7–10 days
Hands	5-0 nylon; 5-0 rapid recommended for <5 years old	7–10 days (10–14 days if over joints)
Feet or sole	3-0 or 4-0 nylon	10–14 days

6. Grasp needle perpendicular to needle driver at junction of proximal to middle third of needle to place first stitch in center of wound bisecting laceration. Grasping the needle incorrectly may result in the needle bending.
7. Use forceps to evert the wound edge while not pinching tissues and insert needle at 90° angle in curvilinear path through the dermis and subcutaneous tissue.
8. Use forceps to secure needle tip, grasping with needle holder to pull through. Leave a 3–4 cm tail so it does not pull back through the skin if there is movement. Repeat on opposite side approximating the tissue.
9. Hold suture at needle end with non-dominant hand, allowing needle to rest on drape. Wrap suture over needle holder once, grasp the tail of suture with needle holder and pull ends in opposite directions. Repeat four times and pull knot to one side. Cut suture with scissor, leaving 1 cm tails.
10. Repeat process with additional sutures until laceration approximated.
11. Wipe off remaining antiseptic solution and cover the repaired laceration with a sterile, non-adherent dressing.

Incision and Drainage

Incision and drainage (I&D) procedures are typically performed when there is an abscess or infected fluid collection in the skin or subcutaneous tissue. Many times these are seen after a failure of treatment with antibiotic therapy; however, I&D alone can be effective in completing treating an infection. Contraindications include very large or deep abscesses in sensitive areas (such as perirectal, palmar, facial) that would like require specialist consultation with general or plastic surgery. Complications can include bleeding or recurrent abscess formation as well as potential nerve damage if I&D is performed near superficial nerves.

Supplies Needed

1. Personal protection equipment: gloves, gown, face shield, surgical cap
2. Sterile drapes
3. 1% lidocaine with epinephrine for local anesthesia (10 mL syringe with 25 gauge needle)
4. Antiseptic skin prep solution (povidone-iodine, chlorhexidine)
5. Incision and drainage kit: #11 scalpel blade with handle, curved hemostat and scissors
6. Wound packing material (iodoform gauze ribbon)
7. NS spray for irrigation
8. Gauze, tape
9. Culture swab

Incision and Drainage Procedure

1. Position patient so that area for drainage is fully exposed and easily accessible. Wash hands and put on non-sterile gloves.
2. Cleanse area of abscess with antiseptic skin prep in an expanding circular motion and drape area to create a sterile field.
3. Infiltrate a wide area around abscess with buffered 1% lidocaine at 12, 3, 6, 9 o' clock positions. Allow 5 min for affect.
4. Incise directly over center of abscess with scalpel, cutting into cavity. Incise parallel to skin fold lines when able. Purulent fluid will drain-use culture swab inside cavity to send for sample, if desired.
5. Extend incision to create opening adequate for drainage and to prevent recurrence. Use gauze to soak up drainage. Use hemostat to gently explore abscess cavity, breaking up any loculations.
6. Irrigate abscess cavity with NS spray until effluent is clear.
7. Consider using packing strip to pack abscess cavity and keep incision open.
8. Place gauze dressing lightly over wound and tape in place.
9. Schedule appointment in 2–3 days for packing removal.

Further Reading

King C, Henretig FM, editors. Textbook of pediatric emergency procedures. 2nd ed. Philadelphia: Wolters Kluwer, Lippincott Williams & Wilkins; 2008.
Practice guidelines for preoperative fasting and the use of pharmacologic agents to reduce the risk of pulmonary aspiration. Anesthesiology. 2017;126:376–93.
Videos in clinical medicine. N Engl J Med. Available at: http://content.nejm.org/misc/videos.shtml.

Chapter 16
Common Testing

Shauna Schord and Alana Painter

Cardiovascular

Electrocardiogram

Pediatric electrocardiogram (EKG) is a screening tool for structural heart disease and can be used in diagnosis of rhythm abnormalities. EKGs may be obtained for patients presenting with chest pain, syncope, and ingestions. While there are several approaches one can take in interpreting a pediatric EKG, evaluating an EKG systematically each time will help ensure familiarity with EKG basics and completeness of the interpretation (see Table 16.1). One approach is discussed below.

- In this approach, the first step is to verify standardization and paper speed on the EKG. Standard paper speed is 25 mm/s. Each small block on the horizontal axis thus represents 0.04 s. The vertical axis measures amplitude of the waveforms. The standard calibration is 10 mm (10 small boxes) equals 1 mV.
- Recall that there is age-related variation in pediatric EKGs. What might be considered a normal heart rate for an adolescent may be considered bradycardia in an infant. Verify patient age to ensure you are correlating the data to age-appropriate norms.
- Next, evaluate the heart rate. This can be done by dividing 300 by the number of large boxes between two consecutive QRS complexes or by counting the number of complexes within the 10 s EKG and multiplying by 6. The P wave is reflective of atrial depolarization. The P wave is normally positive in leads I, II, and aVF if the cardiac rhythm originates from the sinus node.

S. Schord (✉) · A. Painter
Division of Hospital Medicine, Department of Pediatrics, Nationwide Children's Hospital/The Ohio State University, Columbus, OH, USA
e-mail: Shauna.Schord@nationwidechildrens.org; Alana.Painter@nationwidechildrens.org

N. Liao et al. (eds.), *Pediatric Rotations*,
https://doi.org/10.1007/978-3-031-59873-9_16

Table 16.1 Systematic approach to EKG interpretation

1.	Verify standardization and paper speed
2.	Consider normal values for patient age
3.	Evaluate rate and rhythm
4.	Determine axis
5.	Assess intervals (PR, QRS, QT)
6.	Evaluate ST segment

- Determination of the QRS axis can be sought through evaluation of the direction of deflection of the QRS complex in the limb leads. When the most isoelectric QRS in a limb lead is determined, the mean QRS vector is found to be orthogonal to it. If the deflection is positive in lead I and aVF, the axis is roughly normal measuring between 0° and +90°.
- Next, assess the interval durations of the PR, QRS, and QT intervals. The PR interval starts from the beginning of the P wave through the beginning of the QRS complex. The P wave is indicative of atrial depolarization and the PR interval includes atrial depolarization through conduction through the AV node and His-Purkinje system. The P wave is typically 2.5 mm wide and 2.5 mm tall. A wide P wave can represent left atrial enlargement whereas a tall P wave can represent right atrial enlargement. The PR interval varies with age but is usually less than 0.2 s. The QRS duration is 0.08–0.12 s or 2–3 small boxes. A widened QRS may represent bundle branch block or depolarizations originating from the ventricles. The QT interval is shorter at fast heart rates and longer at slower heart rates so the corrected QTc is used that is calculated based on the heart rate. The QTc is equal to the QT interval divided by the square root of the RR' interval. The QTc in children is 350–460 ms. The QTc can be prolonged in genetic long QT syndromes or as a side effect of medications or drug ingestions.

Critical Congenital Heart Disease Screen

Congenital heart defects occur in about 8 out of every 1000 live births. Of these, about a quarter represent critical congenital heart disease—which is likely to require intervention within the first year of life. Critical congenital heart disease screening (CCHD) has been demonstrated to reduce infant mortality from early cardiac death when mandated. The CCHD screen became required in the USA in 2011 when it was added to the Recommended Uniform Screening Panel. The CCHD screen is recommended to be performed after the first 24 h of life, and before the baby is discharged from the hospital. A pulse oximeter is applied to the right hand and one foot to assess pre- and post-ductal saturations. Further evaluation is recommended if either saturation is below 95% or there is a difference of more than 2% between the extremity readings. If hypoxemia is found on the screen, additional testing is needed to identify the source.

Lipid Screen

All children aged 9–11 years are recommended to have a screening lipid profile, sooner if they have risk factors for cardiovascular disease (obesity, diabetes, hypertension, etc.). Pediatric lipid screening aims to identify those patients who need intervention to reduce the risk of cardiovascular disease and its associated risks in adulthood. Dyslipidemia in childhood begins atherosclerosis and premature cardiovascular disease. Pediatric dyslipidemia can occur by dietary mechanisms, secondary to chronic diseases like diabetes mellitus, and from genetic abnormalities in lipid metabolism. Dyslipidemia in the pediatric population includes high total cholesterol, high low-density lipoprotein cholesterol (LDL-C), high non-high-density lipoprotein cholesterol, high triglycerides, or low high-density lipoprotein cholesterol. Screening results are tiered into three categories:

- Normal: Results are within an acceptable range for age. Continue with routine cardiovascular health assessments. Children without identifiable risk factors would be due for a second lipid screen between 17 and 21 years of age.
- Borderline: Recommendations should be given for lifestyle changes to promote heart health. Follow-up testing is tailored to the specific patient but is usually indicated in 1 year.
- Abnormal: Patients with abnormal results require confirmatory testing—two fasting profiles completed 2 weeks to 3 months apart. If dyslipidemia is confirmed, evaluation for secondary causes should be pursued (diabetes mellitus, nephrotic syndrome, hypothyroidism, etc.) through history and physical and targeted laboratory evaluation.

Respiratory

Chest Radiography

Chest radiography is the most commonly used imaging modality for evaluation of the thorax. It may be used in evaluation of acute respiratory distress and is recommended in outpatient evaluation of chronic cough. Chest radiograph interpretation should be approached systematically to ensure completeness (see Table 16.2).

Table 16.2 ABCDE mnemonic for chest radiography

Airway	Trachea, carina, hilar structures
Breathing	Lung fields and pleura
Cardiac	Size, contour
Diaphragm	Position and evaluation of costophrenic angles
Everything else	Bones, soft tissue, devices

After confirming the name of the patient, it is important to evaluate what type of radiograph is being observed. There are several chest radiograph views that can be obtained depending on the nature of the concern. When a patient is able to stand, a posterior-anterior (PA) film is usually obtained, with the X-ray passing through the patient from posteriorly to the film anteriorly placed in front of the chest. When a patient is too ill, such as in an ICU bed, an anterior-posterior (AP) film may be obtained with the patient supine. The X-ray tube is positioned above the patient and a film is placed behind the back to obtain this radiograph. Note that in an AP view, the mediastinal structures and cardiac silhouette will appear wider. Next, evaluate the structures and field of the chest radiograph. The ABCDE mnemonic is a commonly used approach for evaluation of a chest radiograph.

In evaluating the airway, check that the trachea is midline and assess for any narrowing. Count posterior ribs to check for adequate lung expansion, about 10 ribs, and ensure lung volumes are approximately equal. Lung markings should extend all the way to the edge of the pleura. The heart size should be less than 50% of the thoracic width and appropriately positioned. The right hemidiaphragm is slightly elevated compared to the left due to the presence of the liver. Look for clear delineation at the costophrenic angle to evaluate for effusion and ensure no free air is noticed beneath the diaphragm. Observe bony structures for any fractures and assess for presence of tubes, cardiac devices, or soft tissue abnormalities.

GI/Fluid, Energy, Nutrition

Ultrasound

Ultrasound is a useful imaging modality in pediatrics due to the ability to obtain images without radiation or harmful side effects. Ultrasound can be used to evaluate a variety of complaints including abdominal, pelvic, and scrotal pain.

- *Pylorus*—US is used for diagnosis of hypertrophic pyloric stenosis and is considered positive when the pyloric muscle thickness measures greater than 3 mm and the length of the channel is 15 mm or greater.
- *Intussusception*—US is sensitive for diagnosis of intussusception, the telescoping of one segment of bowel into another. A "doughnut sign" is seen when a hypoechoic bowel rim is seen enveloping a hyperechoic central core on transverse section.
- *Appendix*—When the appendix is visualized the diagnostic accuracy of ultrasound for appendicitis is equivalent to CT scan. However, if a normal appendix is not entirely visualized, appendicitis cannot be ruled out with US. The following findings support a diagnosis of appendicitis when seen on ultrasound: a noncompressible tubular structure visualized in the right lower quadrant, diameter of 6 mm or greater, appendix wall thickness of 2 mm or greater, hyperemia, free

fluid in the right lower quadrant, thickened mesentery, presence of fecalith, tenderness with graded compression.

- *Abdominal*—The complete abdominal ultrasound evaluates for structural abnormalities in the liver, gallbladder, kidneys, spleen, and pancreas, as well as for free fluid in the peritoneal cavity.
- *Pelvic/testicular*—Testicular ultrasounds are used to evaluate for testicular torsion, inguinal hernia, hydrocele, epididymitis, and to confirm absence or presence of the testes. Pelvic ultrasound is used to evaluate ovarian structure, and for evidence of ovarian torsion.
- *Renal/bladder*—An ultrasound of the kidneys and bladder is recommended for children less than 12 months who have a first-time febrile UTI. Findings may include hydronephrosis, ureteropelvic junction obstruction, and renal scarring. When abnormalities are noted on ultrasounds following febrile UTI, follow-up imaging is indicated with a voiding cystourethrogram or nuclide cystogram to assess for urinary reflux.

Abdominal Radiography

Abdominal radiography is sensitive for making the diagnosis of free intraperitoneal air or bowel obstruction. Plain film of the abdomen is not recommended for evaluation of functional constipation, instead in most cases a thorough history and physical including evaluation of retained stool in the rectum, should be sufficient to diagnose constipation.

Liver Function Tests

While the terms "liver function tests" or "hepatic function panel" are widely used, they represent a misnomer in that they provide information about injury to the liver but may not specifically capture how the liver is functioning. A typical hepatic function panel (HFP) includes measures of the total protein in the blood, albumin, aspartate transaminase (AST), alanine transaminase (ALT), alkaline phosphatase, and bilirubin. Of these, ALT, AST, alkaline phosphatase, and bilirubin are biochemical markers of liver injury. Elevations in ALT and AST may demonstrate injury to the liver, as these enzymes are released into the bloodstream when hepatocytes are damaged. However, it is important to remember that ALT and AST are also found in other types of cells throughout the body, including cardiac and skeletal muscle. Of the two, ALT is primarily present in the liver and is a more specific marker for hepatocellular injury. Hepatocellular function is measured by albumin and protein levels. Additionally, synthetic function of the liver can be evaluated with measurement of the prothrombin time in a coagulation panel.

CNS

Neuroimaging: Head CT and MRI

Head CT is recommended for pediatric trauma patients with Glasgow Coma Scale scores of less than 14 with normal blood pressure as well as those children with signs concerning for basilar skull fracture (hemotympanum, bruising around the eyes or behind the ear). All children with suspected abusive head trauma should have urgent CT of the head. Neuroimaging also is used in evaluation of headaches with signs of intracranial pathology. Headache symptoms that occur when the child is waking from sleep, worse when lying down, with associated neurologic findings, or with abnormal exam findings such as papilledema or abnormal eye movements suggest an underlying intracranial pathology and should be evaluated with neuroimaging. MRI of the brain is typically recommended due to higher sensitivity and less radiation though CT scan may be needed for urgent evaluation depending upon severity and onset of symptoms.

CSF Studies

Cerebrospinal fluid obtained through a lumbar puncture is tested for cell count (red and white blood cell count and composition), glucose, and protein when there is concern for meningitis or encephalitis. In bacterial meningitis, there is a CSF pleocytosis or increased white blood cell count, low glucose, and elevated protein. In viral meningitis, there is also pleocytosis, however glucose is often normal, and protein is usually mildly elevated. Beyond infectious markers, a measurement of the CSF opening pressure is a surrogate marker of intracranial pressure. An elevated opening pressure can be seen in meningitis as well as idiopathic intracranial hypertension. CSF studies may also demonstrate albuminocytologic dissociation, or an elevation in CSF protein without an associated increase in the WBC count which can be seen during the acute phase of Guillain-Barre syndrome.

Hematologic

Complete Blood Count

A complete blood count measures the white blood cell count, hemoglobin, hematocrit, platelet count, and the size of the hemoglobin and platelet molecules and is a useful tool for the assessment of the cellular immune system. A differential quantifies leukocytes by type (neutrophils, lymphocytes, monocytes, and eosinophils). Alterations in the white blood cell count can be assessed for indications of infection or underlying immune dysfunction while evaluation of the red blood cells tell of oxygen carrying function in the body. Abnormally, low platelets put a patient at increased risk of bleeding; however, platelets also function as an acute phase reactant and can be elevated at times of infection or inflammation.

Iron Studies

All children are recommended to have screening for iron deficiency anemia at 12 months of age, or sooner if risk factors are present. The most common cause of anemia in children is iron deficiency, and iron studies are used to evaluate the patient's iron status. Iron studies include total iron binding capacity, iron saturation, and ferritin. In iron deficiency anemia, hemoglobin is decreased, MCV is decreased, ferritin is decreased, serum iron is decreased, and total iron binding capacity is increased.

Coagulation Panel

If there are concerns about a patient's coagulation status, common coagulation studies may be obtained including activated partial thromboplastin time (aPTT), prothrombin time (PT), and INR. PT and INR assess components of the common and extrinsic clotting pathway by measuring the time it takes plasma to clot when tissue factor is introduced. INR is a standardized measurement calculated by comparing the patient's PT to a standard control PT. PT/INR evaluation is useful in monitoring patients on warfarin therapy, evaluating bleeding, and assessing synthetic function of the liver. The aPTT assesses components of the intrinsic and common pathways. The aPTT is useful in monitoring patients on unfractionated heparin or direct thrombin inhibitors as well as assessing bleeding.

Lead

Toddlers are typically screened for lead toxicity at 12 and 24 months of age. Lead toxicity can result in neurologic sequelae and is treated with chelation.

Renal/Urinary System

Electrolytes

A basic metabolic panel is often obtained when there are questions about a patient's hydration status, electrolytes, and kidney function. It includes sodium, potassium, chloride, bicarbonate, BUN, creatinine, and glucose. A basic metabolic panel is often expanded upon by obtaining calcium, magnesium, and phosphorus.

Urinalysis

Urinalysis measures urine specific gravity, pH, and evaluates various substances in the urine including blood, urobilinogen, white blood cells, red blood cells, squamous epithelial cells, leukocyte esterase, nitrites, and protein. It is used to evaluate urinary tract infection, proteinuria, nephritis, nephrosis, and renal injury.

Blood Pressure Measurement

Blood pressure should be obtained in the upper extremity with an appropriately sized blood pressure cuff, with the patient sitting, relaxed, and the legs uncrossed. Blood pressure norms are determined based on patient sex and height.

Endocrine/Metabolism

Vitamin D

Vitamin D deficiency is common in adolescents, particularly those who live in cooler climates where there is less access to sun exposure. Vitamin D deficiency is also seen in infants and toddlers with malnutrition, and those with hypocalcemia. Screening for vitamin D deficiency in the general population is not recommended but should be considered in patients with risk factors such as low dietary intake or exclusively breastfed infants who are not receiving vitamin D supplementation.

Bone Age

X-rays of the left hand and wrist are obtained to determine a patient's bone age. Bone age X-rays are used to estimate a child's growth potential and adult height. In children with short stature, bone age X-rays can be obtained to determine the presence or absence of accelerated or delayed growth. Bone age is delayed in constitutional delay of growth (normal variant), nutritional deficiency, systemic disease, and growth hormone deficiency. Bone age is normal in familial short stature. Bone age is advanced in precocious puberty and hyperthyroidism.

Hemoglobin A1c

Hemoglobin A1c is a measure of glucose status over a 3-month period of time, and, when elevated, is diagnostic of diabetes mellitus. This test is used to screen for prediabetes and diabetes in obese children and used to track glucose control in patients diagnosed with diabetes mellitus.

Newborn Metabolic Screen

The goal of the newborn screen is to identify potentially life-threatening disorders before they become symptomatic, in order to provide early therapy or/treatment to reduce morbidity and mortality. A blood test is collected in the newborn nursery, after 24 h of life. For out of hospital births, the test is collected at the first clinic visit. Testing includes screening, follow-up, diagnosis, treatment, and outcome tracking for a variety of conditions. Those conditions on the Recommended Uniform Screening Panel are included in every state's test. Specific conditions tested vary by state, but generally include inborn errors of metabolism, endocrinopathies, hemoglobinopathies, immunodeficiencies, and cystic fibrosis. Tandem mass spectrometry allows for mass screening of multiple disorders. The testing is non-diagnostic for the conditions but identifies individuals who require additional testing.

Musculoskeletal

A variety of imaging and laboratory tests can be ordered to evaluate various aspects of the musculoskeletal system. Radiography is helpful in assessing for osseous abnormalities including fractures and lytic lesions. Ultrasound may be obtained to assess for effusion or guide arthrocentesis if indicated.

Skeletal Survey

The skeletal survey is the radiographic evaluation indicated for any child less than 2 years of age in whom child abuse is suspected. The survey includes 21 radiographic views evaluating the skull, ribs, spine, pelvis, long bones, feet, and hands.

Diagnostic yield of the skeletal survey may be improved if repeated in 2 weeks if the initial results are unclear or suspicion of abuse remains.

Reproductive

Testing for Sexually Transmitted Infections (STIs)

Recommendations for screening vary based on gender, sexual orientation, sexual activity, and HIV status. In every state, syphilis, gonorrhea, and HIV are reportable illnesses; in some states, acute HBV, acute HCV, and chlamydia are reportable. Laws about other infections vary by state. Adolescents are able to self-consent for diagnosis and treatment in all 50 states and DC.

- *C. trachomatis*—NAAT urine (preferred for male), vaginal swab (preferred for female), urethral swab, rectal swab, endocervical swab
- *N. gonorrhoeae*—NAAT urine (preferred for male), vaginal swab (preferred for female), urethral swab, rectal swab, endocervical swab, oropharyngeal swab
- *T. vaginalis*—NAAT vaginal swab
- Syphilis—For asymptomatic patients, initial screening with non-treponemal test (RPR or VDRL), if positive confirm with treponemal test (FTA-ABS, TPPA, TP-EIA, or CIA)
- HIV—HIV ½ Ag/Ab combination immunoassay
- HSV—screening asymptomatic adolescents generally not recommended, low specificity, and high false positive rate
- HBV—HBsAg, HBsAb, HBcAb
- HCV—HCV antibody
- People without HIV infection:
  - All people—screening for HIV at least once
  - All females <25 years old who have had sex—annual screening for gonorrhea and chlamydia
  - Males who have sex with males—at least annual screening for HIV, syphilis, chlamydia, and gonorrhea
- People with HIV infection
- Women, and men who have sex with women (MSW):
  - Annually—chlamydia, gonorrhea, trichomoniasis, syphilis
  - First visit—HBV, HCV
- Men who have sex with men (MSM):
  - At least annually—genital chlamydia, rectal chlamydia, genital gonorrhea, rectal gonorrhea, pharyngeal gonorrhea, syphilis
  - First visit—HAV, HBV, HCV

Infectious

Blood, Urine, CSF Cultures

Cultures of bodily fluids including blood, urine, CSF, wound fluid, and lower respiratory fluid are used to evaluate for bacterial infection. Blood cultures are typically monitored for a total of 5 days, and infections are reported as they are observed. If an infection is observed, the lab will perform sensitivity testing to determine which antibiotics the bacteria is sensitive and resistant to.

Inflammatory Markers

C-reactive protein is a marker of acute inflammation. Erythrocyte sedimentation rate is a measure of how long it takes for erythrocytes to settle in solution and is also a measure of inflammation. ESR is later to rise than CRP and remains elevated longer. Ferritin is an acute phase reactant and often obtained in patients with prolonged fever to assist in determining the etiology. Procalcitonin is an acute phase reactant thought to be highly specific for infection.

Group A Streptococcus *Culture*

Group A *Streptococcus* is the most common cause of bacterial pharyngitis in children. When there is suspicion for Group A Strep Pharyngitis, an initial rapid antigen detection test is typically ordered. Since these tests can miss up to 30% of cases, a negative rapid antigen detection test is usually followed with a GAS throat culture.

Respiratory Infection Array

A respiratory infection array uses multiplex PCR (polymerase chain reaction) to detect and identify nucleic acids in a sample of nasopharyngeal fluid obtained via swab. Commonly included pathogens include Adenovirus, Influenza, Respiratory Syncytial Virus, Coronavirus, Rhinovirus, Enterovirus, *Bordetella pertussis*, Human Metapneumovirus, Parainfluenza, Mycoplasma, and *Chlamydophila pneumoniae*. Obtaining a respiratory infection array is typically recommended for cases in which the result is likely to change management or has specific diagnostic importance, like in an immunocompromised patient.

Gastrointestinal Infection Array

A gastrointestinal infection (GI) array uses qualitative PCR to detect and identify nucleic acids from various bacteria, viruses, and parasites from stool samples. Commonly included pathogens include *Campylobacter*, *Clostridium*, *Salmonella*, *Vibrio*, *E. coli*, *Yersinia*, *Shigella*, *Adenovirus*, *Norovirus*, *Rotavirus*, *Sapovirus*, *Cryptosporidium*, *Cyclospora*, *Entamoeba*, and *Giardia*. In cases of acute gastroenteritis of healthy infants and children, a GI array is typically not needed. An array may be considered in an immunocompromised patient or a patient with signs and symptoms concerning for bacterial gastroenteritis in whom treatment is likely to be needed.

Application Exercises

1. A 6-year-old female with chronic constipation presents to the Emergency Department with a one-day history of abdominal pain. She describes the pain as sharp right lower quadrant pain. She has had two episodes of vomiting that was non-bloody and nonbilious since the pain started earlier that day. She has not had a stool in 2 days and her last stool was noted to be hard and painful to pass. On exam, she has RLQ tenderness with guarding.

The next BEST step in management is:

A. Abdominal X-ray
B. CT abdomen with IV and oral contrast
C. Ultrasound appendix
D. Administration of enema

Answer C: The next best step in evaluation of her abdominal pain is an ultrasound to evaluate for appendicitis. She has signs and symptoms including RLQ pain and rebound that are concerning appendicitis and would not be consistent with constipation. Ultrasound is the appropriate first step in diagnosis as it avoids radiation, is lower in cost, and the diagnostic accuracy is equivalent to CT scan when the appendix is visualized.

2. A 6-year-old boy with a normal diet does drink 4–5 glasses of milk per day. He appears pale at his office visit and has tachycardia with normal BP for age. You obtain a CBC to evaluate for anemia. His hemoglobin is 8.0 g/dL, MCV 65 fL (normal 76–96) and MCHC 26% (32–36).

The best test to evaluate for iron stores is:

A. Reticulocyte count
B. Serum ferritin
C. Serum iron
D. Serum total iron-binding capacity

Answer B: While retic count may be low in iron deficiency anemia, the best study to determine total body iron stores is serum ferritin. Low iron body stores may exist with normal hemoglobin (for some time until eventually low RBC production and anemia develop).

3. A 6-year-old boy with short stature and otherwise normal history has been declining in his height SDS (or percentile) over the last 3 years.

The next best step to assess for possible renal tubular acidosis (RTA) is:

A. Arterial blood gas (ABG)
B. Serum bicarbonate
C. Serum creatinine
D. Serum electrolytes

Answer D: While RTA may have low pH (acidemia) on ABG, this finding is not pathognomonic for RTA and even a child with RTA may have normal pH due to respiratory compensation. Likewise, a serum bicarbonate by itself may be due to many possible causes. The first step to evaluate for possible RTA is to determine serum electrolytes: if a normal anion gap metabolic acidosis exists (low bicarbonate with normal anion gap, i.e., between 8 and 14), then RTA is possible and further evaluation should be pursued (e.g., ABG, urine electrolytes). See Chap. 11 for more details.

Further Reading

Hicks JM. In: Soldin SJ, Rifai N, Hicks JM, editors. Biochemical basis of pediatric disease. Washington, DC: AACC Press; 1995. p. 1–16.

Pyle-Eilola AL, Thornton DJ. Chapter 2: Common tests and considerations important in pediatric medicine. In: Jones PM, Dietzen DJ, Haymond S, Bennett MJ, editors. Pediatric laboratory medicine. McGraw-Hill; 2017.

Soldin SJ, Brugnana C, Hicks JM. Pediatric reference ranges. 3rd ed. Washington, DC: AACC Press; 1999.

Chapter 17
Cystic Fibrosis

Michelle Hjelm and Antoinette Wannes-Daou

Background

The earliest reference to cystic fibrosis (CF) in medical texts was around 1595, when salty skin and damage to the pancreas was linked with death in infants and young children. In 1938, American pathologist Dr. Dorothy Andersen described the disorder "cystic fibrosis of the pancreas" based on autopsy findings of children who died of malnutrition. Other physicians referred to the disease as "mucoviscidosis," calling attention to thickened mucus in organ systems such as the lungs and gastrointestinal (GI) tract.

During a heat wave in 1948, emergency room physician Dr. Paul di Sant'Agnese noted infants presenting with dehydration and low serum sodium levels and eventually discovered that the sweat of children with CF had abnormally high concentrations of salt, leading to the gold standard testing for CF diagnosis. In the 1980s, the genetic defect in the Cystic Fibrosis Transmembrane Conductance Regulator (CFTR) was described and began the ongoing process of genetic-based treatments emerging today.

M. Hjelm (✉)
Division of Pulmonary Medicine, Department of Pediatrics, Cincinnati Children's Hospital Medical Center, Cincinnati, OH, USA
e-mail: Michelle.Hjelm@cchmc.org

A. Wannes-Daou
Division of Pulmonary Medicine, Department of Pediatrics, Cincinnati Children's Hospital Medical Center, Cincinnati, OH, USA

Pulmonary and Sleep Medicine, Children's Hospital of Philadelphia, Philadelphia, Pennsylvania, USA
e-mail: Antoinette.WannesDaou@cchmc.org

N. Liao et al. (eds.), *Pediatric Rotations*,
https://doi.org/10.1007/978-3-031-59873-9_17

Pathophysiology

CF is an autosomal recessive disease that affects 1 in 2500–3500 individuals in the USA. Currently, 75% of people with CF are diagnosed before the age of 2 years, and more than 50% of people living with CF are adults. CF is caused by reduction or dysfunction of the CFTR protein which subsequently causes reduction in chloride transport and excessive sodium transport. These abnormal shifts in electrolytes result in loss of water from where it should be creating thick mucus in different organ systems in the body. The most common mutation is the deletion of phenylalanine at position 508, or what is commonly referred to as a F508Del or "delta F508." CFTR is present in upper and lower airways, hepatobiliary system, pancreatic ducts, sweat glands, intestines, and reproductive system, which explains many of the common clinical features of CF (Table 17.1).

Table 17.1 Body systems involved in CF and important pathology

Systems involved	Pathology	Clinical features
Pulmonary	• Dehydration and disruption of mucociliary clearance • Abnormally viscous mucus causes obstruction, chronic inflammation, and bacterial colonization • Superimposed bacterial exacerbations	• Bronchiectasis • Bacterial colonization • Progressive decline of lung function • Major morbidity and mortality
Sinus	• Viscous mucus and bacterial colonization • Inflammation and polyp formation	• Chronic pansinusitis • Nasal polyps
Pancreas	• Exocrine: (a) Progressive blockage of pancreatic ducts by viscous mucus (b) Malabsorption due to absence of pancreatic enzyme • Endocrine: (a) Insulin resistance (b) Decreased insulin production	• Poor weight gain • Steatorrhea • Vitamin deficiencies • Chronic pancreatitis • CF-related diabetes
Intestines	• Deficiency of proteolytic enzymes • Secretion of abnormal mucoproteins by the goblet cells of the small intestine	• Chronic constipation • Distal intestinal obstruction (DIOS) • Meconium ileus
Liver	• Biliary tract obstruction and inflammation	• CF liver disease • Gallbladder disease
Reproductive	• Males: (a) Congenital bilateral absence of the vas deferens • Females: (a) Thick cervical mucus (b) Uterine abnormalities	• Infertility
Behavioral	• CF diagnosis and treatment has psychosocial burden for individuals and their families	• Depression • Anxiety • School issues

Diagnostic Testing

Newborn Screening

Newborn screening (NBS) is a nationwide program to identify babies born with certain genetic health conditions where early intervention and treatment are essential. To date, all 50 states screen newborns for CF on their NBS, but the method for screening may differ from state to state. Most state's CF NBS program begins with a blood test from the baby to check the levels of a chemical made by the pancreas called immunoreactive trypsinogen (IRT). IRT is normally found in small levels in the body. In babies who have CF, IRT levels tend to be high. Some states only test IRT levels on the first blood test. These are called IRT-only states. Other states conduct both an IRT and a DNA test, and these are called IRT-DNA states. The addition of DNA testing can be helpful as IRT levels may be high in the newborn period for other reasons such as if a baby is premature or if there was prolonged delivery, and this is not necessarily indicative of a CF diagnosis.

Gold Standard Testing

Situations to consider testing for CF include:

1. Concerning clinical features: Failure to thrive, recurrent respiratory infections, meconium ileus, liposoluble vitamin deficiency, bronchiectasis, nasal polyps and sinusitis, dehydration with hyponatremia, azoospermia, and chronic pancreatitis.
2. Diagnosis of CF in a first-degree relative.
3. Postnatal confirmation, which is necessary when antenatal test was suspicious for CF.

Current diagnostic testing includes:

- Sweat test—This is the gold standard diagnostic test. Evidence of elevated chloride detected from sweat collected from the skin greater than or equal to 60 mmol/L is most likely consistent with a diagnosis of CF.
- Mutation analysis—This is commonly done in addition to a sweat test to assess for genetic variants in CF. This can be helpful for further prediction of phenotypes, clinical progression, and medication response.

Outpatient Management of CF

The primary goal of the outpatient management of CF is to minimize clinical symptoms and pulmonary function decline while maintaining the best quality of life possible.

Care Centers

Most people with CF are seen at "CF care centers" which are accredited locations of care that include access to multidisciplinary teams. A pediatric pulmonologist is most often the primary medical provider at these centers. The outpatient care at CF centers often includes respiratory therapy, nursing, behavioral health, social work, nutritionists or dieticians, gastroenterologists, otolaryngologists, and endocrinologists. Clinic visits with care teams are recommended quarterly to assess for symptoms and allow for necessary health maintenance activities such as lung function testing and respiratory infection screening. There are well-defined CF care guidelines for newborn, infant, pre-school aged children, school aged children, and adults standardized by the Cystic Fibrosis Foundation (CFF) (Table 17.2).

Table 17.2 Outpatient health maintenance by organ system

Body system	History/exam	Heath maintenance
Pulmonary	Assess sputum, cough, and respiratory symptoms Exam findings: tachypnea, retractions, crackles, wheezing, rhonchi	• Spirometry on each visit—typically looking for evidence of obstruction via the forced expiratory volume in 1 s (FEV1) • Routine respiratory cultures • Imaging if clinical concerns or suspected exacerbation • Assess airway clearance compliance and need for changes • Promote aerobic exercise as adjunct to airway clearance
Sinus	Assess nasal symptoms Exam findings: nasal polyps, mucoid drainage, facial pain/tenderness	• ENT involvement as needed for sinus surgery or nasal polyp removal
GI	Assess for constipation and stooling patterns Assess for reflux symptoms Assess calorie intake, feeding issues Assess for vitamin deficiencies Exam findings: abdominal pain, abdominal tenderness, masses	• Weight and BMI measurements • Yearly comprehensive metabolic panel, coagulation panel, and vitamin levels • Registered dietitian involvement at each visit
Endocrinology	Assess for symptoms of CF-related diabetes (CFRD) Exam findings: weight loss, hair loss, fractures	• Oral glucose tolerance test (OGTT) yearly starting at 10 years of age • DXA bone scan after 8 years of age • Referral to endocrinology as needed if either test is abnormal
Mental health	Screening for depression/anxiety Screening for school issues	Referral to psychology, psychiatry, or school services as needed

Lung Health in CF

A decline in pulmonary lung function is the leading cause of morbidity and mortality for people with CF. Therefore, the care team monitors lung function health with spirometry during clinic visits. Symptoms of a "pulmonary exacerbation" can include a drop in lung function and may suggest the need for an escalation in respiratory care. Baseline testing for certain bacteria such as *Pseudomonas aeruginosa* helps to reduce or eliminate bacterial burden with pathogens that are known to cause a more significant decline in lung function.

Lastly, regular daily mucus clearance or "airway clearance" is important for maintaining and improving lung health. This process includes external or internal vibrations via different devices such as a vest or acapella with nebulized medications to help mobilize mucus out of the lungs. The process of airway clearance can be one of the most time-consuming components of CF care and may take 60–80 min/day.

Nutritional Health in CF

Nutritional health is an important topic in people with CF, as body mass indices between the 50–80th percentiles have been positively correlated with improved pulmonary outcomes. Nutritional issues associated with CF include inadequate calorie intake, reduced absorption of food and vitamins due to impaired pancreatic function, and/or increased caloric demand due to poor lung health or recurrent infections.

One of the main features of CF is exocrine pancreatic insufficiency. Since not all people with CF have exocrine pancreatic insufficiency, screening for this should be performed by obtaining fecal elastase levels. If fecal elastase is low, it suggests the body is not producing enough pancreatic enzymes and supplementation would be beneficial. Supplementation is commonly provided through oral pancreatic enzymes taken prior to each meal.

Emerging Therapies

CFTR modulators are some of the newest genetically targeted medications and are changing the landscape of CF. They are designed to help correct the malfunctioning CFTR protein. People with CF on these medications generally experience a reduction in sweat chloride levels, improvement in lung function, improvement in GI symptoms, and improved quality of life. Unfortunately, not all people with CF are eligible for CFTR modulators because there can be significant side effects (cataracts and liver toxicity) or certain mutations may not be corrected by these medications.

Acute Illness Management in CF

In the era of CFTR modulator therapy, acute illnesses in CF have been reduced, but there are still important considerations for people with CF who present acutely ill (Table 17.3).

The two primary reasons for hospital admission specific for people with CF include pulmonary exacerbation and/or GI exacerbation (Table 17.4).

Table 17.3 Acute illness focused pulmonary and GI review of systems with corresponding physical exam findings

Body system	Question(s)	Common physical exam findings
Pulmonary	Cough or increased work of breathing? Changes of sputum—color, frequency Hemoptysis? Exercise intolerance? Fever? Weight loss?	Persistent cough Dyspnea—tachypnea, retractions Hypoxemia Bloody or thick/greenish sputum Diffuse or localized crackles Decreased breath sounds Rhonchi
GI/abdomen	Stooling frequency? Consistency of the stools? Abdominal pain? Food intolerance?	Abdominal distension Abdominal pain Hypoactive bowel sounds

Table 17.4 Important diagnostic and management considerations for pulmonary and GI exacerbations in CF

	Diagnostic	Management	Therapeutic goal
Pulmonary exacerbation	*Respiratory culture*—sputum, nasopharyngeal/epiglottis sample(s) *Imaging*—chest X-ray or computerize tomography (CT) to assess for pneumonia, bronchiectasis, or pneumothorax *Labs*—signs of acute inflammation or bleeding—CBC, CRP, ESR, Procalcitonin *Spirometry*—forced expiratory volume in 1 s (FEV1)	Antibiotics (a) Covering agents isolated on respiratory cultures (e.g., *S. aureus*, *P. aeruginosa*, *H. influenzae*) while waiting for new cultures results (b) Important to remember that *P. aeruginosa* in people with CF required dual antibiotic therapies or "double-coverage" Increase airway clearance	Improve respiratory symptoms Restore to baseline spirometry/FEV1

Table 17.4 (continued)

	Diagnostic	Management	Therapeutic goal
GI exacerbation	*Imaging*—abdominal X-ray or CT to assess stool burden and intestinal obstruction • Distal intestinal obstruction syndrome (DIOS) is a form of bowel obstruction *Labs*—serum amylase and lipase if concern for pancreatitis	Bowel clean out (a) Osmotic laxatives often have the fastest relief for distal and proximal forms of bowel obstruction that can be seen in people with CF. these are medications such as polyethylene glycol given in boluses or continuously (b) Consider agents per rectum such as saline, bisacodyl, or mineral oil enemas if concern for rectal/lower sigmoid constipation Maintenance hydration Surgery consult if needed Review pancreatic enzymes, hydration, and constipation medications as they can contribute or complicate GI exacerbation	Clear/chicken broth-colored stools by end of clean out Improved abdominal pain, distention Appropriate oral intake with appropriate weight gain for age Maintenance bowel regimen to promote soft, easy to pass stools at home

Medical Emergencies in CF

Respiratory Failure

Respiratory failure is the leading cause of death in CF. People with CF can experience a slow decline in lung function over time leading to chronic elevation in carbon dioxide levels ($pCO_2 > 50$ mmHg) which may not cause acute respiratory symptoms. However, when patients present with acute respiratory distress (tripod, retractions, tachypnea, hypoxemia) with worsening pCO_2 levels, it is important to offer aggressive noninvasive ventilatory support to address this impaired gas-exchange. Some severe situations may require intubation and full ventilator support or extracorporeal membrane oxygenation.

Hemoptysis

Hemoptysis, or coughing up blood, can be a life-threatening complication in people with CF. Bronchial arteries or collateral vessels may enlarge or become inflamed during an acute illness. If these vessels erode or become irritated, this may result in low volume to high volume bleeding into the airway. If major hemoptysis occurs (>200 mL in 24 h), this is a medical emergency and requires further monitoring with consideration of surgical or interventional measures to stop bleeding.

Acute Intestinal Obstruction

During an acute GI exacerbation, the associated intestinal obstruction can be severe enough to warrant emergent surgical intervention including stool evacuation via rectal approach or surgical bowel evacuation with possible bowel resection if there is subsequent tissue necrosis. Surgical procedures on the bowel can increase subsequent risk of adhesions and future obstruction as well as worsen nutritional absorption if significant length of bowel is lost.

Application Exercises

A 12-year-old male presents to CF clinic today for a sick visit. He presents with active respiratory symptoms including increased cough and mucus production for 2 weeks. He has also been losing weight over the past month, per his mother.

On exam, he looks cachectic and tachypneic with coarse breath sounds and crackles at the left lower lung field. His abdomen is soft, non-tender with normoactive bowel sounds. He has a coarse cough that is intermittently productive of thin, green sputum with no evidence of hemoptysis.

1. What acute workup would you recommend to guide your management of this patient?

   Answer: Highly recommended: spirometry, chest X-ray, respiratory culture, nutritional assessment. Consider: chemistry, CBC, CRP.
2. What additional clinical marker would best support an acute diagnosis of pulmonary exacerbation in this patient?

   A. Sweat chloride testing
   B. Respiratory culture
   C. Forced expiratory volume in 1 s (FEV1)
   D. Fecal elastase

   Answer C: Forced expiratory volume in 1 s.
   Explanation of answer choices:

   A. Sweat chloride testing—This test is the gold standard for the diagnosis of cystic fibrosis. This patient has a known diagnosis of CF and obtaining a sweat test would not help to determine the nature of his acute illness.
   B. Respiratory sputum culture—This is a routine care measure that is used to monitor bacterial growth in the airways of people with CF. Most people with CF will have growth on respiratory culture with or without a respiratory exacerbation and growth does not necessarily suggest an acute change in lung health. It is important to use the results of previous and current bacterial growth on respiratory cultures to determine the best antibiotic regimen for an acute exacerbation.
   C. Forced expiratory volume in 1 s (FEV1)—This test is best to diagnose a pulmonary exacerbation. Reduction in lung function by measure of FEV1 is a common clinical tool to determine the severity of a pulmonary exacerba-

tion and whether care should be escalated to an inpatient stay. FEV1 can also be used to monitor improvement during treatment for an exacerbation.

D. Fecal elastase—This is a measure of pancreatic function in the stool which can be helpful to determine whether someone with CF has pancreatic sufficiency (at time of diagnosis or with clinical GI symptom changes), but it is not used for determination of pulmonary exacerbation.

3. What treatment options would you recommend for this patient's pulmonary exacerbation?

   Answer: Increase airway clearance and antibiotics. Given the significant symptom burden this patient is experiencing, his condition warrants inpatient hospitalization with IV antibiotics to cover previous respiratory bacteria that this patient has grown on respiratory cultures. If the patient has a history of *Pseudomonas aeruginosa* growth on cultures, antibiotic coverage should include two different antimicrobial agents to target it.

Further Reading

Cystic Fibrosis Foundation. 2018 Patient registry annual data report. 2019. https://www.cff.org/Research/Researcher-Resources/Patient-Registry/2018-Patient-Registry-Annual-Data-Report.pdf. Accessed 12 May 2020.

Davis PB. Cystic fibrosis since 1938. Am J Respir Crit Care Med. 2006;173(5):475–82.

Dickinson KM, Collaco JM. Cystic fibrosis. Pediatr Rev. 2021;42(2):55–67.

O'Sullivan BP, Freedman SD. Cystic fibrosis. Lancet. 2009;373(9678):1891–904.

Turcios NL. Cystic fibrosis lung disease: an overview. Respir Care. 2020;65(2):233.

Chapter 18
Depression, Anxiety, and Suicide

Alanna Nzoma and Rebekah Shaw

Depression

Background

Depression is a mood disorder that causes a persistent feeling of sadness and loss of interest. Depression can affect how one feels, thinks, and behaves and can lead to a variety of emotional and physical problems. Major depressive disorder (MDD) in children and adolescents is recognized as a serious psychiatric condition with extensive acute and chronic morbidity and mortality. The prevalence of MDD is increasing in teens in the United States. Females are twice as likely as males to be depressed. Research shows that only 50% of adolescents with depression are diagnosed before reaching adulthood.

According to the *Diagnostic and Statistical Manual of Mental Disorders*, Fifth Edition (DSM-V), MDD can be diagnosed if a patient exhibits five or more of the following symptoms almost every day for 2 weeks (although episodes can be considerably longer) and must impair the ability to function normally.

1. Depressed or irritable mood
2. Diminished interest or pleasure in activities
3. Significant weight loss or gain
4. Insomnia or hypersomnia
5. Psychomotor agitation or retardation
6. Fatigue or energy loss

A. Nzoma (✉) · R. Shaw
Department of Pediatrics, University of Michigan, Ann Arbor, MI, USA
e-mail: alannaej@med.umich.edu; rebekash@med.umich.edu

N. Liao et al. (eds.), *Pediatric Rotations*,
https://doi.org/10.1007/978-3-031-59873-9_18

7. Feelings of worthlessness or excessive/inappropriate guilt
8. Diminished ability to think or concentrate
9. Recurrent thoughts of death or suicide, a suicide attempt, or a specific plan

According to the DSM-V, the severity of depressive episodes is based on number, type, and severity of symptoms. Mild cases typically have five symptoms that cause minor impairment whereas severe cases typically have closer to nine symptoms that markedly interfere with daily functioning. Moderate cases will fall somewhere in between mild and severe cases.

It is important to note that other types of depression exist. In the DSM-V, depressive disorders have been separated from bipolar and related disorders, but many of the recommendations regarding identification, assessment, and initial management listed in this chapter can be applied to other forms of depression as well.

History

The United States Preventative Services Task Force (USPSTF) recommends universal screening annually for depression in adolescents ages 12–18 years with a formal, validated, self-report screening tool. While screening tools are helpful in the identification of depression, it is important to follow-up screening with direct interviews with the patients themselves and with caregivers. For resources on how to interview an adolescent alone, refer to Chap. 37.

When obtaining a history, it is important to consider the differential diagnosis as well as the diagnostic criteria for MDD. The mnemonic SIGECAPS can be useful for remembering key signs and symptoms associated with depression.

SIGECAPS

S = *Sleep* referring to sleep changes such as trouble falling asleep, trouble staying asleep, or sleeping more than usual
I = *Interest* referring to loss of interest in things previously enjoyed
G = *Guilt* referring to feeling bad about themselves or feeling like a failure
E = *Energy* referring to fatigue or loss of energy
C = *Concentration* referring to decreased ability to focus on tasks or thoughts
A = *Appetite* referring to either decrease or increase in appetite
P = *Psychomotor retardation or agitation* referring to moving slowly or feeling fidgety and moving more than usual
S = *Suicide* referring to thoughts of wishing they were dead or having thoughts of suicide

In addition to those signs and symptoms outlined in SIGECAPS, adolescents with MDD can also have a wide range of behavioral, physical, and psychological signs and symptoms including:

1. Behavioral signs: school absenteeism, change in school performance, unrestrained behavior (e.g., arguments with family and friends, theft, destruction of property), desire to be alone, withdrawal, or illicit substance use.
2. Physical symptoms: abdominal pain, headaches, or weight changes.
3. Psychological signs: feelings of sadness, hopelessness, or worthlessness.

Whenever interviewing an adolescent, you should always complete a full HEADSSS assessment (refer to Chap. 37) which can be useful in identifying functional impairments associated with MDD.

Additionally, any patient presenting with an emotional problem as a chief complaint or in whom depression is highly suspected despite a negative screening test should be evaluated for MDD.

Risk Factors for Depression

1. Poor school performance or learning disability
2. Frequent somatic complaints
3. Psychosocial adversity (e.g., foster care, adoption, death of a loved one, divorce)
4. Substance use
5. Trauma (e.g., physical or sexual abuse, neglect)
6. Physical illness or chronic disease

   Remember to consider screening for depression in patients with new diagnosis of chronic disease, frequent hospital admissions, prolonged admissions, or not returning to baseline functioning
7. Personal history of prior depressive episode, other psychiatric disorder (e.g., anxiety, bipolar disorder, psychosis, schizophrenia), self-injurious behavior (e.g., cutting), or suicide attempt
8. Family history of depression, suicide, or other psychiatric disorder
9. Previous high-scoring screens without formal mental health diagnosis

Key Focused Review of Systems (ROS)

Complete a full ROS, but below are some key systems. Refer to Chap. 2 for a full ROS discussion.

(a) General—Fatigue? Weight loss or gain? Changes to sleep patterns? Changes in activity?
(b) Head—Headaches? Hair thinning?
(c) Abdomen—Abdominal pain? Constipation? Diarrhea? Changes in appetite?

(d) Skin—Skin dryness? Bruising or bleeding?
(e) Neurological—Agitation? Restlessness? Moving slowly? Irritability? Weakness?
(f) Psychological—Hearing voices? Seeing people who aren't present?

Physical Exam

- Vitals: Monitor for tachycardia or bradycardia
- Weight: Report weight and weight percentile. Compare to previous weights, if available, to assess for weight changes
- General: Describe the patient's overall appearance. Are they well-groomed? Do they appear well-nourished? What is their affect (immediate expression of emotion, e.g., broad, restricted, labile, or flat)?
- Psychologic: Are they responding to external stimuli? Do they appear sad or depressed?
- Head: Assess pupil size and reactivity; examine hair for thinning or dry, brittle hair
- EENT: Assess thyroid size, palpate for lymphadenopathy
- Cardiovascular: Evaluate for tachycardia or bradycardia
- Respiratory: Evaluate for tachypnea or bradypnea
- Abdomen: Palpate to assess for tenderness or masses
- Skin: Assess for dry or moist skin, rashes, bruising, burn, or cutting marks indicating prior self-harm
- Neurologic: Assess cranial nerves, strength, sensation, gait, mental status, psychomotor agitation, or retardation

Work-Up

Laboratory Assessment

Initial work-up of a patient presenting with depression may include a comprehensive metabolic panel, complete blood count with differential, thyroid-stimulating hormone, inflammatory markers such as C-reactive protein or erythrocyte sedimentation rate, vitamin B12, folate, urine drug screen, and urine pregnancy test.

Screening Tools for Depression

As mentioned above, all adolescents aged 12–18 years should be screened annually for depression. Additionally, patients with risk factors for depression should be identified and systematically monitored over time for the development of depression using a targeted depression screening tool. Many practices will use different screening tools as currently more evidence is needed before a specific screening tool can be

Table 18.1 Patient Health Questionnaire-9: Modified for Teens (PHQ-A) (adapted from the American Academic of Child and Adolescent Psychiatry) (available at" https://www.nimh.nih.gov/research/research-conducted-at-nimh/asq-toolkit-materials/asq-tool/phq-9-modified-for-adolescents-phq-a)

	Not at all (0)	Several days (1)	More than half the days (2)	Nearly every day (3)
1. Feeling down, depressed, irritable, or hopeless?	☐	☐	☐	☐
2. Little interest of pleasure in doing things?	☐	☐	☐	☐
3. Trouble falling asleep, staying asleep, or sleeping too much?	☐	☐	☐	☐
4. Poor appetite, weight loss, or overeating?	☐	☐	☐	☐
5. Feeling tired, or having little energy?	☐	☐	☐	☐
6. Feeling bad about yourself—or feeling that you are a failure, or that you have let yourself or your family down?	☐	☐	☐	☐
7. Trouble concentrating on things like schoolwork, reading, or watching TV?	☐	☐	☐	☐
8. Moving or speaking so slowly that other people could have noticed? Or the opposite—being so fidgety or restless that you were moving around a lot more than usual?	☐	☐	☐	☐
9. Thoughts you would be better off dead, or of hurting yourself in some way?	☐	☐	☐	☐
In the **past year** have you felt depressed or sad most days, even if you felt ok sometimes?				
☐ Yes	☐ No			
If you are experiencing any of the problems on this form, how **difficult** have these problems made it for you to do your work, take care of things at home or get along with other people?				
☐ Not difficult at all	☐ Somewhat difficult	☐ Very difficult	☐ Extremely difficult	
Has there ever been a time in the **past month** when you have had serious thoughts about ending your life?				
☐ Yes	☐ No			
Have you ever, in your whole life, tried to kill yourself or made a suicide attempt?				
☐ Yes	☐ No			

recommended for universal use. One instrument used for screening adolescents is the Patient Health Questionnaire-9: Modified for Teens (also called PHQ-A) (Table 18.1).

For younger patients, caregivers can complete the Parent Patient Symptom Checklist-17 (PSC-17) screening questionnaire. In these instances, it is still most helpful to use the caregiver report in conjunction with child reports, as caregiver reports alone have been shown to miss patients with MDD.

Remember that scoring high on a screening tool does not make the diagnosis of MDD. Instead, a positive screen should lead to direct interviews with the patients and families/caregivers. During this interview, you should assess for depressive symptoms based on the diagnostic criteria established in the DSM-V discussed above. To diagnose major depressive disorder, criteria from the DSM-V, must be met and not explained by substance abuse, medication use, or other medical or psychological conditions. Any patient scoring positively on their screening test should also be assessed for other psychiatric disorders.

Differential Diagnosis

Medical conditions that may present similarly to MDD include concussion, hypo- or hyperthyroidism, anemia, autoimmune disease, mononucleosis, and deficiencies in vitamins such as vitamin D or vitamin B12. Other psychological conditions that may present similarly to MDD include persistent depressive disorder and disruptive mood dysregulation disorder. If a patient has a depressed mood for more days than not for 1 year, the diagnosis may be persistent depressive disorder. If a patient is predominantly angry with temper outbursts, the diagnosis may be disruptive mood dysregulation or posttraumatic stress disorder.

Symptoms of bipolar disorder, eating disorders, and conduct disorders may also overlap with MDD. Children and adolescents can have more than one psychiatric diagnosis concurrently; research shows that about three quarters of children with MDD also have anxiety and about half of children with MDD also have a behavior problem.

Management

Management of complex conditions such as MDD is managed most successfully with a proactive, multidisciplinary, and patient-centered approach. Prior to initiating treatment, you should provide education and support to the patient and their family which includes discussing the range of treatment options and assisting the patient and family in arriving at a treatment plan.

In cases of mild MDD, the primary care physician can consider a period of close monitoring with weekly or bi-weekly visits for 5–8 weeks before starting treatment. Evidence has shown that some patients with mild MDD will improve with support and regular symptom monitoring. However, if symptoms persist, in cases of moderate or severe MDD, or MDD with complicating factors such as coexisting substance use, anxiety, or psychosis, patients should be referred to a mental health specialist.

Initial management involves medication management, typically with a selective serotonin reuptake inhibitor (SSRI), and/or psychotherapy. There is currently insufficient evidence to recommend either treatment over the other. Cognitive behavioral therapy (CBT) and interpersonal psychotherapy adapted for adolescents (IPT-A) are first-line psychotherapy recommendations for treatment of MDD in adolescents.

Fluoxetine is recommended as first-line medication for adolescents with MDD. Second-line medication options include escitalopram, citalopram, and sertraline. Once treatment is initiated, you should monitor for symptoms and adverse events. SSRIs typically begin to work within the first 2–4 weeks of initiation, but improvements are seen over the next 8–12 weeks.

Common side effects of SSRIs include dry mouth, constipation, diarrhea, sweating, sleep disturbance, sexual dysfunction, irritability, disinhibition, agitation, jitteriness, headache, appetite changes, and rash. Serious side effects of SSRIs include serotonin syndrome (fever, hyperthermia, restlessness, confusion), akathisia (inability to sit still, urge to move that is out of one's control), and hypomania. All SSRIs have a black box warning for individuals up to age 24 years for increased suicidal thinking and behavior. Although the risk is low, close monitoring for suicidality is recommended by the US Food and Drug Administration (FDA), especially for the first month after starting an SSRI.

If symptoms have improved, continue treatment for a minimum of 1 year. Patients should continue to be monitored for 6–24 months with regular follow-up at least every 3 months. If symptoms have either partially improved or not improved after initial 6–8 weeks of monitoring, you should reassess the diagnosis, consider adding medication, increasing medication dosing as tolerated if already on medication, changing medication if patient is already on maximum dosing, or adding therapy.

All management plans should incorporate the establishment of a safety plan. See discussion in suicide section of this chapter for more information regarding safety planning.

Anxiety

Background

Anxiety is the body's physiological response to stressful stimuli. Anxiety disorders are diagnosed when fears, worries, or anxieties occur outside of the range of normal development or are extreme, causing significant distress or excessive impairment in function at school, home, or social settings. Most adult anxiety disorders begin by early adolescence. The estimated lifetime prevalence of anxiety disorders in the United States is around 20% in men and 30% in women.

Anxiety disorders are some of the most common psychiatric disorders in children and adolescents. Social phobia (social anxiety disorder) is the most common anxiety disorder in teens. This is characterized by excessive fear or worry about being negatively evaluated by others in social situations.

For purposes of simplicity, we will focus on generalized anxiety disorder (GAD) in this chapter. According to the DSM-V, GAD is defined as excessive anxiety and worry that is difficult to control during numerous everyday situations, occurring most days over at least 6 months and affecting various activities (such as school performance). In addition, the anxiety is associated with at least three of the following symptoms:

1. Restlessness or feeling on edge
2. Being easily fatigued
3. Difficulty concentrating or mind going blank
4. Irritability
5. Muscle tension
6. Sleep disturbance (e.g., difficulty falling or staying asleep, or restless unsatisfying sleep)

Finally, the anxiety or worry is not secondary to the direct physiologic effects of a substance (e.g., a drug of abuse, or a medication) or a general medical condition (e.g., hyperthyroidism) and does not occur exclusively during a mood disorder, psychotic disorder, or pervasive developmental disorder. Anxiety disorders, especially GAD, are highly comorbid with other psychiatric conditions. While comorbid depression is the most common, GAD also occurs in conjunction with bipolar, attention deficit/hyperactivity, learning/language, behavior, obsessive-compulsive, eating, and substance-related disorders.

The effect of untreated anxiety is significant, including increasing risk of developing further anxiety disorders, depression, and substance abuse. Decreased academic performance, occupational achievement, and social outcomes are among the long-term social impacts of untreated anxiety. Among adolescents with anxiety, 9% report suicidal ideation.

Anxiety disorders tend to run in families. This is believed to be, in part, related to a combination of genetic predisposition and environmental factors.

History

Physicians will often evaluate for anxiety during a well visit as part of the HEADSSS assessment (see Chap. 37) but also during more focused visits in which a patient or caregiver has a concern about symptoms such as fatigue or abdominal pain. Depending on the age of the child and/or developmental maturity, obtaining the history may include interviews of the child and caregiver together, caregiver alone, or the child alone. With few exceptions, adolescents need to be interviewed alone when discussing mental health concerns (see Chap. 37).

It is important to remember to disclose to the adolescent that significant safety concerns (e.g., suicidal ideation with a plan that puts them in imminent danger) will have to be reported to their caregiver.

Currently, there is no USPSTF recommendation for universal screening for anxiety disorders in children and adolescents. However, freely available general social-emotional screening instruments, such as the Pediatric Symptom Checklist (PSC) can be used systematically to detect signs of anxiety causing psychosocial impairment during routine well-child care.

Symptoms of anxiety are often mentioned as the "chief complaint" during a visit by the patient or caregiver. Children and adolescents with anxiety can also have a wide range of behavioral, physical, and psychological symptoms that one must consider when taking a history.

- Behavioral signs: Avoidance of academic or social activities such as school, camp, or sleepovers, excessive need for reassurance, and poor school performance including inattention, difficulty concentrating, or incomplete school assignments in the allotted time
- Physical signs: headaches, abdominal pain, dramatic presentations of pain, frequent muscle aches and pains, poor sleep, tiredness
- Psychological signs: irritability, feeling tense

To meet the DSM-V criteria, symptoms should be present for at least 6 months and cause significant disturbance across multiple settings, but children with a shorter duration of symptoms or disturbance in a single setting may still need support and treatment. Obtaining history on what stressors or situations contribute to anxiety symptoms is important.

The history for patients with anxiety is similar to the history in patients with depression. See discussion above in the depression section of this chapter for additional history questions and review of systems.

Physical Examination

You should be on the lookout for signs of anxiety including disheveled appearance, poor eye contact, decreased engagement/uncooperativeness, shy demeanor, clinginess, tremor, fidgetiness, restlessness, "nervous" habits (e.g., nail-biting), hypervigilance, pressured or minimal speech, irritability, expression of worry, weak insight, or poor judgment. These signs are not specific to anxiety and may be absent in an anxious person, so their presence may support an anxiety disorder, but their absence does not eliminate one.

Work-Up

Laboratory Assessment

Initial work-up of a patient presenting with anxiety may include a comprehensive metabolic panel, complete blood count with differential, thyroid-stimulating hormone, and urine drug screen.

Screening Tools for Anxiety

Diagnostic evaluation with a screening tool validated for use in children and adolescents is essential prior to beginning treatment. Validated tools include:

- Screen for Child Anxiety-Related Emotional Disorders (SCARED), caregiver, and child versions
- Generalized Anxiety Disorder-7 (GAD-7), teen-adult version (Fig. 18.1)

Differential Diagnosis

Examples of medical conditions that may present similarly to GAD include hyperthyroidism, anemia, asthma, autoimmune disease, or substance use.

Over the last 2 weeks, how often have you been bothered by the following problems	Not at all (0)	Several days (1)	More than half the days (2)	Nearly every day (3)
1. Feeling nervous, anxious or on edge	☐	☐	☐	☐
2. Not being able to stop por control worrying	☐	☐	☐	☐
3. Worrying too much about different things	☐	☐	☐	☐
4. Trouble relaxing	☐	☐	☐	☐
5. Being so restless that it is hard to sit still	☐	☐	☐	☐
6. Becoming easily annoyed or irritable	☐	☐	☐	☐
7. Feeling afraid as if something awful might happen	☐	☐	☐	☐

Total score __ = **Add columns** ________ + ________ +

If you checked off any problems, how difficult have these problems made it for you to do your work, take care of things at home, or get along with other people?

Not difficult at all	Somewhat difficult	Very difficult	Extremely difficult

Fig. 18.1 The Generalized Anxiety Disorder 7-item (GAD-7) scale. (available at https://www.phqscreeners.com)

Management

Reviewing the patient and caregiver preferences on treatment options can increase the likelihood of engagement and adherence to the plan. Treatment for anxiety includes nonspecific recommendations such as activities that decrease stress and improve mood. For example, breathing exercises, meditation, and yoga are useful. Mindfulness and meditation practices are often recommended and may be done via an application on a smartphone. In addition, activities that support well-being including sleep hygiene, healthy eating, regular exercise, predictable routine, and social support are recommended.

Evidence-based treatments for anxiety include CBT and pharmacotherapy (SSRIs or selective serotonin and norepinephrine reuptake inhibitors (SNRIs)). Per the American Academy of Child and Adolescent Psychiatry (AACAP), CBT should be offered as first-line treatment to patients 6–18 years old with social anxiety, generalized anxiety, separation anxiety, specific phobia, or panic disorder. The patient may be exposed gradually to the feared situation to modify the anxiety response through systematic desensitization and habituation. Family-directed interventions can help improve communication skills and problem solving. Additionally, the therapist can assist to create school directed interventions that establish strategies for coping and problem solving in this setting. Treatment plans can also be written into a student's 504 plan or individualized education plan.

> Section 504 requires that school districts provide a free appropriate public education to qualified students in their jurisdictions who have a physical or mental impairment that substantially limits one or more major life activities. An Individualized Education Program (IEP) is a written education plan designed to meet a child's learning needs.

Medication should be considered if the anxiety is moderate to severe. Overall, youth who received antianxiety (i.e., antidepressant) medication did better than those who received placebo and those who received a combination of medication and psychotherapy did the best. AACAP recommends that SSRIs be offered to patients 6–18 years old with social anxiety, generalized anxiety, separation anxiety, or panic disorder. The FDA has approved duloxetine for children 7 years of age and older with GAD. Although some SSRIs have been approved for treating children with depression, SSRIs do not have FDA approval for the treatment of anxiety disorders. There is considerable evidence of their efficacy, and many are used "off-label." Some of these evidence-based SSRIs that are effective and safe in treating children and adolescents with anxiety and/or depression include sertraline, fluoxetine, fluvoxamine, paroxetine, and venlafaxine extended release.

Behavior activation and agitation (e.g., restlessness, insomnia, impulsiveness, aggression) are more common in anxiety than depression and may occur with dose increases. This is one of the reasons slow titration of SSRI dose is recommended. If the activation symptoms are significant, reducing the dose of the medication or discontinuing it is the best management strategy until the symptoms subside. Switching medication is commonly done to find the best balance between anxiety improvement while minimizing side effects.

In pediatrics, we avoid benzodiazepines such as lorazepam, as they are intended for short-term treatment and have an addiction potential when used for longer periods of time. Instead, for intense episodes of anxiety, antihistamines such as hydroxyzine, may be used to reduce anxiety.

The treatment goal for patients with anxiety disorders is to have little or no impairment. Treatment outcome can be measured empirically with screening instruments as well as clinical changes. When to discontinue medication depends on whether the treatment goals were met (i.e., the anxiety is in remission, or there are very few symptoms that cause impairment). In general, experts recommend discontinuing medication 6–12 months after remission has been achieved. This should only be considered in periods of expected lower stress and not when the child is expected to be most anxious. It is important to continue monitoring children once medication has been discontinued to ensure that subtle anxiety symptoms do not return and the child or adolescent has been able to maintain function.

Suicide

Background

Suicidal thoughts, behaviors, and attempts are common among adolescents with depression and anxiety disorders. Suicide is the second leading cause of death for adolescents and young adults aged 10–24 years. It is crucial for the physician to establish an emergency communication mechanism for handling increased suicidality. This mechanism should include a caregiver supporting a safe home environment, warning the patient of the effects of drugs and alcohol on their mood, offering suicide prevention resources, and scheduling appropriate close follow-up. The physician should establish connections with local crisis support and hospital services. It is also helpful to provide the National Suicide Prevention Lifeline, 988.

History

Suicidality may wax and wane. Reassessing adolescents with anxiety and depression or suspected mental health conditions periodically is important. The Ask Suicide-Screening Questions (ASQ) (Table 18.2) is a brief five question screening test specific for suicidality that includes questions to assess acuity of the suicidal ideation and provides guidelines on follow-up depending on the patient's answers.

Table 18.2 The Ask Suicide-Screening Questions (ASQ) (available at https://www.nimh.nih.gov/research/research-conducted-at-nimh/asq-toolkit-materials)

Ask the patient	Yes	No
1. In the past few weeks, have you wished you were dead?	☐	☐
2. In the past few weeks, have you felt that you or your family would be better off if you were dead?	☐	☐
3. In the past week, have you been having thoughts about killing yourself?	☐	☐
4. Have you ever tried to kill yourself?	☐	☐
If yes, how? ______________________ When? ___________________		
If the patient answers yes to any of the above, ask the following question:		
5. Are you having thoughts of killing yourself right now?	☐	☐
If yes, please describe: ________________________		

Risk Factors for Suicidality

It is important for the pediatrician to monitor for risk factors for suicidal ideation including:

- Minority sexual orientation
- Intellectual disability
- History of prior depressive episode, other psychiatric disorder, or suicide attempt
- Family history of depression, suicide, or other psychiatric disorder
- Substance use
- Trauma (e.g., physical or sexual abuse, neglect)

Management

The suicidal adolescent needs to be in treatment including both psychotherapy and pharmacotherapy. See above sections on depression and anxiety for further discussion of treatment modalities. All management plans of adolescents with suicidal ideation should incorporate the establishment of a safety plan. The key components of a safety plan include:

- Restricting access to lethal means (e.g., firearms, alcohol, and both prescription and over the counter medications).
- Providing the adolescent with
  - An emergency contact

    Sometimes the emergency contact is an adult involved in the adolescent's life who is not a caregiver.

The emergency contact should be contacted if the patient deteriorates, becomes actively suicidal or dangerous to others, or experiences an acute crisis associated with psychosocial stressors.

This is especially important during the period of initial treatment when safety concerns are the highest.

- Suicide crisis hotlines available 24 hours a day to call or text for assistance.
- A list of support people who are aware of the adolescents' issues and are willing to be contacted to assist in an acute crisis if needed.

- Developing and discussing an emergency plan for all students who may experience acute suicidal crises while at school.
- Establishing clear follow-up.

Safety contracts should not be used since there is no evidence that they prevent suicide.

According to the AACAP, suicide prevention includes reduced access to firearms and other lethal means for at-risk individuals.

Application Exercises

1. A 13-year-old adolescent boy is admitted to the hospital for abdominal pain that did not improve after administration of multiple medications in the emergency department. His initial laboratory work-up including complete blood cell count was unremarkable. He has been seen in the emergency department four times in the past couple months for similar complaints. On examination, the patient appears thin and non-toxic with normal vital signs for age. The remainder of his examination is unremarkable except for generalized abdominal pain and healing scars noted on the patient's forearms. Upon interviewing him alone, the patient reports that he has felt as though his family would be better off without him.

   Of the following, the best next step in management of this patient would be:

   A. Obtain an MRI of the abdomen
   B. Refer to outpatient psychiatric services upon discharge
   C. Ask the patient if he is having thoughts of hurting himself right now
   D. Provide reassurance that his family is understanding about his medical issues

   Answer C: Suicide is the second leading cause of death for adolescents. The majority of youth who commit suicide were treated in a healthcare setting in the months leading up to their death. For the patient in this vignette, he endorses thoughts that his family would be better off without him. Thus, the next best step would be to screen for suicidal ideation at the time you are seeing him. The ASQ is a validated suicide risk assessment screening questionnaire for adolescents in medical settings. If the answer to any of the screening questions is positive, then a fifth question should be asked: "Are you having thoughts of killing yourself right now?" If the answer to this question is positive, then the patient is considered in imminent risk and safety precautions must be put in place per hospital protocol.

Without more information regarding the patient's current risk of suicide, providing a referral to outpatient psychiatric providers for follow-up or reassuring the patient that his family is understanding of his medical issues is inappropriate. Although the patient is being admitted for abdominal pain, it is likely that his mental health is contributing to his presentation and should be addressed before pursuing additional imaging with an MRI. Additionally, given physical exam findings of generalized abdominal pain with similar presentations recently and unremarkable CBC, the risk of appendicitis is low.

2. A 16-year-old girl presents to your office for her yearly health wellness exam. While reviewing updates from the past year, the patient's mother reports that her grades have recently declined and she has been caught skipping school. Upon review of the patient's growth chart, you notice she has lost approximately 10 pounds since her visit last year. On examination, the patient is noted to be thin-appearing with normal vital signs. The remainder of the examination is normal other than neurologic examination which is notable for flat affect and poor eye contact.

   Of the following, the best next step in evaluation of this patient includes:

   A. Screen for depression with Patient Health Questionnaire-9
   B. Obtain thyroid studies
   C. Have her sign a safety contract
   D. Encourage mom to talk with the school regarding a possible learning disability

   Answer A: This patient is presenting with signs and symptoms concerning for depression. Depression is common in adolescents with girls more commonly affected than boys. Depression can present with various behavioral, physical, and psychological signs including a change in school performance, acting out behaviors, substance use, decreased appetite, weight loss, insomnia, and withdrawal. The United States Preventative Services Task Force recommends screening all adolescents yearly for depression especially those patients presenting with concerning signs and symptoms. Given the patient's behaviors are concerning for depression, they should be screened using the PHQ-9. While the PHQ-9 is only a screening test, it can be useful in determining those patients in whom depression is likely.

   While you should consider other medical causes of behavior change other than depression when making an initial diagnosis, obtaining thyroid studies would not be the next best step. Having patients sign a safety contract has not been shown to prevent suicide and has actually been shown to be harmful to the physician–patient relationship. Given concerning signs and symptoms for depression, having the school evaluate for a learning disability would not be the next best step as the patient would not receive treatment for her depression.

3. You are seeing Sarah, a 12-year-old girl, with no significant past medical history, who comes in for concern of 8 month history of vague abdominal pain. She is in middle school and was formerly very active with sports but is becoming increasingly unwilling to participate and nervous about multiple activities. Sarah's

father has noticed a dip in her school performance and desire to attend school. No social stressors, dietary concerns, safety, or bullying concerns. You obtain further history (including HEADSSS) and screen her with a GAD-7 and PHQ-9 and her symptoms are concerning for moderate anxiety.

What is the best next step to evaluate Sarah?

A. Give Sarah a break from her activities to decrease her anxiety
B. Advise her on appropriate dietary, sleep and stress-relieving habits, refer her for cognitive behavioral therapy, and establish close follow-up
C. Start her on a low dose benzodiazepine before competitions
D. Reassure her family that since her symptoms are not severe, routine follow-up at her next routine health maintenance exam will suffice

Answer B: After obtaining a thorough history and physical and using validated screening tools for anxiety and depression, it is appropriate to begin treatment for any patient who meets the criteria for moderate anxiety.

While you may encourage her parents to connect with the school to help establish support for her learning considering her anxiety (504 accommodations), it is inappropriate at this time to focus on a learning disorder unless there have been previous red flags or signs pointing to this. While SSRI therapy may be indicated, C is incorrect as benzodiazepines are not first-line treatment due to the risk of addiction. D is incorrect since she was found to have moderate anxiety treatment should be started immediately and waiting until her next health maintenance exam is too long.

Further Reading

Bagnell AL. Anxiety and separation disorders. Pediatr Rev. 2011;32(10):440–5; quiz 446. https://doi.org/10.1542/pir.32-10-440.

Cheung AH, Zuckerbrot RA, Jensen PS, Laraque D, Stein REK, GLAD-PC Steering Group. Guidelines for adolescent depression in primary care (GLAD-PC): part II. Treatment and ongoing management. Pediatrics. 2018;141(3):e20174082. https://doi.org/10.1542/peds.2017-4082.

Walter HJ, Bukstein OG, Abright AR, Keable H, Ramtekkar U, Ripperger-Suhler J, Rockhill C. Clinical practice guideline for the assessment and treatment of children and adolescents with anxiety disorders. J Am Acad Child Adolesc Psychiatry. 2020;59(10):1107–24. https://doi.org/10.1016/j.jaac.2020.05.005. Epub 2020 May 18.

Zuckerbrot RA, Cheung A, Jensen PS, Stein REK, Laraque D, GLAD-PC Steering Group. Guidelines for adolescent depression in primary care (GLAD-PC): part I. Practice preparation, identification, assessment, and initial management. Pediatrics. 2018;141(3):e20174081. https://doi.org/10.1542/peds.2017-4081.

Chapter 19
Disordered Eating

Mayya Malakh and Maria S. Skoczylas

Background/Epidemiology

Eating disorders are common in adolescence and peak between 14 and 19 years of age. The general prevalence of eating disorders is estimated to be up to 10% of the population though far fewer seek treatment. Eating disorders encompass a wide variety of disorders including anorexia nervosa (AN), bulimia nervosa (BN), avoidant/restrictive food intake disorder (ARFID), and binge-eating disorder. Incidence is higher in girls and young women. There are two subtypes of AN, restricting type and binge-eating/purging type. Restricting type is diagnosed when, during the last 3 months, weight loss is accomplished through caloric restriction and/or excessive exercise, and the individual has not engaged in binging or purging behavior. In binge-eating/purging type, the individual may use self-induced vomiting or misuse of laxatives, diuretics, or enemas. In adults, tiers of severity are based on BMI: mild (<17.5), moderate (16–16.99), and severe (15–15.99), to extreme (<15). In pediatrics, severity is more difficult to define, but many use the threshold of BMI <10th percentile for age. Patients with eating disorders may have normal or above-normal weights. Severity for BN is defined by the number of episodes of inappropriate compensatory behaviors over several months. The defining features of AN and BN is the development of disordered thoughts and habits surrounding body image, eating patterns, and weight management.

M. Malakh (✉) · M. S. Skoczylas
Department of Pediatrics, University of Michigan, Ann Arbor, MI, USA
e-mail: myamal@med.umich.edu; mshakour@med.umich.edu

N. Liao et al. (eds.), *Pediatric Rotations*,
https://doi.org/10.1007/978-3-031-59873-9_19

Diagnostic Criteria

Summarized DSM-5 Criteria for Anorexia Nervosa

1. Restriction of energy intake relative to requirements, leading to significantly low body weight in the context of age, sex, developmental trajectory, and physical health.
2. Intense fear of gaining weight or of becoming fat, or persistent behaviors that interfere with weight gain, even though patient is at a significantly low weight.
3. Disturbance in the way in which one's body weight or shape is experienced, undue influence of body weight or shape on self-evaluation, or persistent lack of recognition of the seriousness of current low body weight.

Summarized DSM-5 Criteria for Bulimia Nervosa

1. Recurrent episodes of binge eating
   (a) Eating, in a discrete period of time (e.g., within any 2-h period), an amount of food that is definitely larger than what most individuals would eat in a similar period of time.
   (b) A sense of lack of control over eating during the episode.
2. Recurrent inappropriate compensatory behaviors in order to prevent weight gain such as self-induced vomiting; misuse of laxatives, diuretics, or other medications; fasting; or excessive exercise.
3. The binge eating and inappropriate compensatory behaviors both occur, on average, at least once a week for 3 months.
4. Self-evaluation is unduly influenced by body shape and weight.
5. The disturbance does not occur exclusively during episodes of AN.

Summarized DSM-5 Criteria for Avoidant/Restrictive Food Intake Disorder

1. An eating or feeding disturbance (e.g., apparent lack of interest in eating or food; avoidance based on the sensory characteristics of food; concern about aversive consequences of eating) associated with one (or more) of the following:
   (a) Significant weight loss (or failure to achieve expected weight gain or faltering growth in children).
   (b) Significant nutritional deficiency.

(c) Dependence on enteral feeding or oral nutritional supplements.
(d) Marked interference with psychosocial functioning.

2. The eating disturbance does not occur exclusively during the course of AN or BN, and there is no evidence of a disturbance in the way one's body weight or shape is experienced.

History

The pediatric patient is often discovered to have a disordered eating pattern during routine exam or due to concerns brought forward by a caregiver or family member who has noticed a suspicious pattern of behavior. It is important to obtain the history from the patient as well as other family members, as it is common for the patient with an eating disorder to be unaware of the disordered behaviors and to lack emotion or the ability to describe emotions. See Table 19.1 for specific history questions to ask. To help screen for eating disorders, multiple screening questionnaires have been developed including the SCOFF questionnaire, the Eating Disorders Examination-Questionnaire (EDE-Q), and the Female Athlete Screening Tool.

The review of systems must be broad to evaluate for end organ dysfunction that develops with severe malnutrition (Table 19.2).

Table 19.1 History questions to consider when there is a concern for a possible eating disorder

Family concerns	Have you been concerned about your child's eating habits? Have you been concerned about your child's weight?
Weight	What do you think about the way you look? Do you think you need to lose or gain weight? Do you fear gaining weight?
Diet history	What did you eat in the past 24 h? Do you avoid eating with other people?
Exercise	How often do you exercise? What activities? Are you upset if you do not exercise?
Binging/purging	Do you ever feel out of control when you eat? Do you ever vomit intentionally? Do you ever use laxatives?
Reproductive health	Female: When was your last menstrual period? Are your periods regular? Male/Female: How is your sexual drive?
Family history	Are there any family members with eating disorders? Anxiety? Depression?
Social history	HEADSSS (home, education, activities, drugs, sexual activity, suicide/depression, safety)

Table 19.2 Review of systems when there is a concern for a possible eating disorder

System	Symptom
General	Weight loss, fatigue
Pulmonary	Shortness of breath
Cardiovascular	Chest pain, dyspnea on exertion, presyncope or dizziness, palpitations, leg cramps
Gastrointestinal	Abdominal pain, constipation, distension, heartburn
Hematologic	Easy bruising or bleeding
Obstetric/gynecologic/sexual	Menstrual history, sexual drive
Neurologic	Numbness, weakness, dizziness
Endocrinologic	Cold intolerance
Dermatologic	Hair loss, lanugo, sores that will not heal
Psychiatric	Anxiety, depression

Physical Exam

Multiple physical exam findings in eating disorders are attributable to the significantly decreased energy intake or result of other compensatory behaviors. Vital sign instability including bradycardia, hypotension, orthostatic hypotension, and hypothermia are common. Special focus should be placed on parotid gland swelling, enamel erosion, and dental caries which can be more common with purging. The cardiac exam is often notable for bradycardia. The abdomen may demonstrate bloating, distention, or palpable stool. Extremities may be cool to the touch and may show edema, muscle atrophy, or weakness. Skin is often dry and may show lanugo or acrocyanosis. Patients may have comorbid, non-suicidal, self-injurious behavior, and signs of this may be visible on skin examination.

Differential Diagnosis

Differential diagnosis for eating disorders is broad and should be considered based on key features of the patient's history and physical exam.

Vomiting: In cases where vomiting is not self-induced or is present without features such as fear of gaining weight or body-image issues, consider obstructive gastrointestinal pathology such as achalasia or esophageal stricture, central nervous system pathology such as pseudotumor cerebri, central nervous system malignancy or migraine, endocrine etiology such as Addison disease, and other possible causes such as rumination syndrome, cyclical vomiting, and migraine.

Weight loss: For reports of unintentional weight loss, gastrointestinal pathologies to be considered include celiac disease and inflammatory bowel disease, as well as endocrine causes such as hyperthyroidism and Addison disease. Malignancies and autoimmune disorders may also be screened for although they would present with a variety of other concerning symptoms.

Binge eating: Differential includes mood disorders, anxiety disorders, Prader-Willi syndrome, Kleine-Levin syndrome, and nutritional deficiency states.

Coexisting psychiatric disorders: In addition to mood and anxiety disorders, assess for any delusional thoughts around weight gain or eating.

Management

Outpatient vs. Inpatient Management

Treatment of patients who have eating disorders is often challenging, long-term, and requires a multidisciplinary approach. The key aspects of treatment involve managing the patient's malnutrition and addressing associated complications, as well as management of the underlying psychological and psychiatric components of the eating disorder.

Eating disorders are frequently managed on an outpatient basis. A primary care physician can diagnose eating disorders in clinic and initiate treatment including creation of a nutrition plan or referral to a dietitian, scheduling appointments for weight checks and vital sign monitoring, laboratory screening, referral to a therapist and/or psychiatrist, and referral to an adolescent medicine specialist, if available. When outpatient management proves to be ineffective or any of the below criteria for hospitalization are present during the evaluation, the patient may require hospital admission. For medically stable patients requiring intensive eating disorder treatment, a partial hospitalization setting, day treatment program, or a residential facility specializing in eating disorder management may be appropriate options.

Criteria for Hospitalization

- Vital sign abnormalities (in adolescent patients):
  - Bradycardia <50 beats/min
  - Hypotension with blood pressure less than 80/50 mmHg
  - Orthostatic increase in HR (>20 beats/min)
  - Decrease in blood pressure (>10 mmHg)
  - Temperature <35.5 °C
- <75% expected body weight or ongoing weight loss despite outpatient management
- Dehydration

- Electrolyte disturbance (e.g., hypokalemia, hypochloremic alkalosis)
- Acute food refusal; uncontrollable binging/purging
- Medical complications: syncope, arrhythmia
- Acute psychiatric emergencies

Management Approach

A crucial portion of restrictive eating disorders treatment is nutritional rehabilitation, utilizing "food as medicine" to improve a patient's nutritional status. Nutritional rehabilitation involves gradually increasing patient's caloric intake to reach goal daily calories, while monitoring weight, vital signs, and electrolytes to assess for refeeding syndrome (see below). Goal calories may need to be modified to reach weight gain goals. If a patient is not able to finish meals, the remainder of their caloric intake may be given via nutritional drinks either orally or via nasogastric tube.

In the first several days of nutritional rehabilitation, physical activity is significantly restricted to optimize energy conservation. Over the course of the patient's hospitalization, activity is liberalized gradually as the patient's nutritional status improves and vital signs such as bradycardia and orthostatic hypotension normalize. Inpatient admission for eating disorders also involves strict monitoring of the patient's activities, including supervised bathroom use, to ensure no surreptitious binging, purging, exercise, or researching of calories in foods consumed. A patient attendant or another staff member providing strict supervision may be present at the bedside depending on specific hospital policy.

Patients with binge-eating disorders are typically managed on an outpatient basis with intensive psychotherapy and rarely require hospitalization, but these patients may require admission for complications of chronic comorbidities. General approach includes psychotherapy and/or pharmacotherapy to reduce binge-eating behaviors, as well as management of medical comorbidities and lifestyle changes to optimize health.

Electrolyte Management

AN: Refeeding syndrome is a serious potential complication that may occur during the nutrition rehabilitation process in patients with AN. In a patient experiencing prolonged undernutrition, blood glucose concentrations are decreased, resulting in catabolism of fat and protein stores and depletion of intracellular electrolytes, including phosphorus, potassium, and magnesium. During refeeding, insulin is secreted as a result of rising glucose concentration, which causes phosphorus, potassium, and magnesium to move into cells to create adenosine triphosphate (ATP) for metabolism. This may thus cause hypophosphatemia, hypokalemia, and hypomagnesemia, leading to delirium, seizures, arrhythmia, and heart failure. The potential for refeeding syndrome is the reason a patient's calorie intake is gradually increased to reach goal daily calories. During this process, electrolytes are monitored frequently and supplemented orally or intravenously depending on the severity of electrolyte abnormality.

Bulimia: Electrolyte abnormalities, the most common reason for hospitalization in patients with bulimia, are associated with purging behaviors or laxative and/or diuretic abuse. Patients who frequently purge by vomiting may present with hypochloremic, hypokalemic metabolic alkalosis. Patients may also present with hematemesis due to Mallory-Weiss tears from persistent vomiting.

ARFID: Electrolyte abnormalities may be similar to those seen in AN if the degree of food restricting and resulting malnutrition is significant.

Binge-eating disorder: Patients do not typically present with electrolyte abnormalities.

Fluid Management in Malnourished States

Patients who have AN and other eating disorders resulting in malnutrition are at risk of significant fluid shifts, and rehydration should be attempted enterally (orally or via nasogastric tube), if possible. It is important to keep in mind that although patients with AN may have hypotension and appear dehydrated, this is typically a chronic rather than acute state, so immediate resuscitation with intravenous fluids (IVF) is often not warranted. If IVF are started for dehydration (e.g., low urine output or acute kidney injury), they should be given slowly, at ½ to ¾ of maintenance rate due to the potential for relative heart malfunction with resultant fluid overload. Intake and output should be monitored carefully, as some patients may drink water excessively to stave off hunger.

Pharmacotherapy

Restrictive eating disorders (AN, ARFID): Pharmacotherapy may be utilized depending on the patient's comorbidity and specific presentation, for example, significant underlying anxiety or obsessive-compulsive behavior.

Bulimia: There is evidence for fluoxetine, topiramate, and tricyclic antidepressants helping to reduce binging and purging behaviors.

Binge-eating disorders: Topiramate and SSRIs have shown effectiveness in reducing binge-eating behaviors.

Psychotherapy

Common therapies employed in eating disorder management include cognitive behavioral therapy (CBT) focused on recognizing and changing patterns of negative thinking and behavior, dialectical behavioral therapy (DBT) focused on skills for emotional regulation and conflict management, and family-based treatment (FBT) which includes the family in treatment. FBT is currently the most effective for adolescents with AN and has been shown to improve prognosis. Specialized CBT focused on expanding food variety and volume has been shown to be specifically effective for ARFID.

Prognosis

Prognosis for eating disorders is widely variable. For AN, approximately 33% of patients have been shown to achieve recovery by 5 years from the start of treatment initiation although with incorporation of FBT recovery can be up to 50%. Of note, AN significantly increases a patient's chances of dying prematurely with a mortality 5× the mortality of the general population and has the highest mortality rate of any mental illness. In BN, patients have been shown to achieve recovery by 5 years in 33–66% of cases. Mortality in BN is 2× higher than that of the general population. Binge-eating disorder has a wide range of recovery, ranging from 30% to 80%. Not enough data is currently available to give a prognosis for patients with ARFID.

Application Exercises

1. A 15-year-old girl presents to your clinic for her annual well visit. She has been growing appropriately, has a BMI of 24, and is active in volleyball. On your examination, you notice that she has some red, irritated skin on her knuckles. She also has dental caries. Upon a confidential interview without a parent in the room, the patient admits that she is worried she appears larger than her teammates and has been causing herself to vomit after meals for the last 2 months. What laboratory abnormality is this patient most at risk for?

   A. Hyponatremia
   B. Hypernatremia
   C. Hypoglycemia
   D. Hypochloremia
   E. Hyperkalemia

   Answer D: Hypochloremia. This patient has red, irritated skin on her knuckles, and dental caries on your exam caused by self-induced vomiting that she admits to on your interview. Furthermore, she reports concerns about her body image. This presentation is consistent with bulimia nervosa. Patients with bulimia nervosa who induce vomiting are at risk of hypochloremia, as chloride from gastric fluid is lost through emesis. The other answer choices are not electrolyte disturbances typical of bulimia nervosa.

2. A 13-year-old boy's mother brought him into your clinic because she noticed he appeared much thinner than usual while the family was on a beach vacation. His mother reports that he has been significantly more withdrawn lately, avoids family meals saying that he is not hungry, and he sometimes takes his food to his bedroom. The patient's vital signs in clinic: heart rate of 40 beats/min, respiratory rate 14 breaths/min, blood pressure 95/65 mmHg, SpO_2 98%. His weight has decreased by 15 pounds since he was last seen in clinic 6 months ago. He appears thin and his hands and feet are cool to the touch, but his physical exam is otherwise unremarkable. The best next management step is:

   A. Refer the patient for psychotherapy
   B. Arrange hospital admission for nutritional rehabilitation
   C. Have the patient meet with the clinic dietitian to discuss calorie increase in his diet
   D. Ask the patient to return for weight check in 1 week

   Answer B: Arrange hospital admission for nutritional rehabilitation. This patient may have anorexia nervosa. He has had drastic weight loss in the last several months and appears to have been avoiding mealtimes at home, likely to restrict his intake. Notably, he is bradycardic to 40 beats/min and would thus meet criteria for inpatient admission. He will also require the aspects of care provided in other answer options such as weight checks, working with a dietitian and initiating psychotherapy; however, given the apparent severity of his malnourished state, he must first undergo nutritional rehabilitation with careful monitoring for electrolyte imbalances on an inpatient basis.

3. A 17-year-old boy with autism spectrum disorder presents with his father to the clinic after a near-syncopal episode. The patient's father has not noticed any change in behavior and denies financial stressors. On 24-h dietary recall, the patient reports that he ate a slice of pizza yesterday at dinner but otherwise nothing. The patient denies any weight concerns or body-image concerns. Review of systems is unremarkable. He is afebrile with a heart rate of 55 beats/min and blood pressure of 95/55 mmHg. He appears thin and on his growth curve he has decreased from the 50th percentile to the 20th percentile since you saw him 1 year ago. What is the most likely diagnosis?

   A. Food insecurity
   B. Anorexia nervosa
   C. Avoidant restrictive food intake disorder
   D. Celiac disease

   Answer C: The most likely etiology for this patient is avoidant restrictive food intake disorder. Food insecurity is less likely given the social history, and celiac disease is also less likely given the negative review of systems. There is no concern for body dysmorphism; therefore, the diagnosis is not consistent with anorexia nervosa.

Chapter 20
Weight-Faltering in Infants and Children (Failure to Thrive)

Megan E. Coe and Kristin Sundy-Boyles

Background

Poor weight gain or weight-faltering in infants and children has historically been known as failure to thrive since first appearing in textbooks in 1933. Since then, varying terminology and definitions have been used to describe this condition, which makes exact epidemiology difficult to ascertain. Regardless, concern for weight-faltering remains a common occurrence in pediatrics with up to 10% of children affected in the primary care setting and with admissions for weight-faltering accounting for up to 5% of pediatric hospitalizations.

Weight-faltering is not a diagnosis or a syndrome, but rather one of the first symptoms that indicates an infant or child has inadequate nutritional intake or utilization to such a degree that optimal growth and development cannot be properly maintained. This ongoing malnutrition, when severe, not only affects weight gain, but can then sequentially impact linear growth (length or height) and appropriate cranial bone growth (head circumference). If left untreated, long-term outcomes can include impaired cognitive ability (IQ), delay in developmental milestone attainment, and impairment of appropriate immune functioning. Most children, however, have good outcomes with appropriate recognition and intervention.

M. E. Coe (✉)
Department of Pediatrics, Section of Hospital Pediatrics, Nationwide Children's Hospital/The Ohio State University College of Medicine, Columbus, OH, USA
e-mail: megan.coe@nationwidechildrens.org

K. Sundy-Boyles
Department of Pediatrics, Division of Pediatric Hospital Medicine, University of North Carolina School of Medicine, Chapel Hill, USA
e-mail: kristin_sundy-boyles@med.unc.edu

N. Liao et al. (eds.), *Pediatric Rotations*,
https://doi.org/10.1007/978-3-031-59873-9_20

Definitions

Weight-faltering in an infant or child may be an initial presenting problem for the outpatient provider, urgent care, or emergency department, or may be discovered for the first time during an inpatient admission for a related or unrelated illness. Therefore, it is extremely important to review growth and development for all pediatric patients, regardless of care setting and chief complaint for the visit. More commonly, weight-faltering develops over the course of routine well child check-ups with the primary care physician or provider (PCP), during which time growth parameters including weight, length or height, and head circumference are routinely checked. These measurements are used to calculate other important growth parameters such as weight-for-length or BMI.

There is no single, universally accepted definition of weight-faltering in infants or children and in clinical practice, a wide variety of definitions are used. Most often these are based on growth chart trends and percentage of expected weight gain over time. More importantly, weight-faltering is recognized as a multifactorial diagnosis and best practice is to base evaluation of an infant or child's growth over time, with careful consideration of feeding history, developmental milestones, and caregiver concerns.

There is some degree of normal growth variation, either acceleration or deceleration, over time for most infants and children. In one study, about one-third of healthy children crossed two percentiles in either weight or weight-for-length over the first 5 years of life. In the absence of additional concerns from history or physical examination, this may be acceptable.

Commonly used growth chart-based definitions for weight-faltering, using the appropriate chart for gestational age and sex, include:

1. Weight less than the fifth percentile; some sources utilize the second percentile.
2. Weight-for-length less than the fifth percentile; some sources utilize the second percentile.
3. Decrease in growth velocity resulting in weight dropping across two major percentile lines (e.g., a patient with a weight at the 80th percentile is now at the 45th percentile, having crossed the 75th and 50th percentiles).
4. Weight less than 80% of ideal weight for age and sex.

When evaluating a patient who might have weight-faltering, we recommend starting with the patient's appropriate growth chart. From birth through 2 years of age, measurements should be plotted on the World Health Organization (WHO) growth charts. Starting at age 2 years, the Centers for Disease Control (CDC) growth chart should be used. For infants born premature, weight should be plotted on the Fenton Growth chart which begins at 22 weeks and ends at 50 weeks. Once an infant reaches 40 weeks corrected gestational age, weight can be measured in conjunction with term growth charts – corrected age should be used on these growth charts through the first two years of life. For infants with conditions that follow different growth trajectories, specialized growth charts should be used (examples include the

Fenton Growth chart for prematurity and other growth charts for specific syndromic conditions such as Down Syndrome, Turner Syndrome, or Hunter Syndrome which can be easily accessed online).

Consistent measurements over time are needed to appropriately evaluate an infant or child's growth. Growth measurements should always be taken uniformly to increase accuracy and reliability:

1. Weight should be measured at the same time of day, same scale, with similar clothing or, for infants, with no clothes and a clean diaper.
2. Length in infants is measured while lying on their back from the top of the head to the bottom of the heel. Positioning of an infant for this measurement is challenging and typically requires two people to obtain accurate readings. Any measurements that appear inconsistent or surprising should be repeated.
3. Head circumference measurements are done using a paper ruler from the most prominent part of the forehead to the widest part of the back of the head. This is also a challenging measurement to obtain and best practice is to measure three times and take the average of the measurements.

In addition to these definitions, The American Academy of Nutrition and Dietetics along with the American Society for Parenteral and Enteral Nutrition categorize pediatric malnutrition into mild, moderate, or severe based on standard deviations from normal on a set of measurements. A z-score is the number of standard deviations a measurement is from the mean (e.g., a z-score of -2 is two standard deviations below the mean) and is often referenced in the does of registered dietitians who are part of the medical team.

Pathophysiology (Etiology)

Poor weight gain or poor overall growth in infants and children is the physical manifestation of undernutrition. Etiologies can be broadly divided into three categories (see Table 20.1):

1. Inadequate caloric intake.
2. Inadequate nutrient absorption or utilization.
3. Increased metabolic demand.

Infants or children with weight-faltering can have one or more causes or contributing/exacerbating factors that prevent optimal growth and development. Most commonly, the cause in this age group is inadequate oral intake, which is easily uncovered by careful review of a complete history and a thorough physical exam.

When weight is not the first growth parameter affected, this may suggest an endocrinologic etiology (particularly when only length/height is affected), possible infection sequelae (certain TORCH infections), specific growth restriction (premature suture closing, craniosynostosis), or may be a clue to a syndrome or genetic condition.

Table 20.1 Selected etiologies for weight-faltering by category

Inadequate oral intake	Behavior-related feeding issues (oral aversion, texture sensitivity, picky eater) Breastfeeding difficulties Emesis • Gastroesophageal reflux • Pyloric stenosis • Increased intracranial pressure • Malrotation +/− volvulus; other obstruction Excessive low-calorie intake (juice, water) Food insecurity Incorrect formula mixing Insufficient volumes offered (per feeding or cumulative throughout the day) Mechanical feeding difficulties (e.g., cleft lip or palate; other oromotor dysfunction) Neglect or abuse
Inadequate nutrient absorption (malabsorption) or utilization	Chronic gastrointestinal conditions (e.g., celiac disease, inflammatory bowel disease, congenital diarrhea) Cystic fibrosis Inborn errors of metabolism (e.g., glucose–galactose malabsorption) Infectious diarrhea Milk-protein allergy, sensitivity, or intolerance Other food allergy or intolerance
Increased metabolic demand (increased energy requirement)	Chronic lung disease of prematurity Congenital heart disease Congenital and/or chronic infections (TORCH, HIV, tuberculosis) Endocrine disease (e.g., hyper- or hypothyroidism, growth hormone deficiency, diseases or syndromes affecting the pituitary gland and hormones) Renal disease or renal failure Related to syndromic conditions (trisomy 21, turner, Russell-silver) Malignancy

TORCH toxoplasmosis, other agents, rubella (also known as German measles), cytomegalovirus, and herpes simplex virus, *HIV* human immunodeficiency virus

History

Obtaining a thorough history often helps distinguish the etiology as belonging to one of the broad categories mentioned above. As such, it is one of the most important diagnostic tools in determining the cause of weight-faltering in an infant or child. Table 20.2 contains sample questions aimed at uncovering the many contributing factors to poor weight gain.

Table 20.2 Questions to ask in obtaining history of pediatric patient with poor weight gain

Diet/nutrition	Infants <12 months • Feeding method (breastfeeding, bottle feeding with expressed breast milk, formula feeding) • Breast feeding: ask about the experience of breastfeeding (any work with a lactation consultant?); how long does infant nurse from each breast per feeding? Any supplemental expressed breastmilk (EBM) or formula offered? Does mom pump and know how much milk is produced? • Formula: what type/brand – Any changes to formula? If yes, why was change made, and how has the infant been doing since? – Formula preparation: Ask caregivers how they mix the formula (e.g., how many scoops per ounce of water) if not using "ready to feed" bottles – Is the infant on a higher calorie formula concentration (standard is 20 kcal/oz)? • If eating solid foods, ask what types of foods have been introduced and when • Volume and frequency of feeds or frequency of mealtimes, including overnight feeds in newborn and young infants Children older than 12 months • Types of foods typically eaten in a day/week (ask about different food groups specifically) • Ask about frequency of mealtimes (does child eat full meal or "graze" throughout the day?) • Ask about snacks: How often throughout the day, what types of snacks, timing with meals • Ask about introduction of cow's milk or other alternative milk products? How much volume of milk per day? • Any juice or pop/soda intake? (These may take away volume from other nutritional foods)
Feeding difficulty symptoms	• Breast feeding: Any difficulty with latch, suck, or swallow? Does infant fall asleep at breast? Does infant start and stop feeding? • Any coughing, choking, gagging, or other sounds when feeding? • Any irritability or tiredness with feeding? • Does infant seem fatigued during feeding; does infant sweat or turn blue around the lips or face while feeding? • Ask about spit up concerns; can caregivers estimate volume? – Happy spitter vs forceful reflux or emesis – Any arching of the back? Any apparent pain? – Ask if infant or child appears hungry immediately afterwards – Any blood or bile (dark green) in spit up/emesis?

(continued)

Table 20.2 (continued)

Stool history	• Frequency of stool • Consistency or characteristics of stool – Any mucus or stringy stool? – Any blood in the stool? – Any difficulty with passing stool? – Color of stool? • If concerns about constipation brought up: How long in between bowel movements? What is consistency of stool when infant/child does have a bowel movement? Any apparent straining or pain? • Any use of over-the-counter laxatives or stimulant medication for stooling? • Any need for other intervention to help infant or child stool? • If having diarrhea, any environmental exposures or sick contacts? If so, onset and duration of diarrhea?
Environmental and behavioral feeding practices	• Do caregivers have to wake infant to feed? What hunger cues does infant show? • Any oral aversions or is child a picky eater? What foods are difficult to get child to eat? • What is the structure of mealtimes? Sitting at table? Any use of TV or tablets (or other distractions) during mealtimes? • How long does it take to feed? • Any food restrictions for religious or personal preferences?
Prenatal/perinatal history	• Was infant born full term? If premature, how early? • Was infant born AGA (or SGA, LGA)? • Did infant pass stool before 24 hours of life? Any other stooling concerns in infancy? • Any maternal health concerns (including diabetes, iron-deficiency anemia, infections, eclampsia or preeclampsia, etc.)? • Any perinatal complications?
Developmental history	• Is infant meeting developmental milestones? • If child, did they meet all milestones on time? • Any milestone regression?
Family history	• Any siblings? Did siblings have difficulty with weight gain? • What is mother's height and father's height? (Can measure if biological parents present and use this to determine mid-parental height when appropriate) • Any history of GI, heart, renal, lung, etc. disease?
Social history	• Who all lives in home with infant, child? Who is the extended family or support system? • Besides the primary caregivers, does anyone else prepare formula bottles or meals? • Any concerns for safety or Well-being at home? • Do caregivers rely on governmental support [special supplemental nutrition program for women, infants, and children (WIC)] for formula? Any difficulty in the last week or month getting food the family needs?
Previous workup or outpatient management	• How long has infant or child had concern for poor weight? • When was it first noticed? • What workup (if any) has been done? (Labs/imaging; formula changes, etc.) • What changes have been made to breast feeding, formula, mealtimes? • What other changes or trials have the PCP or outpatient provider recommended?

Physical Exam

The general approach to physical examination for an infant or child with weight-faltering is to assess overall development and look for clues that may point towards potential causes of malnutrition. It is helpful to think about the differential as you go through the exam. Most infants with weight-faltering are well-appearing, but early clues to genetic or syndromic conditions can be found with a thorough exam.

A weight-faltering exam is very similar to a newborn exam or a comprehensive exam of an infant or child (see Table 20.3). Performing a thorough head-to-toe exam will keep exam techniques consistent.

Table 20.3 Weight-faltering exam

Body system	What to assess	Possible findings
Head	Head circumference, overall shape; palpate suture lines; assess fontanelle position and size	Microcephaly or macrocephaly; positional plagiocephaly; overriding sutures, craniosynostosis; bulging or sunken fontanelle; small or very wide fontanelle
Ears, eyes, nose	Eye and ear placement and spacing, visual tracking, nasal bridge, philtrum	Hyper- or hypotelorism; epicanthal folds; nasal congestion, nasal polyps or other obstruction; low-set ears; ear pits or tags
Mouth, throat	Visual internal and external inspection, jaw placement; palpate hard palate; assess strength of suck, lip and tongue movement while feeding	Micrognathia; tongue or lip tie; uncoordinated or weak suck; cleft lip and/or palate; bruising or tears; enanthema
Neck	Range of motion, palpation	Torticollis; lymphadenopathy
Chest	Visual inspection of rate and effort of breathing, auscultation	Tachypnea or retractions (other signs of increased work); wheezing; diminished aeration; crackles
Cardiac	Auscultate; palpate pulses: compare left-to-right (upper) and upper-to-lower extremity symmetry; capillary refill, general color, and appearance of extremities	Cyanosis; murmur; asymmetric, delayed, or weak pulses; poor perfusion including delayed capillary refill or mottling
Abdomen	Auscultate, palpate	Distension, hernia, organomegaly, masses
Genitourinary	Visual inspection; palpate testicle location bilaterally	Virilization or ambiguity; undescended testicle
Skin	Visual inspection	Bruising; rashes
Musculoskeletal	Range of motion, visual inspection, palpation of joints	Limb deformities or length discrepancy; joint swelling; tenderness to palpation of muscles or joints
Neuro	Cranial nerves, muscle tone and strength, reflexes, sensation, gross motor milestones	Hypo- or hypertonia, weakness, diminished or increased reflexes, calf muscle pseudohypertrophy

Laboratory and Imaging Assessment or Workup

Studies have shown that routine laboratory or imaging workup is positive in less than 2% of cases where an underlying organic or pathologic condition is the cause of weight-faltering in infants and children. Additionally, the cause of malnutrition is almost always recognized from the history and physical examination. Extensive screening or routine lab testing is not needed in most infants and children with weight-faltering. When the history or physical exam is suggestive of an underlying disease, or if an infant or child without these indications fails to gain weight or improve as expected over time, a tiered and targeted approach can be undertaken. Utilize all prior testing from previous healthcare encounters, including state-mandated newborn screens that cover critical congenital and genetic conditions. As recommended laboratory or imaging evaluation will depend on specific findings in history, review of systems (ROS), and physical exam, the recommendations and considerations for this evaluation are listed in Table 20.4 with corresponding differential diagnosis considerations.

Table 20.4 Key differential diagnosis (etiologies) with history, ROS, and physical exam features that may or may not be present; and evaluation and management considerations

Inadequate oral intake			
Etiologies	History and ROS	Physical exam	Evaluation or management
Breastfeeding difficulties	Maternal description or uncovered with lactation consultant; poor latch, suck, transfer of milk; milk supply concerns	Tongue or lip tie, weak suck, cleft lip and/or palate	Lactation consultation
Mechanical feeding difficulties (e.g., cleft lip or palate; other oromotor dysfunction)	Difficulty with latch or with bottle feeding; excessive noise (air, gurgling) with feeding; milk dribbling out of mouth in excess when feeding		Evaluation by OT or speech; may need enteral tube feeding for all or part of nutritional intake
Insufficient volumes offered (per feeding or cumulative throughout the day) or taken	Compare to estimated caloric need for age (Table 20.5); for newborns and young infants, skipping nighttime feeds		See management section for more details; consider evaluation for nutritional deficiency including vitamins or iron-deficiency anemia; likely will need multivitamin or specific vitamin or iron replacement

Table 20.4 (continued)

Inadequate oral intake			
Etiologies	History and ROS	Physical exam	Evaluation or management
Incorrect formula mixing	Typically excess free water; may also have more powdered formula than needed leading to higher concentration formula; compare reported mixing with formula instructions (most common is 2 oz. of water with 1 scoop of formula)		Higher likelihood of electrolyte imbalances, may consider chemistry panel
Excessive low-calorie intake (juice, pop/soda, water) or milk intake	Large volumes before or in place of meals or nutritious snacks; for children >12 months, recommend less than 24 oz. of milk in 24 hours		If excessive cow's milk intake, consider evaluation for anemia (hemoglobin)
Food insecurity	Consider use of USDA food insecurity survey or other validated survey or questionnaire		Social work consultation
Neglect or abuse	Look for clues in history; may have information from social work or PCP that will raise concerns; no outpatient visits or poor follow-up raises concerns	Overall appearance and hygiene; bruising, musculoskeletal tenderness, refusal to bear weight or use limbs	Social work consultation; consider skeletal survey, possible CT head if concern for non-accidental trauma
Behavior-related feeding issues (oral aversion, texture sensitivity, picky eater)	Refusing nipple/bottle or food in general; pushing food or utensil with tongue; refusal of certain food types; history of "grazing" instead of mealtimes		Consider feeding clinic if available (complex care needs, behavioral treatment); may recommend caregivers keep food diary
Gastroesophageal reflux	Common in infants and not always cause for concern, but can become problematic if losing substantial volume more frequently or over long period of time; sometimes related to overfeeding: Ask about volume and timing of feeds, reflux precautions taken		If signs of severe dehydration, may consider chemistry panel *Severe reflux can be seen in conditions related to cow's milk allergy including allergic eosinophilic gastrointestinal disorders and dietary protein-induced gastroenteropathy

(continued)

Table 20.4 (continued)

Inadequate oral intake			
Etiologies	History and ROS	Physical exam	Evaluation or management
Pyloric stenosis	Forceful emesis; often infant is hungry immediately after emesis; typical age range 3–5 weeks and is rare >12 weeks; more common in first-born and male infants	Olive-shaped mass palpated in epigastric region (rare finding, but more commonly felt when infant has just fed or is in prone position)	Abdominal ultrasound to assess pylorus muscle; if emesis long-standing or signs of severe dehydration, may consider chemistry panel; if pyloric stenosis confirmed, will need surgical consultation and intervention
Increased intracranial pressure	Alteration in consciousness or level of sleepiness; may have correlating history of trauma or fever; vomiting without other viral symptoms; may complain of headache or vision changes if older child	Altered mental status on exam; cranial nerve palsy; optic disc edema; may have bulging Fontanelle; may have macrocephaly	Initial stabilization with consideration of airway, breathing, circulation; head imaging with either CT or MRI
Malrotation +/– volvulus, other obstruction	Vomiting that is persistent or severe, consider obstruction (volvulus) with bilious emesis	Abdominal pain, distension; palpable mass; high-pitched or absent bowel sounds	If concern for volvulus or other obstruction is high: Emergent surgical consultation, obtain X-ray of the abdomen; may consider ultrasound of the abdomen if less convincing of obstruction and more stable

Inadequate nutrient absorption (malabsorption) or utilization			
Etiologies	History and ROS	Physical exam	Evaluation or management
Cystic fibrosis (CF)	Infants or children with CF may present only with GI-related (malabsorption) symptoms; review newborn screening results (screening is done only for most common mutations, a negative newborn screen does not entirely rule out CF). See Chap. 17	Nasal polyps; clubbing (chronic finding); lung findings more likely in older children or more advanced disease: Adventitious lung sounds including wheezing, crackles, rhonchi	Sweat chloride testing; potentially additional genetic testing as directed by pulmonologist with expertise in treating cystic fibrosis

Table 20.4 (continued)

Inadequate nutrient absorption (malabsorption) or utilization			
Etiologies	History and ROS	Physical exam	Evaluation or management
Chronic gastrointestinal conditions (celiac disease, inflammatory bowel disease)	See Chap. 10 for inflammatory bowel disease Celiac classically presents between 6 and 24 months of age after introduction of gluten into diet; may have chronic diarrhea, abdominal distension, and pain; may have vomiting Children with symptomatic celiac often have delayed linear growth	Nasal or oral ulcers, perianal ulcers, or skin tags; with inflammatory bowel disease may see rashes including pyoderma gangrenosum; with celiac, dermatitis herpetiformis	For celiac screening, both TTG and IgA (must be on gluten-containing diet); fecal calprotectin, inflammatory markers; consultation with gastrointestinal specialist for possible upper endoscopy or colonoscopy
Infectious diarrhea	Watery loose stool; may have bloody diarrhea; often frequent or large-volume loss	May have abdominal pain	If unclear etiology, protracted course, or if bloody diarrhea, a stool culture, or PCR panel can be helpful diagnostically
Milk protein allergy, sensitivity or intolerance → FPIES (food protein-induced enterocolitis syndrome) → Food protein-induced proctitis/proctocolitis → FPE (food protein-induced enteropathy)	Non-IgE mediated reactions present with subtle or delayed gastrointestinal symptoms (except in acute cases of FPIES); GER, colic, or constipation may be one of these subtle findings Eosinophilic GI disorders may be mixed IgE and non-IgE reaction IgE-mediated reactions include anaphylaxis, urticaria and angioedema, immediate oral or GI reactions	May have related atopic dermatitis/eczema	Non-IgE mediated testing is very limited IgE-mediated testing should be done in coordination with allergy/immunology consultation

(continued)

Table 20.4 (continued)

Inadequate nutrient absorption (malabsorption) or utilization			
Etiologies	History and ROS	Physical exam	Evaluation or management
Other food allergy or intolerance	May have reflux or vomiting with particular foods; may develop food aversion; may develop urticaria or anaphylactic reaction	May have related atopic dermatitis/ eczema	Allergy testing directed by allergy/immunology consultation; helpful to direct caregivers to keep food diary and related reactions if less subtle findings
Inborn errors of metabolism	Poor feeding, irritability, vomiting, diarrhea, dehydration; developmental delay or regression; onset with change in diet (introduction of protein or carbohydrate); change that coincides with sleeping through the night as infant; older child may have unusual dietary preferences including aversion to carbohydrate or protein; history of sudden infant death in family without explanation; history of consanguinity; review newborn screen	Temperature instability, apnea; ill-appearance may or may not be present	May have clinical decompensation out of proportion to illness presentation; always consider in infants presenting with sepsis-like picture; broad workup can include glucose, chemistry panel, blood gas, lactate and ammonia; more directed testing with consultation of geneticist with specialization in metabolic disease if able

Increased metabolic demand (increased energy requirement)			
Etiologies	History and ROS	Physical exam	Evaluation or management
Congenital heart disease	Fatigue ("wearing out" or becoming sleepy) with feeds; reports of color change or sweating with feeds	Murmur; weak or asymmetric femoral pulses, temporal delay between brachial and femoral pulses; cyanosis	Obtain four-point blood pressure readings, echocardiogram, chest X-ray; consider consultation with cardiology

Table 20.4 (continued)

Increased metabolic demand (increased energy requirement)			
Etiologies	History and ROS	Physical exam	Evaluation or management
Chronic lung disease of prematurity	Correlating history of prematurity and initial or prolonged oxygen requirement; ongoing report of fast breathing or increased effort with breathing may be present or worsen with illness	Tachypnea or respiratory distress	Consider chest X-ray evaluation; consultation with pulmonary
Congenital and/or chronic infections (TORCH, HIV, tuberculosis)	Maternal illness, poor maternal weight gain during pregnancy, fetal anomalies identified during ultrasound	Rashes, low birth weight, microcephaly, eye findings, intracranial calcifications, cardiac abnormalities	Serologic testing with guidance of infectious disease consultation
Endocrine disease (e.g., hyper- or hypothyroidism, growth hormone deficiency, diseases or syndromes affecting the pituitary gland and hormones)	Growth-faltering that is isolated to linear growth with preserved weight along expected percentiles	Appearance of short stature; large or persistently open anterior fontanelle; micro- or macrocephaly	Recommend consultation with endocrinology; consider obtaining TSH, free T4; some hormone testing is less helpful in young infants, defer most testing to specialist recommendation
Renal disease or renal failure	Poor weight gain may be initial sign of renal disease; may have vague pain, fevers or renal tract infections in history; nocturia if child has been potty-trained	May have abdominal mass or pain, edema; hypertension	Chemistry panel, urinalysis; consider renal ultrasound and nephrology consultation
Genetic disorders or etiologies related to syndromic conditions (trisomy 21, turner, Russell-silver)	Family history concerning for specific diseases	Syndromic facies, dysmorphic features, neurocognitive or developmental delay	If not previously diagnosed, genetic testing with consultation to a geneticist; may need additional evaluation of organs (heart, eyes, kidneys, etc.) if a genetic or syndromic condition is suspected

(continued)

Table 20.4 (continued)

Increased metabolic demand (increased energy requirement)			
Etiologies	History and ROS	Physical exam	Evaluation or management
Malignancy	Variable depending on primary malignancy. Fever, fatigue, night sweats, weight loss, pain, swelling or lumps, skin changes, easy bleeding, or bruising	Variable depending on primary malignancy. Lymphadenopathy, swelling, hepato-splenomegaly, abdominal masses, etc.	Recommend consultation with oncology chemistry panel, CBC; LDH, uric acidic; possibly alpha-fetoprotein, urinary testing such as VMA Imaging studies, lumbar puncture, PET scans

Red Flags as an Exception

A small subset of patients with weight-faltering may present with "red flag" symptoms such as altered mental status, lethargy, hypothermia or temperature instability, bradycardia, or hypotension. In these patients, a broad laboratory workup evaluating for infectious and metabolic etiologies is indicated, and these patients should be medically stabilized prior to a more dedicated consideration of the etiology of their poor weight gain.

Key Differential Diagnosis

The differential diagnosis for weight-faltering in infants and children is broad. Most cases in infants and children are due to inadequate nutritional intake which can have multiple contributing factors. Underlying disease or pathologic causes occur less commonly and can often be identified from elements of the history, review of systems, and physical examination. Table 20.4 will help build "illness scripts" by relating various etiologies for weight-faltering with corresponding portions of the history, review of systems, and physical exam. Additionally, we offer considerations in the evaluation or management of these etiologies.

Management

Most patients with poor weight gain in infancy or childhood can be diagnosed and managed in the outpatient clinical setting. Considerations for consultation, specialty referral, and emergency department evaluation or inpatient admission are included in the following section.

Outpatient

On first discovery or presentation of poor weight gain, a thorough history and physical examination should be conducted to determine a likely underlying etiology. During this evaluation, assess for medical stability, concern for abuse, or concern for underlying medical etiology requiring workup that would require referral to an emergency department or direct admission to an inpatient unit. If not such concerns, the following evaluation and management can be done during the clinic visit:

Nutritional and Behavioral Evaluation and Management

- Calculate the 24-h goal volume intake based on caloric needs (see Table 20.5)
- Infant:
  - Review feeding method and correct formula preparation, if applicable
  - Review and document feeding plan with volumes and frequency, including nighttime feeds when necessary
  - Consider lactation counseling in clinic, if possible, or with outside consultant
  - Consider formula supplementation as indicated for breastfeeding mothers
  - Consider fortification of breast milk or increased caloric content of formula to 22 or 24 kcal/oz. if estimated volume intake is below goal
  - Consider hydrolyzed or amino acid-based formula if established diagnosis of milk-protein intolerance or if infant is showing signs of intolerance and is at high-risk of allergy/atopy
- Child:
  - Provide instructions on high-calorie food options and best practices for water and milk intake [limit juice; limit milk intake to less than 24 oz. (700 mL) per 24 h]; recommend routine mealtimes: 3 meals per day with 1–2 snacks per day
- Infant and child:
  - Recommend caregivers maintain feeding log/diary and follow-up in 1 week or earlier if indicated

Table 20.5 Caloric need and target growth rates for age

[a]Caloric need and target growth rates for age	
1–3 month	110 kcal/kg/day with goal 30 g/day weight gain
3–6 months	95 kcal/kg/day with goal 20 g/day weight gain
6–12 months	80 kcal/kg/day with goal 11–15 g/day weight gain
[a]This does not include "catch-up" growth requirements and goals for infants who are undernourished nor does it account for increased caloric needs for acute or chronic illness; these infants may need energy in range of 150–180 kcal/kg/day with goals up to 50–60 g/day weight gain	
12–24 months	80–84 kcal/kg/day with goal growth rate depicted by WHO growth chart

With the next follow-up weight check, review weight gain and whether child meets indications for emergency department referral or inpatient admission. If still not meeting ED or inpatient referral parameters and weight gain is inadequate:

- Review feeding log/diary and calculate intake as percentage (%) of goal
- If able, observe feed in clinic to review technique and/or uncover signs of concern; may consider OT/speech referral
- Fortify breast milk or formula to 24 kcal/oz. if not previously done
- For older children: add Pediasure to meals
- Consideration for nutrition consult, referral to feeding clinic; consider speech or OT referrals as indicated
- If underlying medical disorder now suspected and patient is stable, include evaluation or referral to subspecialists as indicated
- Follow-up in 1 week or earlier if indicated

Diagnostic Evaluation

- Verify normal newborn screen (NBS) results
- Pursue diagnostic studies as indicated from thorough review of history and physical examination (Section on Labs and Imaging, also Table 20.4 "Key Differential Diagnoses")

When to refer a patient for emergency evaluation:

1. Ill-appearance or concern for mental status (poor interaction on exam, appearing sleepy, etc.)
2. Concern for severe dehydration or electrolyte abnormalities
3. Concern for underlying medical disorder requiring prompt medical or surgical evaluation
4. Concern for abuse

When to consider inpatient admission:

1. Severe malnutrition with concern for deterioration
2. Suspected medical disorder requiring inpatient evaluation; this may include the coordination of multiple subspecialists and need for a more extensive laboratory or imaging workup
3. Suspected neglect requiring inpatient evaluation and support
4. Failed outpatient management or concern for appropriateness of outpatient management

   (a) Failure of outpatient management: weight gain persistently <60% of goal despite adherence to feeding and behavioral interventions or insufficient volume intake despite interventions over multiple clinic visits.
   (b) Considerations include caregiver's ability to maintain close follow-up appointments, proximity to clinic, access to resources including food/formula, concern for caregiver–child interaction that may be better monitored inpatient

Inpatient

Regardless of reason for admission, it is essential to repeat a thorough history and physical examination to determine any underlying etiologies for weight-faltering. If there is concern for medical instability, it is important to stabilize and manage these concerns as they present. Additional evaluation and management will depend on the cause for instability or on the suspected underlying etiology. Suggestions are in Table 20.4.

- Calculate 24-h goal volume intake based on caloric needs (see table in outpatient management section)
- Place orders for strict intake/output monitoring and calorie counts if on solid food diet
- Diagnostic evaluation as indicated by H&P assessment
- Consult: nutrition, OT or speech for feeding evaluation, lactation if breastfeeding, and Social Work (SW) with full psychosocial assessment

Goals of admission will depend on the rationale behind admission. Discharge criteria generally include:

- Medical stability
- If diagnostic workup initiated, then all available results considered safe for discharge or, if pending workup, it can be followed up outpatient by the PCP or by the appropriate specialty consultant
- Demonstration of appropriate volume, fluid, and/or caloric intake with weight stable or increased or demonstration of tolerance of supplemental nutritional intake, which may include nasogastric tube feeding (other enteral tube feeding)
- Caregiver education regarding feeding regimen, changes, follow-up
- Caregiver interaction and care appropriate; and all concerns adequately addressed
- PCP follow-up plan in place prior to discharge, including any specialty referrals addressed

Anticipatory Guidance (Caregivers/Families)

As weight-faltering often develops over time, the return to adequate intake and weight gain may also take time, so with these clinical encounters it is important to emphasize high-quality anticipatory guidance so families understand expectations for evaluation, follow-up, and when they need to return to care.

A few key points or answers to commonly asked questions to emphasize:

1. Follow all instructions for recommended feeding regimens, including calorie concentrations (formula) or calorie supplementation. Infants with weight-faltering should feed at least every 3 h or 8 times per day. This may require families to restart nighttime feeds, which can be a challenging adjustment.
2. If an underlying pathologic condition or genetic syndrome is indicated by history or exam and workup was initiated in the outpatient or inpatient setting, it

often does take time for a final diagnosis to be made, which can be frustrating for caregivers. Sharing this expectation at the start of a workup may help alleviate this frustration.

3. There are no "easy fixes" for normal infant reflux except emphasizing good reflux precautions such as frequent burping, avoidance of overfeeding, and keeping an infant upright for 20–30 min after feeding. There are also few medications used in pediatrics to help "stimulate an appetite." These medications are used sparingly and have few studies to support their use, particularly in the infant population.

Families should expect to follow-up in the clinic for weight check-ins more often than they would normally for other well child care. Additional appointments should be made:

- If their child is not meeting their intake goal for more than 1–2 days at a time
- If their child is not having symptomatic improvement after an intervention

Families should seek medical care at an emergency department for more serious weight-faltering related concerns:

- Their infant is refusing all intake for more than 2–3 feeds
- For any hydration concerns such as less than 3 wet diapers per 24-h period
- For alteration in level of awareness or arousal

Application Exercises

A 1-month-old female infant, born at term, is admitted to the general pediatric floor for weight-faltering. At her well child check, her pediatrician noticed that she has still not surpassed her birthweight. On admission, she weighs 2.9 kg, she was 3.1 kg at birth. She is exclusively formula-fed.

After a thorough history and physical exam, you determine that her weight-faltering is most likely due to insufficient caloric intake. The resident team asks you to calculate this infant's goal intake of 20 kcal/ounce formula and feeding schedule for catch-up weight gain.

Steps for calculation/Answer:

1. Catch-up weight gain in the infant period: 120 kcal/kg/day
2. Infants of this age should feed at least every 3 h
3. 120 kcal/kg/day × 2.9 kg = 348 kcal/day
4. $\frac{348\,\text{kcal/day}}{20\,\text{kcal/oz.}} = 17.4\text{ oz./day}$
5. 17.4 oz./day × 30 mL/oz. = 522 mL/day
6. $\frac{522\,\text{mL/day}}{8\,\text{feeds/day}} = \sim 65\text{ mL/feed every 3 h}$

A 5-month-old male infant is admitted to the hospital pediatric service for weight-faltering. He has not gained weight in 2 months resulting in a decrease in weight percentile from the 65th to fifth percentile. He frequently spits up leading to presumed insufficient intake and his pediatrician has already fortified his formula to 22 kcal/oz. Current weight is 5.2 kg. Calculate the goal intake of 22 kcal/oz. formula for catch-up growth in this infant.

Steps for calculation/Answer:

1. Catch-up weight gain in the infant period: 120 kcal/kg/day
2. Infants of this age should feed every 3 h
3. 120 kcal/kg/day × 5.2 kg = 624 kcal/day
4. 624 kcal/day/22 kcal/oz. = 28.4 oz./day
5. 28.4 oz./day × 30 mL/oz. = 851 mL/day
6. 851 mL/day/8 feeds/day = ~105 mL/feed every 3 h

Further Reading

Homan GJ. Failure to thrive: a practical guide. Am Fam Physician. 2016;94(4):295–9.

Jaffe AC. Failure to thrive: current clinical concepts. Pediatr Rev. 2011;32(3):100–7. https://doi.org/10.1542/pir.32-3-100.

Larson-Nath C, Biank VF. Clinical review of failure to thrive in pediatric patients. Pediatr Ann. 2016;45(2):e46–9. https://doi.org/10.3928/00904481-20160114-01.

Schwartz ID. Failure to thrive: an old nemesis in the new millennium. Pediatr Rev. 2000;21(8):257–64. https://doi.org/10.1542/pir.21-8-257.

Tang MN, Adolphe S, Rogers SR, Frank DA. Failure to thrive or growth faltering: medical, developmental/behavioral, nutritional, and social dimensions. Pediatr Rev. 2021;42(11):590–603. https://doi.org/10.1542/pir.2020-001883.

Chapter 21
Fever of Unknown Origin

Chinaemerem Agbakwuru and Michael E. Watson Jr.

Background

Human body temperature is regulated through a complex physiologic feedback loop that maintains normal core body temperature within a relatively narrow window for optimal biochemical functioning. The commonly accepted "normal" human axillary temperature is 98.6 °F (37.0 °C), although temperatures can vary slightly from person to person, or even by time of day. Fever can be seen as an elevation in core body temperature above the normal setpoint as a response to some pathologic process. For most healthy children and adults, a single oral temperature measured >101.0 °F (38.3 °C) constitutes a fever. For infants 0–28 days of life, a rectal temperature >100.4 °F (38 °C) is sufficient for fever. For those considered immunocompromised (e.g., neutropenia), a lower temperature threshold of >100.4 °F (38.0 °C) measured orally at least twice over a 1-h period, is typically considered evidence of a fever warranting further evaluation.

In children, fever is a very common cause for seeking medical care, and acute febrile illnesses make up approximately one-quarter to one-third of outpatient pediatric clinic, urgent care, and emergency department visits. Most febrile illnesses due to common childhood infections last for only a few days. There are some infections, however, where fever may be prolonged and this may be a clue to the diagnosis. Fever of Unknown Origin (FUO) in children is generally defined as a prolonged febrile illness with a temperature >38.3 °C measured on multiple occasions and

C. Agbakwuru
Division of Pediatric Hospital Medicine, Department of Pediatrics, University of Michigan, Ann Arbor, MI, USA

M. E. Watson Jr. (✉)
Divisions of Pediatric Hospital Medicine and Pediatric Infectious Diseases, Department of Pediatrics, University of Michigan, Ann Arbor, MI, USA
e-mail: mewats@med.umich.edu

N. Liao et al. (eds.), *Pediatric Rotations*,
https://doi.org/10.1007/978-3-031-59873-9_21

often present for greater than 8–14 days duration (there is no single standard definition). In addition, an FUO evaluation requires that there is no apparent fever source identified despite careful history taking, physical exam, and preliminary lab studies to exclude other causes of fever.

Fever resolves in approximately 50% of children without identification of a specific cause. For this reason, the diagnosis and management of FUO in children can typically be done in a logical, stepwise approach, often with initial outpatient evaluation to gather information and basic screening labs. Most children evaluated as an outpatient for seemingly prolonged fever are likely to have had multiple, unrelated, sequential, self-limited viral infections. Some children will have recovered and are afebrile and asymptomatic at the time of evaluation. A minority of children will go on to be diagnosed with a serious bacterial infection, malignancy, or rheumatologic disease.

An important distinction from FUO is the term "Fever without a Source" (FWS) which can be used to describe infants and young children with fever of unknown etiology of only a few days duration, and these patients may appear more ill and require more urgent evaluation than patients meeting the usual prolonged duration of FUO. Practically speaking, most children with FWS should be evaluated by at least 5–7 days of persistent fever to consider the possibility of time-sensitive diagnoses such as Kawasaki disease (KD) where treatment with intravenous immunoglobulin by the tenth day of illness is important to reduce the risk of coronary artery complications.

Relevant History Elements to Address

Whether the patient is being evaluated initially in the outpatient clinic or within the inpatient setting, several questions can help provide clues to the etiology of pediatric FWS/FUO:

How Were the Temperatures Measured?

Where did you measure the temperature? Were the temperatures taken by tympanic readings, forehead scans, oral, axillary, or rectal measurements?

The intention of taking a reading is to measure the core body temperature, and rectal temperatures approximate this most closely; most experts recommend that rectal temperatures should be the standard for measuring temperature and diagnosing fever in infants under 3 months of age. Tympanic and oral measurements are less accurate than rectal, and axillary and temporal scans are the least accurate methods of measurement. Having an accurate understanding of how caregivers are measuring temperatures is important as some caregivers may misunderstand what defines a fever, how to measure fevers, and normal temperature variations over the course of a day. In addition, caregivers are sometimes told to add 1–2 °F to the measured temperature as a corrective factor on to temperatures measured in the axilla to better approximate the core temperature which may cloud the evaluation of the febrile child.

What are the Fever Characteristics?

Can the caregivers describe the fever pattern over the course of a day? Does the temperature always remain elevated above normal, or does the fever intermittently resolve either spontaneously or with medication?

The temporal pattern and magnitude of fevers can be helpful to investigate the etiology of fevers. Questions should be asked about the pattern of fevers and whether they occur once daily, multiple times a day, once every few days, or continuously. Fevers are considered *intermittent* when the temperature elevation occurs and then body temperature returns to the normal baseline at least once daily. Fevers that fluctuate, but the temperature always remains above the baseline are called *remittent*. Fevers considered *sustained* are those with minimal fluctuation but remain above the baseline. It is important to confirm when there are fever-free days as this would restart the count on days of continuous fever. Establishing the pattern of fevers may be critical to making an FUO diagnosis, and one of the more important recommendations practitioners can make to family members is to keep a fever diary. A fever diary may be just a calendar in which caregivers record days with fevers and associated symptoms (e.g., fatigue, rash, abdominal pain, mouth ulcers, adenopathy). Having written or electronic documentation can provide more objective examination of the fever pattern than simple memory recall. A fever diary may be very helpful to distinguish a timeframe for periodic or recurrent fevers, some of which may have specific time intervals that can be diagnostic clues.

Certain conditions have more regular and defined intervals between fever episodes. For example, malaria due to infection with *Plasmodium falciparum* may cause fever after 72-h intervals, whereas malaria due to *P. vivax* may cause fever after 48-h intervals. Conditions referred to as periodic fever syndromes occur in clusters of fevers that last 3–5 days recurring on a cycle with roughly specific time periods. For example, the condition periodic fever with aphthous stomatitis, pharyngitis, and adenitis (PFAPA) is a periodic fever condition that occurs every 3–8 weeks. Likewise, the condition cyclic neutropenia is a condition with recurrent severe neutropenia occurring about every 21 days with fevers, mouth sores, and other evidence of infections.

What Potential Exposures to Infectious Agents Exist in the Home and Social Environments?

Are there known sick contacts at home with siblings or caregivers, in the school or daycare environments?

Daycare, preschool, and early grade school years are all times of repeated exposures to other children with viral infections and young children frequently become infected with viral infections several times per year during these years. Having older siblings attending childcare or school with other children may be a risk for infections in younger siblings.

Ask caregivers about exposures to animals, including household pets (e.g., dogs, cats, birds, reptiles, fish), farm animals giving birth (e.g., cattle, lambs), any recreational activities (e.g., hunting, hiking, caving, camping), or household contacts with occupational exposures to animals (e.g., veterinarians or animal technicians).

Any Family History of Infections, Autoimmune Conditions, Inflammatory Bowel Disease, or Malignancy at a Young Age?

A family history of recurrent and invasive infections in childhood could suggest a primary immunodeficiency condition (e.g., chronic granulomatous disease, hyper IgM syndrome, severe combined immunodeficiency). Children with family members with collagen vascular disease, juvenile idiopathic arthritis (JIA), systemic lupus erythematosus (SLE), inflammatory bowel disease (IBD), or a history of malignancy at a young age may be associated with increased risk of these conditions presenting as fevers.

What is the Family Background or Ethnicity?

With regard to certain periodic fever syndromes, the ethnicity of the patient and their family is important and should be explored. Some periodic fever syndromes are hereditary and have an association with certain ethnic groups, such as familial Mediterranean fever (FMF) which may genetically carry in families with Armenian, Arab, Turkish, and Sephardic Jewish ancestry. The hyper IgD syndrome is associated with families with Dutch and French background. Another condition termed tumor necrosis factor receptor-associated periodic fever syndrome (TRAPS) is more common in families of Irish and Scottish descent.

Has There Been Any Ingestion of Raw Meat, Fish, or Unpasteurized Milk?

Infections such as yersiniosis, brucellosis, listeriosis, *Mycobacterium bovis*, giardiasis, or other enteric pathogens, may be associated with fever, usually in association with gastrointestinal symptoms. Ingestion of dirt, also called pica, may be a source of exposure to parasites such as *Toxocara canis*, *Toxocara cati*, or *Toxoplasma gondii* infection.

Has There Been a Travel History to Other Regions, Other Countries, Including Past Residences in Those Locations?

Travel-associated infections may include malaria, endemic fungal infections (e.g., histoplasmosis, blastomycosis, coccidioidomycosis), typhoid fever due to *Salmonella typhi* infection, and tuberculosis. The travel history should include more than the past few months and some infections such as malaria could potentially present years after travel to an endemic area. Travel exposures should include living accommodations, activities, dietary practices, and whether any antimicrobial prophylaxis or travel vaccines were utilized.

What is the Home Water Supply?

Questions should be asked with regard to drinking water sources, including whether water is city-supplied or private well water in more rural areas. Private well water should be regularly tested for potential infectious agents or toxins in the groundwater supply. Home well water may be contaminated with giardia, enteric bacterial pathogens, or other substances that could cause unexplained fever and illness.

What Other Medical Conditions Exist and What Medications are Used?

Caregivers of pediatric FUO patients should be asked about any other medical conditions the patient may have and what medications they may be given, including prescription medications, over-the-counter medications, illicit and recreational drugs, and home remedies tried. Some medications are more likely than others to cause fevers as an adverse effect. Antibiotics (e.g., penicillins, cephalosporins, sulfonamides), antiepileptics (e.g., phenytoin, carbamazepine), anti-arrhythmics (e.g., quinidine, procainamide), and anti-hypertensives (e.g., hydralazine) are common causes of drug fevers. Some clues to possible drug fever include a relatively well overall appearance, a low to normal heart rate despite fever onset (i.e., a relative bradycardia with regard to the temperature), inflammatory markers such as c-reactive protein (CRP) and erythrocyte sedimentation rate (ESR) are usually not elevated in cases of drug fever, and elevation of the relative and absolute eosinophil count.

Etiology and Differential Diagnosis of Pediatric FUO

"When you hear hooves, think horses, not zebras." *A key consideration in the evaluation of pediatric FUO is that the underlying etiology more often represents an unusual presentation of a common disease, rather than a common presentation of an unusual disease.* Infections account for approximately 40–60% of FUO in children. Common infectious causes of pediatric FUO (see Table 21.1) include common

Table 21.1 Common infectious causes of pediatric FUO

Condition	Etiology	Clues to diagnosis
Systemic viral infections	Infectious mononucleosis due to Epstein-Barr virus or cytomegalovirus, adenovirus, human herpes virus-6, human immunodeficiency virus, SARS-CoV-2	Fevers, fatigue, pharyngitis, lymphadenopathy, rashes, hepatosplenomegaly, known sick contacts or exposures
Urinary tract infection (UTI)	*Escherichia coli*, *Proteus* sp., *Klebsiella* sp., *Enterococcus* sp.	Fevers, abdominal pain, dysuria, urinary frequency, urinary urgency, chills, nausea, vomiting, foul-smelling urine, history of previous UTIs
Bone and joint infections	Occult osteomyelitis (*Staphylococcus aureus* most common in children), septic arthritis, *Kingella kingae* in young children	Fevers, limping, inability to tolerate weight-bearing, point-tenderness over bone
Enteric infection	Salmonella species, *Yersinia enterocolitica*, *Yersinia pseudotuberculosis*, *campylobacter jejuni*	Fevers, abdominal pain, diarrhea, bloody stools
Cat scratch fever	*Bartonella henselae*	Cat exposure, particularly kittens, fevers, lymphadenopathy, hepatosplenomegaly, papule at site of initial cat scratch
Respiratory tract infection	Sinusitis, pharyngitis, otitis media, mastoiditis, pneumonia	Fevers, cough, pain with swallowing, nasal congestion, tenderness over face and tenderness behind the ear, tachypnea, shortness of breath
Endemic fungal infection	Histoplasmosis, blastomycosis, coccidioidomycosis	Fevers, weight loss, night sweats, shortness of breath, tachypnea, lymphadenopathy, hepatosplenomegaly
Malaria	Plasmodium species	Recurrent fevers after every 48 h (*P. falciparum*) or after every 72 h (*P. vivax*), night sweats, headaches, myalgias, history of recent travel to malaria endemic area
Less common infections	Tuberculosis, brucellosis, syphilis, Lyme disease, subacute endocarditis	Fevers, weight loss, night sweats, shortness of breath, tachypnea, lymphadenopathy, hepatosplenomegaly, skin rashes, or ulcers

SARS-CoV-2 severe acute respiratory syndrome-associated coronavirus 2, *UTI* urinary tract infection

upper and lower respiratory tract infections, urinary tract infections, and systemic viral syndromes, including infectious mononucleosis due to Epstein-Barr virus (EBV) or cytomegalovirus (CMV). The most common single infectious disease reported in several case series of pediatric FUO patients is mononucleosis due to EBV; children and adolescents with EBV mononucleosis often have prolonged fever and illness duration in association with other symptoms of fatigue, pharyngitis, lymphadenopathy, and hepatosplenomegaly. Beyond EBV, another commonly encountered scenario is children with seemingly prolonged fevers who have unrecognized, sequential viral illnesses. Many common viral infections of childhood can have symptoms that may last 1–2 weeks and even healthy, immunocompetent children in preschool and daycare settings may have as many as 10–14 individual "colds" over the course of a year. To caregivers, it may seem that their child is always sick, but upon further exploration an important clue to sequential illnesses is when there may be short periods of fever and symptom-free time in between the sickness episodes.

Urinary tract infections are frequent causes of FUO and young children may not always report symptoms of dysuria, frequency, or costovertebral angle tenderness. Infants and young children with UTI may simply present with fever, poor feeding, and recurrent emesis. Additional FUO infections considerations include bone and joint infections with osteomyelitis, gastrointestinal infections with one of several enteric bacterial pathogens, cat scratch disease due to *Bartonella henselae* infection. Less common infectious causes of FUO include tuberculosis (TB), brucellosis, Lyme disease due to *Borrelia burgdorferi* infection, chronic sinusitis, and infection with human immunodeficiency virus (HIV).

Beyond infectious causes of FUO, there are several relatively common non-infectious causes of pediatric FUO (Table 21.2) which should be considered, including collagen vascular disease, malignancy, KD, IBD, drug fever, hyperthyroidism, factitious fever, or Munchausen syndrome by proxy, centrally mediated neurologic fever, a periodic fever syndrome, and Kikuchi-Fujimoto disease

Table 21.2 Common non-infectious causes of pediatric FUO

Periodic fever syndromes	PFAPA, familial Mediterranean fever, cyclic neutropenia, tumor necrosis factor receptor-associated periodic syndrome, hyper IgD syndrome
Collagen vascular disease	Juvenile idiopathic arthritis, systemic lupus erythematosus, juvenile dermatomyositis, sarcoidosis
Hyper-inflammatory conditions	KD, MIS-C, HLH
Cardiovascular	Pericarditis, myocardial infarction, deep vein thrombosis
Malignancy	Leukemia/lymphoma, neuroblastoma, osteosarcoma
GI	Crohn's disease, ulcerative colitis, pancreatitis, ischemic colitis
Drug fever	Antibiotics (i.e., penicillins, cephalosporins, sulfamethoxazole), antiepileptics (i.e., phenytoin), methylphenidate, ranitidine, atropine
Neurologic	Cerebrovascular infarcts, traumatic brain injury, seizures
Other conditions	Hyperthyroidism, factitious disorder (Munchausen by proxy)

HLH hemophagocytic lymphohistiocytosis, *KD* Kawasaki disease, *MIS-C* multisystem inflammatory syndrome in children, *PFAPA* periodic fever with aphthous ulcers, pharyngitis, and adenopathy

(histiocytic necrotizing lymphadenitis). While younger children in preschool and daycare are more likely to have FUO from infections, the incidence of autoimmune conditions increases in older children and adolescents. KD should be given consideration after several days of fever due to a need to diagnose KD and initiate treatment within 10 days of fever onset to reduce the risk of developing coronary artery aneurysms. Diagnosis of KD requires at least 5 days of fever, along with associated clinical signs of rash, non-purulent conjunctivitis, oral mucosa changes, cervical adenopathy, and swollen hands and feet. To help remember these features, use the mnemonic "CRASH and Burn" with *C*onjunctivitis, *R*ash, *A*denopathy, *S*trawberry tongue, *H*ands and feet changes and *Burn* with at least 5 days of fever. A recently recognized condition that has emerged since the onset of the COVID-19 pandemic is multisystem inflammatory syndrome in children (MIS-C). An important clue to possible MIS-C is that children with MIS-C typically have a history of infection or exposure with Severe Acute Respiratory Syndrome Coronavirus 2 (SARS-CoV-2) virus in the preceding 2–6 weeks, with an average of 4 weeks. A presentation of MIS-C requires prolonged fever >24 h, lab evidence of inflammation, and clinically significant illness requiring hospitalization with multiple organ systems (≥2) involved (e.g., cardiac, renal, respiratory, hematologic, gastrointestinal, dermatologic, or neurological). There may be significant overlap in the clinical presentations of pediatric patients with KD and MIS-C, so careful inquiry and testing for prior exposure to SARS-CoV-2 virus can be helpful. The definition of MIS-C has evolved over time since the onset of the pandemic, so checking for the most current diagnostic criteria with the Centers for Disease Control is useful (www.cdc.gov). See Chap. 28 Inflammatory Disorders for more information on KD and MIS-C.

Physical Exam Findings

A comprehensive physical exam is an important component in the evaluation of pediatric FUO.

- Examination of a growth chart can help detect trends of impaired weight gain, impaired linear growth or weight loss which may suggest possible chronic infection (e.g., tuberculosis, histoplasmosis), rheumatologic disease (e.g., juvenile idiopathic arthritis), malignancy, or inflammatory bowel disease.
- The overall appearance of the febrile child as irritable or toxic may suggest sepsis due to infection, meningitis, MIS-C, or KD.
- The finding of conjunctivitis may suggest KD, adenovirus, measles, or leptospirosis. A comprehensive eye exam with examination of the retina may identify papilledema, suggestive of increased intracranial pressure due to a possible infectious meningitis or encephalitis or intracranial mass. The eye finding of uveitis may be associated with tuberculosis, toxocariasis and sarcoidosis.
- Sinus tenderness or discharge may correlate with chronic sinusitis.
- The presence of pharyngitis may suggest many viral infections, including EBV or CMV infection, or could be a manifestation of PFAPA.

- A cardiac murmur, gallop, or friction rub may be associated with subacute bacterial endocarditis or pericarditis.
- Enlargement of the liver and spleen, or hepatosplenomegaly, may be associated with infection with one of several hepatitis viruses, HIV infection, EBV, CMV, among others.
- Lymphadenopathy of the cervical, supraclavicular, axillary, epitrochlear, and inguinal nodes should be examined for evidence of possible infection or malignancy.
- The presence of arthritis may suggest possible autoimmune disease with JIA, acute rheumatic fever, or possible underlying osteomyelitis and septic arthritis. Bony tenderness may correlate with osteomyelitis, leukemia, or other malignancy.

Laboratory Assessment and Imaging

The work-up of pediatric FUO has changed over the past several decades. Whereas previous evaluations were based primarily on traditional cultures and serology and were somewhat limited in what could be tested for, more modern-day evaluation of pediatric FUO often includes the use of highly sensitive and specific tests, both via molecular-based lab tests and more advanced imaging modalities. Given more sensitive and specific tests that can exclude many infectious etiologies, the proportion of undiagnosed pediatric FUO cases due to infections has decreased over time, whereas the proportion of those due to autoimmune/autoinflammatory conditions or considered idiopathic has risen. Importantly, the laboratory assessment of a child with FUO should be directed towards the most likely possible etiologies. A random and shotgun approach to ordering lab testing is rarely useful in making the diagnosis and can lead to unanticipated complications, with false positive results that may require additional testing and invasive procedures with potential for harm. Therefore, a logical and stepwise approach to performing a diagnostic evaluation is preferred.

In otherwise healthy-appearing children with a few days of fever and no obvious focus of infection by history and physical exam, initial screening labs might include a complete blood cell count and differential and a urinalysis. If these initial screening labs are normal, then observation for another 48 h may be appropriate. If fever persists longer than 7 days, re-evaluation for signs of KD or MIS-C may be indicated, including additional lab studies with inflammatory markers (i.e., ESR, CRP, ferritin levels), a complete metabolic panel including liver enzyme studies, along with blood and urine cultures. Screening for possible malignancy includes a blood smear, examining for atypical lymphocytes or blasts, and elevations in blood levels of lactate dehydrogenase (LDH), ferritin, and uric acid. Additional testing could be suggested by history and physical exam and could include specific testing for viral syndromes (e.g., EBV mononucleosis), bacterial infections (e.g., cat scratch disease, tuberculosis), stool testing for enteric pathogens (e.g., Salmonella), and possible endemic fungal infections (e.g., histoplasmosis, blastomyces, coccidiomycosis).

Initial imaging studies should include a 2-view chest X-ray to screen for pneumonia, lung infiltrates, mediastinal masses, or enlargement of the cardiac shadow.

Abdominal ultrasound may be obtained to screen for abnormal fluid collections concerning for intraabdominal abscess, masses, or pyelonephritis; ultrasound has advantages of avoiding radiation exposure, being fast and does not usually require sedation. Additional imaging studies may be suggested by history or physical exam and may include magnetic resonance imaging for bones to screen for osteomyelitis or malignancy, bone scan or positron emission tomography/computed tomography scans to screen for anatomic areas of hypermetabolism concerning for infection or malignancy. Additional discussion of lab and imaging studies is shown below (Table 21.3).

Table 21.3 Lab and imaging studies useful for evaluation of pediatric FUO

Complete blood cell count with differential	Leukopenia with many viral infections, thrombocytosis with KD, neutropenia with cyclic neutropenia, pancytopenia with malignancy. Blood parasites may be seen in malaria, babesiosis, and intracellular morulae noted in ehrlichiosis or anaplasmosis
Inflammatory markers	Elevated procalcitonin (>0.25 ng/mL) may indicate a bacterial infection, especially bacterial pneumonia. CRP and ESR are less specific but are evidence of inflammation due to systemic or localized infection, collagen vascular disease, inflammatory bowel disease, other autoimmune condition
Urinalysis and urine culture	Pyuria on urinalysis may suggest UTI, including possible pyelonephritis and/or renal abscess. A urine culture can help establish bacterial etiology. Sterile pyuria may suggest possible KD
Blood cultures	Occult bacteremia (e.g., *Streptococcus pneumoniae* most commonly), endocarditis, salmonellosis
Bone marrow culture	Advanced testing for possible salmonella, TB, brucellosis, endemic fungi, malignancy
Stool cultures and/or PCR for stool pathogens	Identification of enteric bacterial pathogens, Yersiniosis, salmonella infection. PCR and nucleic acid sequence detection, or by antigen detection for giardia, cryptosporidium, *Clostridioides difficile*, adenovirus, rotavirus, norovirus
Respiratory pathogen PCR testing	Identification of SARS-CoV-2, influenza, adenovirus, *Mycoplasma pneumoniae*, *Chlamydophila pneumoniae*, *Bordetella pertussis*
Serology/blood testing	EBV, CMV, Bartonella, interferon gamma release assay for tuberculosis
Plain radiograph	Pneumonia, nodules of TB, endemic fungi, malignancy, joint effusions, bone changes of osteomyelitis may appear >10 days after onset of symptoms
Computed tomography	Evaluation of complicated or chronic sinusitis, lung abscess, liver abscess, hepatosplenic candidiasis or bartonellosis, malignancy
Magnetic resonance imaging	Osteomyelitis (preferred for early diagnosis over plain radiographs), pyomyositis, soft-tissue masses concerning for infections or malignancy
Bone scan, positron emission tomography or tagged white blood cell scan	Occult infection and abscess, osteomyelitis, malignancy

CMV cytomegalovirus, *CRP* C-reactive protein, *ESR* erythrocyte sedimentation rate, *EBV* Epstein-Barr virus, *KD* Kawasaki disease, *PCR* polymerase chain reaction, *SARS-CoV-2* severe acute respiratory syndrome-associated coronavirus 2, *TB* tuberculosis, *UTI* urinary tract infection

Management

Many pediatric patients who appear otherwise well with <5–7 days of fever, yet who are hydrated and behaving appropriately, can be evaluated in the outpatient setting. Empiric antibiotics are not indicated in FUO and may complicate subsequent evaluation delaying the actual diagnosis or causing additional adverse effects (e.g., nausea, diarrhea, rashes). Those with fever in addition to clinical features potentially compatible with KD may require more expedited evaluation and may benefit from inpatient admission to coordinate care and facilitate timely administration of treatments such as intravenous immune globulin, aspirin, and other immunomodulatory therapies.

Many laboratory tests and some imaging studies can be performed in the outpatient setting to reduce unnecessary hospitalization. Hospitalization for inpatient evaluation should be considered for patients who appear acutely ill, require hydration and nutrition, have progression of symptoms, or need fever patterns to be documented under medical supervision (e.g., suspicion of possible factitious fever). Antimicrobial treatment is appropriate when an infection is identified that is susceptible to treatment and the benefits are likely to outweigh the risks of therapy. Approximately 50% of pediatric FUO will self-resolve without explanation and no ongoing issues. In some patients, the evolution or progression of symptoms will give additional clues over time that will aid in the diagnosis of a specific condition that may be treatable. Referral to subspecialists such as Pediatric Infectious Diseases and/or Pediatric Rheumatologist may occasionally be necessary for additional assistance in determining a diagnosis.

Anticipatory Guidance

It is important to educate caregivers about the proper measurement, interpretation and management of fevers, including indications of antipyretic medications. Caregivers of children with prolonged or recurrent fevers are advised to keep a fever diary to help document and track fever occurrences and associated symptoms. This can be reviewed with the physician at subsequent outpatient evaluations to help establish patterns that may give clues to intermittent and recurrent fever syndromes. It is important to educate and reassure caregivers that most pediatric FUO cases self-resolve with no long-lasting effects and that many times no specific diagnosis is identified.

Application Exercises

1. A 5-year-old female has had a fever to 39.7 °C (103.6 °F) once or twice daily for 8 days. Her pediatrician notes on history complaints of body aches and fatigue. Other than fever, there are no abnormal findings on physical exam. Which of the following is the most likely diagnosis at this time?

   A. Bacteremia.
   B. Fever of Unknown Origin (FUO).

C. Fever without a source.
D. Influenza.
E. Rheumatoid arthritis.

Question 1 Answer/Explanation: This 5-year-old currently meets criteria for choice “B”—Fever of Unknown Origin (FUO) having had *intermittent* fevers for *at least 8 days* with *no clear diagnosis or obvious source* at this time. Despite body aches and fatigue, the prolonged time course and otherwise benign physical exam speak against a more urgently ill-appearing child who would likely have already required more emergent evaluation and management more characteristic of answer choices “A”—Bacteremia and “C”—Fever Without a Source. Children with fever without a specific diagnosis and of only a few days (<8 days) duration may be more appropriately labeled as Fever Without a Source (FWS), but it is important to recognize that these patients may actually be more ill and require more urgent evaluation than patients meeting the prolonged duration of FUO. While influenza can be a common viral cause of fever in childhood, lack of localizing symptoms on history/physical exam such as upper respiratory symptoms (i.e., cough, congestion, rhinorrhea, sneezing, tachypnea, increased work of breathing) does not make answer choice “D” the best choice among those listed. Juvenile idiopathic arthritis is a common non-infectious cause of pediatric FUO. However, rheumatoid arthritis is an inflammatory disorder that typically presents later in life around ages 30–50+. Furthermore, much like answer choice D, there are no localizing signs on physical exam (i.e., joint pain, warmth, tenderness, erythema, stiffness) currently to raise increased suspicion for a rheumatologic disorder to the top of the differential.

2. A 6-year-old girl is seen in her pediatrician’s office for 4 days of high fevers despite a normal physical exam. She is currently well-hydrated, is fussy and fatigued, but otherwise seems to be behaving appropriately given her illness. Her fever resolves with a dose of acetaminophen. She is sent home from the pediatrician’s office with anticipatory guidance, including care at home and instructions for when to seek further medical advice. However, by the next morning, after continued fever with worsening aches and fatigue, she is seen in the local emergency room. Her caregivers report she is very fussy and warm to the touch, with flushing of her face, especially red lips. She developed a recurrent cough though is otherwise comfortable breathing room air. She had very little to eat or drink since their office visit and her mother is worried she may be retaining fluids given swollen feet. Physical exam is notable for palpable enlarged lymph nodes on the left side of the neck. A complete blood cell count reveals a WBC of $14 \times 10^3/\text{mm}^3$. Urinalysis is significant for WBC 10/hpf with no nitrites or bacteria present. Urine culture has been obtained and is currently pending. Which of the following is the most likely cause of her fevers?

A. Urinary tract infection.
B. Mononucleosis.
C. Juvenile idiopathic arthritis.
D. Kawasaki disease.

E. Pneumonia.

Question 2 Answer/Explanation: The 6-year-old has had at least 5 days of fever, with associated physical exam findings of oral erythema, cervical lymphadenopathy, and edema of the feet, along with lab features of leukocytosis and sterile pyuria. This presentation best fits Kawasaki disease. Evaluation may have also revealed an erythematous tongue with hypertrophied papillae consistent with the classic strawberry tongue appearance, rash, and/or elevated ESR and CRP. The mnemonic "CRASH and Burn" with *C*onjunctivitis, *R*ash, *A*denopathy, *S*trawberry tongue, *H*ands and feet changes and *Burn* with at least 5 days of fever, helps to remember the key associated clinical features. The cervical lymphadenopathy, cough, fatigue, swelling, and pyuria can all be associated with other infectious and non-infectious causes of prolonged fever in childhood; however, the combination of symptoms in this case best fit a diagnosis of Kawasaki disease. Remember, prompt diagnosis and management with IVIG and aspirin, typically before the 10th day of illness, is important in reducing the risk of coronary artery complication.

3. Which of the following is the best description of typical causes of FUO?

   A. A common presentation of an uncommon disease.
   B. An uncommon presentation of a common disease.
   C. An untreatable disease with increased morbidity.
   D. A relatively serious disease that is usually treatable.

   Question 3 Answer/Explanation: The correct option is answer choice "B". It is most likely for a common disease such as a viral infection with EBV to be the culprit behind fever of unknown origin although the diagnosis may not be as readily apparent initially due to an uncommon presentation. Less common, rare and/or incurable diseases, should be considered in the appropriate clinical setting after more common etiologies are excluded. History, physical exam, and targeted laboratory/imaging data are paramount in helping to identify such illnesses that are less common.

Further Reading

Adam HM. Fever of unknown origin. Point Care Quick Ref. 2020. https://doi.org/10.1542/aap.ppcqr.396074.

Antoon JW, Potisek NM, Lohr JA. Pediatric fever of unknown origin. Pediatr Rev. 2015;36(9):380–90. https://doi.org/10.1542/pir.36-9-380.

Haidar G, Singh N. Fever of unknown origin. NEJM. 2022;386(5):463–77. https://doi.org/10.1056/NEJMra2111003.

Long SS, Prober CG, Fischer M. Principles and practice of pediatric infectious diseases. 5th ed. Philadelphia: Elsevier; 2018.

Marshall GS. Prolonged and recurrent fevers in children. J Infect. 2014;68(Suppl 1):S83–93. https://doi.org/10.1016/j.jinf.2013.09.017.

Chapter 22
Hematology

Kathleen Overholt and Melissa Rose

Anemia

Anemia is one of the most frequent diagnoses seen by physicians and is the most common hematologic abnormality identified in children and infants. With approximately one-third of the world's population (about 2 billion people) and 40–50% of pre-school children diagnosed with some form of anemia, you are guaranteed to encounter this diagnosis during your time as a student on a pediatric rotation. Anemia is associated with increased morbidity and mortality in children and can specifically be associated with poor attention, poor sleep, and impaired neurologic development.

Anemia is the decline in red cell mass or blood hemoglobin concentration that results in a decreased oxygen carrying capacity of the blood. Anemia by itself is not a disease but is a symptom which can be associated with a physiologically diverse group of conditions. Additionally, anemia is often multifactorial, so a thorough history is imperative.

K. Overholt (✉)
Department of Pediatrics, Indiana University School of Medicine, Indianapolis, IN, USA
e-mail: koverho@iu.edu

M. Rose
Department of Pediatrics, The Ohio State University College of Medicine, Columbus, OH, USA
e-mail: Melissa.rose@nationwidechildrens.org

N. Liao et al. (eds.), *Pediatric Rotations*,
https://doi.org/10.1007/978-3-031-59873-9_22

Normal hemoglobin is based on several factors including gender, age, ethnicity, altitude, and genetics. As erythrocytes mature throughout the first year of life, measures of hemoglobin, mean corpuscular volume (MCV), mean corpuscular hemoglobin (MCH), and mean corpuscular hemoglobin concentration (MCHC) change. Additionally, as children grow and develop, changes in these indices fluctuate, particularly with increased testosterone in males, with ultimate steady adult levels reached around age 18 years (Table 22.1).

In assessment of anemia, evaluation should start with a thorough history and physical exam, followed by focused laboratory studies (Table 22.2).

The differential of anemia can be organized in many ways. One useful way of classifying anemia is by relation to decreased production or increased loss/destruction (Table 22.3).

Another way to classify anemia is by cell size using Mean Cell Volume (CV) (Table 22.4). A quick rule of thumb is that lower limit of MCV = 70 + [1 × age in years].

Neonatal anemia has special considerations, particularly due to the normal physiologic nadir that typically occurs by 2–3 months of age. Hemoglobin usually falls

Table 22.1 Normal Hb values in childhood (University of Louisville values, 2023; different labs will have slightly different normal values)

Age	0–3 days	4–7 days	88–60 days	61 days–2 years	2–6 years	7–12 years	13–18 years
Hb (G/dL)	12.6–20.9	11.3–19.8	8.1–13.2	7.2–12.7	11.5–13.5	11.5–15.5	12.0–16.0

Table 22.2 Assessment of anemia in a child

	Category	Issues
1.	History: focus on causes of anemia	Birth history (focusing on jaundice, phototherapy or transfusion, and maternal health); growth and development: symptoms of fatigue, dyspnea, exercise intolerance, dizziness, syncope; diet with emphasis on iron containing foods and milk/tea intake; pica or eating odd items such as ice, clay, dirt, and paper; behavior and sleep; recent infections or travel; bleeding or bruising symptoms including menstrual history in females; gastrointestinal bleeding history in males; joint findings or rash; family history of anemia, jaundice, splenomegaly, need for transfusion, history of autoimmune or blood disease, need for splenectomy or cholecystectomy
2.	Physical exam Focus on severity of anemia	Growth parameters and vital measurements; presence of pallor, jaundice or scleral icterus, systolic ejection murmur; hepatomegaly or splenomegaly; bruising or petechiae; dysmorphic features, especially craniofacial or limb anomalies; signs of systemic disease including rash, joint effusions, or signs suggestive of genetic disease
3.	Laboratory studies Informed by history/physical	Initial labs should be obtained prior to transfusion—complete blood count with differential and reticulocyte count; examination of blood smear for RBC morphology; additional labs, including hemoglobin electrophoresis, iron studies including ferritin, inflammatory markers, folate and vitamin B12, and viral testing, obtained based on history and exam

Table 22.3 Differential of anemia in children based on major mechanism of anemia

Disorders of production	Disorders of RBC loss or destruction F
• Viral suppression • Marrow failure—congenital or acquired aplastic anemia; pure RBC aplasia (diamond Blackfan anemia or transient erythroblastopenia of childhood) • Marrow replacement—malignancy, osteopetrosis, myelofibrosis • Impaired erythrocyte production—anemia of chronic disease, renal disease, malnutrition • RBC maturational disorders—nutritional anemias (iron, folate, vitamin B12, or copper deficiency), lead poisoning, erythropoietic porphyria • Ineffective erythropoiesis: thalassemia • Primary dyserythropoietic anemias, sideroblastic anemia, myelodysplasia (MDS)	• Defects of hemoglobin: sickle cell disease, other structural mutants • Defects in RBC membrane: hereditary spherocytosis, hereditary elliptocytosis • Defects in RBC metabolism: G6PD, pyruvate kinase deficiency • Immune hemolysis: AIHA • Physical damage to RBCs: mechanical/microangiopathic (TTP/HUS/DIC), thermal • Chemical damage to RBCs: oxidants, toxins • Infectious agent-induced damage: malaria • Paroxysmal nocturnal hemoglobinuria (PNH) • Blood loss (acute or chronic)

Table 22.4 Differential of anemia in children based on Mean Cell Volume (MCV)

Microcytic	Normocytic	Macrocytic
• Thalassemia • Anemia of chronic inflammation • Iron deficiency anemia • Hereditary sideroblastic anemia Notes *Lead poisoning is not a cause of microcytic anemia but rather leads to concurrent iron deficiency and is associated with basophilic stippling *Mentzer's index = MCV/RBC count in millions. Mentzer's index >13 indicates iron deficiency and <12 indicates beta thalassemia trait	• Recent/ongoing hemorrhage • Acute or chronic inflammation/renal disease • Acute immune hemolysis • Membrane disorders • Malnutrition • Transient erythroblastopenia of childhood (TEC) • Metabolic defects • Microangiopathic hemolysis (DIC, HUS, TTP) • Paroxysmal nocturnal hemoglobinuria (PNH) • Oxidant exposure	• B12 deficiency/pernicious anemia • Folate deficiency • Reticulocytosis • Bone marrow failure-aplastic anemia, diamond Blackfan anemia (DBA), Fanconi anemia, Shwachman diamond syndrome, MDS • Medications/drugs • Hypothyroidism • Marrow suppression due to infection • Trisomy 21 syndrome • Liver disease • Asplenia

in the range of ~15–20 g/dL at birth, and there is a progressive decline during first 2–3 months of life. For premature infants, the smaller the premature infant, the earlier and deeper the physiologic hemoglobin nadir. In term infants, the Hb nadir (9.5 g/dL) usually occurs by 12 weeks; in premature infants, the nadir (7 g/dL) usually occurs by 6–8 weeks.

Other causes of neonatal anemia include G6PD deficiency, infection, hemolytic diseases of the newborn (such as ABO disease or Rh disease), enzymopathies, or disorders of cell membrane.

Iron Deficiency

Iron deficiency is the leading cause of anemia in children with prevalence of 4.5–9% in pre-school aged children and up to 16% of adolescent females. Clinical presentation is variable and ranges from asymptomatic, to pallor, fatigue, syncope, and pica, to severe cardiovascular collapse.

Children who are high risk for iron deficiency anemia include infants (specifically premature infants and exclusively breast-fed infants), toddlers with excessive milk intake (greater than 20 oz. of whole milk daily), children with restricted diets, menstruating adolescent females, and children and adolescents with inflammatory bowel disease.

Iron metabolism is a highly regulated system. Available iron is either recycled from red blood cell breakdown or absorbed in the duodenum from dietary intake and stored in the liver and reticuloendothelial system until needed. The balance of intestinal absorption is maintained by the hepcidin–ferroportin system. Binding of hepcidin to the membrane transporter, ferroportin, results in the internalization of ferroportin, decreased absorption of iron from the duodenum, and decreased mobilization from iron stores. Production of hepcidin is stimulated in conditions of inflammation and iron overload and suppressed in the context of iron deficiency. See Table 22.5 for common laboratory findings in patients with iron deficiency anemia and Table 22.6 for strategies for management.

Table 22.5 Common laboratory findings in patients with iron deficiency anemia

RBC count	MCV	RDW	Reticulocyte count	Ferritin[a]	TIBC[b]
Low	Low	High	Low	Low	High

[a]Ferritin is an acute phase reactant in patients with ongoing inflammatory conditions; ferritin can be inappropriately high and should be evaluated in context of other laboratory findings
[b]TIBC or total iron-binding capacity is the measure of available transferrin to carry iron from your intestines to where it is needed in the body. The higher this number is, the more seats available on the bus

Table 22.6 Management of iron deficiency anemia in children

1.	Correct imbalance of iron intake, absorption, and iron loss	• Limiting milk intake to less than 18 oz./day • Addressing excessive menstrual bleeding • All adolescent boys with iron deficiency and any child with GI symptoms should be evaluated by gastroenterology
2.	Treat the deficiency with iron supplementation	• Typically, treatment is started at 4–6 mg/kg/day of elemental iron • Dosing can be divided twice daily, given daily, or every other day depending on severity of deficiency and patient tolerance; intravenous iron is available as alternative supplementation if needed • Patients are instructed to take with vitamin C and avoid concurrent milk or other calcium containing products as this blocks absorption
3.	Response to iron therapy	• Anticipated response in reticulocyte count should be seen within 48–72 h, with a 1–2 g increase in hemoglobin within 2 weeks, and return to normal hemoglobin within 1 month • Full course is generally 3 months of consistent use to replete iron stores and a goal ferritin of ≥30
4.	Red blood cell transfusion	• Reserved for Hgb 5 or less, signs of heart failure or cardiovascular compromise, symptoms of syncope or ongoing blood loss • Transfuse 5 mg/kg slowly (over 3–4 h) to avoid cardiovascular compromise as anemia is compensated

Sickle Cell Disease

Sickle cell disease is an inherited hemoglobinopathy caused by mutation in the beta globin chain of hemoglobin. It is the most common inherited disease in the Black population, affecting 1/400 children in the USA, and screening is mandated in all 50 states. Polymerization of the abnormal beta globin chain due to cellular stress causes red cells to adopt a sickle shape resulting in release of free hemoglobin, adherence to the endothelium, clogging of the microvasculature, and tissue ischemia and infarction.

Sickle cell disease comes in many genotypes (i.e., Hb SS, Hb SC, Hb SB + thal, Hb SB0thal, Hb SE, etc.). Please be aware of the patient's "type" of sickle cell. This can be found in the patient's chart or in speaking with the family (Table 22.7).

Sickle cell complications are related to sickle cell disease type and cause serious morbidity and mortality in affected children (Table 22.8).

Table 22.7 "Types" of sickle cell diseases

Type	Baseline hemoglobin (g/dL)	MCV	Reticulocyte count (%)	Severity
HbSS	6–9	Normal	10–25	+++
HbSβ0	6–9	Decreased	10–25	+++
HbSC	9–12	Decreased	5–10	++
HbSβ+	10–13	Decreased	210	+

(Adapted from Quinn CT. Sickle Cell Disease in Childhood: From Newborn Screening Through Transition to Adult Medical Care. Pediatric clinics of North America. 2013;60(6):1363–1381. doi:10.1016/j.pcl.2013.09.006.)

Table 22.8 Sickle cell complications

SC complication	Observations
Vaso-occlusive crisis/ episode (VOC/VOE)	Most common reason for admission in patients with sickle cell disease, but admission is the tip of the iceberg. Most sickle cell pain is treated at home
Acute chest syndrome	New infiltrate on chest X-ray plus fever, chest pain, hypoxia, cough, increased sputum production, dyspnea, tachypnea Etiology infectious: 30–40% cases; also fat embolism, or vaso-occlusion of lung segment (pulmonary infarction)
Stroke	10% of children with Hb SS have overt stroke (20% have silent stroke) prior to age 20 years. Peak incidence 2–6 years
Infection	At risk for infection with capsulated bacteria (due to increasing splenic damage over time)—sepsis, meningitis, pneumonia, osteomyelitis, UTI
Priapism	Unwanted, sustained, painful erection (up to 90% boys by adulthood); low baseline hemoglobin and higher rates of hemolysis are most at risk

Immune Thrombocytopenia

Immune thrombocytopenia (ITP) is the most common acquired bleeding disorder of childhood; this autoimmune disorder is characterized by immunologic destruction of otherwise normal platelets, typically in response to a stimulus. This stimulus is often not directly confirmed but temporally associated with a viral illness/prodrome. Thrombocytopenia is defined as a platelet count $<100 \times 10^9/L$ (yet many laboratories set 2 standard deviation below the mean for platelet counts in the $130–140 \times 10^9/L$ range). In order to study ITP in a standard way, it has been further classified into newly diagnosed (<3 months), persistent (3–12 months) and chronic (>12 months), measured from the time of first low platelet count.

The incidence of ITP in pediatrics is estimated at 2–5 per 100,000, with peak prevalence between the ages 2 and 5 years. The natural history in untreated patients tends to be reduction or cessation of new hemorrhage within 3–10 days and rise in platelet count within 1–3 weeks. Seventy five to 85% of children enter remission by 6 months with specific 1-year remission rates estimated as: < 1 year of age, 74%, 1–6 years of age, 67%, > 10–20 years of age, 62%.

The pathophysiology of ITP involves (1) autoantibody production, (2) increased platelet removal, and (3) reduced platelet production. Antiplatelet antibodies could have multiple target antigens, including glycoprotein IIb/IIIa and Ib/IX, but they are not detectable in up to 50% of patients with ITP and remission can occur despite continued antibody detection; therefore, their clinical/practical use is questionable. Macrophages, particularly in the spleen, express Fc receptors that opsonize platelets for removal. Antibody-mediated reduction of megakaryocyte maturation and phagocytosis suppresses platelet production and release; approximately 40% of patients with ITP have reduced platelet turnover. Several other mechanisms now considered include T cells that are more primed to be platelet reactive, suppression of regulatory T cells, expansion of autoreactive B cell clones, and clearance by complement-mediated pathways. Further work to better define and target these processes is underway, as more targeted therapies are considered.

In assessment of ITP, the history and physical examination is important. ITP is a diagnosis of exclusion. The history should not include persistent fevers, bone or joint pain that would be more consistent with an underlying malignancy or bone marrow infiltration process. There should not be skeletal or soft tissue abnormalities, prompting consideration for underlying bone marrow failure disorder or malignancy, non-petechial rash indicative of lupus or meningococcemia, or pathologic lymphadenopathy that would be characteristic of leukemia/lymphoma. Bleeding scores or Bleeding Assessment Tools have been created to try to consistently describe the bleeding phenotype; the World Health Organization, International Working Group on ITP and modified Buchanan and Adix bleeding scores are examples. Bleeding symptoms can range from nothing, to petechiae, oral petechiae/purpura, bruising with or without hematoma, epistaxis lasting less than or greater than 5 min, hematuria, hematochezia, heavy menstrual bleeding, through internal hemorrhage (brain, lung, muscle, joint, etc.) that could be life threatening or fatal. The mucocutaneous findings are most often seen, with intracranial hemorrhage and life-threatening bleeding reported quite rarely, in up to 0.2% from registries of approximately 2500 children.

For ITP laboratory assessment, the CBC should show normal hemoglobin with normal red blood cell indices and normal white blood cell count with differential. Review of the peripheral blood smear will show normal morphology of these cell lines as well, with few platelets, often with variability in sizes from normal to large and sometimes giant.

The broad differential diagnosis should include microangiopathic hemolytic anemias, such as Thrombotic Thrombocytopenia Purpura, Hemolytic Uremic Syndrome, disseminated intravascular coagulation (DIC), myelodysplastic syndrome/leukemia/lymphoma, lymphoproliferative disorders, infections, medication-induced, and inherited bone marrow failure or thrombocytopenia disorders.

Because of the natural history and rare severe sequelae of ITP, the goal of treatment is to achieve a platelet count that is associated with adequate hemostasis, rather than a normal platelet count. The American Society of Hematology published guidelines for the management of ITP, including sections for pediatric patients with an update in 2019 (Table 22.9). They encourage family-centered collaborative

Table 22.9 American Society of Hematology ITP management guidelines [1]

Newly diagnosed ITP with no or mild bleeding (skin only)	*Suggests against* admission to hospital, in favor of management as outpatient, with referring physician ensuring outpatient follow-up within 24–72 h of diagnosis
	Suggests observation rather than corticosteroids, IVIg or anti-D immunoglobulin, regardless of platelet count
Newly diagnosed ITP who have non-life-threatening mucosal bleeding and/or diminished health-related quality of life (HRQoL)	*Recommends* prednisone 2–4 mg/kg/day with max dose of 120 mg for 5–7 days over dexamethasone 0.6 mg/kg/day with a max dose of 40 mg daily for 4 days, with responses anticipated in 2–14 days with a peak in 4–28 days. Guidelines then suggest IVIg or anti-D immunoglobulin. IVIg dosing recommendations are 0.8–1 g/kg, rounded to the nearest vial size, with time to response of 24–48 h, peaking at 2–7 days. Anti-D therapy is given at 75 mcg/kg, with peak response similar to IVIg
	Suggests use, if not responsive to first-line treatment, of thrombopoietin receptor agonists (TPO-RAs), rather than rituximab, or splenectomy

decision-making, including discussions surrounding health-related quality of life concerns such as medication side effects, access to pediatric healthcare providers, need for surgical procedures, baseline activity levels and risk for injuries, menarche status, as well as symptoms such as difficulty concentrating and fatigue.

Management additionally includes monitoring for bleeding symptoms, such as petechiae (purple "freckles" under the skin), nosebleeds, bleeding from mouth, blood in the urine or bowel movements, "coffee-ground" vomit, severe headache, or changes in behavior. You should also counsel families to avoid aspirin), ibuprofen, or other non-steroidal anti-inflammatory agents, as these impair platelet function and, in the setting of thrombocytopenia, could result in increased bleeding symptoms. There is no consensus regarding recommendations for participation in activities or sports, but these should be discussed prior to participation; close monitoring for bleeding symptoms during activity is also recommended.

Leukocyte Disorders

Pluripotent stem cells are derived from hematopoietic stem cells, arising in the fetal liver, with migration to lymphoid organs, where they differentiate further into myeloid and lymphoid progenitors. From the myeloid progenitor comes erythrocytes, platelets, basophils, eosinophils, neutrophils, monocytes, macrophages and myeloid-related dendritic cells; from the lymphoid progenitor comes dendritic cells, NK cells, T and B lymphocytes.

Total lymphocytes are higher in younger children, decreasing to adult normal values by approximately 10 years of age. T cells are particularly higher in infants and toddlers and B cell values reach a maximum between 2 months and 2 years of age. NK cell numbers remain stable over time. Many individuals of African or

Middle Eastern ancestries have been found to have reduced number of circulating white blood cells, associated with a Duffy-null single nucleotide polymorphism located in the *ACKR1* gene. This genotype leads to increased egress of neutrophils from the circulation into the tissue, resulting in lower circulating neutrophil counts, without an increased risk of infection, viral or bacterial. One study found that approximately two-thirds of Black individuals have the Duffy-null phenotype.

Leukocyte disorders may be qualitative or quantitative. This chapter will focus on quantitative deficiencies, where the cell type is less than two standard deviations below the mean for age. The top three etiologies for these findings include infection, medication side effect, and inherited deficiencies although more specific underlying etiologies will depend on the cell type.

Lymphopenia is often asymptomatic and found at times of illnesses, particularly with acute or recurrent viral infections, fungal and parasitic infections. The infectious differential for lymphopenia is large and includes Epstein-Barr Virus, Cytomegalovirus, Human Immunodeficiency Virus, SARS-CoV-2, influenza virus, Parvovirus, Measles virus, viral hepatitides, *Mycobacterium tuberculosis*, brucellosis, histoplasmosis, and so on. The differential diagnosis for lymphopenia also includes systemic autoimmune diseases, renal failure and protein-losing enteropathy, and iatrogenic causes including medications, radiation, dietary deficiencies such as zinc deficiency or ethanol abuse. Inherited lymphopenias are extremely rare but have a very high susceptibility to sometimes fatal opportunistic infections in infancy or early childhood. Examples include severe combined immunodeficiency, ataxia-telangiectasia, Wiskott-Aldrich syndrome, and cartilage-hair hyperplasia.

Neutropenia is graded in severity based on absolute neutrophil count and may be associated with more specific clinical manifestations based on grade (Table 22.10). Patients with neutropenia are at risk for infections commonly derived from endogenous flora, most notably from the oropharynx, skin and gastrointestinal tract, and therefore, the most common pathogens are *Staphylococcus aureus* and Gram-negative bacteria. Neutropenia may be isolated or associated with an underlying disease, such as mitochondrial or metabolic diseases, immunodeficiencies, autoimmune diseases, nutritional deficiencies, hypersplenism, and intrinsic or extrinsic bone marrow failure or myeloproliferative disorders.

The evaluation of a patient with neutropenia includes a detailed personal and family history for congenital anomalies, malignancy, medication exposures, and infectious history including location, frequency, response to treatment, radiographic

Table 22.10 Grade of neutropenia

Severity	ANC/mm^3	Possible clinical manifestations
Mild	1000–1500	Often asymptomatic, little to no heightened infection risk
Moderate	500–1000	Stomatitis, gingivitis, cellulitis
Severe	<500	Necrotic and ulcerative lesions, especially of the oropharyngeal and nasal tissues, skin, GI tract, vagina and uterus, perirectal abscesses, pneumonia, sepsis *Could be life-threatening

ANC absolute neutrophil count

imaging, complications, and organisms (if known). Perform a physical exam assessment for short stature, abnormal skin, hair or nails, malnutrition, hepatomegaly or splenomegaly, lymphadenopathy, and limb anomalies. Individuals with neutropenia are unable to mount a purulent response, so their infections may present with pain and erythema alone, rather than typical features of local inflammation such as exudate or fluctuance. Due to infectious risk, do not perform rectal temperatures, rectal exams, or administer per rectal medications.

Laboratory workup should include a CBC with differential, with delineation of individual cell line absolute leukocyte counts; these should be evaluated for age-based ranges. Review of the peripheral blood smear should confirm cytopenia and assess for abnormal morphology. Absolute neutrocyte count is calculated by the formula: WBC (cells/μL) × [percent (PMNs + bands) ÷ 100]. If ANC is 1000–1500, patients should be monitored and repeat ANC after 4–6 weeks, with clinical history and exam prompting additional evaluation. If ANC is 500–1000, consider repeat testing before initiating first-level investigations (kidney and liver function tests, C-reactive protein, immunoglobulins, ANA, direct antiglobulin test, and infection studies [cultures, antibody studies]). If ANC is <500 on two samples, obtain first-level testing as above. If neutropenia persists, bone marrow or more targeted assessment of other etiologies should be sought.

Differential Diagnosis of Neutropenia

- Infectious or post-infectious neutropenia: occurs in the first few days of illness and persists for days to weeks; lack of resolution by approximately 6 weeks should prompt further evaluation, including bone marrow aspiration and biopsy.
- Medication-induced neutropenia: can result from direct marrow suppression or immune destruction, may or may not be dose-related, and should improve within 1–2 weeks after cessation. Commonly prescribed medications associated with neutropenia include non-steroidal anti-inflammatory agents (ibuprofen), antibiotics (penicillin and sulfonamides), and anticonvulsant agents, among others.
- Autoimmune neutropenia: results when an infective agent stimulates antibody production that cross-reacts with antigens on the neutrophil surface. Median age of diagnosis is 8 months (range 3–30 months) and median duration is approximately 30 months (6–60 months), where resolution by 4 years of age occurs in ~95% of children. Anti-neutrophil antibody testing has low sensitivity and specificity. Patients may be relatively asymptomatic or develop infections typical of neutropenia, in which case antibiotics should be administered. Granulocyte colony-stimulating factor (G-CSF) may be prescribed to increase bone marrow production, in an effort to decrease infection frequency.
- Cyclic neutropenia: defined as the occurrence of severe neutropenia on at least two separate occasions at approximately 21-day intervals, with nadir spanning 3–6 days. Clinical symptoms of recurrent aphthous stomatitis or abdominal pain/diarrhea may be indicative of cycles of neutropenia. Mutations of the *ELANE*

gene are found in 90–100% of patients with well-documented cyclic symptoms. Obtaining CBC with differential 2–3 times per week for 6 weeks can allow detection of cycling of the absolute neutrophil count, but the other cell lines may also rise and fall. G-CSF may be used to mitigate the nadir; typical dose is ~2 mcg/kg/day, with variable administration most commonly every other day or daily.

- Severe congenital neutropenia: More severe compared to other neutropenia etiologies and presents in infancy with umbilical or other skin, pulmonary or perineal/perirectal infections, recurrent diarrhea, pneumonia, and abscesses of the liver, lung, and subcutaneous tissues. Bone marrow shows maturation arrest at the pro-myelocyte/myelocyte stage. More than 80% of patients will have an identifiable mutation, with autosomal dominant heterozygous *ELANE* mutations being most common. Treatment with G-CSF should be titrated to target a trough ANC >1000/mm^3. The overall risk of developing myelodysplastic syndrome and/or acute myeloid leukemia is 15–25% in these patients, with dose and duration of G-CSF, as well as the mutation itself, as contributing factors. Bone marrow transplant should be strongly considered, especially in the setting of refractory neutropenia, or requiring very high doses of G-CSF for response.

Patients with neutropenia and fever should have a history and physical exam performed, with CBC and calculation of ANC. Blood cultures and empiric antibiotic administration should be strongly considered, particularly in inherited neutropenias. Admission should be prompt in patients with fever and severe neutropenia, moderate neutropenia with severe infection or if clinically ill-appearing with any neutropenia. Outpatient management can be accomplished for those who do not meet above criteria if they have reliable access to medical care and follow-up.

Application Exercises

1. A 4-year-old child is noted to have an HB 9.8 g/dL and MCV 65. She is asymptomatic and has a normal WBC and platelet count. Of the following, the MOST likely cause of this girl's anemia is

   A. Anemia of chronic disease.
   B. Recent hemorrhage.
   C. Thalassemia.
   D. Vitamin B6 deficiency.

   Correct Answer C: Microcytic anemias, as in this girl, include iron deficiency, thalassemia, anemia of chronic inflammation, and sideroblastic anemia. Of these, thalassemia is the only option. Anemia of chronic disease and recent hemorrhage lead to anemia with normocytic anemia (normal MCV) and vitamin B6 deficiency anemia leads to macrocytic anemia (large MCV).
2. A 10-year-old African American boy develops fever, chest pain, cough, and tachypnea. He has new infiltrate on chest X-ray. Of the following complications of sickle cell anemia, the most likely explanation is.

   A. Acute chest syndrome.
   B. Anemic crisis.

C. Stroke.
D. Vaso-occlusive crisis.

Correct Answer A: In a child with sickle cell anemia, acute chest syndrome typically presents with new infiltrate on chest X-ray plus fever, chest pain, hypoxia, cough, increased sputum production, dyspnea, and tachypnea. 30–40% of cases have an infectious etiology; it can also arise from fat embolism, or vaso-occlusion of a lung segment (pulmonary infarction). An anemic crisis is related to an acute drop in hemoglobin, without significant infection, as might be seen with an acute viral-induced suppression of erythropoiesis. Stroke and vaso-occlusive crises do not have fever and acute onset of pulmonary symptoms, such as cough and sputum production.

3. A 4-year-old boy with a history of autoimmune neutropenia (moderate to severe neutropenia) develops fever and cough. He becomes more ill-appearing over the 2 h in the ED. The most appropriate management choice for this boy is:

A. Admission for cultures and empiric IV antibiotics.
B. Admission for cultures and close observation.
C. Cultures and discharge to home for close observation while cultures are pending.
D. Cultures and discharge to home on empiric oral antibiotics.

Correct Answer A: Prompt cultures (blood and urine) and admission for empiric IV antibiotics is the best choice in an ill-appearing child with moderate to severe neutropenia and signs of infection. Starting empiric antibiotics after obtaining cultures is warranted due to this patient's risk of severe infection. Caring for this patient at home is considered too risky and he should be admitted for close monitoring.

Reference

1. Neunert C, Terrell DR, Arnold DM, et al. American Society of Hematology 2019 guidelines for immune thrombocytopenia. Blood Adv. 2019;3(23):3829–66.

Further Reading

Kassebaum NJ, Jasrasaria R, Naghavi M, et al. A systematic analysis of global anemia burden from 1990 to 2010. Blood. 2014;123:615–24.

Mehta B. Leukocyte-related disorders: a review for the pediatrician. Pediatr Ann. 2020;49(1):e17–26.

Ng PC, Long B. Immune thrombocytopenic purpura: pearls and pitfalls. EMDocs Pract Updates. 2016;8:28.

Zanetti R, Feldman B, Porea T. Microcytic anemia. Pediatr Rev. 2021;42(1):41–3.

Chapter 23
Hyperbilirubinemia in the Neonate

Ashleigh Slemmer and Nancy Liao

Background

Neonatal unconjugated hyperbilirubinemia, or jaundice, is a common condition in newborns; up to 60% of term infants and 80% of preterm babies are affected. Jaundice presents as a yellow discoloration of the skin and eye sclera which results from excess of bilirubin. Although jaundice is benign in most cases, specific risk factors and high bilirubin concentrations can result in bilirubin-induced neurologic dysfunction (BIND) and chronic bilirubin encephalopathy (CBE), previously known as kernicterus. CBE is a severe and irreversible neurologic sequela that consists of muscle tone abnormalities, neuromotor signs, neurobehavioral manifestations, and central processing abnormalities such as sensorineural and visuomotor dysfunctions [1].

Pathophysiology

Bilirubin Metabolism

Bilirubin is a product of the breakdown of heme. Heme is first converted to biliverdin by heme oxygenase which is then reduced to unconjugated bilirubin by biliverdin reductase via the reticuloendothelial system. Unconjugated bilirubin is primarily bound to albumin which is transported to the liver where the albumin–bilirubin complex disassociates and the bilirubin is conjugated by uridine diphosphoglucuronosyl transferase (UGT-1A1). Unbound bilirubin is able to leave the vascular space and

A. Slemmer (✉) · N. Liao
Pediatrics, Nationwide Children's Hospital/The Ohio State University College of Medicine, Columbus, OH, USA
e-mail: Ashleigh.Slemmer@nationwidechildrens.org; Nancy.Liao@nationwidechildrens.org

N. Liao et al. (eds.), *Pediatric Rotations*,
https://doi.org/10.1007/978-3-031-59873-9_23

become deposited in tissues such as the brain. Once bilirubin is conjugated in the liver, it is excreted in bile. Once in the colon, bilirubin is reduced by bacterial and intestinal brush border enzymes (β-glucuronidase) to urobilinogens, some of which are reabsorbed via the enterohepatic circulation and others are excreted in the urine and stool.

History

It is important to consider the differential when coming up with questions to ask the patient's family. Below are key components that should be included your history.

When was jaundice first noted? What is the infant's level of irritability? Wakefulness?

Intake and Output

A neonate will excrete bilirubin primarily through the stool and, to a lesser extent, the urine. Therefore, asking about intake and output ("I's and O's") can help to discern your differential diagnosis. A neonate who does not have sufficient intake (for a variety of possible reasons) may not have as much stool output, and therefore does not excrete bilirubin as effectively. Take a detailed feeding and output history (see Chap. 37). Ask specifically about stool color and consistency. Newborn stools transition a lot at this age: ranging from meconium (black and sticky, i.e., "tarry") to yellow/green and seedy to green/brown. Knowing the color and consistency is one of the ways to determine whether the child is getting sufficient intake and if they are excreting bilirubin through stool. Perhaps more importantly, ensuring that the stool is not pale or "clay" colored is vital. Pale stools can indicate cholestasis which would require urgent evaluation for biliary atresia.

Key Focused Review of Systems (ROS)

You should plan to ask a full ROS, but Table 23.1 reviews are some key systems. Refer Chap. 2 for a full ROS discussion.

Birth History

The birth history is an important aspect of every pediatric history, especially for patients less than 1 year of age (see Chap. 38). The most relevant questions for neonatal hyperbilirubinemia are outlined in Table 23.2.

Table 23.1 Focused review of systems for neonatal hyperbilirubinemia

Body system	Question(s)	Reasoning
Head	Birth trauma?	A cephalohematoma is a collection of blood between the periosteum and skull that can occur during delivery and can lead to excess breakdown of heme
Pulmonary	Cough or increased work of breathing?	These can be a sign of sepsis
Abdomen	Stooling frequency? Color and consistency of the stools?	See text
Skin	Rashes or mottling? Bleeding or bruising on your baby?	Significant bruising can lead to excess heme breakdown. Mottling can be a sign of sepsis (i.e., poor perfusion)
Neurological	Fussy or irritable? Has your baby been waking up to feed?	Irritability or increased sleepiness can result from hyperbilirubinemia (neurotoxicity)

Table 23.2 Focused birth history for neonatal hyperbilirubinemia

Questions	Tips, tricks, and examples
Prenatal: – When was your initial ultrasound? – How many prenatal visits did you have? – Number of previous pregnancies? (i.e., gravida, Para)	
What is the patient's gestational age?	*Remember*: Preterm is less than 37 weeks, late preterm is 34–36 weeks 6/7 days, term is ≥37 weeks
Any complications during delivery?	*Examples:* Forceps or vacuum assisted, prolonged rupture of membranes, shoulder dystocia
Did the patient require any resuscitation following delivery? Did they require an NICU stay, and if so, what was the reason?	
What were maternal serology results during pregnancy (if known)? What was mom's GBS status?	*Tip*: Most families will not understand what "serologies" are. It is helpful to ask, "did you have any infections during pregnancy that you were aware of or were told about?" It can also be helpful to specifically ask about GBS status and whether mother was adequately treated, if applicable. *Examples*: Serologies obtained during pregnancy include syphilis (RPR), HIV, gonorrhea, chlamydia, hepatitis B, and rubella immunity *Remember*: Only *some* TORCH infections are tested prenatally (rubella, syphilis, and HIV)

(continued)

Table 23.2 (Continued)

Questions	Tips, tricks, and examples
What is the maternal and patient's blood type (if known)?	*Remember*: ABO incompatibility can cause jaundice *Remember*: In an Rh(D)-negative mother who has been previously exposed to an Rh positive fetus' blood, future pregnancies can be at risk for isoimmune hemolytic disease
Did your child require phototherapy in the newborn nursery or NICU?	*Remember*: Jaundice presenting <24 h of life is more likely to be pathologic

ABO major human blood group system, *GBS* group B β-hemolytic strep, *HIV* human immunodeficiency virus, *NICU* neonatal intensive care unit, *RPR* rapid plasma reagin, *Rh(D)* rhesus factor disease, *TORCH* **t**oxoplasmosis, **o**ther (syphilis, Zika virus, varicella-zoster virus), **r**ubella, **c**ytomegalovirus, **h**erpes simplex virus

Risk Factors for Significant Hyperbilirubinemia

1. Younger gestational age
2. Visible jaundice in the first 24 h
3. Pre-discharge bilirubin near phototherapy threshold
4. Phototherapy required during the birth hospitalization
5. Family history or genetic ancestry of red blood cell membrane defects or glucose-6-phosphate dehydrogenase (G6PD) deficiency
6. ABO incompatibility with positive direct Coombs, known hemolytic disease
7. Parent or prior sibling requiring phototherapy or exchange transfusion
8. Cephalohematoma or significant bruising
9. Trisomy 21
10. Macrosomia in the setting of infant of diabetic mother
11. Exclusive breastfeeding, especially with poor feeding or weight loss

Physical Exam

Vitals: For neonatal jaundice, one should monitor for tachycardia and vital instability (see Chap. 5) as these can be signs of sepsis (see Chap. 34).

Weight: Report the weight percentile and categorization (i.e., small for gestational age (SGA), average for gestational age (AGA), and large for gestational age (LGA). Calculate and report the percent weight loss. It is appropriate for newborns to lose up to 10% of their birth weight over the first few days of life.

$$\textbf{Glucose infusion rate}\ (\text{GIR})\ mg\ glucose/kg/\text{min} = \frac{[\%\ \text{dextrose} \times \text{fluid goal}\ (mL/kg/day)]}{144}$$

See Table 23.3 for a focused exam for hyperbilirubinemia in neonates.

Table 23.3 Focused physical exam for neonatal hyperbilirubinemia

System	Exam	Tips
General	Describe the patient's overall appearance	"Sick or not sick?"
Head	Bruising or cephalohematoma?	A cephalohematoma does NOT cross suture lines (versus caput succedaneum which does cross suture lines)
Eyes	Scleral icterus?	
Cardiovascular	Tachycardia?	May be related to sepsis picture
Respiratory	Respiratory rate? Is there any work of breathing? If so, describe the severity and location	May be related to sepsis picture Focal findings suggest source infection
Abdominal	Soft? Tenderness? Distension? Hepatosplenomegaly?	When evaluating for hepatomegaly, ensure that you begin palpating at the iliac crest and work upwards. You may miss an enlarged liver if you start at the inferior aspect of the costal margin
Skin	Visible jaundice? Bruising?	Jaundice progresses in a cephalocaudal (head to toe) direction however, studies show that visual estimation of bilirubin levels does not correlate well with the actual level. If you are unable to tell if an infant is jaundiced, it can be helpful to press down and blanch the sternum. It is important to keep in mind that recognizing jaundice can be more difficult in babies with darker skin color
Neurological	Fussy or irritable? Inconsolable? Describe their tone Infant reflexes intact?	A floppy baby is very concerning; neonates should have high flexural tone

Laboratory Assessment

There is institutional variation when each of these tests is utilized. Make sure to understand the preferences for testing where you are doing your clinical rotation.

Measuring Bilirubin Levels

Transcutaneous bilirubin (TCB)

- TCB is obtained with a non-invasive meter (that can appear similar to a forehead thermometer) that is placed on the neonate's skin which measures the light transmission through the skin and provides a bilirubin level measurement.
  - Unreliable once phototherapy has been initiated.

Total serum bilirubin (TSB)

- A TSB is a blood test that can be obtained by "heel stick" (utilizing a similar method to a finger stick that patients with diabetes use to check their glucose levels).

Fractionated bilirubin levels

- A fractionated bilirubin level = direct and total bilirubin level. It is important to rule out direct hyperbilirubinemia (direct bilirubin level >1.0 mg/dL).

Other Laboratory Assessments (Table 23.4)

Table 23.4 Other laboratory assessments in neonatal hyperbilirubinemia

Lab test	When to obtain	Purpose
CBC or H&H	Patient requires phototherapy or meets escalation of care threshold[a]	*Hemoglobin*: a low or dropping hemoglobin can be indicative of hemolysis *Hematocrit*: polycythemia can result in increased bilirubin production *Peripheral smear*[b]: fragmented cells, macrocytosis, and polychromasia can be indicative of hemolysis
Blood type and coombs or DAT	Maternal screen not completed, maternal antibody screen was positive, mother has blood group O regardless of Rh(D) status, mother is Rh(D)-negative, patient requires phototherapy, and/or meets threshold for escalation of care[a]	Can be utilized to compare with maternal blood type to determine if there is ABO or Rh incompatibility and possible isoimmune hemolytic disease. There are additional antibodies that can cause isoimmune hemolytic disease which will also be indicated on the coombs (direct antiglobulin) test. A negative DAT does *not* exclude hemolytic disease of the newborn
G6PD assay	Unknown etiology of jaundice and TSB increases despite intensive phototherapy, TSB increases suddenly, or TSB increases after an initial decline. Should obtain if patient meets threshold for escalation of care[a]	G6PD can cause hemolysis of red blood cells
Serum chemistry	Infant meets threshold for escalation of care[a]	Baseline prior to starting IV fluids. Can identify associated hypoglycemia
Serum albumin	Infant meets threshold for escalation of care[a]	Hypoalbuminemia (albumin <3 g/dL) is a neurotoxic risk factor because unbound (free) bilirubin can more readily cross the blood–brain barrier

ABO major human blood group system, *DAT* direct antiglobulin test, *G6PD* glucose-6-phosphate dehydrogenase, *TSB* total serum bilirubin, *Rh(D)* rhesus factor disease

[a]Escalation of care threshold refers to a total bilirubin level that is within 2 mg/dL of the exchange transfusion threshold

[b]An automatic smear is standard on a CBC with differential at most institutions. Usually, you must request a manual smear

Differential Diagnosis

The differential diagnosis for neonatal hyperbilirubinemia is broad (Fig. 23.1). The most important initial step is to determine whether it is a direct (conjugated) or indirect (unconjugated) hyperbilirubinemia. One should then consider whether the etiology is purely physiologic or has a pathologic component. Physiologic jaundice typically occurs on days 2–4 with a peak around days 4–5 and resolution by 2 weeks of life. Physiologic jaundice is not severe enough to require treatment. Pathologic jaundice can occur at any time, but a newborn that develops jaundice within the first 24 h of life is considered pathologic. The rate of rise, or how quickly the bilirubin level is increasing, may suggest pathologic etiology. Generally, a rate of rise ≥0.2 mg/dL/h is considered high.

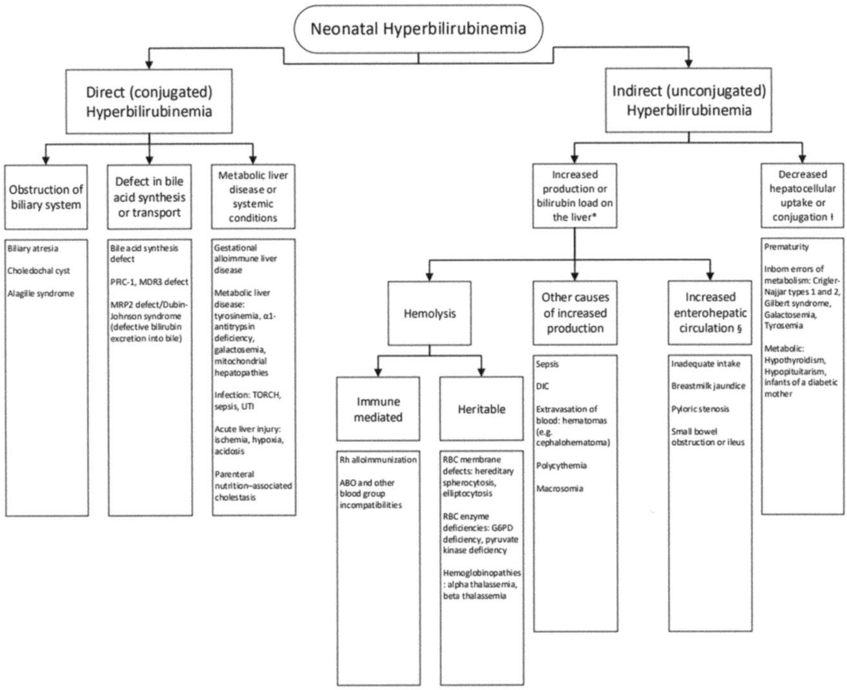

Fig. 23.1 Differential diagnosis of neonatal hyperbilirubinemia. *ABO* major human blood group system, *G6PD* glucose-6-phosphate dehydrogenase, *RBC* red blood cell, *Rh(D)* rhesus factor disease, *TORCH* **t**oxoplasmosis, **o**ther (syphilis, Zika virus, varicella-zoster virus), **r**ubella, **c**ytomegalovirus, **h**erpes simplex virus, *UTI* urinary tract infection. * Bilirubin is derived from the breakdown of red blood cells. Therefore, anything that results in increased breakdown of RBCs will result in higher levels of bilirubin. As compared to adult RBC lifespan of 120 days, neonatal erythrocytes have a shorter lifespan of 60–90 days. ƚ Conjugation of bilirubin in the liver increases the solubility and allows for enhanced elimination from the body. Newborns have decreased UGT-1A1 activity, resulting in the decreased ability to conjugate, and therefore eliminate, bilirubin. § The immature gut microbiota in a neonate results in increased enterohepatic circulation compared to an adult whereby conjugated bilirubin is reduced to urobilinogen by colonic bacteria

$$\frac{\text{Bilirubin level}(\text{most recent}) - \text{Bilirubin level}(\text{previous})}{\text{Time obtained}(\text{most recent}) - \text{Time obtained}(\text{previous})} = \text{rate of rise}(\text{mg per dL per hour}).$$

Suboptimal Intake vs Breastmilk Jaundice

Suboptimal intake hyperbilirubinemia typically peaks around days 3–5 of life and is due to inadequate intake leading to decreased intestinal motility with resultant decreased excretion and increased enterohepatic circulation of bilirubin. Inadequate intake is most commonly related to low maternal breastmilk production but can also include neonates who are exclusively formula fed. This was formerly known as "breastfeeding jaundice."

Breastmilk jaundice typically occurs after 1 week of life and can even persist for months. The mechanism is thought to be due to the inhibition of UDT activity as well as a factor in breast milk that acts similarly to β-glucuronidase and deconjugates bilirubin resulting in increased enterohepatic circulation.

Management

Utilize published nomograms, BiliTool [2] (helpful website, utilizes the American Academy of Pediatrics guidelines), or Northern California Neonatal Consortium (NCNC) Hyperbilirubinemia Treatment Guideline [3]. Phototherapy treatment is based on gestational age, hyperbilirubinemia neurotoxicity risk factors, and the age of the infant in hours. See Fig. 23.2 for thresholds to start phototherapy in infants without neurotoxic risk factors.

Neurotoxicity Risk Factors

Neurotoxic risk factors include: gestational age <38 weeks, albumin <3 g/dL, isoimmune hemolytic disease, G6PD deficiency, or other hemolytic condition, sepsis, and significant clinical instability in the previous 24 h. Infants with neurotoxic risk factors have a lower threshold for starting phototherapy (Fig. 23.3).

Phototherapy

Phototherapy works to decrease bilirubin levels by transforming bilirubin into a water-soluble form that can be eliminated without having to be conjugated in the liver. The keys to optimizing phototherapy include:

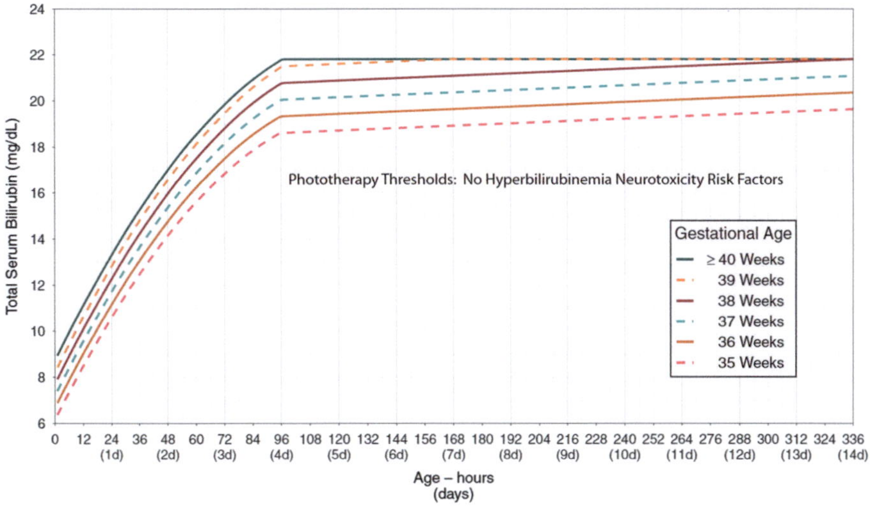

Fig. 23.2 Age-specific nomogram for treatment of hyperbilirubinemia based on total serum bilirubin level, gestational age, and no neurotoxicity risk factors [4]

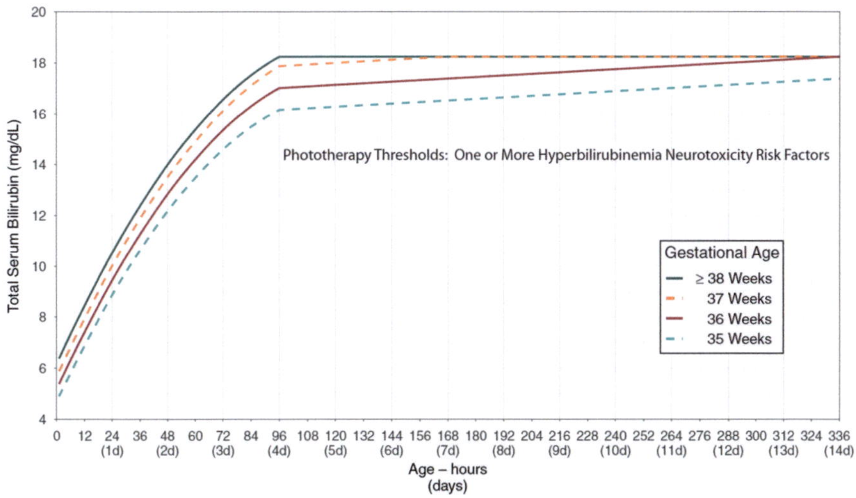

Fig. 23.3 Age-specific nomogram for treatment of hyperbilirubinemia based on total serum bilirubin level, gestational age, and presence of at least one neurotoxicity risk factor [4]

1. Exposing as much skin as possible
   - Most newborns will be in a diaper and an eye shield only
   - Most devices require the infant to be in an isolette so that they will remain warm
2. Limiting the amount of time outside of the lights
3. Adequate hydration and feeding

Escalation of Care

Infants who meet the following criteria require escalation of care:

1. Bilirubin level is above the escalation of care threshold (2 mg/dL below the exchange transfusion level). Refer to AAP Clinical Practice Guidelines for exchange transfusion nomograms [4]. Similar to the phototherapy nomograms, there are two separate exchange transfusion nomograms-based on the presence or absence of neurotoxic risk factors.
2. Infants with rising bilirubin levels despite phototherapy.

Obtain total and direct serum bilirubin, a complete blood count, serum albumin, serum chemistry, and type and crossmatch STAT. Start IV fluid hydration (but should also continue PO hydration if able) and consult the neonatal intensive care unit (NICU). Infants who require exchange transfusion or treatment with intravenous immune globulin for isoimmune hemolytic disease should be transferred to the NICU immediately.

Home Phototherapy

For infants who have been discharged from the birth hospital and later develop jaundice, home phototherapy may be appropriate. Infants must meet the following criteria:

1. ≥ 38 weeks gestational age,
2. ≥ 48 h old,
3. Clinically well and feeding well.
4. No prior phototherapy.
5. No neurotoxicity risk factors.
6. Bilirubin level no more than 1 mg/dL above the phototherapy threshold.

Caretakers must have:

1. Ability to obtain home LED-based phototherapy device without delay.
2. Access to lab for daily TSB recheck.

Phototherapy can be discontinued when the infant's bilirubin level decreases to a level that is at least 2 mg/dL below the phototherapy threshold at the time when phototherapy was initiated. Repeating a bilirubin level after phototherapy is based on risk of rebound jaundice. Infants who are younger than 48 h old at the start of phototherapy, with hemolytic disease, and those with gestational age <38 weeks all are at higher risk of rebound hyperbilirubinemia.
Timing of Rebound Check

- 6–12 h after phototherapy discontinuation
  - Infants with phototherapy before 48 h of life
  - Infants with positive direct antigen test
  - Suspected or known hemolytic disease
- Day after phototherapy discontinuation
  - Infants who received phototherapy at the birth hospital
  - Infants who received phototherapy and the birth hospital and then required readmission for phototherapy
- 1–2 days after phototherapy discontinuation
  - Infants who did not require phototherapy during their birth admission but were readmitted for phototherapy
  - Infants who received home phototherapy

Anticipatory Guidance

Anticipatory guidance for jaundice for caregivers of newborns regardless of setting is important. When discharging the patient, be sure to provide education on the following main points:

1. Ensure that your child is feeding every 3 h, including overnight.
2. Ensure that your child is having adequate wet diapers.
3. Concerning signs: fussiness and irritability, especially if inconsolable; unable to wake for feeds, lethargy.
   - *Remember*: newborns sleep *a lot*, especially in the first week of life, so make sure you clarify the above.
4. Monitor for skin color changes (i.e., worsening of yellowness of the skin).

Application Exercises

You are seeing a 4-day-old Caucasian male infant in your office today for his newborn visit. He was born via vaginal delivery at 38 weeks and 5 days to a 32-year-old G2P2002 mother. There were no complications in pregnancy or delivery. Maternal serologies were negative and her blood type was B+. He spent 28 h in the newborn nursery before being discharged home. His mother is exclusively breastfeeding, and she thinks her breastmilk started to come in the day prior. The infant is feeding every 3 h, including overnight, and he is having about 6 wet diapers and 1 stool per day; stool transitioned to a yellow-seedy color and consistency this morning. The parents express to you that they were thankful their newborn did not need phototherapy in the newborn nursery like their previous child had.

On exam, he appears jaundiced but is overall well appearing. He is down 8% from birth weight. Serum bilirubin is obtained and resulted at 22 mg/dL. CBC is within normal and reticulocyte count is 1.5%.

1. Of the following, what is the most likely etiology for the infant's jaundice?

   A. Sepsis.
   B. G6PD deficiency.
   C. Suboptimal intake hyperbilirubinemia.
   D. Hemolysis secondary to ABO incompatibility.

   Answer: C. Suboptimal intake hyperbilirubinemia.

   Given that mom has just recently had her milk come in, in conjunction with the weight loss being at the higher end of acceptable, it is most likely that the largest contributor to jaundice is suboptimal intake hyperbilirubinemia, formerly known as "breastfeeding jaundice." An infant who is septic would not be well appearing and may have some abnormalities on CBC—such as elevated white count and/or elevated platelets. With hemolytic conditions, we would expect to see increased reticulocyte counts. Since 1.5% is within normal range, ABO incompatibility and G6PD deficiency would be less likely. G6PD deficiency is of highest prevalence in people of African, Asian, or Mediterranean descent.

2. Does this level necessitate phototherapy?

   Answer: This infant requires phototherapy. This child should be assessed for need for phototherapy on the "no neurotoxic risk factors" graph. The threshold to start is 21 mg/dL based on his gestational age of 38 weeks and current age of 4 days.

References

1. Wusthoff CJ, Loe IM. Impact of bilirubin-induced neurologic dysfunction on neurodevelopmental outcomes. Semin Fetal Neonatal Med. 2015;20(1):52–7. https://doi.org/10.1016/j.siny.2014.12.003.
2. BiliTool™. https://bilitool.org/. Accessed 9 Dec 2021.
3. NCNC Hyperbilirubinemia Treatment Guidelines. https://www.phototherapyguidelines.com/. Accessed 2 Jan 2022.
4. Subcommittee on Hyperbilirubinemia. Management of Hyperbilirubinemia in the newborn infant 35 or more weeks of gestation. Pediatrics. 2004;114(1):297–316. https://doi.org/10.1542/peds.114.1.297.

Chapter 24
Infectious Diseases: Common Inpatient Considerations

Guliz Erdem, Christopher Ouellette, and Cristina Tomatis Souverbielle

Skin and Soft Tissue Infections (Cellulitis/Abscess)

Background

Skin and soft tissue infections (SSTI) result from microbial invasion of the skin and its supporting structures, involving the skin, subcutaneous fat, fascial layers, or musculotendinous structures. SSTIs can be purulent or non-purulent. SSTIs are classified as simple (uncomplicated) or complicated (necrotizing or non-necrotizing). Simple infections include cellulitis, erysipelas, impetigo, ecthyma, folliculitis, furuncles, carbuncles, abscesses, and trauma. Complicated and severe infections can show signs of systemic inflammation and extension into deep tissues, including deep abscesses, decubitus ulcers, and necrotizing fasciitis. SSTIs are most frequently caused by Gram-positive pathogens and especially by *Staphylococcus aureus*.

Pathogenesis

Most SSTIs occur de novo or follow a breach in the skin. Any microbial pathogen that gains entry to the skin can potentially cause SSTI. *S. aureus* and Group A streptococci are responsible for most community acquired SSTIs [1].

G. Erdem (✉) · C. Ouellette · C. Tomatis Souverbielle
Ohio State University, Nationwide Children's Hospital, Columbus, OH, USA
e-mail: guliz.erdem@nationwidechildrens.org

N. Liao et al. (eds.), *Pediatric Rotations*,
https://doi.org/10.1007/978-3-031-59873-9_24

Diagnosis

The diagnosis of SSTIs is predominantly clinical. Patients will experience erythema, warmth, edema, and pain over the affected site. Fever is common. Tense overlying edema and bullae can be seen with rapidly evolving and severe SSTIs. Patients with necrotizing fasciitis may have pain disproportionate to the physical findings with rapid progression of infection. Cultures from purulent drainage and deep tissue should be done on all SSTIs when possible. A complete blood count, C-reactive protein (CRP) level, liver and kidney function tests should be ordered for patients with severe infections. If necrotizing fasciitis is considered, magnetic resonance imaging (MRI) can support the diagnosis.

Management

- Simple infections such as impetigo and folliculitis: Topical treatments with mupirocin, retapamulin.
- Completely drained abscesses without significant surrounding cellulitis: antibiotic treatment may not be necessary.
- Cellulitis and incompletely drained abscesses and while culture results are pending: treatment of common pathogens, including methicillin-resistant *S. aureus* (MRSA) infection should be initiated. For methicillin susceptible staphylococci (MSSA) infections, treatment with a first-generation cephalosporin is suggested.
- Abscesses associated with extensive cellulitis (usually larger than 5 cm in diameter), rapid progression, poor response to initial drainage and lesions involving certain body sites including the face, hands, and genitalia are treated with systemic antibiotics.

Retropharyngeal Abscess (RPA)

Background

A retropharyngeal abscess (RPA) is an abscess occupying the space between the posterior pharynx and the prevertebral fascia [2]. RPA is most commonly seen in children under the age of five and usually follows an upper respiratory infection (URI). In older children, RPA can be caused by trauma to the posterior pharynx. The infection may extend from retropharyngeal space to alar and prevertebral space.

Although rare, if not diagnosed and treated in time, RPA can lead to upper airway obstruction and asphyxiation.

Pathophysiology

In younger children, the lymph nodes within the retropharyngeal space are not yet involuted and URIs can lead to suppurative adenitis within the space. This can later lead to phlegmon and abscess formation. As the retropharyngeal abscess grows in size, it results in gradual upper airway obstruction and eventually asphyxiation if left untreated. Typical microorganisms identified from RPAs include *Streptococcus pneumoniae, Streptococcus pyogenes*, *Staphylococcus aureus*, *Fusobacterium*, *Haemophilus* species, as well as respiratory anaerobic organisms.

History/Diagnosis

In addition to URI history and fever, symptoms associated with airway obstruction will become common (Table 24.1).

If clinically stable, lateral neck radiographs may be obtained during inspiration with the neck held in normal extension. Inflammation will be demonstrated by an increase in the depth of the prevertebral space. The upper limit of normal prevertebral space is 7 mm at C2 and 14 mm at C6 in children. If clinically feasible, ultrasound (US) or computerized tomography (CT) of the neck should be obtained to identify the extent of the infection.

Table 24.1 Signs of RPA

Fever
Dysphagia
Odynophagia
Inability to tolerate oral secretions
Neck stiffness
Torticollis
Refusal to extend neck due to pain or discomfort
Change in voice, "hot potato voice," muffled voice
Trismus
Neck swelling, cervical lymphadenopathy
Chest pain (if mediastinal extension)
Respiratory distress (stridor, tachypnea, retractions).

Treatment/Management

All patients need to be evaluated by otolaryngology to determine if there is a need for surgical incision and drainage. Factors that have been associated with an increased need for surgical incision and drainage include an abscess with a cross-sectional area greater than 2 cm^2 and symptoms for greater than 2 days. All patients should have close airway monitoring when undergoing treatment of RPA, especially during the first 24–48 h of therapy.

In patients without severe respiratory distress or airway compromise, intravenous antibiotics can be first-line treatment for 24–48 h. Ampicillin/sulbactam or clindamycin are typically recommended for initial treatment. If the patient has severe disease such as extension to the mediastinum, the addition of vancomycin is recommended. Parenteral antibiotics should be continued until patients are clinically improved and afebrile for 24 h. After patients demonstrate clinical improvement and remain afebrile, they may be transitioned to oral antibiotics. The differential diagnosis and complications of an RPA are noted in Tables 24.2 and 24.3.

Table 24.2 Differential diagnosis of retropharyngeal abscess

Foreign body in airways
Pneumonia
Mediastinitis
Parapharyngeal abscess
Peritonsillar abscess
Odontogenic infection or abscess
Sialadenitis
Epiglottitis
Pharyngitis

Table 24.3 Complications of retropharyngeal abscess

Airway obstruction
Bronchial erosion
Mediastinitis
Sepsis
Acute respiratory distress syndrome
Cranial nerve palsies
Esophageal perforation
Erosion into carotid artery or jugular vein

Orbital Cellulitis

Background

Orbital cellulitis is an infection involving the muscle and fat located within the orbit. The most important distinguishing feature of orbital cellulitis from other local infections is the presence of ophthalmoplegia, the presence of pain with eye movement, and/or proptosis [3]. Orbital cellulitis also typically cause eyelid swelling with or without erythema; however, these findings are also seen in preseptal cellulitis which is a less serious condition. The diagnosis of orbital cellulitis can be confirmed by CT and/or magnetic resonance imaging (MRI). Without prompt diagnosis and proper treatment, orbital cellulitis can lead to loss of vision, subperiosteal abscess, orbital abscess, and intracranial extension of the infection.

Pathophysiology and Etiology

Orbital cellulitis often originates from bacterial rhinosinusitis. Infections of the teeth, middle ear, face, and dacryocystitis or trauma and surgery can also lead to orbital cellulitis as well. As such, common organisms include *S. aureus* (including methicillin-resistant *S. aureus* [MRSA]), *Streptococcus pneumoniae,* other *Streptococci* and Gram-negative bacilli.

Diagnosis

Fever, pain with eye movements, proptosis, and ophthalmoplegia with diplopia are typical signs of orbital cellulitis. Chemosis is common; however, it may also be seen in severe cases of preseptal cellulitis. Eyelid erythema may or may not be present. An ophthalmologist should evaluate the patients for extraocular movements, visual acuity, and to assess for proptosis. In addition, an otolaryngologist can be consulted for evaluation of patients with extensive rhinosinusitis. Peripheral leukocytosis with a predominance of neutrophils and elevated CRP are also seen but nonspecific. Trends in CRP results can be utilized to determine when to discontinue antimicrobial treatment. Although low yield, it is recommended to obtain blood cultures for common bacterial pathogens.

Further imaging should be considered when

- Proptosis
- Limitation of eye movements
- Pain with eye movements
- Double vision
- Vision loss
- Edema extending beyond the eyelid margin
- Signs or symptoms of central nervous system (CNS) involvement
- Inability to examine the patient fully (patients less than 1 year of age)
- Patients who do not begin to show improvement with intravenous treatment in 24 h

Management

- An ophthalmologist should evaluate the patients for extraocular movements, visual acuity, and to assess for proptosis.
- An otolaryngologist can be consulted for evaluation of patients with extensive rhinosinusitis.
- Initiate antibiotics to cover common organisms. The typical initial antibiotic recommended is ampicillin/sulbactam and if a clear nidus from skin is present, the addition of clindamycin could be considered.
- For patients with uncomplicated orbital cellulitis, it is suggested that antibiotics be continued until all signs of orbital cellulitis have resolved. The duration of antibiotic therapy usually ranges from 2 to 3 weeks though patients with severe ethmoid sinusitis and bony destruction of the sinus at least 4 weeks is recommended. Smaller abscesses can be followed clinically with repeat imaging unless there is concern for vision impairment.
- Surgery is almost always indicated in patients with intracranial extension of the infection. Other indications for surgery are failure to respond to antibiotic therapy, worsening visual acuity or pupillary changes, or evidence of an abscess especially if the abscess is greater than 10 mm in diameter. Surgery may also be indicated to obtain cultures.

Croup (Laryngotracheitis)

Background

Laryngotracheitis, otherwise known as croup, is a common respiratory tract infection of young children (typically 6–36 months of age) and predominantly diagnosed during the fall and early spring months. While typically a self-limited illness, those with more severe respiratory tract infection or underlying airway abnormalities may have significant respiratory distress requiring additional interventions or hospitalization.

Pathophysiology

Laryngotracheitis is caused by a variety of respiratory viruses with seasonal variation. Parainfluenza virus (PIV, type 1 in particular) is the most common cause of croup and is most often diagnosed in the fall months. PIV types 2–4 also may cause croup, though type 3 is more frequently implicated in severe disease and occurs in the springtime months. Respiratory syncytial virus (RSV) and adenoviruses are also relatively common causes of croup. Less frequent causes of croup include influenza, picornaviruses (rhinovirus, enteroviruses), and coronaviruses including SARS-CoV-2 [4, 5].

The signs and symptoms of laryngotracheitis are directly related to the pathophysiology of the disease process. Specifically, viral infection results in edema (swelling) of the upper airway. As young children have a smaller airway, a small amount of edema within the airway can lead to symptomatology, hence the predisposition to disease in younger populations or those with congenital or acquired abnormalities of the upper airway. In young children, the narrowest portion of the airway is the cricoid ring. As one ages, the narrowest portion of the airway becomes the vocal cords. As the narrowest portion of the airway is what generates the turbulent airflow (and thus symptomatology), young children develop croup, whereas older patients tend to develop a near equivalent process which is "laryngitis." As the airway becomes narrowed due to edema, the resultant turbulent airflow creates the characteristic high-pitched, inspiratory sound known as "stridor." Biphasic stridor can occur; however, this is generally in the setting of severe upper airway compromise and impending airway failure.

History

It is important to consider the differential diagnosis in a patient presenting with signs and symptoms consistent with croup (see Table 24.4) and the following questions would be key components of the history:

Table 24.4 Focused history for croup

Body system	Question(s)	Reasoning
Constitutional General	Fever Prior history of similar symptoms?	Fever is common in children with croup and can help differentiate it from structural abnormalities or foreign-body aspiration History of croup can be a clue to recurrent disease, especially in the setting of other viral symptoms (cough, congestion, rhinorrhea)
HENT	History of intubation or airway abnormality? Drooling? Rhinorrhea, congestion?	History of intubation or airway abnormality? Typically, not present, would suggest epiglottitis or retropharyngeal abscess Often present in the setting of viral illnesses, such as croup

(continued)

Body system	Question(s)	Reasoning
Pulmonary	Symptom onset? Cough (and quality of cough)? Voice quality? Stridor? Increased work of breathing? Positioning with symptoms? Anything that improved symptoms?	Onset is usually gradual. A rapid symptom onset of stridor without other symptoms suggests a foreign-body aspiration A "bark-like" cough (think of the bark of a seal) is characteristic of croup More frequently hoarse. A muffled or "hot potato" voice is suggestive of epiglottitis or retropharyngeal abscess Stridor (inspiratory) is common in croup Suggestive of greater degree of symptomatology The stridor present is often *not* positional, in contrast to some other upper airway abnormalities (i.e., laryngomalacia) Cool air, or humidified air, may temporarily improve symptoms of croup
Abdomen	Belly breathing?	Additional sign of increased work of breathing

Birth History

In a patient with croup, the neonatal history can be particularly important. Specifically, infants who required intubation (for any reason, including prematurity or endotracheal suction due to meconium aspiration) may develop subglottic stenosis. This airway abnormality can increase the risk of symptomatic croup requiring intervention.

Family History

Family history is generally non-contributory apart from a familial history of croup which increases risk of croup threefold.

Risk Factors for Croup

1. Age: peak incidence between 6 and 36 months of age, mostly ≤6 years of age.
2. Epidemiologic history: seasonality (typically fall months, occasionally see in early spring), exposures to other ill contacts (daycare exposure, siblings, other individuals with "laryngitis").
3. History of upper airway abnormalities (subglottic stenosis, vascular malformations, etc.)

Table 24.5 Focused physical examination for croup

System	Exam	Tips
General	Describe the patient's overall appearance Positioning	"Sick or not sick?" "Tripoding" or "sniffing position" is often suggestive of epiglottitis or retropharyngeal abscesses
EENT	Alar flaring	If present, may suggest increased work of breathing
Cardiovascular	Tachycardia	May be related to sepsis picture, but also potential medication effect
Respiratory	Respiratory rate Is there any work of breathing? If so, describe the severity and location Stridor? If so, would clarify if present at rest	If tachypneic, it is suggestive of increased work of breathing. Similarly, retractions would signify increased work of breathing. As it is an upper airway obstruction, suprasternal retractions may be prominent Stridor is a classic feature of croup. Stridor at rest, especially in the setting of increased work of breathing, signifies significant symptomatic disease
Abdominal	Abdominal breathing	An additional marker of respiratory distress, especially if present with other features

Physical Exam

Vitals: make note of the respiratory rate, heart rate, and oxygen saturations. As this is an upper airway obstruction, oxygen saturations should remain normal; hypoxemia, if present, is an indicator of severe disease. During the acute evaluation, vitals should be monitored for instability, though continuous monitoring is generally not required apart from those with severe disease. See Table 24.5 for a croup focused physical exam.

Laboratory Assessment

Croup is a clinical diagnosis, and laboratory/radiographic assessment is not necessary in the setting of uncomplicated disease. A thorough history and physical examination will obviate the need for additional diagnostic workup, resulting in cost-effective practice of medicine.

However, in patients with severe respiratory compromise, with an atypical course, or for whom the diagnosis remains uncertain, laboratory and imaging workup can help narrow the differential diagnosis. In patients with croup, leukocytosis is common. Electrolytes are typically normal in absence of concomitant dehydration. Respiratory viral testing by polymerase chain reaction can identify an etiologic agent; however, directed antiviral therapy remains limited (and often unnecessary) aside from infection with influenza and SARS-CoV-2 requiring hospitalization. Plain X-ray imaging of the neck can provide additional diagnostic guidance if the diagnosis is unclear. Specifically, croup will have evidence of a "steeple sign" where narrowing of the subglottic airway creates a pitched appearance of the airway like a steepled roof. This differentiates it from other airway findings such as bacterial tracheitis (ragged appearance of the tracheal wall) and epiglottitis (thumb sign due to inflamed epiglottis).

Differential Diagnosis

The differential diagnosis of croup is extremely broad, ranging from mild anatomical issues without substantial compromise (e.g., laryngomalacia) to severe lower respiratory tract illnesses that can be life-threatening (e.g., epiglottitis). See Table 24.6 for a broad infectious and non-infectious differential diagnosis listing.

Table 24.6 Differential diagnosis of infectious and non-infectious etiologies mimicking croup

Infectious considerations	
Diagnosis	Clinical/laboratory/radiographic features
Bacterial tracheitis	Rough cough, ill appearance, highly febrile, "ragged" airway on neck X-ray
Epiglottitis	Ill appearance, muffled (hot potato) voice, highly febrile, edematous epiglottis (if visualized), tripod positioning, thumb sign on neck X-ray
Retropharyngeal abscess	Ill appearance, muffled (hot potato) voice, posterior pharyngeal edema/erythema, posterior pharyngeal edema/gas on lateral neck X-ray

Non-infectious considerations	
Diagnosis	Clinical/laboratory features
Foreign-body aspiration	Acute onset stridor, concern for ingestion of foreign body, radiopaque body seen on imaging, afebrile
Laryngomalacia	Positional (worse supine, improves when prone), no fevers
Post-extubation stridor	Usually noted after prolonged periods of intubation once the endotracheal tube is removed. Treated with steroids and inhaled epinephrine (if needed)
Inhalational injury (thermal, chemical)	History of inhalational injury (e.g., house fire), visualized soot or caustic injuries in nasopharyngeal tissues
Vascular malformations of airway (e.g., hemangioma)	Noted recurrent "croup" that responds well to racemic epinephrine, though less responsive to steroids, and is present during non-seasonal months. May also see other cutaneous vascular malformations
Vascular ring	Stridor that is neither positional nor responsive to typical croup management; potential issues with swallowing/choking on foods. May see diagnosis with upper GI due to vascular impingement of esophagus
Vocal cord paralysis	Stridulous sounds secondary to laryngeal nerve trauma (i.e., surgery) or neurologic disease (i.e., Guillain-Barre syndrome)
Laryngeal web	Recurrent stridor episodes, noted on direct visualization
Allergic reaction (angioedema)	Concomitant oropharyngeal edema, urticaria, wheezing, potential history of severe allergic reactions
Laryngeal papillomatosis	Noted on direct visualization, typically after recurrent episodes of croup. Maternal history of human papilloma virus

Management

Supportive management is the mainstay of therapy with laryngotracheitis. Most cases are self-resolving in nature without additional interventions. Simple interventions that can be done at home for children with mild symptoms (intermittent bark-like cough without stridor at rest or increased work of breathing) include having the child breathe in cool air. In the fall, exposure to the cool nighttime air can decrease symptoms. In warmer weather, opening a freezer door and letting the child breathe in this cool air from a safe distance can often be temporarily effective. Humidified air (such as a steamy bathroom) may have a similar effect. For a child with a more symptomatic cough who does not have stridor at rest, a single dose of oral dexamethasone (0.6 mg/kg, max dose 16 mg) or oral prednisolone (1 mg/kg) can help alleviate symptoms. For children with moderate to severe symptoms, corticosteroids [typically a single dose of oral or IV dexamethasone 0.6 mg/kg (max dose: 16 mg)] are necessary to reduce airway edema. As the effects of the steroids are not instantaneous, children with stridor at rest, those with concomitant increased work of breathing, benefit from inhaled epinephrine. Inhaled epinephrine is effective as it causes vasoconstriction of upper airway vessels reducing edema, with an onset of action of about 10 min. However, this is a temporizing measure, and steroids should be given concomitantly. Lack of response to inhaled epinephrine, especially to multiple doses, should raise question to the correct diagnosis. Multiple doses of inhaled racemic epinephrine can increase the risk of "rebound" symptoms whereby the airway edema becomes more pronounced as the medication effects wear off. This should be considered when determining treatment options for symptomatic patients.

In patients who continue with significant symptomatology despite the above interventions, alternative management strategies include the use of Heliox [oxygen (O_2) and helium (He) mixture]. Non-invasive and invasive positive pressure ventilation are rarely required, but sometimes utilized in cases of severe disease.

Acute Osteomyelitis

Background

Acute osteomyelitis is an inflammatory process involving the bone and bone marrow caused microorganisms that spread through the bloodstream, fractures, or surgery. The overall incidence of osteomyelitis in the United States is mostly unknown, but reports show it to be as high as 1 in 675 US hospital admissions each year or about 50,000 cases annually. Boys contract the disease 1.2–3.7 times more often than do girls. Approximately 25% of children with osteomyelitis are younger than 2 years old, and 50% are younger than 5 years [6].

Pathophysiology

Bone can get infected via the hematogenous route of infection through bacteremic seeding from a distant source of infection, contiguous spread from surrounding tissue and joints, or direct inoculation of bone from trauma, surgery and in the presence of foreign bodies. The well-perfused metaphysis of the long bones are usually the initial site of infection and are usually affected by hematogenous spread. Most common organisms spread this way are *Staphylococcus aureus*, group A streptococcus, *Kingella kingae* (young children <5 years). Other specific organisms to consider are: if water exposure/trauma-related infection: *Pseudomonas* sp., *Aeromonas* sp., other environmental Gram negatives; if mud/significant dirt exposure or foreign body involved: again, environmental Gram negatives, anaerobes, fungal organisms.

Symptoms of osteomyelitis are influenced by the age of the child and the etiologic agent. In newborns, the thin cortex is a poor barrier and infection can easily progress to the soft tissues and other bones. Newborns are usually irritable and have pain when the affected area is touched. In older infants, the cortex is thicker, and the periosteum is slightly denser. Consequently, the infection spreads less often to the soft tissues of the extremity. In infants and young children, pain is usually accompanied by limping because osteomyelitis occurs more commonly in the lower extremities. Pseudoparalysis may occur. In older children, the infection rarely ruptures or spreads to the outer cortical lamellae resulting with more focal findings. Due to this, point tenderness is often sharply circumscribed. Osteomyelitis can affect any part of the skeleton but occurs mostly in long bones with the femur and tibia the most common sites.

History/Signs and Symptoms

Patients can present with severe constitutional symptoms including high fevers (39–40 °C), pain, erythema, swelling, and warmth at the site of infection. Pain may be dull with or without motion. In subacute presentations, some patients may have generalized malaise, mild pain over several weeks with minimal fever, or other constitutional symptoms. Acute osteomyelitis may also present as septic arthritis, especially if the metaphysis of the bone is within the infected joint capsule. See Table 24.7 for an osteomyelitis focused exam.

Table 24.7 Focused history for osteomyelitis

Body system	Symptom	Reasoning
Constitutional	Fever	Fever is variable but usually present
	Appetite	May have malaise
Extremity/area concern	Continuing to have age-appropriate activity	Limited movement
	Pain	Localized pain is more common beyond toddler years
Other	History of trauma, fracture (open vs. closed), foreign body, water/dirt exposure	Different mechanism of injury can lead to different presentation of disease, and different exposures may hint us about organisms involved

Table 24.8 Focused physical examination for osteomyelitis

System	Exam	Tips
General	Describe the patient's overall appearance	"Sick or not sick?"
Extremities	Positioning Pain Edema or erythema Involvement of joint Pulse	How is the child holding their body: What is the position of the extremity and is there pseudoparalysis? Careful examination of any area of concern. Look for associated joint swelling, erythema, or tenderness

Physical Exam

Vitals: Especially in patients with possibility of critical illness and dissemination of the infection, abnormal vital signs can be the first clues alerting you to the critical nature of the infection. See Table 24.8 for a focused exam for osteomyelitis.

Laboratory Assessment and Diagnosis

Laboratory data is usually nonspecific in patients with osteomyelitis. There may or may not be leukocytosis, and the erythrocyte sedimentation rate (ESR) and CRP are usually elevated. The CRP level correlates with clinical response to therapy and may be used to monitor treatment. If blood cultures are positive, they can be helpful in timely identification of the pathogen. Clinically, the most useful studies are plain radiographs and MRI. Radiographs could be used to rule out other potential causes of symptoms such as a cancer metastasis or underlying fractures. Finding in

Table 24.9 Infectious and non-infectious differential diagnosis of osteomyelitis

Infectious diagnosis	Non-infectious diagnosis
Septicemia—systemic signs of infection, ill appearance, bacteremia, elevated WBC	Fractures—deformity or radiographic abnormalities
Cellulitis—soft tissue edema but not true bone tenderness	Scurvy-other features of vitamin C deficiency present, skin findings
Septic bursitis—inflammation of bursa but not joint itself	Rheumatic fever—migratory arthralgias
Myositis—muscle inflammation/infection, myalgias present, not true bone tenderness	Toxic synovitis—low inflammatory markers, preceding illness 1–2 weeks prior
Thrombophlebitis	Chronic recurrent multifocal osteomyelitis—Resolving with NSAIDS, no other signs of infection

radiographic studies can include soft tissue swelling, osteopenia, osteolysis, bony destruction, and nonspecific periosteal reaction, you usually see these after at least ~2 weeks if illness. Rarely, Brodie's abscess, which is a well-circumscribed lytic lesion, may be seen. MRI has the highest sensitivity and specificity to detect early bone infection within 3–5 days of disease onset. A negative MRI is sufficient for the exclusion of disease if symptoms have been present for at least 1 week. The use of intravenous contrast does not improve the detection of disease but helps provide the distinction between a phlegmon, necrotic tissue, and abscess. A CT scan is ordered primarily to determine the extent of bony destruction (especially in the spine) to guide biopsies or in patients with contraindications to MRI.

If possible, an open bone biopsy is preferred over percutaneous biopsy. Cessation of antibiotics 48–72 h before open bone biopsy may increase microbiological yield. Bone cultures may be positive regardless of prior antibiotic therapy because these infections occur in areas of infection-induced infarction or necrosis, but still, it is ideal especially in chronic/indolent cases, or when suspecting atypical or hard to grow organisms. *Staphylococcus aureus* (SA) is the most common cause of acute osteomyelitis and methicillin-resistant SA (MRSA) infections should be considered. After SA, group A streptococci is the next most common cause. Rarely in younger children *Kingella kingae* infections can be seen. See Table 24.9 for a differential diagnosis of infectious and non-infectious etiologies mimicking osteomyelitis. It is important to know that some of these diagnoses can be seen along with osteomyelitis.

Differential Diagnosis

Management

The initial antimicrobial therapy should have potent activity against MRSA and group A streptococci. Surgical debridement of the infection, if feasible, is as important as the prolonged antimicrobial treatment. In areas where community

Table 24.10 Complications of osteomyelitis

Septic arthritis
Pathological fractures
Sinus tract formation
Bone deformity
Systemic infection
Septic thrombophlebitis
Contiguous soft tissue infection

acquired MRSA (CA-MRSA) is common, either vancomycin or clindamycin (if >90% of CA-MRSA isolates are clindamycin susceptible) should be included in the initial empiric therapy for CA-MRSA. Vancomycin should be reserved in critically ill patients and patients that clindamycin cannot be administered. If MRSA is not a concern, cephalexin or amoxicillin/clavulanate would cover well MSSA and streptococci. In ill-appearing children, antibiotic treatment should not be delayed. Switching to oral therapy is an acceptable option when the following criteria have been met: ideally an organism has been identified to best target therapy (but not always required), the patient can swallow the appropriate medication, and the patient has a clear clinical response to intravenously administered antibiotics. The recommended duration of treatment for osteomyelitis is 4–6 weeks of antibiotic therapy to achieve acceptable cure rates and decrease the risk of recurrence.

Some complications which may arise with osteomyelitis are listed in Table 24.10.

COVID-19

Background/Pathophysiology

Children of all ages can experience a COVID-19 infection and transmit the virus to others. The number of cases is likely underestimated. The incidence increases with increasing age. Transmission can occur within a household, in large gatherings, educational or childcare settings, etc. Masking and vaccination policies decrease transmission. Children from underrepresented racial and ethnic groups, similar to adults, appear to be disproportionately affected, likely due to underlying health and socioeconomic conditions. COVID-19 hospitalization rates in children have varied throughout the pandemic. Reinfection can occur, especially with the newer variants.

Transmission is human to human, through inhalation of infected droplets. Fomite transmission is very low. Airborne transmission is a significant concern when patient is receiving an aerosol generating procedures (AGP). The virus infects and replicates mainly in the respiratory tract; the incubation period is 2–14 days. Transmission is possible from 2 days prior to the start of symptoms until day 10 after the onset symptoms (after day 10 the risk is substantially lower, but not zero). Asymptomatic transmission can occur as well.

Table 24.11 Acute COVID-19 signs and symptoms

Symptom	Overall frequency	Comment
Fever	60–70%	
Cough	35%	
Rhinorrhea	16%	More common in infants
Diarrhea	13%	
Dyspnea	10%	More common in infants
Sore throat	9%	More common over 10-year age group
Vomiting	6%	
Asymptomatic	15–40%	More common in 1–10 year age group

History

Respiratory symptoms are similar in children and adults, but disease appears to be milder in children, though severe cases and deaths have been reported. There is a wide spectrum of disease, for which high level of suspicion especially during high community transmission rates, is needed. Common symptoms [7] are listed in Table 24.11. Symptoms usually last a few days to 2 weeks, but post-acute COVID-19 symptoms and long COVID-19 symptoms (including neurologic or neurocognitive symptoms) may occur in children as well (more widely described in adults).

Less frequent symptoms include myocarditis, pulmonary embolism, or deep vein thromboembolism (DVT). Loss of smell and taste are uncommon in children.

Shortly after the initial peak rates of acute COVID-19 infection in children were noted in 2020, we started seeing an increase in Kawasaki disease-like presentations, with some specific characteristics, associated with a recent infection or exposure to COVID-19 (usually 4–6 weeks prior to presentation). This was later named the multisystemic inflammatory syndrome related to COVID-19 or MIS-C. This is a post-infectious phenomenon, characterized by a multi-system hyper inflammatory response that can lead to heart failure, coronary abnormalities/aneurisms, and secondary cardiac or thromboembolic events. See Chap. 28, section on MIS-C.

Physical Examination

Signs vary from asymptomatic, mild congestion or upper respiratory infection symptoms to severe respiratory distress, hypoxemia, and respiratory failure. Hypotension/shock can occur if the patient has myocarditis or an MIS-C type presentation. Dehydration from vomiting and diarrhea are more common in certain variants. Rash, conjunctivitis, other mucosal or skin changes can be seen with MIS-C.

Table 24.12 Common laboratory and imaging findings in acute Covid illness

Laboratory analyses	Associated findings
CBC with differential	Lymphopenia 32%, associated with severity
D-dimer	Elevated
CRP	May be normal or elevated
Liver enzymes	Elevated
Lactate dehydrogenase, ferritin, interleukin 6, 10	Elevated
Creatinine, BUN	Elevated, signs of acute kidney injury
Brain natriuretic peptide (BNP), troponins	Elevated
Imaging	
Echocardiogram	Decreased heart function
Chest X-ray	Perihilar thickening, multifocal interstitial or alveolar infiltrates, lymphadenopathy, pleural effusion, pericarditis
Chest CT angiography	Pulmonary embolism, multifocal pneumonia

Laboratory Assessment/Imaging

To confirm the diagnosis of a COVID-19 acute infection, a positive viral test is required, both antigen and molecular-based testing are available. Molecular tests are more sensitive and specific, but less widely available. Rapid tests can have false positives and false negatives results. A high index of suspicion is needed in the appropriate setting. See Table 24.12 for common laboratory and imaging findings in acute Covid illness.

Differential Diagnosis

1. Other respiratory viral infections
2. Bacterial pneumonia
3. Gastroenteritis
4. Kawasaki disease
5. Sepsis/septic shock

Management

Management depends on severity of the disease.

For mild to moderate cases: Patient is otherwise stable, without hemodynamic compromise or need for oxygen supplementation, symptomatic relief is recommended with antipyretics/anti-inflammatory drugs. Preemptive antiviral treatment is reserved for patients who are at high risk for progression to severe disease (such as immunocompromising condition or treatment, chronic heart and lung conditions, obesity) with remdesivir or paxlovid (nirmatrelvir and ritonavir combination), according to age and eligibility.

For severe cases: Patient requires hospitalization, oxygen therapy. Treatment with steroids (dexamethasone) and the antiviral medication remdesivir are indicated. Remdesivir is now FDA approved for patients ≥28 days and with weight ≥3 kg for 5–10 days though if a patient rapidly improves, they can receive less days of therapy. If there is co-infection and/or a question if a COVID infection is causing acute or chronic symptoms, consultation with an infectious disease specialist for treatment considerations is of benefit. Most of the information on treatment is extrapolated from adult data.

Due to emerging variants of the virus, monoclonal antibodies have decreased effectiveness and currently they are not recommended for treatment. Tixagevimab and cilgavimab combination (EVUSHELD) is a long-acting monoclonal antibody product for pre-exposure prophylaxis against COVID-19 that was reserved for immunocompromised individuals or those for whom vaccination is contraindicated. It is not currently authorized for emergency use in the United States until further notice by FDA. This is because it is unlikely to be active against certain SARS-CoV-2 variants, projected to be responsible for more than 90% of current infections in the US.

Masking and isolation decreased risk of transmission to others, refer to CDC Guidance for COVID-19 for the most up-to-date recommendations.

Vaccines

Covid vaccines are now approved and recommended for ages 6 months and up. Bivalent boosters are also approved and should be recommended to all patients. They have been shown to be effective in reducing risk of severe disease, hospitalization, and covid-19-related complications.

Application Exercises

1. You are seeing a 2-year-old female patient who was noted to have a red pimple on her right buttock 1 day ago. Since yesterday, she has been fussy and felt warm. This morning her mom noticed that the area with pimple grew to the size of an egg and the patient has been very upset throughout her diaper change. Her mom thinks that she is avoiding urinating due to pain. She reports that patient had a similar pimple last year, but it resolved with the use of an antibiotic ointment. The patient is otherwise a healthy child. The patient's father has had skin staph infections in the past possibly related to his diagnosis of severe eczema. Exam is notable for a fluctuant tender mass on the right buttock with 5 cm of surrounding erythema.

   What would be the best approach for this patient?

   A. Perform incision and drainage; send wound culture, but do not initiate antibiotics pending results.
   B. Initiate clindamycin IV and admit for observation

C. Perform incision and drainage; send wound culture and initiate clindamycin PO as outpatient
D. Initiate topical antibiotic ointment

Correct answer is "c." Most younger children have significant area of cellulitis surrounding the abscess and if this continues even after abscess is fully drained a short course of antibiotics is recommended. If there is no residual abscess and/or cellulitis, drainage may be sufficient.

2. A 10-year-old patient with a recent history of cough, runny nose, and low-grade temperatures, now resolved, now presents with acute cheek and forehead erythema. About a day ago, she noticed erythema of her right cheek and forehead which quickly became tender and bright red. The erythema is now surrounding her eye and her eyelids are edematous. She is obviously uncomfortable and does not want anyone touching her face or eye. Her conjunctivae appear red. You do not observe any limitation in her eye movements.

   How would you approach this patient?

   A. Obtain urgent ophthalmology consultation
   B. Obtain urgent ENT consultation
   C. Start ampicillin/sulbactam IV and consult ophthalmology
   D. Start vancomycin IV and consult ophthalmology

   The correct answer is "c." Although patient's full examination is not provided, they appear to have progressing infection and should be started on treatment and evaluated by ophthalmology. In the case of severe infection, vancomycin should be added in addition to ampicillin/sulbactam treatment.

3. You are seeing a 2-year-old male with a history of prematurity for onset of bark-like cough, fevers (Tm 101 °F), and mild inspiratory stridor at rest. He was born at 27 weeks gestation requiring admission to the NICU for intubation and mechanical ventilation, but did not have bronchopulmonary dysplasia. It is currently October, and the family notes that his cough had begun that evening with progression of his symptoms prompting presentation. Incidentally, they note that his stridor had improved slightly on the brief walk from the car to checking in to the emergency department though it is back to what it was before. There is no significant family history, and the child is without any other medical comorbidities.

   On exam, the child is resting in the father's arms. Vitals are notable for mild tachypnea (respiratory rate: 42 breaths/min), SpO_2 98% on room air. Heart rate is in upper range of normal at 140 beats/min. He is mildly ill appearing, but non-toxic in nature. Noted stridor at rest, with minimal/intermittent retractions, which is more notable when he is upset/crying. The remainder of his examination is unremarkable.

   (a) What risk factors does this patient have for croup?
   (b) What is the next best step in his management?

   A. Obtain AP and lateral neck X-rays
   B. Inhaled epinephrine alone
   C. Inhaled racemic epinephrine and oral/IV dexamethasone

D. Observation and anticipatory guidance
E. Direct laryngoscopy

Answers: This child has several classic history and epidemiologic risk factors for croup. Specifically, his prior history of intubation as a premature infant may predispose to development of subglottic stenosis, and thus risk for symptomatic disease. His age is typical for children with croup, and the seasonality (late fall) is quite typical for this disease process.

Correct answer: C (inhaled racemic epinephrine and oral/IV dexamethasone). His clinical history is very consistent with croup. This child likely has moderate disease given his stridor at rest with some questionable concerns of retractions at baseline and non-toxic appearance. For moderate croup, inhaled epinephrine and oral/IV dexamethasone should be administered. (A) is incorrect as the laboratory or imaging assessment is not required in the setting of a patient with uncomplicated laryngotracheitis, as is this case. (B) is incorrect as inhaled racemic epinephrine is not used alone—it is always given with corticosteroids concomitantly as the effect racemic epinephrine is temporary, whereas steroids have a longer lasting effect of airway edema resolution. (D) is incorrect in this setting given the stridor at rest—this indicates a greater disease severity necessitating pharmacologic intervention. (E) is incorrect as the clinical presentation is quite consistent with croup and not of recurrent nature to warrant substantial concern for upper airway abnormality. However, should recurrences be noted in his future, laryngoscopy may be indicated given his prior history of intubation to evaluate for subglottic stenosis or other airway abnormalities predisposing to symptomatic disease.

4. You are seeing a 4-year-old previously healthy male who has been refusing to walk since yesterday. In the days before this, his mother noticed that he was not as active as usual and he had a decreased appetite. The child is resting in the mother's arms and is very irritable when you try to carry him to the hospital bed. Vital signs are notable for temperature to 103 °F, mild tachypnea, and SpO_2 99% on room air. On physical examination, he is avoiding moving his right leg with slight erythema and edema at the distal end of femur. He is tender when you palpate the area. The remainder of his examination is unremarkable.

   Which is the most sensitive imaging needed for this patient?

A. MRI with and without contrast of R femur and hip
B. XR of R hip
C. Hip ultrasound
D. No need for imaging, clinical exam is good enough

Answers:

Correct answer: A.

X-rays are helpful for initial assessment, mainly for ruling out fractures, or other bone lesions but osteomyelitis can be missed early especially in the course, you need at least 2 weeks to start seeing bone changes concerning for osteomyelitis in XR. A normal XR does not completely rule out osteomyelitis. MRI is the most sensitive imaging and should always be ordered with contrast to evaluate abnormal enhancement, or presence of collections. This patient may need surgical involvement for obtaining cultures from affected bone as well as drainage if it is needed. Antibiotics could be held till a radiologic and surgical decision are made but, in most instances, starting coverage for MRSA will not affect the culture result in a short period of time as the bacterial load will be significant within the bone tissue.

5. You are seeing a 10-month-old infant in your office for fever and upper respiratory infection symptoms. The patient has a temperature of up to 38.5 °C and been congested for 2 days but otherwise acting and eating normally. The patient has a 12-year-old brother with juvenile idiopathic arthritis on anti-TNF treatment who is currently unvaccinated. What is the appropriate management for both of the children and what would you advise family?

   - The 10-month-old infant is healthy and well appearing with mild disease. He is now eligible for vaccination (which can be done as soon as his isolation period ends) and can be managed at home.
   - His 12-year-old brother is immunocompromised and at high risk for severe disease so he could be a candidate for monoclonal antibody therapy for prophylaxis vs. treatment if he develops symptoms. Also eligible for vaccine, but if given antibody therapy he needs to wait for 90 days because it can interfere with immune response.
   - General advice for family would include maintaining isolation/quarantine precautions as directed by the most recent Center for Disease Control guidelines Vaccination is recommended for everybody eligible in household even if they have had COVID-19 disease.

References

1. Stevens DL, Bisno AL, Chambers HF, Dellinger EP, Goldstein EJ, Gorbach SL, et al. Practice guidelines for the diagnosis and management of skin and soft tissue infections: 2014 update by the Infectious Diseases Society of America. Clin Infect Dis. 2014;59(2):e10–52.
2. Akhavan M. Ear, nose, throat: beyond pharyngitis: retropharyngeal abscess, peritonsillar abscess, epiglottitis, bacterial tracheitis, and postoperative tonsillectomy. Emerg Med Clin N Am. 2021;39:661–75.
3. Baiu I, Melendez E. Periorbital and orbital cellulitis. JAMA. 2020;323(2):196.
4. Committee on Infectious Diseases AAoP, Kimberlin DW, Barnett ED, Lynfield R, Sawyer MH. Parainfluenza viral infections. In: Red book: 2021–2024 report of the Committee on Infectious Diseases. American Academy of Pediatrics; 2021.
5. Malhotra A, Krilov LR. Viral croup. Pediatr Rev. 2001;22(1):5–12.
6. Woods CR, Bradley JS, Chatterjee A, Copley LA, Robinson J, Kronman MP, Arrieta A, et al. Clinical practice guideline by the Pediatric Infectious Diseases Society and the Infectious Diseases Society of America: 2021 guideline on diagnosis and management of acute hematogenous osteomyelitis in pediatrics. JPIDS. 2021;10(8):801–44.
7. Yasuhara J, Kuno T, Tagaki H, Sumitomo N. Clinical characteristics of COVID-19 in children: a systematic review. Pediatr Pulmonol. 2020;55:2565–75.

Chapter 25
Infectious Diseases: Common Outpatient Considerations

Lindsay Cameron and Anna Rueda

Infectious Pharyngitis

Background

Pharyngitis is inflammation of the pharynx and/or surrounding anatomic structures that results in sore throat. Viruses (Adenovirus, Coxsackie virus, SARS-CoV-2, etc.) are the most common cause of pharyngitis in all age groups [1]. The most common bacteria causing pharyngitis is *Streptococcus pyogenes* or Group A Streptococcus (GAS), which accounts for 20–30% of pharyngitis in children aged 5–15 years and most often occurs in winter and early spring. GAS infection is a rare cause of pharyngitis in children less than 3 years of age. Less common bacterial causes include: *Fusobacterium necrophorum*, Groups C and G Streptococcus, *Arcanobacterium haemolyticum*, *Corynebacterium diphtheria*, *Neisseria gonorrhoeae*, *Yersinia enterocolitica, Mycoplasma pneumoniae*, and *Chlamydia pneumoniae*. The incidence of epiglottitis has decreased significantly since the introduction of the vaccination against *Haemophilus influenzae* type B. Bacteria in the oropharynx (including GAS, other oral streptococci, *Staphylococcus aureus*, and oral anaerobes) are often implicated in causing retropharyngeal, lateral pharyngeal, or peritonsillar abscesses.

L. Cameron (✉)
Texas Children's Pediatrics, Texas Children's Hospital, Houston, TX, USA
e-mail: lahatze1@texaschildrens.org

A. Rueda
Division of Academic General Pediatrics, Department of Pediatrics, Baylor College of Medicine, Houston, TX, USA
e-mail: Anna.Rueda@bcm.edu

N. Liao et al. (eds.), *Pediatric Rotations*,
https://doi.org/10.1007/978-3-031-59873-9_25

History

In a child who presents with pharyngitis, the most important questions to ask the patient and/or parent/caregiver are timing of onset and associated symptoms. Most children with pharyngitis will have some associated fevers. Low-grade fevers are more often associated with viral syndromes, and higher fevers are more often bacterial in etiology. Children who present with more indolent symptoms and have associated nasal congestion or rhinorrhea, cough, and fatigue are more likely to have a viral illness. Children who present with an abrupt onset (within hours) of pharyngitis symptoms with high fever, drooling, and respiratory distress will need to go to the emergency room. Children who have high fevers with an associated muffled voice (or a "hot potato voice"), significant neck swelling, or refusal to swallow are more likely to have a deep neck infection such as a retropharyngeal, lateral pharyngeal, or peritonsillar abscess.

Physical Exam/Differential Diagnosis

The physical exam of a child who presents with a sore throat must begin with an overall clinical assessment. If the child's pharyngitis illness occurred abruptly, if he/she is toxic appearing (as outlined above), or if he/she is in respiratory distress (due to impending upper airway obstruction), then Emergency Medical Services (EMS) should be contacted urgently. A minimal exam can be performed to alert incoming EMS providers of the appearance of the child. The child should be kept calm while awaiting transfer to a tertiary facility (this includes not placing any objects in a child's mouth for an examination). Etiologic examples include: (1) children who are ill-appearing with difficulty breathing due to a thickened pharyngeal membrane and significant anterior cervical lymph node swelling from diphtheria, (2) adolescents who present ill-appearing in respiratory distress due to severe neck pain and swelling with edematous pharyngitis from Lemierre syndrome, and (3) children who are toxic in appearance with high fever, inspiratory stridor, and are drooling from epiglottitis.

Children with pharyngitis may present to the clinic while febrile with dry mucus membranes. Pharyngeal inflammation can range from mild erythema to beefy red with edema, ulcerations, and/or exudate. Specific findings may help in distinguishing between infectious etiologies. Viral pharyngitis due to Adenovirus can present with pharyngeal erythema and edema with associated follicular conjunctivitis ("pink eye") and anterior cervical lymph node swelling. Coxsackie virus (an enterovirus) causes herpangina or "hand, foot, and mouth disease" which often manifests as oral ulcerations in the mouth and posterior oropharynx and a vesicular rash on the hands, feet, and buttocks. Epstein-Barr virus (EBV) or infectious mononucleosis ("Mono") presents with posterior cervical lymphadenitis, erythema, edema, and exudate of the posterior oropharynx with or without splenomegaly. SARS-CoV-2 (COVID-19) causes pharyngeal erythema in approximately 50% of children, and in those with mild illness this may be accompanied by nasal congestion. Some children with COVID-19 present with chilblains (perino-like lesions) of the toes, ("COVID toes"). See Chap. 24 for additional information on COVID-19 infection. Herpes Simplex Virus (HSV) causes gingivostomatitis which results in ulceration of the lips and mouth and blisters of the lips and anterior mouth. These patients can also have inflamed, swollen gingiva. Children with GAS pharyngitis often present with fevers, exudative pharyngitis and tonsillitis, petechiae of the palate, and anterior cervical lymphadenitis. Those with a pharyngeal abscess (retropharyngeal, lateral pharyngeal, or peritonsillar) are often ill-appearing with high fever and difficulty swallowing. On exam, they will have marked swelling of the affected tissue. For example, those with a peritonsillar abscess often have an asymmetrical, fluctuant, swelling in the posterior soft palate with a deviated uvula away from the affected side.

Laboratory Assessment/Imaging (Workup)

The child's history and physical exam will guide the diagnostic workup. In those who are toxic appearing or have localized swelling in the posterior oropharynx, imaging is often necessary to evaluate the upper airway and to assess for an abscess that would benefit from surgical drainage. These patients need urgent treatment; therefore, imaging is usually obtained at the hospital. Viral respiratory testing is not necessary to support a diagnosis of adenoviral conjunctivopharygitis syndrome or a Coxsackie virus-associated illness. Rapid antigen or PCR testing is recommended in those with suspected COVID-19; this will guide infection control recommendations (isolation or quarantine). HSV viral culture or PCR testing can be obtained to confirm a diagnosis of gingivostomatitis. In those with suspected EBV illness, heterophile antibody testing ("monospot" testing), and/or EBV-specific serology can be obtained. Heterophile antibody testing can be falsely negative in children less than 4 years of age; therefore, serologic testing is often more helpful in this age group. GAS testing is recommended in children (over age 3) who present with acute pharyngeal or tonsillar inflammation without viral symptoms like cough, congestion, and rhinorrhea. Those less than 3 years old should only be tested if they are symptomatic and they have been exposed to an individual with confirmed GAS infection. Testing includes rapid antigen diagnostic testing (RADT) and culture. RADT results are available in minutes and cultures take 24–48 hours. Often, dual swabs are obtained, and a culture is sent to the lab only if the RADT test is negative.

Management

The management of most viral causes of pharyngitis is supportive care. This includes children with mild COVID-19 illness, and otherwise healthy children with HSV stomatitis, both of which are self-limited conditions. Some children with recurrent HSV stomatitis (often at times of concurrent illness or stress) are treated with chronic suppressive antiviral treatment. In those with confirmed or suspected GAS pharyngitis, the recommended treatment is either penicillin (orally for 10 days or one IM injection of benzathine penicillin) or oral amoxicillin for 10 days [1, 2]. Those who have a non-anaphylaxis allergic reaction to penicillin can be treated with 10 days of cephalexin. In those with a true penicillin allergy, recommended agents include: 10 days of clindamycin, 10 days of clarithromycin, or 5 days of azithromycin. The main goal of treatment of GAS pharyngitis is to prevent the development of rheumatic fever [3].

Anticipatory Guidance (For Parents/Families)

It is important for parents and families of children with pharyngitis to know what to expect (a self-limited illness) and when to anticipate clinical improvement. It is also important for the family to be aware of potential complications from the child's illness (dehydration from limited oral intake or clinical worsening). Clinical resolution of symptoms from a Coxsackie illness will take 7–10 days. This is short compared to an EBV-associated illness, during which the pharyngitis and cervical lymph node swelling may resolve in the same time period, but the associated fatigue can last weeks to months. Following appropriate treatment for GAS pharyngitis, children often improve rapidly (in 24–36 hours) after the initiation of antibiotics. Children with GAS pharyngitis should stay home from school for 24 h after the initiation of antibiotic therapy [1, 2].

Acute Otitis Media

Background/Pathophysiology

Acute otitis media (AOM) is one of the most common infectious diagnoses that is encountered in the pediatric outpatient setting. Most AOM occurs in children between the ages of 6 and 24 months, but it remains common into the early school-age years. AOM is an important diagnosis to consider when a patient in this age group presents with fever. While most AOM infections are not severe, some infections, if untreated, can progress to complicated infections (i.e., mastoiditis, intracranial extension (with associated meningitis), inner ear damage with resultant hearing loss, and speech delay. There are several risk factors that make infants and young children more susceptible to developing AOM. One factor is that their eustachian tubes are shorter and in a more horizontal position than older children or adults which leads to difficulty in fluid drainage in the nasopharynx during an upper respiratory infection (URI). Fluid stasis in the middle ear leads to bacterial overgrowth and resultant infection. In addition, young children have immature immune systems and are often exposed to other young children often carrying infections. This places them at risk of developing recurrent infections. On average, young children can develop up to 10–12 URIs per year, causing an increased risk of fluid in the eustachian tube and therefore an increased risk of AOM. Other risk factors for AOM include bottle feeding, prematurity, incomplete pneumococcal vaccination, secondhand smoke exposure, exposure to young siblings, daycare attendance, obesity, and craniofacial anomalies [4]. Studies show that bacteria and/or viruses are detected in 96% of middle ear fluid collected from children and young infants with signs and symptoms of AOM (66% had bacteria and viruses detected, 27% had bacteria alone, and 4% had virus alone) [5]. Since the introduction of the PCV13 and PCV20 vaccines (which have led to a decrease in the prevalence of pneumococcal infections), the most common types of bacteria that cause AOM in all ages are nontypeable *Haemophilus influenzae, Moraxella catarrhalis*, and *Streptococcus pneumoniae* (listed in order of most to least common).

History and Exam

An accurate history and physical exam will assist with the appropriate diagnosis and treatment plan for a child with AOM. Table 25.1 provides tips on questions to ask and how to examine a patient based on their age.

AOM can only be diagnosed with visualization of the tympanic membrane (TM). In order to properly TM, obstructive cerumen should be removed. When the TM is in view, look for a *loss of the typical landmarks* seen on a healthy TM (i.e., cone of light, malleus, pars flaccida), as well as a change in color from a pearly gray transparent membrane to an opaque, yellow, and/or red appearance. It is important to note if the membrane is bulging or retracted, Fig. 25.1 shows a normal TM (image a), TM with

Table 25.1 History and exam tips for suspected AOM

Age	History questions	Exam tips
Infant 6 months–11 months	Increased fussiness? Poor feeding? Changes in sleep habits? Fever, if so how high? Ear drainage? Medications given?	Best to lay supine on the table and examine each ear by turning head to the side. Ask the child's caregiver to hold the child's arms and body.
Toddler 12 months–3 years	Touching, tugging, rubbing of one or both ears? If so, duration? Changes in sleep habits? Fever, if so how high? Medications given?	Best to have patient sitting on a caregiver's lap in a side hug-like position so that the child's inside arm and the side of the child's head is pressed against the caregiver's body, and the outside arm is being held by the caregiver's arm/s.
Preschool child or older 3 years +	Does he/she have pain of one or both ears? Waking at night with ear pain? Fever if so, how high? Medications given? Are these treatments providing relief?	Patient can sit upright on the exam table. They are less fearful if you explain briefly that you are going to look inside of their ears with a light. You can show them the otoscope and let them touch it first (3–4 year olds may still need to use the toddler exam above).

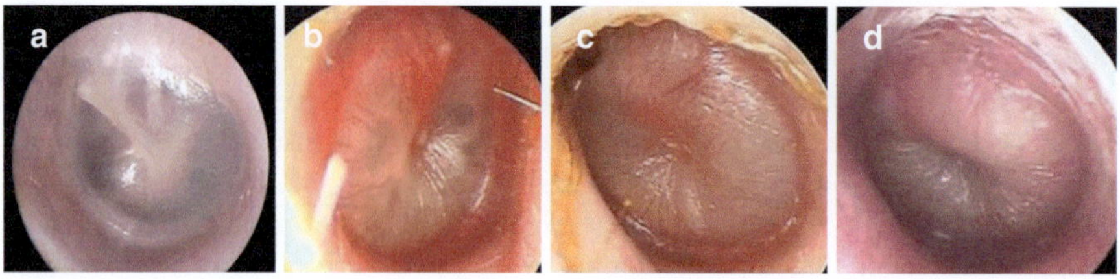

Fig. 25.1 (**a**) Normal tympanic membrane (**b**) AOM with mild bulging of TM (**c**) acute otitis media with moderate bulging of TM (**d**) AOM with severe bulging of TM

mild bulging (image b), TM with moderate bulging (image c), and a TM with severe bulging (image d). A pneumatic otoscope (an otoscope with a bulb that blows air into the ear canal) can help to assess mobility of the TM. Loss of landmarks, bulging of the TM with an opaque effusion, erythema, and lack of mobility are all signs of AOM. A bulging TM with impaired mobility is the best predictor of AOM [5].

Key Differential Diagnoses

The two main differential diagnoses for AOM are otitis media with effusion (OME) and acute otitis externa (AOE). OME is the presence of fluid behind the ear without signs of infection or inflammation. OME can either precede an AOM, for example, initially sterile fluid that later becomes infected, or it can be fluid that persists behind the TM after the bacterial infection has been treated. Acute otitis externa is a bacterial infection of the external ear canal. It causes thick, clumpy, white, and/or yellow discharge to build up in the canal and the surrounding area becomes erythematous, edematous, and painful. Acute otitis externa is often accompanied by pain with movement of the ear pinna or when pressure is applied to the tragus. See Table 25.2 for differences in findings for these three diagnoses.

Laboratory/Imaging (Workup)

AOM is a clinical diagnosis. Laboratory studies and/or imaging are only necessary to diagnose a complication due to progression of infection from the middle ear.

Management

The factors that aid in the decision of treatment are the duration and severity of symptoms, otorrhea, age of the patient, and if the infection is unilateral or bilateral. Any child who has AOM with otorrhea and/or severe symptoms (i.e. fever or

Table 25.2 Comparison of ear exam findings based on diagnosis

Exam findings	Normal findings	Acute otitis media (AOM)	Otitis media with effusion (OME)	Acute otitis externa (AOE)
Color of TM	Pearly gray	Yellow/moderate-severe redness, increased vascularity	Clear, white, or yellow	Pearly gray or white (if TM visible)
Contour	Neutral	Bulging	Neutral or retracted	Varies
Translucency	Translucent	Cloudy	Cloudy or clear with air fluid levels	Translucent or opaque
Mobility	Mobile	Immobile	Immobile	N/A
Ear canal	Normal, clear	Normal, fluid seen in canal only if perforation of TM	Normal, clear	Thick white/yellow clumpy discharge
Pull on pinna/push on tragus	No pain	No pain	No pain	Pain

moderate to severe otalgia) should be treated with antibiotics. If the child is <2 years old and has bilateral AOM, they also should always receive antibiotic treatment; whereas if they are >2 years old with bilateral AOM, it is up to the clinician's discretion to treat or watch and wait. It is also up to the clinician's discretion to treat or watch and wait in any child ≥6 months with unilateral AOM without severe symptoms [5]. The first-line treatment is high-dose amoxicillin (80–90 mg/kg/day divided BID). There are two circumstances when amoxicillin is not recommended; these include: (1) the child who has had treatment for AOM with high dose amoxicillin in the last 30 days or (2) the patient who has otitis-conjunctivitis syndrome (eye discharge plus AOM). In these two cases, high-dose amoxicillin-clavulanate (Augmentin) is recommended. Additionally, if a patient does not improve after 48 h on high-dose amoxicillin alone, then, it is recommended to switch to amoxicillin-clavulanate (Augmentin). In case of a penicillin allergy, use acceptable alternative regimens. Regarding duration of treatment, the AAP guidelines recommend 10 days for children <2 years old, 7 days for children 2–5 years old, and 5 days for children or adolescents ≥6 years old. Keep in mind guidelines are recommendations, and you may see variation in practice among providers.

Anticipatory Guidance (For Parents/Families)

Families should be advised to complete the full course of antibiotic prescribed and to return to clinic if there has been no clinical improvement or clinical worsening within 48 h of starting treatment.

Urinary Tract Infections

Background/Pathophysiology

Although a urinary tract infection (UTI) can occur at any age, UTI is more common under the age of 2 years old [6]. Among children ages 2–24 months with fever of unknown origin, UTI is the cause in 5% of cases [7]. The incidence of UTI spikes at various time points: (1) during infancy for girls and boys; (2) around the time of toilet training and (3) at the onset of sexual activity in adolescent girls [8]. Boys that are <1-year old and uncircumcised and girls who are <2 years old are at highest risk for UTIs [7]. The most common organism to cause a UTI is *E. coli* followed by other Gram-negative enteric pathogens such as *Klebsiella, Proteus, Enterobacter*, and *Citrobacter*. Common Gram-positive organisms that cause UTIs are *Staphylococcus saprophyticus* and *Enterococcus*.

UTIs develop when bacteria from the perineum and/or rectum travel up the urethra and replicate in the urine within the bladder. This leads to inflammation of the bladder (cystitis) and bacteriuria; further ascension into the ureters and to the kidneys can then lead to infection of the renal parenchyma (pyelonephritis) or even the development of a renal abscess. Risk factors for the development of UTIs are described below. Females have shorter urethras than males making a shorter distance to travel to the bladder and therefore easier to develop infection. It is thought that school-age girls may develop UTIs due to improper/inadequate hygiene when toileting, although there is no hard evidence for this assumption. Constipation is a risk factor for development of UTIs; compression of the urethra and pressure on the bladder from a full rectum/descending colon can lead to abnormal bladder mechanics, incomplete emptying of the bladder, urinary stasis, and then bacterial growth [8]. Sexually active adolescent girls may develop UTIs due to introduction of bacteria into the urethra during sexual activity. Children who have anatomic abnormalities of the genitourinary tract, including hydronephrosis and vesicoureteral reflux, are also at higher risk of developing upper tract UTIs (pyelonephritis).

History and Physical Exam

The history that leads a clinician to suspect a UTI varies based on the age of the patient (Table 25.3).

Key Differential Diagnoses

In toddlers and preschool children, dysuria can be a result of inflammation or infection of the skin in the GU area near the urethral opening. In males, infection of the glans or foreskin (balanitis and balanoposthitis, respectively), and in prepubertal

Table 25.3 History and physical exam for suspected UTI

	History questions	Exam findings
Infants	Fever? ≥39 °C (102.2 °F)? Fussiness? Poor feeding? Lethargy? Changes in urine color/odor?	No other focal findings to explain fever Typically normal GU exam
Toddlers	Fever? If in diapers: stop and cry and/or hold the diaper area when urinating? Changes in color/odor of urine? If potty trained: Urinary hesitancy and increased frequency? Urinary accidents? +/− Hematuria	No other focal findings to explain fever Typically normal GU exam
School age and adolescents	Pain with urination (dysuria)? Urinary hesitancy and increased frequency? Hematuria? Fever? Abdominal pain? Back pain? Vaginal discharge, what color? Any odor? Rash, itching, or burning of the skin in GU area?	Usually, normal exam Could have: • Lower abdominal or suprapubic tenderness • CVA tenderness if it has pyelonephritis/renal involvement No GU exam needed unless patient has discharge, burning, itching, or rash

females, external irritation of the vulva and labia, called vulvovaginitis, can cause painful urination. None of these diagnoses have associated fever, urinary frequency, urgency, or hematuria, and a urine culture (if sent) would be negative. In post-pubertal adolescents with GU symptoms, sexually transmitted infections (STIs) that cause urethritis (including gonorrhea or chlamydia) should be considered and ruled out by further testing. Although STIs often present with lower abdominal pain, dysuria, and/or GU discharge, they can also be asymptomatic.

Laboratory Assessment/Imaging (Workup)

To diagnose a UTI, a clean urine sample needs to be collected. For infants and young children who are not toilet trained, urinary catheterization with a sterile technique is recommended. Older children and adolescents can provide a midstream clean catch sample. These collection techniques ensure that the sample is not contaminated with bacteria present on the skin from the surrounding area. After proper collection of the urine, the first test to perform is a urinalysis (UA). A rapid dipstick UA is used most often in the outpatient setting. The presence of nitrites, leukocyte esterase, and/or blood, with associated lower urinary tract symptoms is suggestive of a UTI. A UA with microscopy can be sent to the lab which includes detection of

Table 25.4 Indications for imaging related to UTIs [9]

Indications for a renal ultrasound	• Children <2 years with first febrile UTI • Any child with recurrent febrile UTIs • Any child with a UTI and family history of renal or urologic abnormalities, hypertension (HTN), poor growth • Any child who is not improving with the appropriate antibiotic treatment
Indications for a voiding cystourethrogram (VCUG)	• Children of any age with recurrent UTIs • Children with first febrile UTI and – Abnormalities on renal ultrasound **or** – Temperature ≥39 °C plus bacteria other than *E. coli* **or** – Poor growth or HTN

bacteria and/or WBCs in the urine. A symptomatic patient with positive nitrites or leukocyte esterase on a UA or WBCs or bacteria on microscopy is very likely to have a UTI; therefore, empiric antibiotics should be started while awaiting the results of the urine culture. However, it is possible that the UA can be falsely negative in a patient with a UTI. This is especially true in younger children who void more frequently and cannot verbalize typical UTI symptoms; therefore, it is best to send both a UA and urine culture for these patients. The typical definition of a positive urine culture is presence of ≥50,000 colony forming units (CFU)/mL on a catheterized specimen and ≥100,000 CFU/mL on a clean catch specimen, of a single uropathogen. Evidence of infection on the UA and a positive urine culture provides a definitive diagnosis of a UTI.

Imaging to evaluate for underlying anatomic abnormalities of the kidneys or genitourinary tract is necessary in some children. Specific circumstances and the indications for advanced imaging are summarized in Table 25.4. If an abnormality is found on advanced imaging, the child should be referred to Urology for further evaluation and management.

Management

The goals of antibiotic treatment for a UTI include: treating the acute infection, preventing ascending infection, and reducing likelihood of future renal damage [7]. If a patient is well appearing and tolerating oral fluids, empiric oral treatment outpatient is appropriate; otherwise, a patient should be admitted for parenteral antibiotics until they clinically improve. Empiric treatment usually consists of a second or third generation cephalosporin (i.e., cefixime or cefdinir), however depending on the local patterns of antimicrobial susceptibility testing, a first generation cephalosporin (i.e., cephalexin), amoxicillin-clavulanate (Augmentin), or trimethoprim-sulfamethoxazole (Bactrim) are appropriate alternative empiric antibiotic agents. If the child has a history of recurrent UTIs, it is good practice to base the empiric treatment choice on past urine culture results. The time course of treatment depends on the location and severity of the infection. Simple cystitis (isolated to the bladder only) is treated for a shorter duration than pyelonephritis (upper tract infection) or those with complicated infections. The most recent AAP UTI treatment guidelines from 2011 recommend a minimum duration of treatment of 7 days for cystitis and up to 14 days for pyelonephritis or more severe infections. The European Association of Urology guidelines from 2016 recommend at least 3–5 days of antibiotic treatment for cystitis and 7–14 days for pyelonephritis. Once the culture results identify the causative bacteria and its susceptibility information, the initial antibiotic is either continued (if deemed appropriate) or changed based on bacterial resistance patterns. In most situations, a child with cystitis who is receiving an appropriate antibiotic should improve within 48 hours. Children with more complicated infections, including pyelonephritis, often take longer to respond to antibiotic therapy.

Anticipatory Guidance (For Parents/Families)

Families should be advised to return if there is no clinical improvement or clinical worsening within 48 h of starting antibiotic treatment. It is also important to educate patients and families to complete the full course of antibiotic treatment. Age-appropriate education on toileting/GU hygiene and avoiding preventable risk factors (i.e., treatment of constipation) can reduce the risk of recurrent UTIs.

Periorbital and Orbital Cellulitis

Background/Pathophysiology

This section will focus on bacterial causes of periorbital and orbital cellulitis. The orbital septum is a thin membrane separating the eyelids from the eye and the deeper structures of the eye. *Periorbital* (aka preseptal) cellulitis is a bacterial infection that occurs *anterior* to the orbital septum including the eyelids and surrounding soft tissues. *Orbital cellulitis* is a bacterial infection *posterior* to the orbital septum involving the orbit and deeper structures of the eye. It is important to identify and treat both types of these infections promptly. It is imperative to know how to distinguish the two clinically. Orbital cellulitis is more severe, requires hospitalization, and sometimes surgical management; whereas periorbital cellulitis can be managed as an outpatient. Periorbital cellulitis is often caused by an overlying skin cellulitis. Orbital cellulitis can occur as a complication of periorbital cellulitis, extension from the sinuses or mouth, or rarely due to hematogenous seeding of the area. Bacterial pathogens implicated in causing periorbital or orbital cellulitis are outlined in Table 25.5.

Table 25.5 Common causes of periorbital and orbital cellulitis [10]

Initial source of infection	Causative organisms
Rhinosinusitis (most often ethmoiditis)	*S. milleri* group (including *Streptococcus anginosus*) *S. pneumoniae*, nontypeable *H. influenzae*, *Moraxella catarrhalis*
Infection near the eye from insect bite, impetigo, eczema, or hordeolum	*S. aureus*, *S. pyogenes,* MRSA, *S. epidermidis*
Dacryocystitis	*S. pneumoniae, nontypeable H. influenzae, S. aureus, S. pyogenes, pseudomonas*
Dental abscess	Mixed oral flora; aerobic and anaerobic organisms

History and Physical Exam

An astute medical student should be able to perform the history and the physical exam simultaneously in cases of pediatric eye infection. This is so that one can triage the severity of symptoms and determine the next best step in management promptly. Both orbital and periorbital cellulitis can present with unilateral edema, erythema, and tenderness of the eyelid. If a patient presents to clinic and cannot open their eye to allow for examination due to severe edema or if the child is ill appearing, they should be referred to the emergency room for further evaluation. If the patient has proptosis, ophthalmoplegia (restricted movement of eye muscles), pain with eye movement, and/or chemosis, these are all signs and symptoms consistent with orbital cellulitis and will also need urgent evaluation in the emergency room and prompt ophthalmologic consultation. Edema, erythema, and warmth of the eyelid alone indicate that the diagnosis of periorbital cellulitis is most likely, and further questioning and exam can be performed to determine the source of the infection. Based on the information in Table 25.5, history of recent viral URI symptoms, skin infections near the eye, insect bites, or dental concerns should be solicited.

Key Differential Diagnoses

Other differential diagnoses to consider with eyelid edema, include: (1) allergic reaction: often has a known trigger, unilateral or bilateral swelling, associated pruritus, erythematous, not painful, no fever, resolves with antihistamine treatment; (2) hypoproteinemia causing fluid retention: non-painful bilateral eyelid edema without erythema or pain, fluid retention also seen in other dependent parts of the body, no other signs or symptoms of infection; (3) thyroid disease: bilateral exophthalmos, other findings of hyperthyroidism such as goiter, tachycardia, diarrhea, sweating, and anxiety; (4) malignancy involving the eye or orbital space such as retinoblastoma, lymphoma, or rhabdomyosarcoma (can present very similarly to orbital cellulitis and can be differentiated based on fundoscopic exam and imaging with commuted topography (CT)).

Laboratory Assessment/Imaging (Workup)

No labs or imaging are needed for periorbital cellulitis. For orbital cellulitis, the diagnosis is best confirmed with CT scan with contrast or MRI of the orbit with and without contrast. The additional assessment of findings on radiography such as bony destruction and the size of subperiosteal abscesses can allow clinicians to more accurately determine those patients requiring surgical intervention [11]. The most reliable cultures are those from orbital abscesses and sinus aspirates; blood cultures are infrequently positive in orbital cellulitis; however, in any ill or toxic-appearing child, they should be obtained prior to starting antibiotic therapy [11].

Management

A well-appearing patient with uncomplicated periorbital cellulitis can be treated outpatient with 7–10 days of oral antibiotics. If the etiology is a local skin infection such as impetigo, insect bite, or hordeolum, initiating an antibiotic that covers Staphylococcal and Streptococcal species is recommended. Antibiotic options include dicloxacillin or cephalexin; if MRSA is suspected, clindamycin or trimethoprim-sulfamethoxazole with amoxicillin is recommended. If the etiology is rhinosinusitis or a dental infection, amoxicillin-clavulanate is the first-line treatment. Table 25.5 lists the typical causative organisms that are targeted.

A patient who is ill or toxic appearing and/or has orbital cellulitis will require hospitalization and parenteral (IV) antibiotics. They may transition to oral antibiotics after demonstrating at least 48 hours of clinical improvement. In these cases, a second or third generation cephalosporin plus vancomycin for MRSA coverage and metronidazole is recommended. Once discharged, these patients should complete a minimum of a 14-day course of antibiotic treatment; the total duration will depend on clinical response to therapy. Any case of complicated orbital cellulitis will require involvement of ophthalmology and otorhinolaryngology.

Anticipatory Guidance (For Parents/Families)

If the child is being treated as an outpatient, families should be advised to return to clinic if symptoms worsen or fail to improve after 48 h of antibiotic treatment or if the patient cannot tolerate the medication. For those who required hospitalization, it is important to follow up with their primary care physician within a few days of discharge to ensure that they are continuing to improve.

Toxic or Transient Synovitis

Background/Pathophysiology

Toxic or transient synovitis is characterized by hip pain and limitation in movement of the joint, which resolves slowly over time. This diagnosis is relatively uncommon, and typically affects children between the ages of 3 and 8 years old. Boys are more often affected than girls (ratio of 2:1). The trigger of the process is thought to be infectious; however, post-traumatic and allergic causes also occur [12].

History

Approximately 30–50% of children have preceding upper respiratory tract symptoms. Children will present with associated low-grade fever, limp, and unilateral hip pain (in 95% of cases). Their symptoms last approximately 1 week. Very few children have symptoms that last up to 4 weeks.

Physical Exam

Most children have low-grade fevers and are nontoxic in appearance. They may refuse to bear weight or limp and will have point tenderness and limitation in range of motion of the affected hip.

Laboratory Assessment/Imaging (Workup)

Recommended evaluation includes obtaining a complete blood count (CBC) with differential, C-reactive protein (CRP), and an erythrocyte sedimentation rate (ESR). Most children with toxic/transient synovitis have a normal white blood cell count, normal CRP, and normal ESR. Often radiographs (X-rays) of the affected hip are normal. Magnetic resonance imaging (MRI) will reveal a joint effusion, which may show enhancement. If the laboratory studies are concerning, often these children undergo a diagnostic joint aspiration. Joint fluid is sent for cell count with differential, Gram stain with culture and PCR testing (if available).

Key Differential Diagnosis

In children who present with a limp or refusal to bear weight and a history of fever, it is important to exclude a serious bacterial infection (septic arthritis or osteomyelitis). Children with septic arthritis or osteomyelitis often present with high fevers, are often ill-appearing, and have an elevated WBC and CRP. Children with toxic/transient synovitis often have a preceding viral illness, are well appearing, and have normal laboratory studies. In some cases, an MRI with and without contrast of the affected hip can help distinguish between these two diagnoses. Additional diagnoses to consider include a fracture (often visualized on X-ray) and avascular necrosis of the femoral head (visualized on MRI).

Management

Most children are managed conservatively with the administration of nonsteroidal anti-inflammatory (NSAID) medications. They are allowed to return to normal activity as soon as tolerated.

Anticipatory Guidance (For Parents/Families)

Most children experience rapid and full recovery. Recurrence can occur in up to 15% of children. Future recurrences are also self-limited with expected full recovery. A very small percentage of children ($\leq$2%) may develop Legg–Calvé–Perthes disease which is an avascular necrosis of the femoral head (on the affected side).

Infectious Rashes [1, 13]

Pediatric rashes are a common presentation in the outpatient setting. They are often infectious in etiology. See Table 25.6 for an overview of common infectious rashes.

Table 25.6 Common infectious rashes

Infectious organism	Common disease name(s)	Systemic symptoms	Rash description	Management
Coxsackie virus (an enterovirus)	Hand-foot-and-mouth disease	Fever, oral ulcers, odynophagia	Macular rash with fluid-filled blisters	Symptomatic: Acetaminophen, nonsteroidal anti-inflammatory drugs (NSAIDS), magic mouthwash

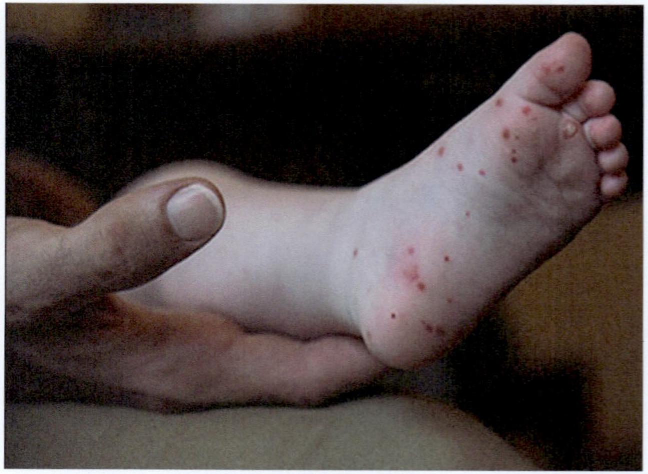

Infectious organism	Common disease name(s)	Systemic symptoms	Rash description	Management
Parvovirus B19	Fifth disease, erythema infectiosum	Low-grade fever, malaise, sore throat, headache and nausea, arthralgias (8%)	"Slapped cheek" rash (several days after symptom onset), pink papules and macules in lacy/ reticular pattern (+pruritus) (2–4 days)	Symptomatic: NSAIDS Antihistamines

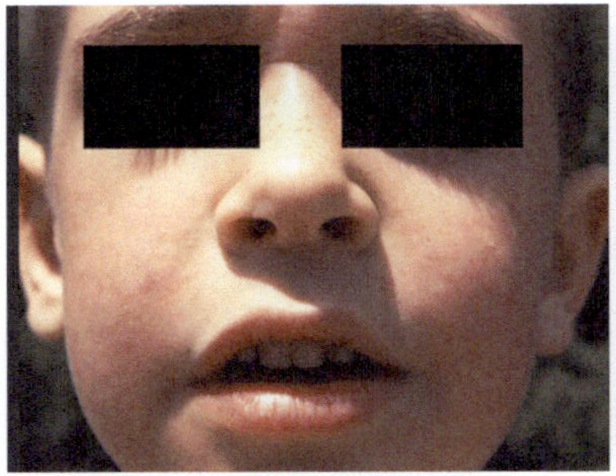

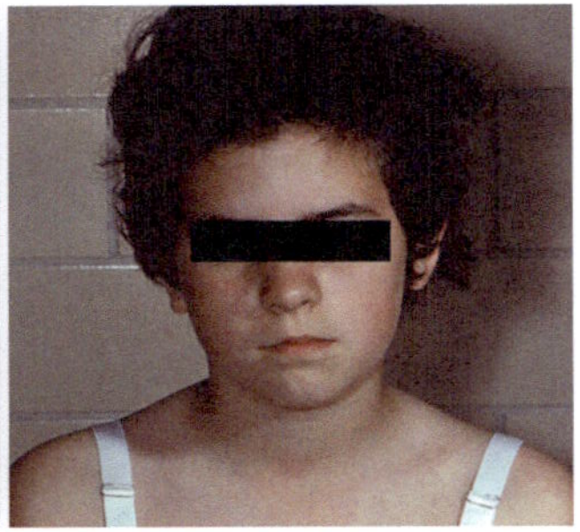

Human herpes virus-6 (HHV-6)	Roseola	Abrupt onset high-fever (1–5 days), URI congestion, mild cough, diarrhea, associated with febrile seizures	Macular or maculopapular rash appears after fever resolution, starts on trunk and spreads peripherally (1–2 days)	Self-limited, no treatment

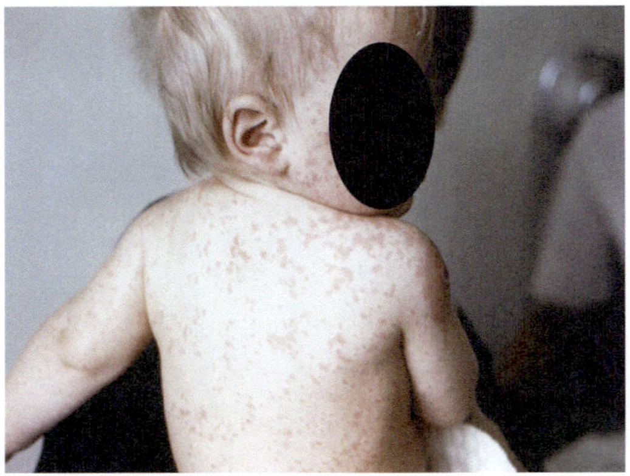

(continued)

Table 25.6 (continued)

Herpes simplex virus 6, 7 (HHV-6, HHV-7)	Pityriasis rosea	Mild URI symptoms, pruritus (50%)	Herald patch (appears first) oval shaped, rose colored with a peripheral scale (weeks later): Truncal rash of smaller lesions in Christmas tree pattern, lasts 2–12 weeks	Self-limited, no treatment

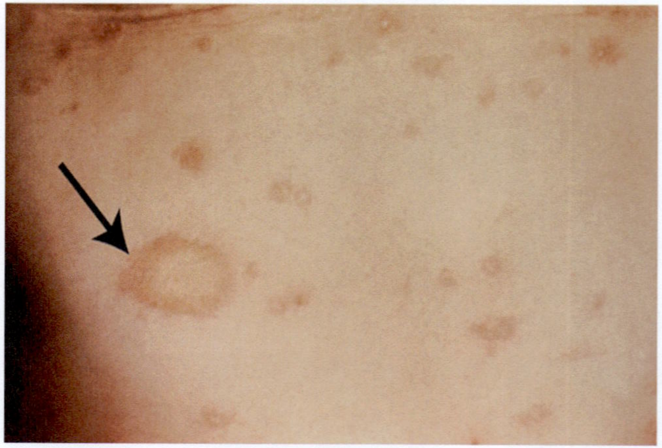

Dermatophytes Microsporum and Trichophyton	Tinea capitus (scalp), corporis (body), pedis (feet), manus (hands), nails (unguium)	Posterior occipital lymphadenopathy	Scaling or circumscribed alopecia and broken hair follicles	Oral grisefulvin or turbinafine for capitis or moderate/severe corporis; topical antifungal for mild corporis

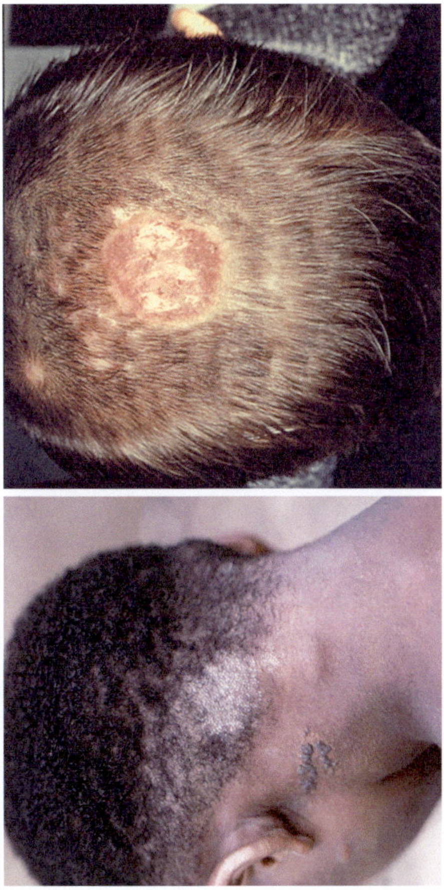

Immunodeficiencies [14, 15]

Frequent and recurrent infections or infections with more unusual bacterial/fungal/viral etiologies may present when a patient has an immunodeficiency. See Table 25.7 for review of the most common types of immunodeficiencies seen in the pediatric population.

Table 25.7 High yield immunodeficiencies review [14, 15]

	Immune cell deficiency/defect	Genetic inheritance	Signs and symptoms	Common infections	Treatment
Bruton's X-linked Agammaglobulinemia (XLA)	B-cell deficiency in number and function All subtypes of Igs are low	X-linked (males) Defect in Btk gene	Recurrent sinopulmonary infections: sinusitis, otitis media, pneumonia Gastroenteritis present at 6–9 months of life	Encapsulated bacteria, fungal, parasitic, viral (enterovirus)	IVIG Antibiotics
Common variable immunodeficiency (CVID)	B-cell defect Low IgG and/or IgA IgM	Sporadic or autosomal dominant	Recurrent sinopulmonary and GI infections Autoimmune cytopenias Most present later in life 20s/30s	Encapsulated bacteria, viral (Norovirus, CMV), parasites Giardia)	IVIG
IgA deficiency	B cell defect Very low or no IgA	Sporadic	Majority are not symptomatic If symptoms: sinopulmonary and GI infections	Same as XLA and CVID	IVIG, if symptomatic
DiGeorge syndrome (DS)	T-cell deficiency Complete DS-absent thymus/parathyroid [Partial DS-hypoplastic thymus/parathyroid]	Sporadic or AD Deletion of 22q11.2	Complete: Seizures due to hypocalcemia recurrent infections, poor growth, cardiac/facial/palate abnormalities	Opportunistic infections: bacterial, fungi, viruses, GVHD	Thymic transplant Bone marrow transplant
Severe combined immunodeficiency	Caused by one of a variety of known genetic defects: All have absent/low T cells, some have B cell and/or NK cell deficiency	X-linked or AR depending on defect	Diarrhea, sepsis, otitis media, skin infections Presents in the first few months of life, not compatible with life without treatment	Opportunistic infections: bacterial, fungi, viruses	Bone marrow transplant, gene therapies are in development

(continued)

Table 25.7 (continued)

	Immune cell deficiency/defect	Genetic inheritance	Signs and symptoms	Common infections	Treatment
Wiskott-Aldrich syndrome	T and B cell dysfunction	X-linked, mutation of WASP, a protein involved in immune function	Thrombocytopenia, hematochezia, bruising, bleeding after circumcision Eczema Recurrent sinopulmonary infections	Opportunistic infections: bacterial, fungi, viruses	Bone marrow transplant, gene therapies are in development
Chronic granulomatous disease	Phagocyte disorder—can ingest but not kill catalase + organisms	X-linked or AR	Recurrent pneumonia, lymphadenitis, osteomyelitis, hepatic abscess Granulomas of skin, GI and GU tracts	Bacteria and fungi; *S. aureus, aspergillus, Serratia, Nocardia, Burkholderia cepacia*	Antimicrobials and interferon gamma until bone marrow transplant

References

1. American Academy of Pediatrics. Red Book: 2021–2021 report of the committee on infectious diseases. 32nd ed; 2021.
2. Shulman ST, Bisno AL, Clegg HW, et al. Clinical practice guideline for the diagnosis and management of group a streptococcal pharyngitis: 2012 update by the Infectious Disease Society of America. Clin Infect Dis. 2012;55(10):1279–82.
3. Gerber MA, Baltimore RS, Eaton CB, et al. Prevention of rheumatic fever and diagnosis and treatment of acute streptococcal pharyngitis. Circulation. 2009;119(11):1541–51.
4. Rosa-Olivares J, Porro A, Rodriguez-Varela M, Riefkohl G. Otitis media: to treat, to refer, to do nothing: a review for the practitioner. Pediatr Rev. 2015;36(11):480–8.
5. Lieberthal AS, Carroll AE, Chonmaitree T, et al. The diagnosis and management of acute otitis media. Pediatrics. 2013;131(3):e964–99.
6. Okarska-Napierała M, Wasilewska A, Kuchar E. Urinary tract infection in children: diagnosis, treatment, imaging—comparison of current guidelines. J Pediatr Urol. 2017;13(6):567–73.
7. Roberts KB, Subcommittee on Urinary Tract Infection, Steering Committee on Quality Improvement and Management. Urinary tract infection: clinical practice guideline for the diagnosis and management of the initial UTI in febrile infants and children 2–24 months. Pediatrics. 2011;128(3):595–610.
8. Jackson EC. Urinary tract infections in children: knowledge updates and a salute to the future. Pediatr Rev. 2014;36(4):153–64.
9. Shaikh N. Urinary tract infections in infants older than 1 month and young children: acute management, imaging, and prognosis. In: Post TW, editor. UpToDate. Waltham: UpToDate; 2022.
10. Hauser A, Fogarasi S. Periorbital and orbital cellulitis. Pediatr Rev. 2010;31(6):242–9.
11. Williams K, Allen R. Paediatric orbital and periorbital infections. Curr Opin Ophthalmol. 2019;30(5):349–55.
12. Clark M. Overview of causes of limp in children. In: Post TW, editor. UpToDate. Waltham: UpToDate; 2022.
13. Allmon A, Deane K, Martin KL. Common rashes in children. Am Fam Physician. 2015;92(3):211–6.
14. Cooper MA, Pommering TL, Korányi K. Primary immunodeficiencies. Am Fam Physician. 2003;68(10):2001–8.
15. Dosanjh A. Autoimmunity and immunodeficiency. Pediatr Rev. 2015;36(11):489–94.

Chapter 26
Inflammatory Diseases

Katrina Foo and David Roofeh

Juvenile Idiopathic Arthritis

Epidemiology/Pathophysiology

Juvenile idiopathic arthritis (JIA) occurs in 1 in 1000 children. The distribution of disease varies based on subclassification as defined in Table 26.1. The cause of juvenile idiopathic arthritis remains unknown. These subgroups have different clinical characteristics; each likely has a different pathogenesis and different responses to therapy. Both the innate and adaptive immune systems have been implicated in the pathogenesis.

Clinical Manifestations

By definition, all patients with JIA must have symptoms for a minimum of 6 weeks beginning before the age of 16 years. These patients show a summating burden of arthritic joints (arthritis involving a series of joints, developing over time, without previously involved joints remitting). This is in distinction to a migratory pattern of arthritis, where one joint becomes involved, and another joint remits spontaneously.

K. Foo (✉)
Department of Pediatrics, Rutgers Robert Wood Johnson Medical School, New Brunswick, NJ, USA

D. Roofeh
Department of Internal Medicine, Rutgers Robert Wood Johnson Medical School, New Brunswick, NJ, USA

N. Liao et al. (eds.), *Pediatric Rotations*,
https://doi.org/10.1007/978-3-031-59873-9_26

Table 26.1 Epidemiology and clinical manifestations of Juvenile Idiopathic Arthritis (JIA) by subtype

Subtype of JIA	Distribution of disease	Specifics of each subtype
Systemic	10–15%	*Epidemiology*: Any age *History*: Fever (usually 1–2 times per day at the same time of day) for at least 2 weeks *Exam*: Rash—salmon pink, transient, migratory, usually occurs with fever. Arthritis—can be preceded by fever, rash by days/months; has a variable presentation but eventually is a chronic polyarthritis
Oligoarthritis	30–60%	*Epidemiology*: Peak age 2–4 years old. Girls much more commonly affected than boys *History*: Morning limp with refusal to walk but minimal pain *Exam*: Arthritis—<4 joints are swollen in the first 6 months of diagnosis; generally large joints such as knees. Slit lamp exam may reveal anterior uveitis (inflammation of the anterior chamber of the eye) as it is most common in this subtype of JIA
Polyarthritis with RF positive	5–10%	*Epidemiology*: Peak age late childhood or adolescence. Girls more commonly affected than boys *History*: No fever. Fatigue and poor appetite *Exam*: Arthritis—≥5 joints are swollen; generally symmetric joint swelling of small joints in the hands/feet. Subcutaneous nodules may be present
Polyarthritis with RF negative	10–30%	*Epidemiology*: Peak age 2–4 years old. Girls more commonly affected than boys *History*: No fever. Fatigue and poor appetite *Exam*: Arthritis—≥5 joints are swollen; generally symmetric joint swelling of small joints in the hands/feet
Psoriatic arthritis	2–15%	*Epidemiology*: Peaks at both age 2–4 and 9–11 years. Girls more commonly affected than boys *History*: Psoriatic rash (plaques, silvery scale) *Exam*: Arthritis—generally asymmetric oligoarthritis. Rash—psoriatic rash. If rash not present can be diagnosed by two of the following: family history of psoriasis in first degree relative, swelling of digits (dactylitis), nail pitting (onycholysis)
Enthesitis-related arthritis/juvenile spondyloarthropathy	20%	*Epidemiology*: Peak age late childhood or adolescence. Boys more commonly affected than girls *History*: Patients may complain of back pain (inflammatory spinal pain) in addition to arthritis pain *Exam*: Arthritis—most often of the lower extremity joints. Enthesitis (inflammation of the tendon and ligament attachments) most often of the heels and knees

RF rheumatoid factor

Arthritis patterns may be divided into oligoarthritis (1–4 joints) and polyarthritis (≥5 joints). Patients/caregivers describe joint stiffness typically worst first in the morning, gelling phenomenon (stiffness worsening with inactivity), and potentially an abnormal gait attributed to pain. Children may report improvement with increased activity or taking warm showers. Extra-articular manifestations vary by subset. For patients with arthritis who do not fit a specific type of JIA, they may be diagnosed as JIA undifferentiated which has variable features and includes 11–21% of JIA patients.

Laboratory Assessment/Imaging

Laboratory exams can be helpful in diagnosing JIA but must be taken into consideration with the supportive findings of the clinical manifestations. All patients with JIA should be tested for anti-nuclear antibody (ANA) by immunofluorescence, as well as rheumatoid factor (RF). RF is helpful in dividing the subtypes of polyarticular JIA. Erythrocyte sedimentation rate (ESR) and c-reactive protein (CRP) suggest an inflammatory state and may be used to track response to therapy over time. Absence of elevated ESR and/or CRP does not exclude JIA. X-rays are rarely useful in establishing the diagnosis of JIA. In patients with long-term, chronic disease, radiographs may be helpful in detailing disease and prompting escalation of therapy. Slit lamp examination should be performed at the time of diagnosis of JIA and then at regular intervals depending on the risk for chronic anterior uveitis; patients with a positive ANA are at particularly high risk for chronic anterior uveitis.

Differential Diagnosis

The diagnosis of JIA is generally not made with symptoms less than 6 weeks; other diagnoses should be considered for patients who do not meet this timeline. Overall, inflammatory arthritis should prompt consideration for a systemic cause: possible etiologies include infection (e.g., septic arthritis, tuberculosis, osteomyelitis), hematologic disorders (e.g., sickle cell disease, hemophilia), malignancy (e.g., leukemia, sarcoma), auto-inflammatory (e.g., familial Mediterranean fever), and other rheumatic diseases (e.g., inflammatory bowel disease-related arthritis, reactive arthritis, psoriatic arthritis, systemic lupus erythematosus, vasculitis). Any patient who presents with a large joint monoarthritis (e.g. knee), especially in the setting of fever, requires arthrocentesis to rule out infection and malignancy. The diagnosis of transient synovitis should be considered in patients presenting with large joint monoarthritis, especially those with a recent viral illness.

Management

Nonsteroidal anti-inflammatory drugs (NSAIDs) are appropriate monotherapy in those with oligoarthritis with low disease activity. For patients with active disease, NSAIDs are best used as adjunctive therapy with immunosuppressive medication. Disease-modifying antirheumatic drugs (DMARDs) are used to reduce inflammation and consequent bone erosion that leads to chronic disability. DMARDs include conventional DMARDs such as methotrexate, leflunomide, and sulfasalazine as well as biologics such as various monoclonal antibodies (e.g., adalimumab, abatacept, tocilizumab, rituximab). Glucocorticoids are effective in rapidly improving pain and swelling; short-term therapy is used in the initial phase of the disease when DMARD therapies are initiated and for flare episodes.

About 50% of patients with oligoarthritis may achieve remission (no active disease, without medication for 12 months or more). Patients with arthritis involving the cervical spine, the hips, ankles, and wrists, especially with elevated inflammatory markers and X-rays confirming bony erosions, portend a worse outcome. Patients with systemic JIA should be monitored closely, as uncontrolled disease may lead to macrophage-activating syndrome.

Henoch-Schönlein Purpura

Epidemiology/Pathophysiology

Henoch-Schönlein purpura (HSP), also referred to as IgA vasculitis, is the most common systemic vasculitis of childhood, affecting 10–20 per 100,00 children. HSP primarily occurs between 2 and 10 years of age with a peak incidence at 4–7 years old. There is a male predominance in childhood and a seasonality with most cases occurring in the fall/winter months.

HSP is a necrotizing small-vessel vasculitis with characteristic IgA deposition on direct immunofluorescence. The etiology of HSP remains unknown. Many cases of IgA vasculitis occur following a respiratory infection, suggesting that infection leads to inappropriate activation and deposition of IgA.

Clinical Manifestations

The classic tetrad occurring in up to 80% of cases includes (1) palpable purpura, (2) arthritis, (3) abdominal pain, and (4) renal disease. The appearance of these symptoms can be variable and can develop over time. Additionally, not all patients will

Table 26.2 Clinical manifestations of Henoch-Schönlein purpura

Clinical manifestation	Physical exam
Palpable purpura	Typically occurs in pressure-dependent areas like the lower extremities and buttocks. Lesions vary in size from minor petechiae to large ecchymoses
Arthritis	Occurs in most patients (60–84%). Commonly symmetric involving ankles and knees with characteristic signs of inflammation (warmth, tenderness, swelling)
Abdominal pain	Usually described as a diffuse, crampy, colicky pain which may be non-localizing
Renal disease	While 50% of patients may have renal involvement, this is usually asymptomatic. Elevated blood pressure may be the only physical exam finding

demonstrate the tetrad of clinical manifestations. The diagnosis is made based on the single mandatory finding of palpable purpura plus one of the three remaining clinical manifestations. See Table 26.2 for clinical manifestations of HSP.

Laboratory Assessment/Imaging

A normal complete blood count (CBC) and coagulation panel may help exclude a bleeding diathesis as the cause of the purpuric skin rash. Serum IgA levels are often elevated in HSP but are not specific for the disease and have little diagnostic value. Markers of inflammation (e.g., ESR, CRP) point toward a systemic inflammatory disease, but are non-specific for HSP.

HSP is a clinical diagnosis; a skin biopsy is not necessary to make the diagnosis. If done, skin biopsy confirms the diagnosis showing small-vessel leukocytoclastic vasculitis with IgA deposition in vessel walls on immunofluorescence.

Evaluation of renal involvement is important. Rise in serum creatinine reflects a decline in glomerular filtration. Urinalysis will detect hematuria and proteinuria. A urine protein-to-creatinine ratio helps to quantify the degree of proteinuria. A renal biopsy is indicated for patients with concern for nephritic or nephrotic syndrome. Biopsy confirms renal involvement with IgA immune complex deposition in the renal mesangium.

Differential Diagnosis

The diagnosis of HSP is made based on the presence of palpable purpura plus an additional clinical manifestation. For a patient with atypical presentation of HSP, a broader differential diagnosis should be considered based on the clinical manifestation. In patients with purpura, infectious etiologies such as meningococcemia, disseminated gonococcemia, thrombocytopenia secondary to viral illness, and rickettsial diseases should be considered as well as hematologic/oncologic disorders such as immune thrombocytopenia purpura, disseminated intravascular coagulopathy, and leukemia. Systemic lupus erythematosus and hypersensitivity vasculitis are two systemic vasculitis diseases to also consider in patients with purpura. For patients with arthralgia/arthritis, the differential could include JIA, septic arthritis, serum sickness, or trauma to the joint. Abdominal pain includes a very broad differential; however, some diagnoses to consider are gastroenteritis, constipation, appendicitis, mesenteric adenitis, inflammatory bowel disease, pelvic inflammatory disease, pregnancy, ovarian torsion, and obstruction. See Chap. 10 for further discussion of abdominal pain. In the case of hematuria, other disorders to consider are post-streptococcal glomerulonephritis, urinary tract infection, interstitial nephritis, nephrolithiasis, hemolytic uremic syndrome, and acute tubular necrosis.

Management

Skin lesions typically last 3–10 days and require no specific treatment. Arthritis responds to nonsteroidal anti-inflammatory drugs. GI bleeding and edema may require systemic glucocorticoids. For greater than 95% of patients with renal involvement, the resolution is rapid and complete. These patients with self-limited disease do not require treatment. Frequent monitoring with urinalysis and blood pressures are advised until resolution occurs. For those with progressive renal disease, glucocorticoids have not been clearly demonstrated as a disease modifying drug. Nevertheless, aggressive treatment with high-dose glucocorticoid alongside immunosuppressive agents (e.g., azathioprine, mycophenolate mofetil, cyclophosphamide) is indicated for those with poor prognostic factors which include proteinuria greater than 1 g/day, nephrotic syndrome, or crescentic glomerulonephritis with more than 50% of glomeruli with crescents.

The onset is acute, and resolution may be rapid and complete in most patients within 1 month. Duration of disease ranges from 6 to 16 weeks. In cases of protracted disease, almost all children will have complete recovery by 2 years. Despite its self-limited course, all patients diagnosed with HSP should be followed for 6 months with urinalysis and blood pressure checks to monitor for renal involvement. HSP can reoccur after its initial occurrence; however, the second episode is generally less severe than the first.

Kawasaki Disease

Epidemiology/Pathophysiology

Kawasaki disease (KD), the second most common systemic vasculitis of childhood, generally occurs in children between the ages of 6 months to 7 years with a peak incidence between ages 2 and 3 years. There is seasonal variability.

KD is a clinical diagnosis of unknown etiology that is characterized by inflammation of small-to-medium sized arteries leading to multisystem involvement and potential complication of coronary artery aneurysms.

Clinical Manifestations

The hallmark of KD is fever for 5 contiguous days. The fever is generally acute in onset and greater than 102 °F (>39 °C). A thorough fever history is critical as it is the key qualifying finding for making the diagnosis of KD. Patients must have four of the five clinical manifestations to be diagnosed with KD (Table 26.3). These findings do not have to be present at time of diagnosis and may be reported in history of the clinical course. In addition to the diagnostic clinical findings, many patients will have other symptoms including irritability, myalgias, arthralgias, arthritis, and gastrointestinal complaints. Patients with incomplete KD have the component of fever with only two or three of the clinical findings.

Laboratory Assessment/Imaging

All patients with the diagnosis of KD should undergo an echocardiogram to evaluate for coronary artery aneurysms. An echocardiogram is performed at the time of diagnosis, 1–2 weeks later and 5–6 weeks after hospital discharge. While the echocardiogram is necessary as part of the workup for KD, it should not be a reason to delay treatment.

Table 26.3 Clinical manifestations of Kawasaki disease

Clinical manifestation	Physical exam
Bilateral conjunctivitis	Occurs in approximately 90% of cases and is a non-exudative, limbic sparing conjunctivitis. Specifically, this appears as a white clearing around the iris with surrounding erythema of the conjunctiva.
Mucous membrane changes	The mucous membrane changes manifest as oral mucosal changes with pharyngitis, red swollen tongue with prominent papillae (strawberry tongue), and red, cracked, swollen lips as the most common presentations.
Cervical adenopathy	Cervical adenopathy is the least common criterion. It is usually a unilateral, nonfluctuant, nontender, anterior cervical adenopathy that exceeds 1.5 cm in diameter.
Rash	Rash can take many forms; it is most reported as erythematous, maculopapular, truncal. A morobiliform, erythema multiforme, and erythoderma rash have also been reported.
Changes in distal extremities	The distal changes have a biphasic pattern. Early changes, within the first 7–10 days, will present as swelling, induration, and erythema of the hands and feet. Later findings generally occur 2–3 weeks after onset of fever and result in periungual peeling from the fingers and toes.

Laboratory studies are not a necessary component of the diagnostic criteria for KD; however, they are strongly considered in patients who do not meet the classic criteria for KD (e.g., incomplete KD). In patients with suspected incomplete KD, laboratory evaluation includes inflammatory markers, CRP and ESR.

If inflammatory markers are elevated (CRP ≥3 mg/dL or ESR ≥40 mm/h), CBC, comprehensive metabolic panel (CMP), urine studies, and an echocardiogram are performed.

If there are ≥3 of the following seven findings, then the patient is diagnosed with incomplete KD and treatment should be pursued:

- Anemia for age
- Platelet count $\geq 450 \times 10^3/\mu L$ ($\times 10^9/L$) after seventh day of fever
- Albumin level ≤3 g/dL
- Elevated alanine transaminase
- White blood cell (WBC) count of ≥15.0/μL
- Urine ≥10 WBC/HPF with no bacteria
- Positive echocardiogram findings

Differential Diagnosis

With fever as the hallmark of diagnosis, the differential diagnosis of KD predominately includes infectious etiologies. Some common clinical mimickers of KD are adenovirus, enterovirus, Epstein-Barr virus (EBV), and measles. It is possible to have the diagnosis of KD regardless of concomitant infections. The conjunctivitis and desquamation of skin in KD can suggest Stevens-Johnson syndrome (SJS) or Toxic Epidermal Necrosis (TEN). Blistering and skin necrosis are not seen with KD and favor the diagnosis of SJS or TEN. An erythodermic rash in KD can be similar to that seen in toxin-mediated syndromes such as toxic shock syndrome or staphylococcal scalded skin syndrome. However, the toxin-mediated syndromes tend to have visceral organ involvement such as renal insufficiency, which is uncommon in KD. Systemic juvenile idiopathic arthritis (JIA) symptoms can also overlap with KD.

Management

Treatment for KD focuses on prevention of its most serious complication: coronary aneurysms. Treatment should be administered within the first 7 days of illness and at the latest by the tenth day of fever to prevent the development of coronary aneurysms. The primary treatment for KD is high-dose intravenous immune globulin (IVIG) and aspirin. Initially, medium (30–50 mg/kg/day) to high-dose (80–100 mg/kg/day) aspirin is given. Once IVIG has been administered and appropriate response with defervescence achieved, aspirin is stepped down to antithrombotic dosing (3–5 mg/kg/day) and continued until the patient is cleared by a pediatric cardiologist to discontinue; in patients who have not developed coronary aneurysms, aspirin is typically stopped when the ESR/CRP have normalized and thrombocytosis has resolved. Patients can continue with fever for up to 36–48 h after administration of IVIG as a reaction to the IVIG. Fever past 36–48 h is generally considered KD refractory to the first dose of IVIG, and a second dose of IVIG is given. Steroids and immune-mediated therapies such as infliximab have been used in addition to IVIG for those refractory to the first dose of IVIG.

Children with KD should be monitored for fever up to 7–10 days after receiving IVIG. Recurrence is rare but seeking evaluation is important given the cardiac risk with KD. Note that patients should not receive live vaccinations such as mumps, measles, and rubella or varicella 11 months post-IVIG due to the potential for decreased immune response to the vaccine as a result of receiving IVIG. It is important for patients to be closely monitored by a cardiologist following treatment as coronary aneurysms are the most serious complication of KD.

Multisystem Inflammatory Syndrome in Children

Epidemiology/Pathophysiology

Multisystem inflammatory syndrome in children (MIS-C) was first reported April 2020 in the United Kingdom and has been documented worldwide following the SARS-CoV-2 pandemic (hereafter COVID-19). The median age of onset is 8 years, but cases have been reported in both infants and young adults. The true incidence is unknown at this time. Obesity is the most commonly identified medical comorbidity, occurring in 30% of cases.

MIS-C is a constellation of symptoms following COVID-19 infection, consequent to a dysregulated immune response. The pathogenesis is suspected to be a super antigen phenomenon: the SARS-CoV-2 spike protein and endogenous antigens create an immunologic milieu such that a hyperinflammatory response to the initial infection leads to a massive expansion of T-cells propagating multisystem inflammatory dysfunction. The immune dysregulation spans both the innate and adaptive immune systems with evidence of elevated inflammatory markers, interferon gamma, and autoantibodies directed against self-antigens.

Clinical Manifestations

For the diagnosis of MIS-C to be considered, patients must meet three necessary clinical criteria:

1. Unremitting fever ≥38 °C
2. Current or past COVID-19 infection

3. At least two of the clinical features which include: rash, gastrointestinal symptoms (e.g., vomiting, diarrhea, abdominal pain), edema of the hands/feet, oral mucosal changes, conjunctivitis, lymphadenopathy, or neurological symptoms (e.g., altered mental status, focal deficits)

If patients fulfill all three of these criteria, further workup is conducted to evaluate for a possible diagnosis of MIS-C.

About half of MIS-C patients fulfill criteria for typical or atypical Kawasaki disease (KD). Distinguishing between these is critical as treatment protocols defer for the two diagnoses (Table 26.4).

The clinical features of MIS-C found on physical exam include:

1. Rash: A non-vesicular rash that can be polymorphic, maculopapular, or petechial
2. Gastrointestinal symptoms such as non-specific abdominal pain
3. Edema of the hands/feet
4. Mucosal changes such as red and/or cracked lips, strawberry tongue, or erythema of the oropharyngeal mucosa
5. Conjunctivitis that is bilateral and non-exudative
6. Lymphadenopathy
7. Neurological symptoms such as altered mental status, focal deficits, stiff neck, or papilledema

Severe MIS-C can occur with severe cardiac and neurocognitive dysfunction. Patients may present with features of shock at least in part due to cardiac

Table 26.4 Distinguishing multisystem inflammatory syndrome in children from Kawasaki disease

Distinctive to MIS-C	Overlapping features of MIS-C and KD	Distinctive to KD
– Presents in temporal contiguity with COVID-19 infection – Broader age range with older median age of 8 years old – Can consider diagnosis after 3 days of fever – Often presents as gastrointestinal symptoms (nausea, vomiting, diarrhea, and abdominal discomfort) – Severe cardiac dysfunction and shock more common in MIS-C – Cardiac dysfunction frequently manifests as ventricular dysfunction – Lab findings of lower platelet counts, lower absolute lymphocyte counts and higher CRP levels as compared to KD	– Fever – Mucocutaneous features – Conjunctival injection – Rash – Swollen and/or erythematous hands and feet – Cervical lymphadenopathy	– Younger age (median age is 3 years old) – Consider diagnosis after 5 days of fever – Gastrointestinal and neurological symptoms are less common – Most common cardiac manifestation is coronary artery aneurysms

CRP c-reactive protein, *KD* Kawasaki disease, *MIS-C* multisystem inflammatory syndrome in children

dysfunction; symptoms can include somnolence, lethargy, irritability, confusion, and respiratory distress. Severe neurological symptoms may include encephalopathy, meningismus, confusion, and irritability.

Laboratory Assessment/Imaging

The American College of Rheumatology recommends a stepwise workup for MIS-C, see Fig. 26.1.

Tier 1 workup: CBC, CMP, ESR, CRP, ferritin
Tier 2 workup: brain natriuretic peptide, troponin, procalcitonin, prothrombin time, partial thromboplastin time, d-dimer, fibrinogen, lactate dehydrogenase, urinalysis, cytokine panel, triglycerides, blood smear, electrocardiogram, COVID-19 serologies

Concerning labs (must have criteria 1 and 2):

1. CRP ≥3 mg/dL or ESR ≥40 mm/h
2. At least one of the following:

   Absolute lymphocyte count (ALC) <1000/μL
   Platelets <150,000/μL
   Sodium <135 mmol/L
   Neutrophilia
   Hypoalbuminemia

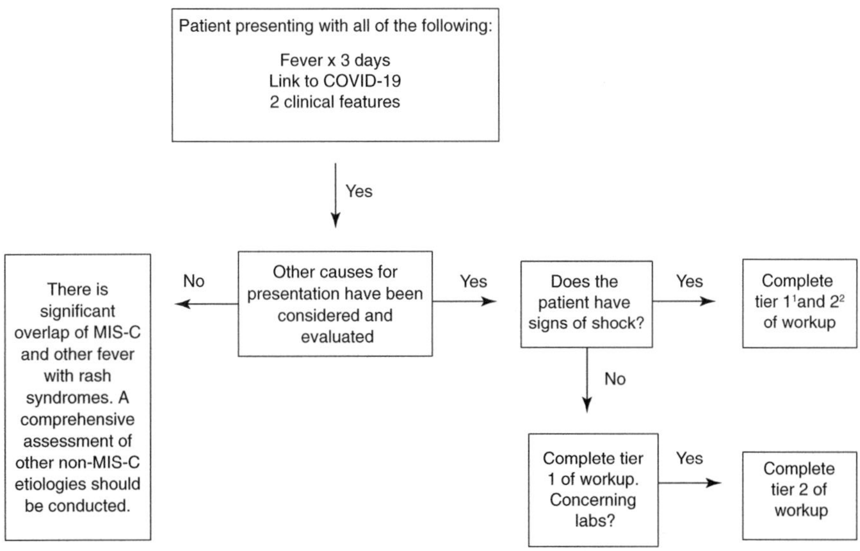

Fig. 26.1 Diagnostic workup for MIS-C. (Adapted from the American College of Rheumatology Clinical Guidelines for Pediatric Patients)

Differential Diagnosis

Immunologic diseases such as KD, macrophage activation syndrome, systemic lupus erythematosus, and systemic JIA should also be considered. Viral infections may be considered based on the pattern of symptoms:

Fever and exanthem: adenovirus, enterovirus, parvovirus, measles
Fever and conjunctival injection: measles and adenovirus
Gastrointestinal involvement: adenovirus, enterovirus, rotavirus, and Norwalk virus
Multisystemic and cardiac involvement: EBV, human immunodeficiency virus, influenza, echovirus, coxsackieviruses, and cytomegalovirus

Aside from viral infections, bacterial infections such as staphylococcal or streptococcal infection presenting with toxic shock syndrome should also be considered.

Management

All patients with MIS-C should be hospitalized and monitored for disease feature development and complications. Early subspecialty consultation may include cardiology, rheumatology, infectious disease, hematology, or neurology depending on organ involvement. Patients with suspected bacterial sepsis or toxic shock should receive broad-spectrum antibiotics until bacterial infection is ruled out.

Treatment for MIS-C includes IVIG (if patient meets KD criteria) and IV methylprednisolone for 5–7 days or until CRP normalizes followed by oral prednisone tapered over 2–3 weeks. Treatment refractory disease should be escalated to include a biologic immunosuppressant, specifically high-dose anakinra or infliximab. Tocilizumab has ongoing trials for safety and efficacy.

MIS-C patients should have electrocardiograms performed every 48 h while hospitalized and if conduction abnormalities are identified, they should be placed on continuous telemetry; a Holter monitor should be considered during outpatient follow-up. An echocardiogram should be performed at diagnosis and follow-up as an outpatient. For patients with coronary artery aneurysms, pediatric cardiology should discuss the need for anticoagulation therapy. For those with significant left ventricular dysfunction during the acute phase of illness, cardiac magnetic resonance imaging should be considered 2–6 months after diagnosis. Imaging suggesting ongoing inflammatory disease may impact decisions regarding long-term immunosuppressive therapy.

For disease prevention: as of the fall of 2022, the Center for Disease Control recommends COVID-19 vaccination for all people aged 6 months and older. The majority of patients who receive timely supportive care make a full recovery. Most children with MIS-C with severe cardiac manifestations can expect clinical recovery within 30 days.

Application Exercises

1. A 5-year-old girl presents to your clinic for evaluation of 3 days of abdominal pain and knee pain. On examination, she is afebrile with an HR of 110 and a BP of 120/70. She has diffuse abdominal pain with palpation, bilateral swelling of her knees, and a petechial rash on her buttocks.

   What is the next best step in evaluation of this disease?

   A. Complement levels
   B. Skin biopsy
   C. Urinalysis with a protein-to-creatinine ratio
   D. Antistreptolysin titers

   Answer C: Urinalysis with protein-to-creatinine ratio. This patient has an elevated blood pressure for her age which warrants further evaluation for renal involvement in the setting of HSP. Up to 50% of patients with HSP will have renal involvement. Though the minority of patients will have progressive renal disease, it is important to screen for these patients with urinalysis and a protein-to-creatinine ratio. Patients with progressive renal disease will require kidney biopsy and possible further treatment with steroids or immunosuppressive agents. Though a skin biopsy can be helpful in confirming the diagnosis of HSP, it is not necessary as HSP is a clinical diagnosis. Complement levels (C3 and C4) may be helpful in distinguishing HSP from other vasculitic processes such as systemic lupus erythematosus or antineutrophil cytoplasmic antibody vasculitis, but neither test is useful to diagnose HSP. Similarly, antistreptolysin O titers can distinguish HSP from post-streptococcal glomerulonephritis but is not a laboratory test specific to HSP.

2. An 18-month-old male presents to the ED for 6 days of fever. Per his mother, the patient has had a fever every night ≥38 °C. On day 3 of illness, the patient had a diffuse erythematous rash that has now resolved. Today in the ED, the patient has a temperature of 39 °C. The remainder of the vital signs are within normal limits. On exam, the patient is very fussy with dry cracked lips, a bright red tongue, and swollen hands. The remainder of the clinical exam is unremarkable.

   A. Does this patient qualify for IVIG?
   B. What other clinical features does this patient require to meet the diagnosis of Kawasaki Disease?
   C. Are there any lab tests you would want to order to further evaluate this patient?

   Answers:

   A. This patient does not meet the clinical criteria for Kawasaki disease. While he has had greater than 5 days of fever, he has only met 3 of the 5 diagnostic criteria for the disease.
   B. The two clinical features that the patient has not developed are enlarged cervical lymph node and limbic sparing conjunctivitis. While he does not cur-

rently have a rash, the history of the rash does count toward the diagnosis of Kawasaki disease.

C. While the patient does not meet the diagnosis for typical Kawasaki disease, his fever duration as well as having three of the five diagnostic criteria, does raise suspicion for incomplete Kawasaki disease. The patient should undergo an ESR, CRP, CBC, CMP, urinalysis, and echocardiogram to evaluate for the possibility of incomplete Kawasaki disease.

3. A 10 year-old female presents to your office for the second time in 7 weeks for knee and ankle pain. She has not had a fever and the parents do not recall any rash. No recent injury. On exam, she has right knee and left ankle swelling and redness. Her initial X-rays from her first presentation were negative. Which one of these statements is most accurate regarding the likely diagnosis for this patient?

A. A normal ESR or CRP would make the diagnosis of JIA unlikely
B. NSAIDs are appropriate treatments for patients with high activity disease
C. A positive ANA would exclude the need for an evaluation by ophthalmology
D. This patient has a 50% chance of achieving remission

Answer D: This patient has a 50% chance of achieving remission.

This patient likely has JIA oligoarthritis subtype based on her age, duration of arthritis, and location of arthritis. Patients with oligoarthritis JIA have a 50% chance of achieving remission of which is defined as no active disease and off of medication for 12 months or more.

While inflammatory markers such as ESR and CRP may indicate an inflammatory state and be helpful in monitoring response to treatment, neither of them are necessary to make the diagnosis of JIA, and a lack of elevated inflammatory markers does not exclude this disease. For patients with highly active disease, NSAIDs are not appropriate as monotherapy. These patients should receive immunosuppression in addition to NSAIDs to manage their disease. Patients with oligoarthritis JIA who are ANA positive are at significant risk for developing chronic anterior uveitis; all patients with the diagnosis of JIA should undergo initial slit lamp examination by ophthalmology followed by regular intervals as designated by the rheumatologist and ophthalmologist.

Further Reading

Henderson LA, Canna SW, Friedman KG, Gorelik M, Lapidus SK, Bassiri H, et al. American College of Rheumatology clinical guidance for pediatric patients with multisystem inflammatory syndrome in children (MIS-C) associated with SARS-CoV-2 and hyperinflammation in COVID-19. Version 2. Arthritis Rheumatol. 2021;73:e13–29.

Leung AKC, Barankin B, Leong KF. Henoch-Schönlein purpura in children: an updated review. Curr Pediatr Rev. 2020;16(4):265–76.

Prakken B, Albani S, Martini A. Juvenile idiopathic arthritis. Lancet. 2011;377(9783):2138–49.

Reid-Adam J. Henoch-Schonlein purpura. Pediatr Rev. 2014;35(10):447–9.

Son MBF, Newburger JW. Kawasaki disease. Pediatr Rev. 2018;39(2):78–90.

Chapter 27
Medical Devices

Stephanie Kwon and Hilary Lin

Background

You will encounter many children assisted by technology on the inpatient wards. This assistance can come in the form of supplemental oxygen or mechanical ventilation with or without tracheostomy, gastrostomy and jejunostomy tubes, semi-permanent venous catheters, enterostomies, and urostomies. There are many reasons why a child may require such assistive devices and include conditions relating to sequelae of prematurity; neuromuscular disorders; genetic syndromes; congenital anomalies; and complications of injury, infection, and illness. The technology may be temporary or permanent depending on the child's underlying diagnosis.

Enteric Tubes

Nutrition is an essential component to the growth and development of children. The enteral tract is the preferred route to provide nutrition. Enteric tubes can deliver nutrition directly into the stomach or jejunum when oral intake is not possible. Common indications for enteric tube placement include inability to safely eat by mouth, increased metabolic demand, congenital upper gastrointestinal or airway

S. Kwon (✉)
Pediatric Hospital Medicine, Medical University of South Carolina, Charleston, SC, USA
e-mail: kwonst@musc.edu

H. Lin
Pediatric Hospital Medicine, Children's Hospital of Orange County, Orange, CA, USA
e-mail: Hlin1@choc.org

N. Liao et al. (eds.), *Pediatric Rotations*,
https://doi.org/10.1007/978-3-031-59873-9_27

malformations, and chronic inadequate oral intake. There are a variety of enteric tubes and sizes (based on the tube diameter in French scale) available. The decision of which tube to use is dependent on indication and duration of use.

Oral and Nasal Tubes

Oral and nasal tubes are generally used for temporary enteral feeding requirements or in anticipation of a more permanent enteric tube. These include orogastric (OG), nasogastric (NG), and nasojejunal (NJ) tubes. Oral and nasal tubes can be placed at bedside by a trained healthcare professional. Following placement, the tube is secured with adhesive tape on the cheek. These tubes can easily be dislodged so it is important to evaluate the need for a more secure, long-term option for providing enteral nutrition.

Gastrostomy Tubes

For patients who require a long-term enteric tube for nutrition, gastrostomy tubes (G-tube) are preferred as the risk of dislodgement is decreased and replacement does not need to be confirmed using radiography. See Fig. 27.1 for a type of low

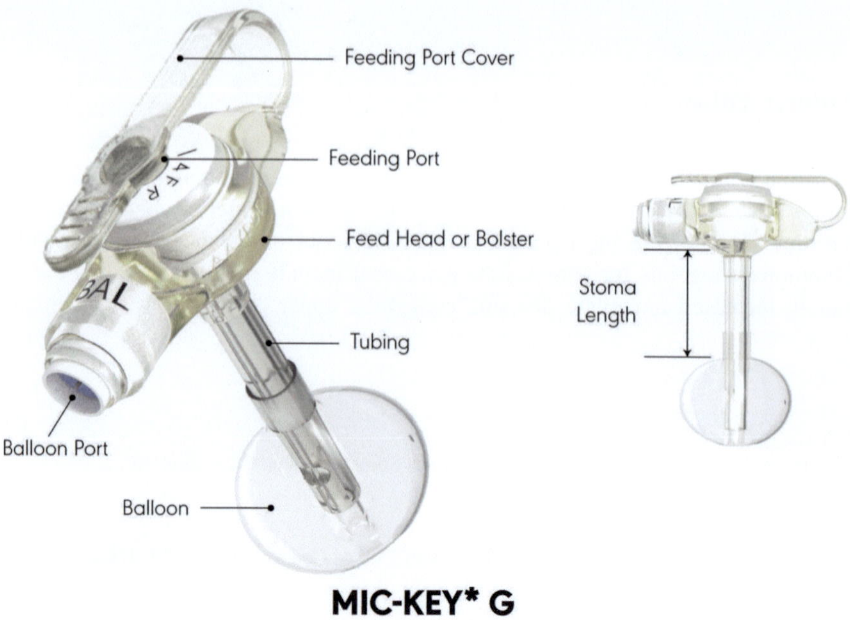

Fig. 27.1 MIC-KEY™ low profile gastrostomy tube. (Used with permission from Avanos Medical, Inc.)

profile G-tube commonly used in children. G-tube placement is performed surgically, percutaneously, or endoscopically. Prior to placement, upper gastrointestinal (UGI) series should be considered in symptomatic patients (emesis or intolerance with gastric feeds) to evaluate anatomic abnormalities, like malrotation, or degree of reflux to determine the most appropriate approach to placement of G-tube and need for fundoplication. After the G-tube is placed, enteral feeds are usually initiated within 24 h and titrated up to goal feeding regimen as tolerated. Caregivers will receive training on how to care for and administer enteral nutrition through the G-tube.

Common Complications with Gastrostomy Tubes

Gastrostomy tube dislodgement is a common complication which necessitates quick resolution because the stoma can close within 1–2 h of dislodgement. Tube dysfunction includes tube leakage, which should be evaluated by a radiologic contrast study, and tube blockage which can usually be resolved by flushing with water, saline, or carbonated drink. Repeated irritation or infection can cause granuloma tissue to develop which is treated with silver nitrate, topical steroid application, and/or protective dressing. Systemic infections from the gastrostomy tube are uncommon. Local peristomal infections can be treated with topical antimicrobials.

Tracheostomies

A tracheostomy is a procedure whereby an artificial opening (stoma) is created in the anterior trachea to establish an airway. The procedure is performed by an otolaryngologist.

Indications

Tracheostomies may be indicated for a variety of reasons. These include structural abnormalities of the upper airways (e.g., subglottic stenosis, laryngeal anomalies, or craniofacial anomalies) or lower airways (e.g., severe tracheo-bronchomalacia). Some children may receive a tracheostomy if there is a need for long-term ventilation, such as following a head or spinal injury. Tracheostomies may also be indicated if there is a need for airway protection, underlying neuromuscular disease, or to facilitate clearance of secretions.

Tracheostomy Tubes

Pediatric tubes can be either cuffed or uncuffed and come in various sizes. See Fig. 27.2 for a type of commonly used tracheostomy tubes. Selection of tube size depends on the size of the child's airway and the indication. For instance, a ventilator-dependent child may need a larger diameter tube. Appropriate sizing is important because an oversized tube may cause mucosal injury, bleeding, fistula formation, or tracheal stenosis. Cuffed tubes allow for a seal if the child requires mechanical ventilation and prevents aspiration of refluxed stomach contents into the lungs. Uncuffed tubes encourage spontaneous breathing and allow for improved vocalization. Using a Passy-Muir valve helps promote speech. It attaches to the outside opening of the tracheostomy tube. When the child breathes in, the valve opens, and the air is then forced up through the vocal cords and out of the mouth, allowing sounds to be made.

Management of the Tracheostomy Tube

Immediately after the tracheotomy surgery, the child is kept sedated and paralyzed to prevent accidental decannulation. The first tracheostomy change occurs between postoperative days 3 to 7 and is typically done by the surgeon. Sutures that were placed in the operating room to help with reinsertion of the tube in an immature stoma ("stay sutures") are removed. Now, routine trach care begins. Home care involves routine tube changes every 2–4 weeks, humidification to decrease mucous plugging, and suctioning of secretions. Tracheostomy tube ties are the bands that go around the neck and help hold the tracheostomy tube in place.

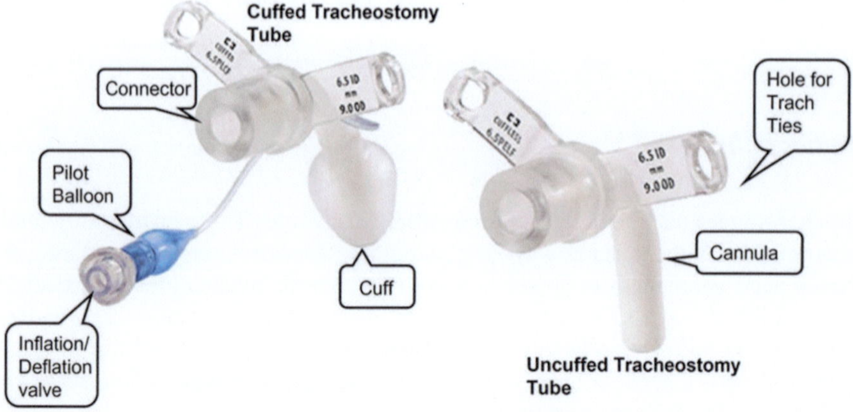

Fig. 27.2 Tracheostomy tubes (Shiley™ neonatal and pediatric tracheostomy tubes). (©2023 Medtronic. All rights reserved. Used with the permission of Medtronic)

Complications

Complications can be divided into early (within the first 7 days of placement) and late (any time after). In the early postoperative period, you'll want to watch out for bleeding, subcutaneous air dissection, pneumothorax, pneumomediastinum, and injury to the recurrent laryngeal nerve. Long-term complications include recurrent tracheitis, suprastomal obstruction, tracheal ulceration or granuloma, persistent tracheocutaneous fistula, and hemorrhage such as when there is erosion into the innominate artery, though this is rare. Patients with tracheostomies may experience repeated respiratory infections with colonized organisms or those that bypass the upper airway defense mechanisms. Cannula obstruction from secretions and accidental decannulation can occur and are airway emergencies. If a child with a mature tracheostomy loses their airway, the tracheostomy tube should be quickly and expertly replaced with the same size or a size smaller tube. All children should always have a spare tracheostomy tube with them, and a caregiver trained in how to replace it in close proximity.

There can also be complications from the tube itself. If the child has a cuffed tube, the caregiver will need to take care to prevent overinflation, which may lead to airway trauma. The trach ties can lead to pressure ulcers and should be inspected several times a day. The tube itself can also form pressure ulcers around the stoma, under the chin, or on the chest if the tube is positioned inappropriately.

Intentional Decannulation

Decannulation may occur when the indications for a tracheostomy are no longer present. Exact criteria vary by center, but there are several general criteria the child must meet. First, the child must have a period without ventilation support for 2–4 months and no evidence of ongoing aspiration that would preclude decannulation. A flexible laryngoscopy should then document the absence of complications that may interfere with breathing such as granuloma tissue, severe stenosis, or vocal cord abnormalities. If these criteria are met, the indwelling tube is replaced with successively smaller tubes. Once the child is breathing comfortably with the smallest available tube in place, the tube is removed and the stoma is covered.

Ostomies

An ostomy is a surgically created opening between a hollow organ and the outside via a stoma.

Intestinal Ostomies

Intestinal ostomies can be created anywhere along the intestinal tract to allow the diversion of feces through the stoma into a pouch that is secured to the abdomen with adhesive. The most common types are ileostomy and colostomy. Indications for ostomy vary based on age of patient. In the neonatal period, ostomies may be indicated in patients with anorectal malformation, necrotizing enterocolitis, Hirschsprung disease, intestinal malrotation/volvulus, or atresia along the gastrointestinal tract. In children and adolescents, ostomies may be indicated in inflammatory bowel disease, neurogenic bowel, trauma, or bowel perforation. The majority of intestinal ostomies are reversed within a few months to years.

Urinary Diversion

Some children do not have effective bladder evacuation. Routine catheterizations and pharmacotherapy like anticholinergics or botulinum-A toxin are often the first-line treatment options and can delay and sometimes obviate the need for surgical interventions. If these treatment options fail or are not possible, surgical procedures are considered. Ultimately, the goal of treatment is to preserve renal function and prevent recurrent urinary tract infections. Urinary diversion can be subdivided into two categories: continent and incontinent.

Urostomies

A urostomy is a form of incontinent urinary diversion. This approach is less commonly used and was more popular a few decades ago, prior to the institution of clean intermittent catheterizations, medications, and surgical approaches allowing for continence. However, this is a good option for those whose social circumstances may preclude strict compliance to a catheterization regimen.

A urostomy typically uses an ileal conduit, whereby a small piece of the ileum is detached from the rest of the small intestines. The ureters are then removed from the bladder and connected to this detached portion of the ileum. One end of the ileum is sewn closed, and the other end is brought to the front of the abdominal wall to form the stoma. This forms a small pouch that will hold urine. The output cannot be controlled, so a collection pouch must be worn continuously.

Mitrofanoff

A mitrofanoff procedure allows for urinary continence by creating a channel that can be catheterized channel, most commonly using the appendix. One end of the appendix is attached to the bladder, with the other portion terminating in the umbilicus or in the lower abdominal wall. The child or caregiver can then use this channel to intermittently catheterize. If the appendix is not available or inappropriate to use, other structures have been used including a ureter, ileum, or fallopian tube. Common reasons for children to undergo either procedure include conditions such as a neurogenic bladder, epispadias-exstrophy complex, or bladder outlet obstruction.

Complications

For any surgery involving the bowel, there is a risk for ileus, adhesions, and bowel obstruction.

For the Mitrofanoff procedure, the most common complication is stomal stenosis. Other complications include leakage, conduit stricture, difficulty with catheterization, and prolapse. Any time that a portion of the small intestine is used as a conduit, there will be mucus output which is naturally produced by the intestines. This is an expected finding.

Central Venous Catheters

There are many reasons why a child may have a central venous catheter. Some children need them if they are receiving chronic infusions. Some children require frequent blood draws and will have a line placed if they have difficult peripheral access. Others may not be able to tolerate enteral feeds, such as those with intestinal failure from short gut syndrome and need intravascular access for parenteral nutrition and other hyperosmolar solutions that are caustic to peripheral veins and pose a greater risk of tissue injury if there is extravasation.

There are several types of central lines. Non-tunneled central venous catheters are inserted directly into the desired vessel such as the internal jugular, subclavian, and femoral veins. These are for more short-term use (7–10 days). Peripherally inserted central catheters (PICCs) are inserted into a peripheral vein and threaded into a central vein. These are generally recommended for short- to medium-term use (4 weeks–6 months). Tunneled lines (e.g., port-a-caths) are placed at a distant site and tunneled subcutaneously before entering the vessel. While a tunneled line requires general anesthesia to place, its advantages are a decreased risk of infection and greater stability with less risk of accidental dislodgement. These are recommended if the child will require access for months to years.

Complications

Central lines are not without risk. Early, or insertion-related complications, include pneumothorax or hemothorax, accidental arterial puncture, hematoma, and arrhythmias. Late complications include occlusion, dislodgement or migration, and infection. If a child with a central line develops a fever, chills, or hypotension, you will need to evaluate for a central line-associated bloodstream infection (CLABSI). Ideally, this is done by obtaining peripheral and central line cultures simultaneously to differentiate between a line-associated versus a systemic infection. Central lines may also become occluded if a fibrin sheath develops around the intravascular portion of the catheter. This can sometimes be overcome with fibrinolytic therapy. Children with a central line may also develop a symptomatic thrombus in the catheterized vein. A duplex ultrasound is the initial diagnostic study to evaluate for such a complication and if present, treatment requires systemic anticoagulation.

Further Reading

Bakewell C, Corlett C, Sharrard A, Howarth LJ, Lee AC. Current trends in paediatric enteral tube feeding. Paediatr Child Health. 2021;31(8):308–15.

Browning JD, Stephany HA. Advances in pediatric urinary diversion. Urol Clin N Am. 2018;45:123.

Glader LJ, Palfrey JS. Care of the child assisted by technology. Pediatr Rev. 2009;30(11):439–45. https://doi.org/10.1542/pir.30.11.439.

Mattei P, Nichol PF, Rollins I, Muratore CS. In: Mattei P, Nichol PF, Rollins I, Muratore CS, editors. Fundamentals of pediatric surgery: ileostomy and colostomy. 2nd ed. Cham: Springer International Publishing; 2017.

Triplett A, Zeller K, Potisek NM. Indwelling lines. Pediatr Rev. 2021;42(2):106–8. https://doi.org/10.1542/pir.2020-002303.

Chapter 28
Medications and Fluid Management

Melissa Rodriguez Rodriguez, Brianna Glover, and Sarah Varghese

Medications and Weight-Based Dosing

Background

Similar to adults, pharmacokinetics defines how pediatric medications are administered. Pediatric patients, unlike adults, however, are in a constant state of change and development. These physiological changes are unique in pediatrics and impact drug metabolism and its effects throughout the body. Examples of this can be seen in fluctuations in total body water (TBW), body fat percentage, and drug-binding proteins. TBW will be in higher proportions in newborns at ~75% TBW and decrease in adulthood to ~20–30% TBW. In contrast, body fat percentage can be around 16% in a neonate yet increases to ~25–50% in adults, with variations based on age and sex. Finally, circulating proteins that carry out drug binding in the plasma are reduced in neonates and do not reach adult values until infancy.

M. R. Rodriguez
Division of Hospital Medicine, Department of Pediatrics, Emory University School of Medicine/Children's Healthcare of Atlanta, Atlanta, GA, USA

Puerto Rico Woman and Children's Hospital, Bayamon, Puerto Rico
e-mail: melissa.n.rodriguez.rodriguez@emory.edu

B. Glover · S. Varghese (✉)
Division of Hospital Medicine, Department of Pediatrics, Emory University School of Medicine/Children's Healthcare of Atlanta, Atlanta, GA, USA
e-mail: brianna.patrice.glover@emory.edu; sarah.varghese@emory.edu

N. Liao et al. (eds.), *Pediatric Rotations*,
https://doi.org/10.1007/978-3-031-59873-9_28

As such, dosing medications in a fixed way, as is done in adult medicine, can lead to adverse drug reactions (ADRs) in children and adolescents. Traditionally, ADRs are either Type A (dose-dependent and predictable) or Type B (not dose-dependent and unpredictable) reactions. In pediatrics, a true incidence of ADRs is hard to estimate. This is likely due to a lack of recognition by parents combined with underreporting by healthcare professionals. That said, ADRs account for up to 10% of pediatric admissions to children's hospitals.

Many different methods have been described for the initial selection of a drug dose in pediatric patients. The majority of these use total body weight (mg/kg) or total body surface area (mg/m^2) dosing as ways to reflect the developmental and physiological changes seen in pediatrics. Selection of drug dosing based on total body weight or body surface area will usually lead to a similar plasma concentration of any given drug. The major exception to this depends on a drug's volume of distribution (VD). If the drug's VD exceeds the extracellular fluid space, then a total body weight-based approach is preferred. In contrast, if the drug VD is equal to the extracellular fluid space, then a body surface area-based dosing is better.

It should be noted that higher weight in children can also alter drug pharmacokinetics. Overweight in pediatrics is defined as a BMI-for-age above the 85th percentile but below the 95th percentile, while obesity is a BMI-for-age above the 95th percentile. Currently, limited literature and data exist on dosing medications in obese or overweight pediatric patients. These individuals will usually have a higher proportion of lipids which can lead to a higher volume of distribution for lipophilic medications. The volume of distribution for hydrophilic medications is also altered in relation to the amount of lean body mass, blood volume, and total body water the individual possesses. The Pediatric Pharmacy Advocacy Group has made some recommendations for medication dosing in overweight and obese pediatric patients. In general, weight-based dosing can be used in patients <18 years of age who are <40 kg. When children are ≥40 kg, weight-based dosing can be used as long as the total dose or dose per day does not exceed the recommended adult dose for the same medication.

The Importance of Milliliters (mL) vs Milligrams (mg) When Prescribing Medications

In pediatrics, medications are usually prescribed with the amount of milligrams (mg) a patient should take per dose. That said, most medications come in oral solutions where the milligrams are distributed in a certain amount of milliliters (mL). Most parents are good at remembering the amount of milliliters their child takes of a certain medication, but practitioners should be cautious in using milliliters and milligrams as a 1:1 conversion when prescribing.

For example, you are prescribing acetaminophen for fever in an 8-year-old patient who weighs 22 kg. Acetaminophen usually comes in a 160 mg/5 mL solution, and you want to prescribe 15 mg/kg every 6 h as needed. For this patient,

Step 1: 22 kg × 15 mg/kg = 330 mg per dose
Step 2: 160 mg ÷ 5 mL = 32 mg in each mL
Step 3: 330 mg ÷ 32 mg/mL = 10 mL per dose

As such, for this patient, 10 mL per dose accounts for the 320 mg the patient needs to achieve an antipyretic effect. Conversely, 10 mg of acetaminophen would be significantly underdosed for this patient's weight. As in this example, milliliters should be rounded to the nearest half or whole milliliter to ease measuring and administration by parents.

Common Pediatric Medications and Their Dosing

The conversion of medications between milliliters and milligrams can lead to medication dosing errors. It is important to review this with parents when prescribing medications. When ordering home medications at the time of inpatient admission, make sure to conduct a review and double check doses in milliliters as well as

Table 28.1 Common medications and dosing in pediatrics

Medication classes	Weight-based dosing and interval	Max dose
Fever/pain		
(a) Acetaminophen (b) Ibuprofen	(a) 10–15 mg/kg every 4–6 h (b) 10 mg/kg every 4–6 h	(a) 650 mg/dose; 4000 mg/day (b) 400 mg/dose; 2400 mg/day
Nausea		
(a) Ondansetron (b) Metoclopramide (c) Promethazine (d) Diphenhydramine	(a) 0.1–0.15 mg/kg every 8 h (b) 0.1–0.2 mg/kg every 6 h (c) 0.25–0.5 mg/kg every 4–6 h (d) 0.6–1.25 mg/kg every 6 h	(a) 8 mg/dose (b) 10 mg/dose (c) 25 mg/dose (d) 50 mg/dose
Antibiotics		
(a) Amoxicillin ± clavulanic acid (b) Ampicillin ± sulbactam[a] (c) Clindamycin (d) Cephalexin (e) Ceftriaxone[a] (f) Vancomycin[a]	(a) 45–90 mg/kg/day divided twice or thrice daily (b) 200–400 mg/kg/day divided every 6 h (c) 30–40 mg/kg/day divided every 8 h (d) 25–100 mg/kg/day divided every 6–8 h (e) 50–100 mg/kg every 24 h (f) 40–80 mg/kg/day divided every 6–8 h	(a) 1000 mg/dose (b) 2000 mg/dose (c) 600 mg/dose (d) 1000 mg/dose (e) 2000 mg/dose (f) 2000 mg/dose

[a] IV form only

milligrams with parents. Table 28.1 below includes some of the most commonly used medications in pediatrics. This is not a comprehensive medication list. Many medications have varying dosing ranges and intervals which are often influenced by treatment indication. One such example is the use of high-dose amoxicillin which is 90 mg/kg/day; however, this dose is divided twice daily for acute otitis media and three times daily for pneumonia in order to maintain effective antibiotic levels within the targeted site.

Fluid Selection

Dehydration

Dehydration is a common reason for pediatric patients to be hospitalized. Commonly, fever and gastrointestinal and respiratory illnesses can lead to increased insensible losses. This in turn can lead to hypovolemia and electrolyte disturbances which can be detrimental to a patient's health.

A patient's history of present illness, vital signs and physical exam can provide clues to their degree of dehydration. History may elicit the presence of emesis, diarrhea, decreased oral intake, or decreased urinary output. Tachycardia is usually an early sign of dehydration in pediatrics with hypotension being a late and more ominous sign of severe dehydration. Physical exam findings consistent with dehydration can include delayed capillary refill, decreased skin turgor, weak pulses, dry mucous membranes, and sunken anterior fontanelles in infants. Table 28.2 reviews common signs of mild, moderate, and severe dehydration.

Table 28.2 Clinical classification of dehydration

Signs of dehydration	Mild	Moderate	Severe
Mental status	Alert, conversating	Listless, tired	Lethargic
Pulse rate	Normal	Slightly increased	Markedly increased
Pulse quality	Normal	Weak	Thready
Capillary refill	Normal (<2 s)	~2–3 s	>3 s
Blood pressure	Normal	Normal	Normal to decreased
Eyes	Normal	Deep set	Sunken
Tear production	Present	Decreased	Absent
Fontanelle (infant)	Flat	Sunken	Very sunken
Urine output	Normal to decreased	Mild oliguria	Severe oliguria, anuria
Skin turgor	Normal	Decreased	Tenting
Skin (to touch)	Normal	Dry	Clammy
Mucous membranes	Moist	Dry	Parched
Thirst	↑	↑↑	↑↑↑
Percent dehydration	<5%	5–9%	≥10%

In general, mild dehydration can be managed with enteral fluid replacement. Moderate to severe dehydration usually requires parenteral fluid replacement with the use of intravenous fluids.

Phases of Rehydration

For patients requiring intravenous fluids, there are distinct phases to consider in terms of rehydration. The components of each of these will be discussed at more length in this chapter. In general, phase one or the resuscitative phase is when parenteral fluids are required to restore intravascular volume and avoid end organ injury. This is usually achieved with a bolus or large infusion of fluids over a short amount of time. This is followed by phase two, the titration phase, where once the patient is stabilized, they can be transitioned to maintenance intravenous fluids. The rate of fluids can be adjusted to account for any new or ongoing losses. Phase three, the maintenance phase, is where a balance is achieved between physiological needs and both sensible and insensible losses. Finally, in phase four, the convalescent phase, the patient has a good ability to hydrate themselves and regulate their losses, and as such intravenous fluids can be stopped.

Fluid Types

There is a diverse array of enteral and parenteral fluid solutions which vary in the composition of electrolytes. The differences are outlined in Tables 28.3 and 28.4. In terms of intravenous (IV) fluids, 0.9% NaCl (normal saline or NS) and Lactated Ringer's (LR) are considered isotonic solutions as they have a similar sodium concentration to that of plasma (135–144 mEq/L). On the contrary, 0.45% NaCl (½ NS) and 0.225% NaCl (¼ NS) are considered hypotonic solutions.

Historically, hypotonic IV fluid solutions were preferred for maintenance intravenous fluid therapy. However, many hospitalized patients are at risk for developing hyponatremia. This is thought to be secondary to elevated arginine vasopressin (AVP) hormone release secondary to pulmonary (i.e., pneumonia), central nervous system (i.e., meningitis) diseases as well as pain, stress, hypovolemia, and medications. As these are common factors and conditions in hospitalized pediatric patients,

Table 28.3 Composition of commonly used parenteral fluids

Parenteral fluid	Na (mEq/L)	K (mEq/L)	Cl (mEq/L)	HCO_3 (mEq/L)
Lactated Ringer's (LR)	130	4	109	28
NS (0.9% NaCl)	154	0	154	0
½ NS (0.45% NaCl)	77	0	77	0
¼ NS (0.225% NaCl)	34	0	34	0

Table 28.4 Composition of commonly used oral rehydration solutions (adapted from The Harriet Lane handbook)

Oral fluids	Na (mEq/L)	K (mEq/L)	Cl (mEq/L)	HCO_3 (mEq/L)	Dextrose (g/100 mL)
Apple juice	0.4	26	0	0	11.9
Ginger ale	3.5	0.1	0	3.6	9
Milk	22	36	28	30	4.9
Powerade	18	2.7	0	0	5.8
Pedialyte	45	20	35	0	2.5

it is not surprising that the administration of hypotonic intravenous fluids can precipitate hyponatremia. As such, the Clinical Practice Guideline: Maintenance Intravenous Fluids in Children by the American Academy of Pediatrics recommends that isotonic solutions be used for intravenous fluids in patients 28 days to 18 years of age to decrease the risk of hyponatremia.

Isotonic fluids are typically used for initial fluid resuscitation. However, when starting a patient on maintenance intravenous fluids, the addition of dextrose and potassium should also be considered. The addition of dextrose helps with preventing hypoglycemia in patients with poor caloric intake. It also aids with preventing catabolism or starvation ketosis. In general, most pediatric patients will do well with the addition of 5% dextrose. The exception to this is neonates as they typically have low glycogen storages and are at higher risk of hypoglycemia. Children with metabolic disorders may also require higher levels of dextrose concentrations depending on their disease and degree of dehydration. In general, up to 12.5% of dextrose can be administered in a peripheral IV. Higher dextrose concentrations require central line access to avoid irritation to the peripheral vasculature. In terms of potassium, 1–2 mEq/kg/day can be administered as long as the patient is not suffering from hyperkalemia, oliguria/anuria, or kidney issues. The most common composition of maintenance fluids ordered on hospitalized children is D5 + 0.9% NaCl (NS) + 20 mEq KCl.

Complications of Intravenous Fluid Use

Normal saline or 0.9% NaCl is the most commonly used and studied isotonic fluid in pediatrics. Administration of this solution is similar to the administration of any other drug in that potential complications and side effects must always be considered. The most common complications include hypernatremia, acidosis, and fluid overload. Hypernatremia, while rare, can occur in patients receiving 0.9% NaCl, particularly if they're experiencing significant free water losses. This can be remedied by use of hypotonic solutions. Given the amount of chloride in a 0.9% NaCl solution (154 mEq/L), patients can develop a non-anion gap metabolic acidosis secondary to hyperchloremia due to excessive renal bicarbonate elimination. Discontinuing an infusion of these fluids or switching to fluids with a lower chloride content can resolve this issue in patients with adequate renal function. Not all patients on intravenous fluids require constant laboratory monitoring of electrolytes, but those on prolonged therapy or with risk factors to develop these electrolyte disturbances should be closely monitored. A chemistry profile (complete metabolic panel [CMP] or basic metabolic panel [BMP]) can be utilized to assess the degree of electrolyte derangements. If hypernatremia or hyperchloremia are identified, electrolytes should be monitored until the derangements are corrected.

Finally, pediatric patients receiving intravenous fluids are at risk for fluid accumulation leading to volume overload. Patients with underlying chronic conditions such as congestive heart failure, hepatic failure and chronic kidney disease are at even higher risk for this. Therefore, patients on intravenous fluid therapy should have strict intake and output recorded while receiving fluids. Other clinical factors such as increasing weight, auscultated crackles on the respiratory exam and facial or peripheral edema can indicate fluid overload. These clinical findings should guide the decision to decrease rate of fluids being administered or consider cessation of fluid therapy.

Fluid Calculations

Moderate to severe dehydration can be treated with the use of parenteral or intravenous fluids. The amount of fluid used in each of the phases of rehydration (resuscitative, titration, maintenance, and convalescent) is different.

Resuscitative Phase

In general, when a patient presents with clinical signs and symptoms of moderate or severe dehydration, they will require a bolus, a rapid and large infusion of fluids, to restore their intravascular volume. This is typically achieved with the use of 0.9% NaCl or lactated ringer's solution, without addition or dextrose or potassium. A typical fluid bolus volume is 20 mL/kg with a maximum of 1000 mL per bolus. Smaller aliquots of 5–10 mL/kg are used if there is concern for fluid overload or reduced cardiac function. A bolus is typically administered quickly through the IV via an IV pump over 30 min to 1 h. During instances of severe dehydration or shock, a push-pull method using a syringe can be used to deliver fluid much more quickly over 5–10 min. Each time a bolus is given, the patient's clinical condition and vital signs should be reassessed. In general, improvement in heart rate, urine output, pulse quality, among others, are signs of a good response. Patients can receive repeat boluses, up to a limit of 60 mL/kg. At that time, if the patient is not having a response to fluid therapy, there should be an evaluation for other medical conditions, i.e., septic shock, adrenal crisis, or heart failure and consideration of the use of vasopressors.

An example of this is an 11-year-old who weighs 35 kg and presents to the emergency department with parched mucous membranes, tachycardia for age and sunken eyes after multiple days of vomiting and diarrhea at home. The emergency physician decides to administer a bolus with 0.9% NaCl. The patient would require a bolus of 700 mL given the following calculation:

$$\text{Example of bolus calculation} : 35\,\text{kg} \times 20\,\text{mL} / \text{kg} = 700\,\text{mL}$$

Titration and Maintenance Phase

Once patients have been successfully resuscitated with fluids, many will require continued intravenous fluids to account for ongoing losses, such as emesis or diarrhea. The Holliday-Segar Method, also known as the 4-2-1 rule, estimates maintenance fluid requirements. It approximates insensible and urine losses in a fixed weight category as seen in Table 28.5. It can then be used to calculate the maintenance fluid rate for any patient up until the maximum maintenance fluid rate of 100 mL/h is achieved. See Table 28.6 for an example calculation using the 4-2-1 rule.

Using the previous example, once the 11-year-old who weighs 35 kg has been resuscitated with fluids in the emergency department, he will require admission for maintenance intravenous fluid therapy in the setting of ongoing vomiting and diarrhea. His calculated hourly fluid rate with the 4-2-1 rule is as follows (Table 28.6):

Assuming this patient has normal potassium levels and good renal function, the best maintenance fluid choice to order for him on admission would be D5 + 0.9% NaCl (NS) + 20 mEq KCl to run at 75 mL/h.

If the ongoing losses are significant, many clinicians will choose to run the fluid at 1.5 times the maintenance rate to account for the replacement of ongoing losses

Table 28.5 Holliday-Segar/4-2-1 Method for estimating fluid requirements

	Water requirement	
Body weight	Hourly (100 mL/h maximum)	Daily (2400 mL/day maximum)
First 10 kg	4 mL/kg/h	100 mL/kg/day
Second 10 kg	2 mL/kg/h	50 mL/kg/day
Each additional 1 kg	1 mL/kg/h	20 mL/kg/day

Table 28.6 Example of 4-2-1 rule calculation

First 10 kg: 10 kg × 4 mL/kg/h	40 mL/h
Second 10 kg: 10 kg × 2 mL/kg/h	20 mL/h
Remaining 1 kg: 15 kg × 1 mL/kg/h	15 mL/h
Total kg: 35 kg	**Total fluid rate: 75 mL/h**

as well as the initial fluid deficit. However, you can systematically account for the volume of ongoing losses by measuring the output of emesis and diarrhea and replacing the volume with an isotonic fluid in a 1:1 ratio. Furthermore, a child's fluid deficit can be calculated using the percent dehydration in Table 28.2 and the equation below.

$$\text{Fluid deficit}(\text{mL}) = \%\ \text{dehydration} \times \text{weight}(\text{kg}) \times 10$$

This fluid deficit can then be added to the maintenance fluid rate, with the goal of the first 50% of the deficit being replaced in the first 24 h. Using Table 28.2 and the signs and symptoms identified in the vignette, the 11-year-old who weighs 35 kg is 10% dehydrated. Below outlines the addition of his fluid deficit into his maintenance fluid rate:

Step 1: Fluid deficit (mL) = 10 % dehydration × 35 kg × 10 % = 3500 mL
Step 2: Residual fluid deficit to replace : 3500 mL − 700 mL bolus = 2100 mL
Step 3: Only replace the first 50 % of the fluid deficit in the first 24 h (1050 mL or 44 mL/h)
Step 4: Adjusted maintenance fluid rate = 75 mL/h + 44 mL/h = 119 mL/h

If the clinician instead chose to run the maintenance fluids at 1.5 times the maintenance rate without this formal calculation, the 1.5 times maintenance rate in this patient would be 113 mL/h which is comparable to the 119 mL/h calculated.

Convalescent Phase

As a patient's oral intake improves and ongoing losses decrease, intravenous fluids can be discontinued. Intravenous fluids should be treated as an ongoing medication administration. The maintenance of an IV catheter should also be recognized as an ongoing intervention with risks such as IV infiltration. IV infiltration is where the fluids accidentally leak out of the vein and into the surrounding tissues. Thus, cessation of intravenous fluids should be considered frequently.

Application Exercises

1. You are discharging a 13-month-old female who weighs 10 kg from the emergency department who presented with fever. You want to prescribe ibuprofen every 6 h which comes in an oral solution of 100 mg/5 mL. What is the amount of mL you will tell the family to administer?

   A. 100 mL
   B. 20 mL
   C. 5 mL
   D. 10 mL

Table 28.7 Solution to application exercise using 4-2-1 rule for calculation of maintenance fluids

First 10 kg: 10 kg × 4 mL/kg/h	40 mL/h
Second 10 kg: 10 kg × 2 mL/kg/h	20 mL/h
Remaining 1 kg: 5 kg × 1 mL/kg/h	5 mL/h
Total kg: 25 kg	**Total fluid rate: 65 mL/h**

Answer C: The pediatric dose of ibuprofen is 10 mg/kg so 10 mg/kg × 10 kg = 100 mg. The oral solution has 100 mg/5 mL or 20 mg/1 mL. Dividing the 100 mg dose by 20 mg in each mL = 5 mL.

2. An 8-year-old previously healthy male who weighs 25 kg presents to the emergency department after 2 days of profuse vomiting. He appears tired with dry mucous membranes, decreased skin turgor, and weak pulses. You decide to administer a bolus. What is the most appropriate order?

   A. 500 mL of 0.45% NaCl (½ NS)
   B. 500 mL of 0.9% NaCl (NS)
   C. 1000 mL of 0.9% NaCl (NS)
   D. 500 mL of 0.225% NaCl (¼ NS)

   Answer B: Isotonic fluids such as 0.9% NaCl (NS) or Lactated Ringer's (LR) are used for parenteral fluid bolus administration. The volume of a bolus is calculated at 20 mL/kg, which in this case 20 mL/kg × 25 kg = 500 mL.

3. The same 8-year-old male who weighs 25 kg from question #2 is now being admitted to the hospital. What will you order for his maintenance fluids?

   A. 0.9% NaCl at 65 mL/h
   B. D5 + 0.9% NaCl (NS) + 20 KCl at 25 mL/h
   C. Lactated Ringer's at 25 mL/h
   D. D5 + 0.9% NaCl (NS) + 20 KCl at 65 mL/h

   Answer D: The rate of 65 mL/h is calculated in Table 28.7 below using the 4-2-1 rule. The most commonly used composition of maintenance fluids is D5 + 0.9% NaCl (NS) + 20 KCl.

Further Reading

Feld LG, Neuspiel DR, Foster BA, Leu MG, Garber MD, Austin K, et al. Clinical practice guideline: maintenance intravenous fluids in children. Pediatrics. 2018;142(6):e20183083.

Hughes HK, Kahl LK. Fluids and electrolytes. In: The Harriet Lane handbook. 21st ed. Philadelphia, PA: Elsevier; 2018.

Kliegman R. Pediatric drug therapy. In: Nelson textbook of pediatrics. 21st ed. Philadelphia, PA: Elsevier; 2020.

Matson KL, Horton ER, Capino AC. Medication dosage in overweight and obese children. J Pediatr Pharmacol Ther. 2017;22(1):81–3.

Rauch DA, Gershel JC. Fluids and electrolytes. In: Caring for the hospitalized child: a handbook of inpatient pediatrics. Elk Grove Village, IL: American Academy of Pediatrics; 2018.

Chapter 29
Oncology

Tim J. Porea

Overview

The term "childhood cancer" encompasses a diverse group of diseases with a scope much different from the cancers that adults face. In addition to a different spectrum of pathophysiology, childhood cancer is much less common than adult oncologic conditions with approximately 15,000 children and adolescents diagnosed with cancer each year. Thus, cancer is a rare condition in children. While cancer is a devastating diagnosis, tremendous strides have been made over the years in improving the management of many childhood malignancies. Today approximately 85% of children diagnosed with cancer can be expected to survive their disease. To become a survivor, patients and their families face many medical, emotional, and psychosocial hurdles. Cancer affects the entire family so careful attention must be paid to more than just the patient. In addition, survivors may face a lifetime of challenges due to their disease and its treatment. Even though most students will not become pediatric oncologists, almost everyone will end up caring for childhood cancer patients or adult survivors at some point in their career. Because of this, it is important to have an understanding of what these patients go through in their treatment. Despite an overall favorable survival rate, certain forms of childhood cancer still have poor outcomes and, overall, cancer remains the number one cause of death by illness in childhood.

T. J. Porea (✉)
Department of Pediatrics, Texas Children's Cancer and Hematology Center, Baylor College of Medicine, Houston, TX, USA
e-mail: tjporea@texaschildrens.org

N. Liao et al. (eds.), *Pediatric Rotations*,
https://doi.org/10.1007/978-3-031-59873-9_29

Meeting a Childhood Cancer Patient as a Medical Student

The initial evaluation of an undiagnosed patient should take the same format as a new patient evaluation for any condition. A history and physical exam will lead to a differential diagnosis and evaluation plan. When the team comes to a point where an oncologic process is suspected, the family and patient (in an age-appropriate manner) must be told honestly what is being considered. Using the word "cancer" or "tumor" is uncomfortable for non-oncologists but must be done if you are seriously considering such a diagnosis. If you are planning to admit the patient to an oncology floor, transfer to another facility for an oncologic evaluation, or have an oncologist see the patient, it is crucial that the family knows what you are considering. When you disclose your suspicions, the family will no doubt have many questions and fears. It's best to initially give them a few minutes to process what you've told them before moving on in the discussion. This silence can be unnerving, but you should take your cues regarding moving on from the family. You will not be able to answer most of their initial questions, but they will at least not be surprised by who they meet next.

If you are rotating on an oncology team caring for patients who are already diagnosed, it's not uncommon for trainees to be intimidated by patients and their families. They have very complex diseases and treatments, and you'll feel like the parents know more than you do about their child's disease. They do! Don't shy away from this but use their knowledge as an opportunity to learn. If you have free time, ask parents how their child presented at initial diagnosis as a way for you to learn varied presentations. Also ask them what medications work for them in various situations or how they usually take a medication. A good example is with anti-emetics. There are several different drugs and formulations (liquid, pill, dissolvable tablet). Over time, a patient and their family will find a regimen that works best for them. Ask the patient/family if they have found one that works best for them and use that. Don't just presume to use "what we always use."

Anticipatory Guidance for Cancer Patients

Patients and families deserve honest, up-to-date information. Students may well not be able to answer many of their questions—it is never wrong to say "I don't know but I'll find out." Families should be told that no information will be kept from them—good or bad. They and their child will go through many ups and downs during therapy. Support through other oncology families and support groups can be very helpful in offering guidance on how to handle the challenges of oncology treatment and side effects. And if treatment is unsuccessful the medical team will stand by them with support and resources for end-of-life care.

A discussion of every possible tumor is beyond the scope of this chapter. However below are discussed the primary tumors seen in children.

Leukemias

1. *Background*: Leukemia is the most common childhood cancer diagnosis. There are two main pediatric subtypes—Acute Lymphoblastic Leukemia (ALL) and Acute Myeloid Leukemia (AML) with ALL being more common with a ratio of 4:1. Leukemias are caused by a clonal expansion of white blood cell blasts within the bone marrow. There are a myriad of genetic abnormalities within the blasts that are used in risk stratification for prognosis and treatment. Leukemias can be seen at any age though for ALL there is a peak in presentation in preschool age children.
2. *History*: Patients often present with nonspecific symptoms. There may be symptoms of thrombocytopenia or anemia such as bleeding, bruising, petechiae, and/or pallor. Not uncommonly patients may also have symptoms related to an increase in blasts in the marrow cavity causing bony pain. In pre-verbal children, this can manifest as refusal to bear weight, limp, or generalized fussiness.
3. *Physical exam*: Patients may have signs of extramedullary hematopoiesis including lymphadenopathy and hepatosplenomegaly. A testicular exam should be performed as this is also a potential site of leukemic involvement. Involved testicles will be firm and painless and are often unilateral.
4. *Laboratory assessment/imaging (workup)*: The patient with suspected leukemia should have a complete blood count (CBC). When abnormalities of 2 or 3 of the main cell lines (red cells, white cells, and platelets) are seen the diagnosis of leukemia should rise higher on the differential list. A full chemistry panel with a focus on intracellular substances including potassium, creatinine, phosphate, and uric acid (all may be elevated in tumor lysis- see oncologic emergencies section) should also be ordered. A prothrombin time and partial thromboplastin time (PT/PTT) should be obtained as some new patients will be coagulopathic. And all should have a chest X-ray (CXR) to evaluate for mediastinal mass (common in T-cell ALL) before they are sedated for any procedures. Peripheral blood flow cytometry can often confirm the diagnosis, but all patients will need a bone marrow aspirate and biopsy to collect all samples required for diagnosis. All newly diagnosed patients will need a lumbar puncture to evaluate for central nervous system (CNS) disease.
5. *Key differential diagnosis*: Patients with aplastic anemia, a bone marrow failure syndrome, can also present with cytopenias.
6. *Management*: Treatment of both ALL and AML is highly dependent on risk stratification including cytogenetic analysis of the blast cells. It consists of multidrug chemotherapy given via a variety of routes including intrathecal therapy. Patients with AML are more likely to have a need for bone marrow transplantation while most ALL patients are managed with standard chemotherapy alone. Treatment for ALL generally lasts about 3 years with the majority of time being outpatient. AML treatment is typically more intense, all inpatient, and can be completed in about 6 months if no transplant is needed.

Lymphomas

1. *Background*: Lymphomas are caused by a malignant transformation of lymphoid cells. They are divided into Hodgkin Lymphoma (HL) and Non-Hodgkin Lymphoma (NHL) categories. Within each of these there are various subtypes. Epstein-Barr virus infection has been implicated in the development of some lymphomas, and there may be an association between some immunodeficiencies and lymphomas. The classic histopathologic finding for HL is the Reed-Sternberg cell.
2. *History*: Lymphomas can present in a variety of ways. Many of these depend on the specific location of adenopathy, which is typically painless. One may see asymptomatic peripheral masses in the neck, axilla, or groin. Internal adenopathy could manifest with respiratory symptoms or superior vena cava (SVC) syndrome (neck swelling and venous distension) from mediastinal disease as well as constipation or other abdominal complaints from abdominal disease. Occasionally, lymphomas may involve the marrow so children could present like a new leukemia patient. In taking the history, one should ask about the classic B-symptoms of HL including fevers, night sweats, and unexplained weight loss. If present, these will increase the stage of the patient's disease.
3. *Physical exam*: The exam should focus on all areas of potential adenopathy. Additional focus on respiratory and head and neck exams is warranted.
4. *Laboratory assessment/imaging (workup)*: Like a new leukemia patient the child with suspected lymphoma should have a CBC and a full chemistry panel to assess for tumor lysis. A PT/PTT should also be obtained. Imaging includes a CXR at the outset. Full staging will involve computerized tomography (CT) scans of the neck, chest, abdomen, and pelvis. Eventually, patients will also have a positron emission tomography (PET) scan looking for nodal areas with increased metabolic activity. Excisional biopsy is preferred over any type of needle biopsy for confirmation of the diagnosis.
5. *Key differential diagnosis*: Lymphadenopathy has a broad differential diagnosis. Lymphadenopathy is much more likely to be related to an infectious etiology than a malignancy. Other possibilities include autoimmune diseases and storage diseases. Lymph nodes less than 1 cm in size are rarely pathologic for malignancy.
6. *Management*: Treatment of HL consists of systemic chemotherapy with the potential to add localized radiation therapy in advanced stage disease. Patients with NHL are often treated more like ALL patients with systemic chemotherapy, including intrathecal therapy, but usually without radiation.

Neuroblastoma (NBL)

1. *Background*: NBL is the most common extracranial solid tumor in children. It arises from neural crest cells. As such it can manifest anywhere along the sympathetic chain of the nervous system though is most commonly seen involving the adrenal gland. It often metastasizes to the bone marrow. It is most commonly seen in the pre-school age range.
2. *History*: The NBL presentation will be dependent on the location of the primary tumor. In this way, they are similar to lymphomas and can present with symptoms of abdominal pain and fullness or mass effect causing airway compression and SVC syndrome. Paraspinal tumors can cause symptoms of spinal cord compression such as weakness, bowel/bladder dysfunction, or paralysis. Marrow involvement of NBL can present like a new leukemia patient with bony pain, refusal to walk or bear weight and symptoms of anemia or thrombocytopenia.
3. *Physical exam*: A focus on the abdominal exam is important in a suspected NBL patient. Other unique physical exam findings are the possibility of proptosis or Horner's syndrome (ptosis and miosis) in a tumor of the head and neck. NBL patients may also have a paraneoplastic syndrome called opsoclonus-myoclonus (rapid eye movements and involuntary muscular jerking movements). Lastly, they may have bluish skin nodules with infiltration of NBL cells.
4. *Laboratory assessment/imaging (workup)*: Initial basic labs consisting of a CBC and general chemistries should be obtained. Urine catecholamines (homovanillic acid and vanillylmandelic acid) are makers that may be elevated in NBL and should be sent before any tumor excision. Practically speaking in the emergency center, the first imaging study of an abdominal mass is likely to be an ultrasound. Following this, NBL patients will eventually have CT scans of the chest, abdomen and pelvis, and a meta-iodo-benzyl-guanidine (MIBG) scan for staging purposes. Bilateral bone marrow aspirates and biopsy are also indicated as part of the staging evaluation.
5. *Key differential diagnosis*: Given its common location in the abdomen NBL must be differentiated from Wilms tumor. Often the new NBL patient is described as the "sick" looking patient with an abdominal mass as opposed to patients with Wilms tumor who are often asymptomatic.
6. *Management*: The outcome of NBL can vary widely. Treatment can range from excision only all the way up to extensive chemotherapy regimens including monoclonal antibodies, high dose chemotherapy with autologous stem cell rescue, and radiation therapy including radioactive MIBG therapy.

Wilms Tumor (WT)

1. *Background*: WT is the second most common abdominal tumor in children and is a tumor intrinsic to the kidneys. It most commonly manifests as a unilateral renal mass but may occasionally present bilaterally. It is also primarily a tumor of pre-school age children. WT can be seen in patients with syndromes such as Beckwith–Wiedemann, isolated hemihypertrophy, and WAGR (Wilms tumor, Aniridia, Genitourinary malformations, and a Range of developmental delays).
2. *History*: WT frequently presents asymptomatically in pre-school children. It is often picked up incidentally on a routine well-child exam. Alternately, a parent or other relative may feel an abdominal mass when bathing a toddler.
3. *Physical exam*: The general exam of a patient with new WT is often only notable for the palpable abdominal mass. Palpation should be done gently to avoid breaking the renal capsule and spilling tumor cells into the abdomen. Because of its renal origin a blood pressure should be checked as hypertension is possible.
4. *Laboratory assessment/imaging (workup)*: In addition to routine bloodwork, a urinalysis should be checked for hematuria. As with NBL, the initial radiology imaging obtained is likely to be an abdominal ultrasound. Following this ultrasound, other studies will include a CT scan of chest, abdomen, and pelvis. A dedicated Doppler ultrasound of the kidney including the inferior vena cava (IVC) is important before surgery to look for tumor growth up into the IVC.
5. *Key differential diagnosis*: As previously noted the major differential diagnosis in a patient with an abdominal mass is NBL. Distinguishing between these two will require tumor biopsy or resection.
6. *Management*: Initial management is surgical. For a unilateral tumor, the entire kidney will be removed to avoid breaking the renal capsule and spilling tumor cells into the abdomen. Again, similar to NBL, if the tumor is small enough the patient may not need any further therapy. A larger tumor will require chemotherapy and potentially radiation therapy for metastatic disease.

Bone Tumors: Osteosarcoma (OS) and Ewing's Sarcoma (ES)

1. *Background*: The two most common bone tumors in children often present in the second decade of life.
2. *History*: Many bone tumors will present with nonspecific symptoms of pain or soreness in the area of the tumor. These symptoms are often mistaken for and managed as musculoskeletal injuries in a physically active adolescent. Thus, diagnosis can be delayed for months until a radiographic evaluation is eventually initiated. Patients with ES may also present with systemic symptoms such as fever, weight loss, and fatigue.
3. *Physical exam*: The exam is often unremarkable. One may see swelling or a mass over the affected tumor area but not always.

4. *Laboratory assessment/imaging (workup)*: General blood work is typically unrevealing. Plain radiographs of the symptomatic location are the initial imaging obtained. Following this, MRI of the affected location as well as chest CT and technetium whole body bone scan to look for metastatic disease are indicated. Both tumor types are diagnosed via needle biopsy. If a diagnosis of ES is determined, the patient will also need staging with bilateral bone marrow aspirates and biopsies.
5. *Key differential diagnosis*: The differential between OS and ES can often be determined based on tumor location. OS has a predilection for the distal ends of long bones with the distal femur being the most common location. ES is seen in the diaphysis of long bones and also in flat bones such as ribs, scapula, and pelvis. A minority of ES patients may also have tumor arising in the soft tissues around bones.
6. *Management*: Both diagnoses are treated with upfront chemotherapy followed by definitive resection of their tumor. The in vitro tumor response to chemotherapy determined at tumor resection is a major prognostic factor. Depending on the location of the primary tumor, a joint replacement or an amputation may be required. Following definitive tumor resection, the patient will receive subsequent chemotherapy as well. ES is radiation sensitive though radiation is typically reserved for tumors that are considered unresectable, such as extensive pelvic tumors.

Central Nervous System (CNS) Tumors

1. *Background*: Brain tumors as a group form the second largest number of cancers in children after leukemias. They are a heterogeneous mix of tumors, locations, and outcomes. Histologic types range from low-grade tumors such as juvenile pilocytic astrocytomas (JPA) to more aggressive lesions such as medulloblastomas or glioblastomas. Diffuse intrinsic pontine gliomas (DIPG) are a tumor in the brainstem with a dismal prognosis. Some centers include retinoblastoma in their CNS tumor treatment teams.
2. *History*: Given their varied locations, CNS tumors may present with a variety of symptoms. These can include headaches, seizures, clumsiness, nausea/vomiting, abnormal gait, and coordination. Headaches in particular with morning vomiting are a classic CNS tumor presentation. In infants, loss of developmental milestones should also raise concern for a CNS tumor.
3. *Physical exam*: A complete neurologic examination should be performed in any child suspected to have a CNS tumor. Increased intracranial pressure (ICP) can lead to the Cushing triad of bradycardia, hypertension, and abnormal respirations. In infants, enlarging head circumference warrants concern for a CNS tumor. Well-child visits in infancy and early childhood should always include evaluation for a red reflex in both eyes as a screen for retinoblastoma.

4. *Laboratory assessment/imaging (workup)*: Most patients presenting in an emergency center with symptoms concerning for a CNS tumor will undergo a CT scan of the head initially. Advantages for an initial CT scan include that it is less expensive, quicker and may be able to be completed without sedation even in young children. If the CT scan confirms the presence of a mass, the child will eventually need a more detailed MRI of the brain and spinal cord to look for drop metastases down the spine. Infants with leukocoria should be referred to ophthalmology for a sedated examination under anesthesia.
5. *Key differential diagnosis*: Since CNS tumors cause increased ICP other conditions on the differential diagnosis include things that also elevate intracranial pressure. These include other lesions causing hydrocephalus, or CNS bleeds.
6. *Management*: Patients with a CNS tumor will be managed by a team including oncology, neurosurgery, radiation oncology, and neurology. Complete excision of the mass is the goal but not always possible. Given their location in the brainstem, DIPGs cannot even be safely biopsied. Diagnosis of DIPG is usually made radiographically. Depending on the final pathology, treatment can range anywhere from monitoring only after complete excision (in the case of JPA) to various combinations of chemotherapy and/or radiotherapy. Medulloblastoma is the primary CNS tumor that can spread down the spinal column. For this reason, these patients' radiation will include spinal treatment in addition to radiation of the primary tumor. A newer radiation technology used for many brain tumors is proton radiation therapy. Proton therapy is a more targeted treatment with less damage to surrounding tissue than conventional radiation. Retinoblastoma treatment used to involve enucleation for all patients. More modern treatments with modalities such as laser or cryotherapy, and systemic or intravitreous chemotherapy have decreased the need for enucleation in many infants.

Oncologic Emergencies

Fever and Neutropenia

Cancer treatment often causes patients to be neutropenic (Absolute Neutrophil Count (ANC) of 1000 or less). The lower the ANC the higher the risk for serious bacterial infections. The resulting inability to fight infection makes any fever a medical emergency and a sign of a potentially life-threatening infection. Different institutions may have varied definitions of what they consider fever so check with your local hospital. Bacterial sources of infection are typically from the patient's own flora as opposed to being community acquired. The presence of a central line increases risk for Gram-positive skin organisms. Translocation of gut bacteria is possible leading to a wide spectrum of Gram-negative infections.

- *History*: The team should assess when the last chemotherapy was given and when fever began. Also ask about other symptoms like nausea, vomiting,

diarrhea, new rashes, pain, or swelling/redness/drainage anywhere. Inquire about recent travel or invasive procedures.
- *Physical exam*: A detailed physical should be performed to include assessing for signs of shock (tachycardia, hypotension, prolonged capillary refill, altered mental status). One should also assess for mucositis, look over the entire body for signs of redness, swelling or drainage, and assess the external peri-rectal region for the same. No internal rectal exam should be performed in a neutropenic patient. If a central venous catheter is in place look for redness, tenderness, or swelling at this site.
- *Diagnostic evaluation*: Minimum laboratory studies should include a CBC, chemistry panel to look at renal and hepatic function, and blood cultures from all central line lumens as well as a peripheral site. The patient with respiratory symptoms should have a CXR. Procedures that could disrupt a mucosal barrier like a catheterized urine collection are contraindicated.
- *Management*: Priority in initial management should address any signs of shock to include giving fluid boluses as indicated. The gold standard for initiation of empiric intravenous antibiotics is to have the first dose administered within 60 min of initial presentation. Institutions may have varied specific antibiotic policies so check with your hospital regarding initial empiric coverage. In general, all will begin with a third or fourth generation cephalosporin. If there are signs of shock, Gram-positive coverage may be broadened with the addition of vancomycin. And with any signs or symptoms of gastrointestinal compromise such as tenderness to abdominal palpation or peri-rectal pain anaerobic coverage with metronidazole may be indicated. Further definitive management will be determined by any positive cultures that arise. All patients with fever and moderate to severe neutropenia (ANC < 500) will typically be admitted for observation. Some institutions may have protocols that allow for outpatient management of febrile patients who have mild neutropenia (ANC 500–1000).

Tumor Lysis Syndrome (TLS)

TLS can be a life-threatening condition seen when cancer cells break down, either spontaneously or with the initiation of chemotherapy. The highest risk period is during the diagnostic process and initial days of treatment. Release of intracellular uric acid, potassium, and phosphorus can lead to elevated serum levels of all, as well as hypocalcemia. These derangements can lead to acute renal failure, cardiac arrhythmias, seizures, and potentially death. Patients most at risk are those with new leukemias and non-Hodgkin lymphoma. It is crucial to maintain a high index of suspicion in patients being evaluated for these cancers.

- *History*: There is no specific historical information to obtain.
- *Physical exam*: Part of assessing the overall risk for TLS is assessing potential tumor burden. The patient with hepatosplenomegaly or large lymphadenopathy will be at higher risk due to a larger tumor burden.

- *Diagnostic evaluation*: A higher peripheral white blood cell count also implies a higher tumor burden, and thus increased the risk of TLS. Close monitoring of uric acid, potassium, phosphorus, and calcium should occur, as well as watching creatinine for signs of kidney injury.
- *Management*: Maintain vigorous hydration to promote adequate urine output. Patients are often begun on 1.5 × maintenance rate with close monitoring of input/output. Prophylaxis with allopurinol can help to decrease uric acid production. If uric acid is markedly elevated, the use of rasburicase can rapidly decrease uric acid levels. Hyperkalemia is initially managed by prevention (no potassium in iv fluids) and then standard options such as the use of kayexalate, insulin, albuterol, or loop diuretics to promote excretion. Evaluate for arrhythmias in the hyperkalemic patient. Hyperphosphatemia is managed by increased hydration, dietary restrictions, and phosphate binders. In cases of severe electrolyte disturbances, dialysis may be needed.

Mediastinal Mass

Mediastinal masses may be seen in a variety of tumors. The differential diagnosis can vary with the location. Anterior mediastinal masses are more commonly seen with lymphomas and some leukemias (particularly T-cell ALL) while posterior mediastinal masses can be associated with solid tumors such as neuroblastoma and germ cell tumors. The primary concerns with mediastinal masses at diagnosis are the risk of airway compression and respiratory failure as well as cardiac dysfunction.

- *History*: Areas on which to focus include signs of respiratory compromise such as orthopnea, cough, shortness of breath, or wheezing.
- *Physical exam*: Auscultate for decreased breath sounds or wheezing. Focus on the neck for signs of superior vena cava syndrome such as neck swelling or venous engorgement. Look for other palpable lymphadenopathy that could be a target for biopsy.
- *Diagnostic evaluation*: A plain chest radiograph should be performed in all suspected leukemia or lymphoma patients as a starting point. If a mass is seen, then further imaging with computerized tomography (CT) scans of the neck and chest are warranted. Mediastinal masses should also prompt concern for tumor lysis syndrome with evaluation and management as previously described.
- *Management*: Initial management includes an index of suspicion for respiratory decompensation. The patient may not be able to lie fully flat in either their hospital bed or for scans. If airway compromise is a concern, observation in a critical care unit may be necessary. In patients with respiratory failure intubation will not be helpful as the mass will be below the level of the endotracheal tube and extracorporeal membrane oxygenation (ECMO) may be needed. A multidisciplinary approach to obtaining tissue through a biopsy is crucial. This will include discus-

sion with anesthesia, surgery, and interventional radiology to determine the safest anatomic location for a biopsy. It may be inadvisable to fully sedate the patient and a peripheral biopsy may be performed with local anesthesia if a lymph node group is available. Definitive treatment requires tissue diagnosis. In the case of respiratory failure though emergent treatment may have to begin before confirmation with therapy directed at the most likely diagnosis based on anatomic location. This could include potentially chemotherapy or radiation therapy. Avoid giving steroids without the involvement of an oncologist. Administration of steroids can kill tumor cells making diagnosis challenging and leading to tumor lysis syndrome.

Spinal Cord Compression (SCC)

SCC can manifest either at initial tumor presentation or as a component of relapse. It is an emergency due to risks of long-term paralysis, sensory loss, or dysfunction of continence. Many tumor types can cause SCC including neuroblastoma, Ewing sarcoma, other sarcomas, or metastatic central nervous system tumors.

- *History*: Symptoms may include weakness and motor deficits, back pain, sensory abnormalities and sphincter deficits. If the lesion is high enough, respiratory distress may be seen due to paralysis of the diaphragm.
- *Physical exam*: A thorough neurologic exam should be performed on anyone with SCC symptoms.
- *Diagnostic evaluation*: While plain radiographs may be the initial imaging performed, they may be falsely reassuring. Definitive evaluation for SCC should include MRI of the entire spine.
- *Management*: Definitive treatment will depend on the pathologic diagnosis. Initial management is often with emergent intravenous dexamethasone. This is not geared toward treating the tumor but rather decreasing edema around the mass. Steroids should not be given without discussing with oncology. Following this, definitive management will require a multidisciplinary team discussion including oncology, neurology, neurosurgery, and radiation oncology. Treatment options include laminectomy for decompression and tissue diagnosis, chemotherapy based on the presumed tumor type and emergent radiation therapy. All options have pros and cons that must be weighed by the team.

Supportive Care

Improved outcomes for pediatric cancer patients over the years have come from advances in supportive care as much as therapeutic regimens. Recognition and early management of oncologic emergencies is crucial. Other items to be aware of include:

1. Transfusion support. Pediatric cancer patients frequently need blood products as a result of either their disease itself or chemotherapy-induced cytopenias. Individual institutions will have standardized thresholds for transfusion of red cells and platelets. Platelet counts will likely need to be higher on days of surgical procedures. Blood products are irradiated to prevent graft versus host disease in immunocompromised individuals.
2. Infection prevention. The most common infectious prophylaxis in cancer patients is to prevent *Pneumocystis jirovecii.* Regimens can include the use of trimethoprim-sulfamethoxazole or pentamidine. Certain high-risk patients may also receive prophylaxis for other bacterial, fungal, or viral infections throughout their treatment.
3. Nutrition. Children undergoing cancer therapy are at high risk for malnutrition so monitoring nutritional status is crucial. Dieticians can help work with patients and families to offer various enteral supplements though there will be times when patients will not be able to tolerate any oral intake. In these situations, parenteral nutrition may be employed. For some head and neck cancers when prolonged interruptions in oral intake are anticipated, a gastrostomy tube may be placed to minimize the need for parenteral nutrition.
4. Fertility preservation. Chemotherapy and radiation therapy may impair future fertility at any treatment age. Research is ongoing into methods of fertility preservation for varied ages. Methods can include sperm banking as well as cryopreservation of ovarian or testicular tissue. It is crucial to discuss fertility risks at the outset of treatment for any age patient.

Psychosocial Care

Cancer is a devastating diagnosis to give any child and family. Patients and families lose all sense of normalcy and independence once a diagnosis is made. Because of this children's oncology centers place great emphasis on supporting the patient and entire family throughout treatment (which may last years) and beyond. No treatment team is complete without social workers and child life experts who provide invaluable support. These specialists can help families access supportive networks and financial assistance. They assist with return to school strategies. And they can help to involve patients with peer support groups and specialized camps designed to allow patients to experience activities similar to their peers in a safe environment designed for their needs. Medical students can learn a great deal from the psychosocial team. If their schedules allow, volunteering at a residential camp as a cabin counselor can be a tremendous learning opportunity as well. Seeing patients with significant medical needs outside the hospital can give students a great appreciation for what patients and families go through on a daily basis at home. Interacting with patients at camp also allows the student to realize that cancer is a disease which can be managed and overcome despite the many hurdles placed in the path of patients.

Survivorship

Cancer survivors are at risk for any number of long-term complications from their diseases and treatment. Because of this they will need regular education regarding these risks and monitoring for the rest of their lives. Late complications can be seen in any organ system so detailed follow-up with a practitioner aware of oncology complications is important. Adult habits like smoking, use of alcohol or other drugs and poor exercise routines can exacerbate end organ dysfunction. Psychosocial late effects can include challenges with depression, securing insurance coverage and employment, maintaining relationships and even the ability to live independently. While not an exhaustive list, late effects of note by disease can include:

1. Leukemias: Neurocognitive and developmental difficulties from intrathecal chemotherapy. Osteonecrosis due to frequent steroid chemotherapy for ALL. Cardiac dysfunction from anthracycline chemotherapy. Obesity, metabolic syndrome, secondary malignancies, and growth disturbances.
2. Lymphomas: Infertility and gonadal failure from cyclophosphamide. Secondary malignancies either from chemotherapy or in the radiation field if they received radiation. Infection due to chemotherapy that targeted B-cells. Cardiac dysfunction from anthracyclines. Pulmonary fibrosis from bleomycin.
3. Neuroblastoma: Infertility, secondary malignancies, cardiac dysfunction, hearing loss, pulmonary dysfunction, endocrinopathies.
4. Wilms tumor: Maintaining and monitoring the health of the remaining kidney is crucial. Secondary malignancies in a radiation field.
5. Bone tumors: Cardiac dysfunction. Hearing loss from cisplatin chemotherapy. Secondary malignancies in the radiation field if a patient with ES receives this treatment. If a prosthesis has been placed, this hardware can become loose or infected over time. And patients may have functional limitations related to their tumor location or prosthesis.
6. CNS tumors: These survivors have high risks of neurocognitive difficulties, and the psychosocial challenges listed above. They are more likely to have been treated with radiation and thus carry a risk of a secondary malignancy. Also due to their radiation they may have endocrine dysfunctions from pituitary damage.

Summary

Caring for pediatric oncology patients and their families can be very rewarding. Treatment requires meticulous attention to the patient and entire family. Patients may experience complications in any organ system so students will be exposed to them on every subspecialty on which they rotate. And finally, cancer in children is not a death sentence but rather a complex condition that requires a multidisciplinary team approach to ensure the best possible outcomes. Long-term follow-up of survivors is crucial.

Application Exercises

1. Pediatric Oncology Tumors Matching Test

A. Leukemias	1. Usually present with nonspecific pain/soreness in local area
B. Lymphoma	2. Second most common cancer in childhood
C. Neuroblastoma	3. Most common childhood cancer
D. Wilms Tumor	4. Elevated levels of catecholamines
E. Bone Tumors	5. Usually present with non-tender adenopathy
F. CNS Tumors	6. Arise only in the kidneys

Answers: A. 3; B. 5; C. 4; D. 6; E. 1; F. 2

2. Tumor Lysis Syndrome can be seen with some forms of lymphoma (and high white count leukemias). The characteristic lab abnormalities of TLS include all except:

   A. Elevated myoglobin
   B. Elevated phosphorus
   C. Elevated potassium
   D. Elevated uric acid

   Answer A: Elevations in potassium, phosphorous, and uric acid are common in TLS. There may also be elevations of creatinine and BUN. Myoglobin is not characteristic since TLS is a not a primary muscle disorder.

3. The gold standard for management of the child with shock and neutropenia is

   A. Empirical antibiotics started within 60 min of initial presentation
   B. Gastrointestinal decompression
   C. Provision of granulocyte-stimulating factor
   D. Rapid administration of WBC infusions

   Answer A: It is standard for rapid administration of empiric antibiotics once a child with shock and neutropenia. While gastrointestinal decompression may be required for severe ileus, this is avoided as much as possible to minimize irritation of the gastrointestinal tract. Granulocyte- stimulating factor may be used in children with neutropenia, but it is not part of acute management of neutropenia. WBC infusions are not an effective treatment of neutropenia.

Further Reading

Allen-Rhoades W, Whittle S, Rainusso N. Pediatric solid tumors in children and adolescents: an overview. Pediatr Rev. 2018a;39:444–52.

Allen-Rhoades W, Whittle S, Rainusso N. Pediatric solid tumors of infancy: an overview. Pediatr Rev. 2018b;39:57–67.

Buhtolarov I. Pediatric lymphoma. Pediatr Rev. 2017;38:410–23.

Kaplan J. Leukemia in children. Pediatr Rev. 2019;40:319–31.

Pehlivan K, Paul M, Crawford J. Central nervous system tumors in children. Pediatr Rev. 2022;43:3–15.

Chapter 30
Murmurs

Kaitlin L'Italien

Background

Our goal in this chapter is to give you the contextual knowledge regarding pediatric murmurs so that when you hear them for the first time, you can recognize the sounds and understand their significance. Before beginning, it is important to stress the fact that reading a chapter about murmurs is akin to reading a chapter about Beethoven's Symphony No. 5; we will describe the components, the background and the sounds, but nothing replaces the learning that takes place from listening to the murmur. This chapter will enrich your understanding, but you need to listen to learn. Thankfully, there are many free resources that are available with just a quick Google search. A few particularly great resources to practice listening to heart murmurs are through the University of Michigan, University of Washington, and Johns Hopkins' Murmur Quiz. We highly recommend using these resources to deepen your understanding.

If you are feeling insecure about your listening skills, you are not alone. Multiple academic studies have shown that physicians only become good at identifying heart murmurs through practice. While studies have shown at baseline most physicians are not very good at identifying murmurs, it has also been shown that with dedicated practice, people can make significant improvements. Barrett et al. showed accuracy improved from 13.5% to 85% among medical students who listened to 500 repetitions of 4 common murmurs. Finley et al. showed accuracy in diagnosis of murmurs improved from 75% to 95% after just a 1 h dedicated lesson.

One of the most important skills a pediatrician can develop is the ability to accurately distinguish innocent versus pathologic pediatric murmurs. While much

K. L'Italien (✉)
Department of Pediatrics, Nationwide Children's Hospital/The Ohio State University College of Medicine, Columbus, OH, USA
e-mail: kaitlin.litalien@nationwidechildrens.org

N. Liao et al. (eds.), *Pediatric Rotations*,
https://doi.org/10.1007/978-3-031-59873-9_30

education focuses on identifying specific pathologic murmurs, it is not actually a helpful way to grow confidence in murmur identification. Why? Despite the fact that 1% of babies born will be affected by congenital heart disease, given the increasing likelihood of prenatal referral and diagnoses, and the role of the pulse oximetry screening, pediatric providers are far more likely to hear an innocent murmur for the first time compared to a pathologic murmur. Innocent murmurs are very common (80% of children will have an innocent murmur at some point in their life), and it is more useful to focus on the innocent murmurs as these will be heard time and time again. If you can reliably recognize the four most common innocent murmurs of childhood, you are in very good shape.

While this chapter's focus is on interpretation of pediatric murmurs, this involves more than just auscultation. Determining how concerned you are about a murmur involves synthesizing elements from the history as well as the complete cardiac exam, as described next.

History

The critical elements of a pediatric cardiac history vary by age, as we are typically worried about different cardiac pathology in neonates versus older children and teens. In neonates, we are most concerned about identifying critical congenital heart disease. History should include a detailed review of prenatal concerns as well as any perinatal complications. After birth, questions related to feeding, energy, work of breathing, as well as growth are very important. At older ages, the most significant elements of the history will focus upon cardiac symptoms—chest pain, syncope, pre-syncope, palpitations, dyspnea, and especially those symptoms that are worse with exercise.

The Pediatric Cardiac Exam

The cardiac examination includes *observation*, *palpation*, and *auscultation*. While we present them as separate assessments, an experienced provider usually develops their own routine which assesses the visual, tactile, and listening components of the exam at the same time.

Observation

Begin your assessment of your patient by simply *observing the patient at rest*. Does the child show any signs of distress? Is she/he ill appearing? Does she/he appear well nourished? Small or large for stated age? This is where you start to get a sense for whether this is a generally healthy, or potentially unwell child.

Next look at the *facial features* and *overall impression* of the child. Are there any signs of a syndrome? Many genetic syndromes have characteristic congenital heart disease associated with them. It is worth spending some time being able to recognize the physical features of Down, Turner, Noonan, Williams, Alagille, 22q11 deletion syndrome, as well as the common types of congenital heart disease seen in each syndrome.

Next assess *work of breathing*. It is important to minimize stressors to the patient during this assessment, as a toddler who is having a tantrum or starting to get nervous will have a reactive type elevated work of breathing. Often it is helpful to assess work of breathing for an infant or toddler who is being held comfortably in their caregiver's arms. Ask the parent to assist in removing the clothes/blanket from the child just enough to reveal their chest and abdomen. From here you will be able to assess respiratory rate, and effort of breathing. Look for retractions-subcostal, intercostal, suprasternal. Also look for signs of nasal flaring or grunting respirations. While respiratory viruses in infants can often cause increased work of breathing, in a child without signs of an infection an increased rate and effort of breathing may be a sign of congenital heart lesion causing excessive blood flow to the lungs. This abnormal distribution can be seen in left to right shunting lesions, like ventricular septal defects (VSD), large atrial septal defects (ASD), atrioventricular septal defects (AVSD), patent ductus arteriosus (PDA), or more complex congenital heart disease lesions resulting in a greater proportion of blood flow to the lungs versus the body.

Next, observe for any *signs of cyanosis*. Before we get into where and how to assess, let's take a moment clarify a few things about cyanosis. Cyanosis is defined as a bluish discoloration of the skin and/or mucous membranes. Cyanosis usually becomes apparent with the amount of deoxyhemoglobin is in the range of 3–5gm/dL, which roughly equates to an O_2 saturation of around 85%. The more deoxyhemoglobin, the lower the O_2 saturations, the deeper, and more obvious the cyanosis.

Cyanosis can be described as central or peripheral. *Central cyanosis*—evident everywhere on the body—is due to either a heart or a lung problem. One of the best places to assess central cyanosis is on the oral mucosa—the tongue and gingival tissues. *Peripheral cyanosis* is due to decreased blood flow to a particular part of the body leading to increased O_2 uptake from the tissues and increasing the amount of deoxyhemoglobin leading to the bluish appearance in the extremities and/or periorally. This is most commonly due to peripheral vasoconstriction secondary to cold temperatures, dehydration, or stress, but it also can be due to poor peripheral perfusion due to shock.

For cyanosis, it is important to identify where it is located on the body. Most newborns will have signs of acrocyanosis, or peripheral cyanosis of the hands or feet. This is usually not a worrisome sign. Go ahead and look at the fingers and toes, are there any signs of digital clubbing? Digital clubbing is a result of long-standing hypoxemia and is characterized by a bulbous enlargement of the distal phalanx leading to an increase in the anteroposterior and lateral diameter of the nails.

If you have a child in no distress with no significant increased work of breathing, but who is cyanotic and desaturated, this is more suggestive of a cardiac etiology of the cyanosis as opposed to pulmonary; children with a respiratory etiology of hypoxia typically present with more work of breathing than if there is a cardiac reason for the hypoxia.

An experienced pediatrician can usually assess each of these things within a few moments of observing the patient. For students/trainees, it's OK to take your time and really look for the presence or absence of each of these things. These are all part of a thorough pediatric cardiac exam and should be reported as pertinent positive and negative findings.

Palpation

Begin by placing your hand with your thumb parallel to the left sternal border. Here you will be able to appreciate any increased or hyperdynamic precordial motion. If you rotate your hand to be perpendicular to the sternal border, the heel of your hand should be touching the left sternal border and your fingers should now extend over the point of maximal impulse (PMI) of the left ventricle. Make a note whether the PMI is displaced or where expected. If the heel of your hand is lifted with each beat this indicates a right ventricular heave or lift and can be a sign of an increased pressure or volume load on the right ventricle.

Detection of *arterial pulses* is next. For infants, it is wise to palpate brachial and femoral pulses. Appropriate assessment of femoral pulses can take practice but is worth doing as part of every infant exam. Only if you get a sense of what is a "normal" femoral pulse would you be confident in picking up *reduced or delayed femoral pulses which is an important sign of a coarctation of the aorta.* In older children and teens, it is appropriate to palpate radial and either dorsalis pedis or posterior tibialis pulses. Again, do this on every patient so that you get a sense of normal timing versus a delay, which again, can indicate a missed coarctation of the aorta. *Bounding pulses* are seen in conditions in which the arterial upstroke is increased and then abruptly decreases, like *patent ductus arteriosus or significant aortic insufficiency*. While palpating pulses, it is reasonable to assess for any lower extremity edema; however, it should be noted that lower extremity edema due to cardiac dysfunction is extremely rare in children.

It is extremely important to *palpate the liver and spleen* in all patients. Assessing for where the liver is relative to the costal margin can give important information regarding hepatic congestion due to heart failure and/or elevated right heart pressures. It is important to note that heart failure in infants and children is often subtle and does not typically present with fluid retention in the extremities as in adults. Most often heart failure in children is picked up by an astute provider finding hepatosplenomegaly in a patient with otherwise vague and non-specific findings.

Auscultation

General

The auscultation portion of the exam is not just about listening for murmurs, but rather should be a systematic assessment of the heart sounds. *Evaluate the first and second heart sounds, then listen for additional sounds during systole, followed by listening for any diastolic sounds.*

It is reasonable to *listen in the four primary auscultation locations:*

- **Aortic area** at the right upper sternal border in the 2nd intercostal space
- **Pulmonic area** at the left upper sternal border in the 2nd intercostal space
- **Tricuspid area** at the left lower sternal border at the 4th intercostal space
- **Mitral are**a along the left mid-clavicular line at the 5th intercostal space

However, most cardiologists listen in many more places than the traditional four auscultation sites when listening to children. Unlike heart disease in adults, in which most start with normal heart structure and function, but then develop valvar or coronary issues over time, heart disease in kids is much more varied. Often it is advisable to *listen in multiple places along the left sternal border, the axillae and back.* It is also advisable to listen to both while the patient is supine as well as sitting and/or standing. Additionally, in small babies and kids, pathologic sounds may be heard in multiple areas, and attention to where it is loudest or most prominent can help to determine the etiology.

It is useful to begin the auscultation exam by listening at the left sternal border and to get a *baseline assessment of rate and rhythm.* Many children have a prominent "sinus arrhythmia," which is a reflex causing a slight increase in heart rate in inspiration and decrease in heart rate during expiration. Take care to distinguish this respiratory variation in heart rate from other types of rhythm abnormalities, like premature ventricular contractions.

S1 and S2

At the beginning of systole, we hear the closure of the mitral and tricuspid valves and this *first heart sound* is often called "S1". *The second heart sound*, comprised of the closure of the aortic and pulmonic valves, gives us "S2". S2 is actually comprised of two separate components, with the *aortic valve (A2)* closing slightly faster than the *pulmonary valve (P2)*. The splitting of this second sound is more prominent during inspiration, as it takes a little longer for the pulmonary valve to close. The slight delay in pulmonary valve closure is thought to be due to a combination of more blood filling the right ventricle in inspiration, leading to a slightly longer ejection time, as well as the lower pressure within the pulmonary artery and able to accommodate more blood prior to the pressure increasing above the threshold for valve closure. A2 is louder than P2, and often P2 can only really be heard well at the pulmonic area. Because kids' heart rates are generally much faster than adults, it can sometimes be hard for trainees to appreciate the splitting of S2. Additionally, there are particular types of congenital heart disease in which S2 does not demonstrate physiologic splitting. This can be heard in certain types of single ventricle congenital heart disease due to absence of either the aortic or pulmonary valves, or in transposition of the great arteries (TGA) due to altered position in the chest of the great vessels. If S2 is fixed and/or widely split it can be a sign of an atrial septal defect, even in the absence of a notable flow murmur.

S3 and S4

A *third heart sound (S3)* may be heard in early diastole at the end of the rapid filling of the ventricle. Some healthy kids and adolescents may have an S3. In the absence of any other signs or symptoms of cardiac disease, this can be considered a normal variant and would be called a "physiologic S3". The *fourth heart sound (S4)* may be heard in late diastole, just prior to S1. It is caused by the atrial contraction sending blood into a stiff or non-compliant ventricle. This can happen with systemic hypertension, cardiomyopathy, among others.

Murmurs

Murmurs are often described using the following five characteristics:

1. Intensity
2. Pitch (or frequency)
3. Timing
4. Location
5. Effect of position change

Qualitative words are also commonly linked to particular types of murmurs (like "musical," "blowing," "harsh," "vibratory"). Though many cardiologists do not like the use of qualitative descriptors, as they can mean different things to different people, they are commonly used both in clinical practice as well as on written assessments.

Intensity

The intensity or "loudness" of a systolic murmur is commonly conveyed by using the Levine Scale of murmur intensity.

- Grade 1: murmur softer than the heart sounds
- Grade 2: murmur about as loud as the heart sounds
- Grade 3: murmur louder than the heart sounds
- Grade 4: murmur louder than the heart sounds and associated with a palpable thrill
- Grade 5: very loud murmur heard with stethoscope barely touching chest
- Grade 6: murmur heard even without the stethoscope on the chest

Diastolic murmurs are sometimes graded on the same scale, but others use a scale of 1-4/4. Generally innocent murmurs tend to be softer, usually 1–2/6, rarely 3/6 and never associated with a thrill. Given that thrills are vibratory, they are actually best appreciated with the less-sensitive parts of the hand (i.e., not fingertips). Bases of fingers are the preferred way to palpate a thrill.

Pitch

The pitch of a murmur may be described as low-, medium-, or high-pitched sound. In general, innocent murmurs tend to be lower pitched, while pathologic murmurs are more commonly high pitched.

Timing

The timing of the murmur usually involves identifying when in the cardiac cycle the murmur is heard: *systolic, diastolic,* or *continuous*. A general rule of thumb is that all murmurs heard in diastole are pathologic (a venous hum is the rare exception). Most innocent murmurs, as well as the most common pathologic murmurs of childhood, are systolic.

Systolic Murmurs

Systolic murmurs are typically described as either holosystolic/S1 coincident murmur, or ejection/crescendo-decrescendo murmur. Classically, the murmur of a VSD or mitral regurgitation has been described as a holosystolic murmur. However, this is sometimes confusing for learners as the murmur may not always last through all of systole. But what is implied by the term holosystolic is that the murmur starts immediately upon onset of systole. In other words, a way to think about a holosystolic murmur or S1 coincident murmur is that we cannot hear S1 as a distinct sound before the onset of the murmur. The murmur starts with S1 and indicates either mitral or tricuspid regurgitation, or a ventricular septal defect.

Ejection or crescendo-decrescendo murmurs begin after S1, and we can usually hear the first heart sound separately, then the murmur begins shortly thereafter and gets louder then softer prior to hearing S2. In pediatrics, these murmurs most commonly occur due to narrowing of either semilunar (aortic or pulmonary) valves. Ejection murmurs that are benign can display this pattern; especially in the neonatal period, significant aortic or pulmonary valve stenosis may also display this pattern. Semilunar valve stenosis can progress rapidly in the first few weeks of life and what is thought to be mild narrowing can progress rapidly, depending upon the substrate.

Diastolic Murmurs

Diastolic murmurs are very rare in pediatrics and difficult to hear for an untrained ear given the higher heart rate in children and short diastolic period. Native aortic valve or pulmonary valve regurgitation that is significant enough to be able to hear it (at least moderate or above) is very rare. Most diastolic murmurs heard in a pediatric population are due to prior cardiac intervention, such as a transannular patch repair of tetralogy of Fallot (TOF) or aortic or pulmonary balloon valvuloplasty, in which the patient has been left with significant semilunar valve regurgitation.

Continuous Murmurs

A continuous murmur is one that is heard in both systole and diastole. The most common continuous murmur is the murmur of the patent ductus arteriosus (PDA). This is the sound of the blood moving through the residual PDA and flowing from the aorta to the main pulmonary artery. It is commonly described as a "machine-like" murmur. While a PDA murmur can be a normal transitional murmur in a neonate within the first 1–3 days of life, a PDA murmur that persists into infancy indicates that the ductus did not close and should be evaluated by a pediatric cardiologist.

Location

The location at which a murmur can best be heard is typically noted, as well as whether the murmur radiates to any location. Radiation typically refers to the sound heard along the line that the blood flows. Classically, aortic stenosis will radiate to the neck, and peripheral pulmonary stenosis to the axillae.

Effect of Position Changes

Determining in which position a murmur is best heard can be helpful in distinguishing pathologic from benign. Most innocent murmurs are best heard in the supine position. Pathologic murmurs can usually be heard well in any position. The murmur of hypertrophic obstructive cardiomyopathy is louder when standing.

Innocent Murmurs

There are four very common innocent murmurs of childhood; *Still's murmur, peripheral pulmonary branch stenosis (PPBS or PPS) murmur, venous hum, and functional flow murmur.* See Fig. 30.1 for locations of these murmurs. Some sources will report an arterial supraclavicular murmur and a mammary soufflé as innocent murmurs of childhood, and while reasonable to know that these murmurs exist, they are relatively uncommon. If time and care is taken to develop skill in identifying, the four most common innocent murmurs of childhood, you will have a good foundation to be able to tell the difference between a murmur that needs further workup and evaluation by a cardiologist, versus one that is benign.

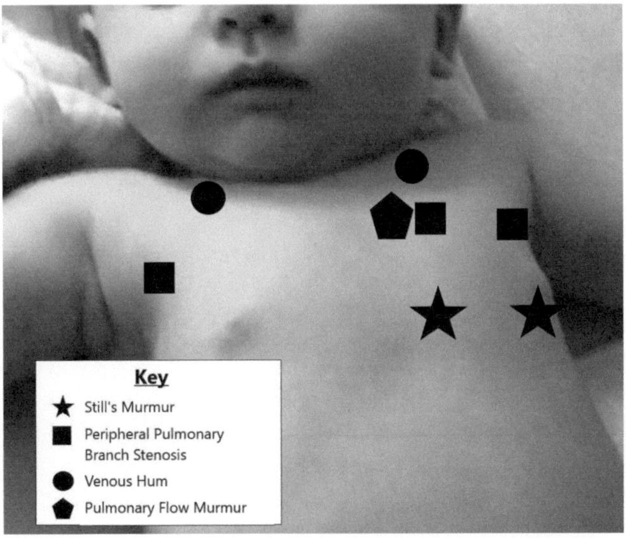

Fig. 30.1 Auscultation sites of the four common innocent murmurs of childhood

Still's Murmur

Still's murmur is the most common, and the most easily recognizable and reassuring of the pediatric murmurs. A Still's murmur is classically heard in kids between 2 and 6 years of age (though can be heard in newborns through teens) and is described as "vibratory," or "musical." To many individuals, a Still's murmur resembles the sound of plucking an upright bass (instrument)—low pitched and almost more a vibration than sound. While there is no single consensus on the etiology of a Still's murmur, there have been studies which have demonstrated a few anatomic and physiologic situations in which a Still's murmur can be heard. A Still's murmur has been shown to be associated with patients with mitral valve chordae that cross the left ventricular outflow tract. A Still's murmur has also been shown to be more common in patients with increased contractility of the left ventricle and reduced elasticity of the aorta as well as can be elicited in a structurally normal heart after administration of dobutamine. Importantly, there is no pathology related to the Still's murmur, nor any association with any long-term cardiac issues.

Still's Murmur Fast Facts

Age of patient	2–6 years old most common, neonate to teen possible
Location	Left lower sternal border, or apex (see Fig. 30.1)
Timing	Mid-systolic
Intensity	1–3/6
Quality	Vibratory, musical
Modifiers	Louder with increased cardiac output
Differential diagnosis	VSD, left ventricular outflow tract obstruction

Peripheral Pulmonary Branch Stenosis Murmur

The murmur of peripheral pulmonary branch stenosis (PPS) occurs due to the abrupt increase in the amount of blood moving through the branch pulmonary artery as the baby transitions from fetal circulation to post-natal life. In utero, most of the blood that passes through the right side of the heart moves from the main pulmonary artery through the ductus arteriosus and out to the aorta. Less than 10% of the right ventricle output goes through the branch pulmonary arteries in fetal circulation. And as we like to say in pediatric cardiology—no flow, no grow. So, when the ductus arteriosus closes shortly after birth, the relatively small branch pulmonary arteries are now responsible for carrying much more volume than before, and we can hear a murmur corresponding to the flow of blood through these relatively small vessels. They will grow and by 6 months of age we should no longer be able to hear a PPS murmur.

PPS Murmur Fast Facts

Age of patient	Infant up to 6 months old
Location	Left upper sternal border with radiation to axillae (see Fig. 30.1)
Timing	Mid-systole
Intensity	Soft, usually 1–2/6
Quality	Ejection, "whoosh"
Modifiers	Increases with increased cardiac output
Differential diagnosis	Pulmonary valve stenosis, ASD, left or right pulmonary artery stenosis, coarctation

Venous Hum

The venous hum murmur is the main exception to the rule that all murmurs heard in diastole are pathologic. The venous hum is a common innocent childhood murmur that can be heard in systole and diastole (continuous murmur). It is caused by turbulence of the blood returning to the heart from the head and neck vessels. And unlike most other childhood murmurs, this murmur can only be heard while sitting up and disappears when laying supine or turning head in the direction of the vessels causing the murmur. Even though venous hums are very common, many people have not heard one due to the fact that they may not listen in the correct location to hear it. In fact, when you try to hear one, you can almost always hear one on every patient between the ages of 3 and 8 years old. The venous hum is best heard in the right or left mid-clavicular region, while sitting or standing, and disappears when supine.

Venous Hum Fast Facts

Age of patient	3–8 years old
Location	Infraclavicular (see Fig. 30.1)
Timing	Continuous
Intensity	1–3/6
Quality	Low pitched, rumble
Modifiers	Disappears when supine, turning towards the murmur or jugular compression
Differential diagnosis	Pulmonary arteriovenous malformation, patent ductus arteriosus

Pulmonary Flow Murmur

Given the pulmonary valve is the closest to the chest wall, in certain conditions we are able to hear the sound of the blood passing through a normal valve. This murmur is more commonly heard in people with thin chest walls, and/or in certain conditions which increase the turbulence of the blood passing through the valve, like anemia (less viscous blood = more turbulent flow), or increased cardiac output in the setting of illness, fever, stress, etc. It should be noted that if a pulmonary flow murmur is heard across multiple visits and the patient is not ill or anemic, a congenital heart lesion that increases pulmonary blood flow (like an atrial septal defect) or a mild pulmonary valve stenosis should be ruled out.

Pulmonary Flow Murmur Fast Facts

Age of patient	Any age, but common in teens
Location	Left upper sternal border (see Fig. 30.1)
Timing	Systolic
Intensity	1–3/6
Quality	Ejection
Modifiers	Increased with increased cardiac output
Differential diagnosis	Pulmonary stenosis, atrial septal defect

Pathologic Murmurs

In general, there are some red flags that can help determine if a murmur is due to a structural heart problem. We will review some features that are commonly associated with pathologic murmurs, and then spend some time discussing the most common congenital heart disease lesions and the murmurs associated with the conditions.

Murmur Red Flags

- Holosystolic/S1 coincident
- Diastolic murmurs
- Grade 3/6 or higher
- Harsh in quality
- Associated with abnormal heart sounds (split S2, systolic click, etc.)
- Associated with other clinical concerns (i.e., failure to thrive, cyanosis, increased work of breathing, etc.)
- Louder when standing

Ventricular Septal Defect

VSDs are the most common type of congenital heart disease. Classically, a VSD murmur is described as a harsh, holosystolic/S1 coincident murmur heard loudest at the left lower sternal border. A VSD murmur can vary in intensity but is usually at least 2/6 and often louder. VSD murmurs may be difficult to hear immediately after birth as the pulmonary vascular resistance (PVR) has not yet fallen. When the PVR is high, the pressures within the right ventricle remain high, and there may not be much of a pressure gradient to cause flow from the left to right ventricle across the VSD. However, as the PVR falls over the first few days and weeks of life, more flow will go across the VSD and the murmur will become more obvious.

Atrial Septal Defect

The murmur of an atrial septal defect is a bit tricky because the intensity of a murmur usually depends upon the pressure difference across the defect. Because there is usually very little difference in pressure between the left and right atrium, we don't actually hear the sound of the blood moving across the ASD. Instead, we hear the sound of the extra blood that has moved from the left to right side of the heart through the ASD as the blood passes through the pulmonary valve. This often creates a pulmonary flow murmur. Because the right ventricle is pumping extra blood, it takes longer to leave the heart and creates a delay in the pulmonary component of S2. This causes a prominently split and sometimes "fixed split" S2. A classic description of an ASD would be a 2/6 ejection murmur at the left upper sternal border with a fixed split S2.

Patent Ductus Arteriosus

The murmur of a PDA is a continuous murmur best heard at the left upper sternal border and left infraclavicular region. It is often described as a "machine-like" murmur, and it almost sounds like pistons moving to and fro (Think of the sound of a train starting up). While it too varies in intensity, it is usually 2/6 or louder.

Pulmonic Stenosis

The murmur of pulmonary stenosis is typically described as a harsh ejection murmur heard best at the left upper sternal border, with radiation to the back. The intensity depends both upon the degree of narrowing, as well as the distal pressures (the

PVR), but is usually 2/6 or louder. More severe narrowing generally causes a high-grade murmur. Elevated PVR can make a pulmonary stenosis murmur not as loud as it otherwise would be, because the sound intensity depends upon the pressure difference across the defect. Elevated PVR means not as much of a pressure difference compared to the right ventricle, and therefore not as loud of a sound.

Aortic Stenosis

The murmur of aortic valve stenosis is typically described as a harsh ejection murmur heard best at the right upper sternal border with radiation to the neck. Again, the intensity depends upon the degree of narrowing, generally with louder murmurs associated with worse narrowing. It should be noted though in critical valve stenosis, when there is little if any blood flow across the valve, the murmur may be very hard to be heard due to so little volume moving across the defect. Often a valve click can also be heard in early systole.

Application Exercises

1. Case 1

   Term female born to G2P2 Mom presents for 1-month well-child exam. Birth weight was 3.5 kg, and there were no perinatal complications. Breast feeding was not going well, so Mom is supplementing with formula. She has no concerns.

   Vitals signs:

   Weight: 3.9 kg, Temp: 37.6°C, Pulse: 135, Respiratory Rate: 40, Blood Pressure: 85/53, SpO_2: 99% on room air

   Exam:

   General: no acute distress, no cyanosis, non-syndromic

   HEENT: moist mucous membranes, fontanelle soft

   Resp: normal respiratory effort, with symmetric aeration and no crackles/wheezes

   CV: Normal rate and rhythm. Normal point of maximum impulse (PMI). Soft, 1–2/6 systolic ejection murmur at left upper sternal border (LUSB) with radiation to bilateral axillae, normal brachial/femoral pulses, capillary refill 3 sec

   Abd: Soft, non-tender non-distended. No hepatosplenomegaly.

   Which of the following demonstrates the next best step in management of this condition?

   A. Outpatient referral to a Pediatric Cardiologist
   B. Obtain chest X-ray and EKG
   C. Reassure family and follow-up to ensure it resolves by 6 months of age
   D. Direct patient to ER for urgent workup

   Answer: C

   A. Incorrect. The clinical vignette is describing the murmur of PPS, and in the absence of any other clinical concerns, no additional testing or evaluation is necessary. It is important to ensure that the murmur resolves by 6 months of age. If not, then evaluation by a pediatric cardiologist would be advised.

B. Incorrect. The clinical vignette is describing the murmur of PPS and no additional diagnostic testing is necessary at this time. CXR and EKG have low yield in helping to detect congenital heart disease as an outpatient, and if there were true clinical concern for congenital heart disease, an evaluation by a pediatric cardiologist would be the preferred next step in management.

C. Correct. The clinical vignette is describing a murmur of PPS in an otherwise well baby. PPS resolves by 6 months of age, and therefore, the murmur should no longer be heard. If the murmur was heard beyond 6 months of age, a pediatric cardiology referral would be needed.

D. Incorrect. The clinical vignette is describing the murmur of PPS in an otherwise well baby. No additional testing or workup is needed at this time.

2. Case 2

You are the attending physician rounding in the well-baby nursery at your local community hospital. The nurse calls to tell you that the mother of Baby Girl A would like to be discharged. Baby Girl A is a 1-day-old ex 39-week-F born via normal spontaneous vaginal delivery to an experienced G6P6 mom. She passed her pulse oximetry screening on the first try with oxygen saturation of 97%. On your exam, you note a well-appearing, non-syndromic neonate with normal respiratory effort and acrocyanosis in hands and feet. Upon auscultation, you appreciate a 2/6 harsh systolic ejection murmur, loudest at the left upper sternal border. No hepatosplenomegaly, belly soft, and normal brachial and femoral pulses.

What is the next step in management of this patient?

A. Because the pulse oximetry screen was normal, allow baby to be discharged home with her mother as asked, with outpatient cardiology follow-up
B. Obtain an echocardiogram prior to discharge
C. Place lines and start prostaglandins
D. Obtain a blood gas and CXR

Answer: B

A. Incorrect. While the pulse oximeter is reassuring, the exam findings suggest pulmonary valve stenosis. Because the pulmonary vascular resistance may not have fallen yet, and the ductus arteriosus may not have closed yet, the murmur intensity may be falsely lowered, and the blood saturation bolstered by an open ductus. It is important to clarify the degree of pulmonary stenosis prior to discharge, to ensure that the patient would maintain saturations in the setting of a closed ductus, and to determine the appropriate timing of follow-up.

B. Correct. You are hearing a murmur of pulmonary stenosis, and it is important to define the degree of stenosis and whether the ductus arteriosus has closed yet. If not, the patient's saturations may fall dramatically upon ductal closure, and you would want to ensure that you were not putting the child at risk. Pulmonary valve stenosis is associated with other more complex congenital heart lesions, like tetralogy of Fallot, and it is useful to clarify the anatomy prior to discharge from the hospital to ensure appropriate family education and timing of follow-up. If you were at a hospital that had a pediatric cardiologist available, a consultation with them may also be an appropriate next step.

C. Incorrect. It would be unusual for a patient with critical pulmonary valve stenosis to pass the pulse oximetry screen with such high saturations, even if the ductus was not yet closed. Typically, a diagnosis is sought prior to starting interventions for ductal-dependent heart disease. An exception would be a baby that presented in extremis for whom every second counts; in a baby who is otherwise moribund, if congenital heart disease is on your differential diagnosis, it is reasonable to start prostaglandins while completing a workup to define the anatomy.

D. Incorrect. If the child had hypoxia of unclear etiology, a blood gas and chest XR would be very helpful in distinguishing a cardiac versus pulmonary etiology of the hypoxia. A hyperoxia test in which a baby is given FiO_2 of 100% for 10 min, and then an arterial blood gas is drawn, can be extremely helpful in distinguishing a cardiac versus pulmonary etiology of hypoxia. If the PaO_2 remains <50 mmHg after the 10 min of 100% O_2, this is associated with a cyanotic congenital heart lesion. If the PaO_2 >150 mmHg, it is likely a pulmonary problem. PaO_2s of 50–150 mmHg is a bit of a gray area, but is commonly associated with congenital heart disease called "mixing lesions." In this child with normal saturations, a blood gas and CXR is not needed at this time.

Further Reading

Barrett MJ, Lacey CS, Sekara AE, Linden EA, Gracely EJ. Mastering Cardiac Murmurs: The power of repetition. Chest. 2004;126:470–5.

Finley JP, Caissie R, Nicol P, Hoyt B. International trial of online auditory training programme for distinguishing innocent from pathologic murmurs. J Paediatr Child Health. 2015;51(8):815–9.

Frank JE, Jacobe KM. Evaluation and management of heart murmurs in children. Am Fam Physician. 2011;84(7):793–800.

Menashe V. Heart murmurs. Pediatr Rev. 2007;28(4):e19–22.

Shaddy RE, Penny DJ, Feltes TF, Cetta F, Mital S. Moss & Adams' heart disease in infants, children, and adolescents: including the fetus and young adult, vol. 1. 10th rev. ed. Philadelphia: Wolters Kluwer; 2022.

Chapter 31
Pneumonia

Y. Katharine Chang and Christine Mikesell

Background

According to the World Health Organization, pneumonia and lower tract respiratory infections account for 14% of all deaths in children under age 5 in 2019. In developed countries, pneumonia accounts for <1% of pediatric deaths, but can represent a large burden of disease in the pediatric population, with significant morbidity.

Pathophysiology

Most cases of community-acquired pneumonia are preceded by a prodromal respiratory infection, often viral in etiology, triggering an immune response that leads to the alveoli and interstitial spaces filled with white blood cells, cellular debris, and fluid. This inflammatory response makes the lung parenchyma more vulnerable to invasion by bacteria or viruses, resulting in pneumonia. Clinically, the presence of mucus, fluid, and cellular debris in the airways results in an increase in airway resistance. As the airways become obstructed, the distal airways may collapse, increasing the ventilation/perfusion mismatch and resulting in hypoxemia. The pattern of airway obstruction determines the typical findings of pneumonia seen on physical exam (Table 31.1). Pneumonia can be complicated by effusions, empyemas, and abscesses within the lung parenchyma.

The most likely infectious etiology of pneumonia differs depending on the age of the patient (Table 31.2). Bacterial pneumonia is more common in developing countries than in developed countries; in the United States, most pneumonia in young

Y. K. Chang (✉) · C. Mikesell
Department of Pediatrics, University of Michigan Medical School, Ann Arbor, MI, USA
e-mail: yilingc@med.umich.edu; cemikese@med.umich.edu

N. Liao et al. (eds.), *Pediatric Rotations*,
https://doi.org/10.1007/978-3-031-59873-9_31

Table 31.1 Types of pneumonia by anatomic location

Type	Physical findings	Etiology	Pathophysiology
Lobar pneumonia	– Focal findings – Diminished breath sounds – Rub	Bacterial ≫ viral	– Alveoli within one lobe filled with neutrophils, exudate, usually bacteria – Consolidation with fibrinous fluid and cellular infiltrate and no air – Stiff lungs due to thickening of alveolar walls and pleura
Bronchopneumonia	– Patchy, focal findings, especially in dependent areas	Viral ≫ bacterial	– Inflammation throughout bronchi and alveoli – Smaller airways filled with exudate
Interstitial pneumonia	– Non-toxic appearance – Diffuse, often unremarkable findings on auscultation	Atypical bacterial	– Inflammation within alveoli and interstitial spaces – Lymphocytic infiltrate – Alveoli filled with hyaline membranes
Miliary pneumonia	None	Tuberculosis Histoplasmosis	– Commonly due to hematogenous spread of pathogen – Widespread lesions

Table 31.2 Most common infectious agents with pneumonia in developed countries by age

Age group	Viruses	Bacteria
Neonate	Cytomegalovirus Herpes simplex virus	*Escherichia coli* Group B streptococcus
1 mo–3 mo	Respiratory syncytial virus (RSV) Influenza A and B Parainfluenza 1, 2, 3 Human metapneumovirus Rhinovirus Adenovirus	Group B streptococcus Enteric Gram-negative bacilli *Streptococcus pneumoniae* *Bordetella pertussis* *Chlamydia trachomatis* *Staphylococcus aureus*
3 mo–5 yrs	RSV Influenza A and B Parainfluenza 1, 2, 3 Human metapneumovirus Rhinovirus Adenovirus	*S. pneumoniae* *Mycoplasma pneumoniae* *C. pneumoniae* *S. aureus* Non-typeable *Haemophilus influenzae*
≥5 yrs	Influenza A and B	*S. pneumoniae* *M. pneumoniae* *Chlamydophila pneumoniae* *S. aureus*

children is caused by viruses. It can be difficult to distinguish between viral and bacterial pneumonia based upon screening labs and radiologic findings, so history and physical exam findings are central to making a diagnosis.

History

The presentation of pneumonia can vary greatly in severity depending upon how widespread the disease is, the infectious etiology, and other various patient factors. Typical symptoms include cough, tachypnea, sputum production, and systemic symptoms such as fever, decreased energy, loss of appetite, and difficulty sleeping. Other conditions affecting the patient's clinical status must also be assessed, such as hydration, mentation, and respiratory distress. It is not unusual for patients to complain of abdominal pain with a lower lobe pneumonia or neck stiffness with an upper lobe pneumonia. A chronologic history may make it easier to elucidate if the patient's pneumonia is more likely to be viral or bacterial in etiology.

History of Present Illness

- When did symptoms start? What symptoms were first? What symptoms were next?
- Is there fever? When did it start?
- Any cough? Any change in severity or quality of the cough?
- Any difficulty breathing or distress?
- Are the symptoms waxing and waning, or have they been steadily worsening over time?
- Any preceding events, like choking episodes or environmental exposures?

Because many pneumonias are preceded by a prodromal viral illness, it is helpful to understand whether the patient is experiencing a new-onset illness or the result of an evolving illness. Patients who have symptoms of a respiratory illness and develop acute worsening, with respiratory distress, worsening cough, and new or renewed fever, are more likely to have an initial viral illness followed by a secondary bacterial pneumonia. Patients with viral pneumonias frequently present with an upper respiratory illness, with symptoms like rhinorrhea and nasal congestion, accompanied by lower respiratory tract symptoms, such as cough and shortness of breath, that begin at the same time or shortly after onset of illness. Atypical pneumonias are often called "walking pneumonias," as patients are well enough to go about their daily activities but have persistent respiratory symptoms that do not improve over the course of a week or two, as expected. Understanding the time course of illness also helps distinguish between pneumonia and sequential viral upper respiratory illnesses, asthma exacerbations, or aspiration events.

Past Medical History

- Any risk factors (Table 31.3)?
  - Patient factors: age < 2 years, prematurity, lack of immunization, malnutrition
  - Environmental factors: tobacco exposure, school or daycare exposure, crowded living conditions
  - Underlying conditions that impact the immune system or effective airway clearance: cystic fibrosis, asthma, diabetes, sickle cell disease, bronchopulmonary dysplasia, primary or secondary immunodeficiency, brain injury or hypotonia
- Any recurrent or unusual infections or history of other invasive infections?
  - Should prompt evaluation for immunodeficiency

Family History

- Any family members with inheritable immunodeficiencies or pulmonary conditions?

Social History

- Daycare or school attendance? Older siblings?
- Any sick contacts?
- Contact with individuals living in institutionalized settings? Contact with individuals with recent travel history?
- Living conditions: Crowded housing? Infested living space? Reliable water and heating/cooling? Access to transportation and healthcare?

Table 31.3 Risk factors for severe or bacterial pneumonia

Risk factor	Examples
Socio-economic status	Crowded conditions in the home, lack of access to healthcare
Cardio-pulmonary disorders	Asthma, bronchopulmonary dysplasia, congenital heart disease
Impaired airway clearance	Neuromuscular disorders, GI disorders such as TEF or GERD, impaired muco-ciliary clearance from cigarette smoke exposure
Congenital anomalies	Lung abnormalities such as CPAM, TEF
Immunocompromise	Sickle cell disease

CPAM congenital pulmonary airway malformation, *GERD* gastroesophageal reflux disease, *GI* gastrointestinal, *TEF* tracheoesophageal fistula

Questions on social history help determine possible pathogenic etiologies of the illness once you have made a diagnosis of pneumonia. Children who are in daycare sometimes have a known exposure to a specific viral illness. A diagnosis of atypical pneumonia caused by Mycoplasma must be considered in school-aged children and sometimes in younger children with school-aged siblings. Tuberculosis is endemic in some parts of the world and among people who live in institutionalized settings. It is helpful to explore the patient's living conditions to appreciate the likelihood of factors that might affect the patient's overall health and the ability to seek medical care.

Review of Systems

- Any preceding or recent illnesses?
- Nasal congestion, rhinorrhea, ear pain, sore throat?
- Any eye discharge or redness?
- Headache, neck stiffness?
- Any gastrointestinal symptoms?
- Is the patient drinking sufficiently? Urinating?
- How is the patient acting? Playful? Listless? Irritable or lethargic?

The questions on review of systems help round out the clinical picture, as well as ruling in or out other conditions on the list of differential diagnoses.

Physical Exam

Physical exam findings on patients with pneumonia can also vary greatly (Table 31.4). Signs on physical exam depend on the location and cause of the pneumonia and whether there are complications or comorbid conditions. Fever, tachypnea, hypoxemia, as well as cough and increased work of breathing, are all highly suggestive of pneumonia in the correct clinical setting. Tachypnea alone is insufficient to make a diagnosis of pneumonia, but pneumonia is unlikely in the absence of tachypnea. Increased work of breathing, hypoxia, and a toxic appearance are common in more severe disease. In addition, patients with pneumonia are at risk for sepsis and should be monitored for worsening tachycardia and hypotension.

Table 31.4 Physical exam findings in patients with pneumonia

System	Physical sign	Tips/significance
General	Overall appearance	• Does the child appear sick or not sick? • In distress or comfortable?
HEENT	Tympanic membranes	• Secondary bacterial infections following viral upper respiratory infections, including acute otitis media
	Nasal flaring	• Indicates increased work of breathing
	Nasal congestion	• Viral etiology or preceding viral trigger; possibly due to comorbid sinusitis
	Mucous membranes	• Patients often dehydrated due to decreased intake and increased insensible losses
	Lesions in oropharynx	• Possible signs of viral etiology, such as vesicles on palate or ulcers in mouth
Heart	Tachycardia	• Associated with sepsis, dehydration, hypoxia; sepsis can be bacterial or viral in etiology
Lungs	Respiratory rate	• Too fast suggests respiratory distress • Too slow suggests impending respiratory failure • Absence of tachypnea helps rule out pneumonia
	Grunting	• Effort to increase end-expiratory pressure; sign of increased work of breathing
	Adventitious sounds	• Rales/crackles = suggestive of an area of consolidation • Rhonchi = presence of mucus • Wheeze = bronchospasm in the setting of asthma or viral/atypical bacterial pneumonia
	Decreased breath sounds	• Due to consolidation
	Focal findings	• Focality of any of the above could indicate an area of consolidation or atelectasis; if the area is fixed, more likely to be associated with bacterial pneumonia; if it is shifting, more likely to be associated with viral etiology
	Egophony	• E to A change caused by limits on some sound frequencies traveling through solid or fluid-filled areas of lung; suggestive of effusion or empyema but can be heard in any area of consolidation
	Friction rub	• Suggestive of effusion or empyema
Chest	Retractions	• Occur in subcostal, intercostal, and suprasternal areas; indicate accessory muscle use; sign of increased work of breathing
	Dullness to percussion	• Suggests consolidation under area being percussed as sounds are dull when traveling through dense tissue
	Splinting	• Pain associated with pneumonia or effusion causes decreased respiratory effort
Abdomen	Abdominal breathing	• Significant use of abdominal muscles during respiration is a sign of increased work of breathing
	Abdominal pain	• Common symptom of pneumonia so abdominal pain does not rule out lung pathology
Extremities	Warm or cool	• Poor perfusion associated with sepsis or dehydration

Table 31.4 (continued)

System	Physical sign	Tips/significance
Skin	Rash	• Some viral respiratory illnesses may have associated exanthems
	Mottling or cyanosis	• Possible signs of sepsis, severe hypoxia, severe dehydration
Neurologic	Alertness	• Neurologic status is a good marker for brain perfusion—too little blood flow results in too little oxygen

Table 31.5 Significance of laboratory findings

Inflammatory markers	High: Difficult to differentiate between bacterial or viral; elevated procalcitonin and CRP may be more common in bacterial infections Normal: Less likely to be bacterial
WBC	Elevated neutrophils: More likely to be bacterial Elevated lymphocytes: More likely to be viral
Blood culture	Rarely positive in most community-acquired pneumonia Consider obtaining in hospitalized children or suspected complicated pneumonia
Respiratory viral PCR panel	May reveal a viral or, on some tests, an atypical bacterial cause
Sputum culture	Very difficult to obtain in children so rarely obtained

CRP C-reactive protein, *PCR* polymerase chain reaction

Workup

Laboratory Assessment

Labs are not necessary for outpatient management of pneumonia. Consider labs for hospitalized patients, especially those at risk of bacteremia or further clinical deterioration. While screening laboratory data rarely fully differentiates viral from bacterial pneumonia, there are some differences that can aid in diagnosis and medical decision-making. Table 31.5 outlines some significant findings on common laboratory testing.

Imaging

Pneumonia is a clinical diagnosis and does not need to be confirmed with imaging. Imaging studies may be helpful, however, if there is suspicion for a complicated pneumonia or to monitor disease progression. Of note, radiologic findings tend to lag behind a patient's clinical progress. Moreover, chest X-rays may not show the true extent of disease if the patient is dehydrated.

Standard imaging begins with a 2-view chest radiograph to evaluate for pattern and extent of disease. Further imaging is dictated by the concern for a more complicated pneumonia. Ultrasonography or computed tomography scan may be indicated to better visualize pleural effusions, empyemas (purulent pleural effusions), or lung abscesses, as well as causes of respiratory difficulty that may not be due to pneumonia.

Key Differential Diagnoses

Since the presentation of pneumonia can be highly variable, the list of differential diagnoses is extensive (Table 31.6). It includes foreign bodies, congenital or acquired anatomic abnormalities, malignancy, rheumatologic disease, among other conditions. Keep in mind that it is possible for some of these diagnoses to be comorbid with pneumonia or even a predisposing factor for the development of pneumonia.

When making a diagnosis of pneumonia, it is important to consider the etiology of the infection, including viral, typical bacterial, atypical bacterial, and aspiration. Each of these has common findings on history and physical exam that can help establish the infectious etiology and thus the appropriate management (Table 31.7).

Management

Management of the patient with pneumonia begins with deciding if the patient's clinical status warrants admission to the hospital. Inpatient treatment is not needed for all pediatric patients with pneumonia; many do quite well with empiric antibiotics at home, careful anticipatory guidance, and close follow-up, if needed.

Table 31.6 Differential diagnoses for pediatric pneumonia

Anatomic	Autoimmune	Malignant	Other
• Congenital pulmonary airway malformation • Bronchogenic cyst • Congenital lobar emphysema • Pulmonary sequestration • Congenital diaphragmatic hernia	• Systemic lupus erythematosus • Granulomatosis with polyangiitis • Sarcoidosis	• Lymphoma • Metastatic tumor • Lung tumor	• Bronchiolitis • Asthma • Aspiration • Inhaled irritants • Atelectasis • Heart failure • Renal failure • Intra-abdominal processes • Chylothorax

Table 31.7 Differential diagnosis by pathogen

Etiology	Key H&P findings
Viral	• Gradual onset • Prolonged non-productive cough • URI symptoms • Headache, malaise, sore throat, low-grade fevers • Minimal physical exam findings
Typical bacterial	• May have a viral prodrome • Higher fevers • Cough • Focal findings on auscultation
Atypical bacterial	• Similar to viral • Tend to be older (5+ years old) • Less common than viral
Aspiration	• Similar to bacterial • In a child with risk for aspiration—neurologic disease, hypotonia, dysphagia

URI upper respiratory infection

Criteria for Admission

- Age:
  - Neonates and infants under 3 months of age should be admitted due to the risk of rapid deterioration.
  - Hospitalization should be carefully considered for infants between 3 and 6 months of age, but may not be required.
  - Decision to admit children over 6 months of age will depend on clinical status.
- Clinical criteria:
  - Hypoxia
  - Increased work of breathing
  - Periods of apnea
  - Poor oral intake or dehydration
  - Complicated pneumonia
  - Comorbid conditions that increase risk of severe disease, such as asthma or hypotonia
  - Failure of outpatient management
- Social/environmental factors:
  - Inability of caregivers to follow up as directed
  - Lack of access to care in case of worsening illness

Disease-specific management depends upon the infectious etiology, but all patients require basic supportive care including respiratory support, supplemental oxygen, fluid and nutritional support, pulmonary clearance techniques, fever control, and respiratory isolation as needed.

Table 31.8 Empiric therapy for uncomplicated inpatient community-acquired pneumonia

	Fully immunized	Underimmunized	Atypical
Target pathogens	*S. pneumoniae*	*S. pneumoniae* plus *H. influenzae* type B	*M. pneumoniae* *C. pneumoniae*
Parenteral antibiotics	Ampicillin 2nd line: Ceftriaxone or Levofloxacin if allergic	Ceftriaxone 2nd line: Levofloxacin	Azithromycin (if unable to take oral)
Oral antibiotics	Amoxicillin or Clindamycin if allergic 2nd line: Levofloxacin	Amoxicillin-clavulanate 2nd line: Levofloxacin	Azithromycin (same bioavailability as IV) 2nd line: Doxycycline if allergic

Patients with viral pneumonia typically do well with supportive care alone. In the case of influenza, antiviral agents such as ribavirin or oseltamivir may be recommended for certain high-risk patients.

As bacterial and viral pneumonia cannot be distinguished from each other based upon radiologic and basic laboratory data, many patients receive empiric antibiotics. There may be clues in the patient's history or physical exam that help guide antibiotic choice by raising the index of suspicion for specific pathogens causing disease. In the absence of such information, empiric antimicrobial treatment is determined based on the most common causative organisms for that age group, typically including *S. pneumoniae*. Moreover, whenever antimicrobial therapies are considered, the choice of medication is focused on identifying the most narrow-spectrum agent that can achieve appropriate tissue penetration with good patient compliance (Table 31.8).

Complications

Patients who are not improving as expected—typically within 48–72 h after initiating antibiotics—or who have clinical deterioration on appropriate antibiotics should be evaluated for complications.

Complicated pneumonias are more likely to be bacterial than viral in infectious etiology. They are more likely to present with a worse clinical status and result in hospitalization, longer length of stay, and greater antibiotic use. Abscesses, pleural effusions, and empyemas are collections of fluid and inflammatory debris within the lung or intrapleural space that may impede healing and the expected resolution of pneumonia; they represent the most common complications of pneumonia. Patients with these conditions may require procedures such as a pleural tap or chest tube placement to sample and culture the fluid or to facilitate drainage of infected fluid. In the case of a loculated or septated empyema, the use of a fibrinolytic agent may facilitate drainage, helping to avoid more invasive treatment, as well as reducing morbidity and length of stay.

In some instances, it is prudent to consult a specialty service while managing a pediatric patient with pneumonia. Patients with effusions, empyemas, or abscesses should have a surgery consultation. An infectious disease expert should be consulted when patients present with an unusual or unexpected infectious agent or when they have a complicated or prolonged clinical course. Patients with repeated episodes of pneumonia or other pulmonary conditions, such as persistent asthma, primary ciliary dyskinesia or cystic fibrosis, should be seen and followed by a pulmonologist.

Anticipatory Guidance

While there is a wide range of clinical presentations for patients with pneumonia, in general, even patients with complicated pneumonia do well if diagnosed early and treated appropriately. Pediatric patients with pneumonia require close, outpatient follow-up. Key points to highlight with families include:

- Long-term pulmonary complications, even in the setting of a very complicated pneumonia, are unusual.
- It is important to complete the entire course of antibiotics, if prescribed.
- Continue to encourage rest and fluids until the patient is feeling better.
- Children will naturally become more active and playful as they improve.
- Seek medical attention for:
  - signs of respiratory distress
  - persistent or renewed fever
  - worsening cough
  - inability to drink enough to maintain hydration or any signs of dehydration
  - persistent irritability or fatigue
  - no improvement or looking sicker after a couple of days

Application Exercises

1. A previously healthy, 4-year-old boy presents to the outpatient pediatric office with a 3-day history of cough, nasal congestion, and fevers to 38.5 °C. On exam, the patient has mild tachypnea, diffuse rhonchi, focal right-sided rales, and no signs of increased work of breathing. The patient attends daycare and several other children in the class have been ill recently with similar symptoms. Mom reports that the patient has been eating and drinking well and has been active when he is afebrile.

   What is the next best step?

   A. Provide reassurance
   B. Obtain chest X-ray
   C. Order blood work

D. Start oral antibiotics
E. Admit to the hospital

Answer D: This patient's presentation is consistent with a focal pneumonia. The focality of the findings points towards a bacterial etiology, but it is not truly possible to distinguish between viral and bacterial causes. Given the possibility of a bacterial infection, empiric oral antibiotics are indicated, with good anticipatory guidance and close follow-up. First-line antibiotic choice would be amoxicillin. Reassurance alone at this time would not be appropriate since the patient has an infection that requires treatment, and without it, he is at risk for developing severe or complicated disease. Further workup, such as imaging and laboratory studies, are not necessary, as community-acquired pneumonia is a clinical diagnosis, which can be made based on history and physical exam findings that are consistent. Moreover, imaging may lag clinical symptoms and be unrevealing at this early stage. Since the patient is well-appearing at this time and has not had tried any outpatient therapy, admission to the hospital is not indicated.

2. The patient initially seems to improve, but 2 days later, he has worsening cough, increased work of breathing, and continued fever to 39.5 °C. The patient is not eating or drinking as much as usual, and he is less active than before. On exam, the patient is listless and tachypneic. He has intercostal and subcostal retractions noted, and he is using his abdominal muscles with each breath. He has bilateral rhonchi, and you note a rub and markedly diminished breath sounds on the right side.

   What is the most likely cause of the patient's symptoms?

A. New viral infection
B. Asthma exacerbation
C. Empyema
D. Myocarditis
E. Congestive heart failure

Answer C: A return or persistence of fever, accompanied by worsening symptoms, several days into the course of illness raises the suspicion for a complication of the initial pneumonia. The exam findings are consistent with an intrapleural fluid collection, which could be either an effusion or an empyema. A new viral infection is possible, but given the short timeframe between initial presentation and worsening, the patient is more likely to be experiencing a complication of the initial problem, rather than a new problem. Myocarditis is also possible and may manifest with many of the same signs and symptoms; it should be considered, but again, the patient is more likely to have complicated pneumonia than a new infection. Congestive heart failure is unlikely to present with persistent fever and is frequently accompanied by edema, which this patient does not have. At this time, the patient requires further workup, including imaging and blood work, and may require hospitalization for further treatment and monitoring.

3. The patient is sent to the emergency department for further workup and consideration for admission. He is given intravenous fluids for dehydration. The patient's pulse oximetry demonstrates desaturations to 88%, which improve to 93% on supplemental oxygen per nasal cannula. Blood work and chest X-ray are completed, which reveal an elevated white blood cell count with a predominance of neutrophils, elevated inflammatory markers, and bilateral infiltrates with a moderate right-sided effusion on chest X-ray. Blood cultures are pending. The patient remains febrile, tachycardic, and tachypneic.

   What are indications for admission?

   A. Hypoxia
   B. Dehydration
   C. Persistent vital sign abnormalities
   D. Need for parenteral antibiotics
   E. All of the above

   Answer E: The patient warrants inpatient admission for all of the above reasons, starting with the need for supplemental oxygen to remain normoxemic. Given the patient's poor oral intake and signs of dehydration on presentation, he requires continued fluid support until he can demonstrate the ability to remain hydrated on his own. Patients with pneumonia, especially complicated pneumonia, are at risk for sepsis and vital sign abnormalities should be monitored closely. Since the patient has a worsening clinical status in spite of appropriate oral antibiotics, he requires parenteral antibiotics and possible drainage of the effusion for improved control of his infection. In light of the moderate-sized effusion, the patient should undergo further imaging, such as ultrasound or computed tomography (CT), to delineate the extent and nature of the pleural fluid, and he would benefit from consultation with a surgeon. Furthermore, an Infectious Diseases specialist could also be helpful in determining type and duration of antimicrobial treatment for this complicated pneumonia.

Further Reading

Antibiotic Stewardship Program. Antibiotic treatment guidelines for pneumonia in pediatric patients. Michigan Medicine; 2021, accessed 21 September 2022, https://www.med.umich.edu/asp/pdf/pediatric_guidelines/PNA_PEDS.pdf.

de Benedictis FM, Kerem E, Chang AB, Colin AA, Zar HJ, Bush A. Complicated pneumonia in children. Lancet. 2020;396(10253):786–98.

Messinger AI, Kupfer O, Hurst A, Parker S. Management of pediatric community-acquired bacterial pneumonia. Pediatr Rev. 2017;38:394–409.

Sattar SBA, Sharma S. Bacterial pneumonia (Updated 2021 Dec 28). In: StatPearls. Treasure Island, FL: StatPearls Publishing; 2022. Available from: https://www.ncbi.nlm.nih.gov/books/NBK513321/.

Chapter 32
Poisonings and Intoxications

Christopher E. Gaw and Anna K. Weiss

Background

Pediatric patients may be exposed to a wide variety of poisoning hazards. Many substances—including medications, recreational drugs, household consumer products, and environmental chemicals and gases—can have toxic effects on the human body depending on the magnitude or duration of exposure. Memorizing the toxic effects of substances and their associated treatments is a daunting—and perhaps impossible—task, particularly as the landscape of available substances is ever-changing. As you begin learning about pediatric poisonings, focus instead on general principles, which will help you understand patterns of illness in poisoned children.

Epidemiology

Poison Control Centers across the United States receive over one million calls annually regarding toxic exposures in children and adolescents less than 20 years of age. Children under the age of 6 comprise over half of these exposures. The typical

C. E. Gaw (✉)
Division of Emergency Medicine, Department of Pediatrics, Nationwide Children's Hospital/The Ohio State University, Columbus, OH, USA
e-mail: Christopher.Gaw@nationwidechildrens.org

A. K. Weiss
Division of Emergency Medicine, Department of Pediatrics, Children's Hospital of Philadelphia, Philadelphia, PA, USA
e-mail: weissak@chop.edu

N. Liao et al. (eds.), *Pediatric Rotations*,
https://doi.org/10.1007/978-3-031-59873-9_32

mechanism of exposure and exposure substance changes throughout a child's development:

- Young infants have limited gross and fine motor skills. Thus, they are typically accidentally or intentionally exposed to a medication or substance by a caregiver.
- Older infants and toddlers develop increasingly sophisticated motor skills and oral exploratory behaviors. These children often accidentally expose themselves to substances such as medications and household consumer products within their reach.
- Older children and adolescents may experiment with different substances. Exposures in this age group are often intentional and involve over-the-counter, prescription, or recreational drugs. Among adolescents, behavioral health concerns such as depression, suicidality, and substance use disorders account for a subset of these intentional ingestions.

Pathophysiologic Considerations

Toxic substances can have wide and varying effects on the body, and these substances affect children differently compared to adults. Table 32.1 summarizes several important pediatric pathophysiologic differences to consider when caring for a poisoned patient.

Table 32.1 Pediatric poisoning pathophysiologic considerations

Pathophysiologic consideration	Implication
Weight	Exposure to the same amount of a substance may be more toxic for a child than for an adult due to smaller weight and size
Body surface area (BSA) to weight ratio	In children, a higher BSA-to-weight ratio can lead to increased absorption of a substance through the skin
Metabolic rate	Substances that affect respiratory drive can lead to acidosis, hypoxemia, and respiratory failure sooner in children than adults
Heart rate compensation	To maintain cardiac output, children preferentially increase heart rate rather than stroke volume. Thus, drugs that prevent tachycardia (e.g., beta-blockers) may have significant consequences on hemodynamics
Neurodevelopmental maturity	The developing nervous system of children may respond to certain drugs differently than the nervous system of adults (e.g., paradoxical agitation from benzodiazepines)

History

The approach to taking a poisoning-focused history is similar to that for many other chief complaints. Remember to ask about medications, allergies, and the patient's past medical and family histories. There are several unique aspects of the history of present illness and social history to be sure to review with the family in suspected poisoning cases.

Substance Exposure Questions

Asking focused exposure questions is critical to identifying the magnitude, timing, and severity of a child's exposure to a substance (Table 32.2).

Symptoms and Review of Systems Questions

Children who are poisoned may present with a variety of symptoms. Be prepared to ask a thorough review of systems (refer to Chap. 2 for a full review of systems discussion). As you identify the symptoms a child is exhibiting, make sure to focus on these key aspects:

Table 32.2 Poison exposure history questions

Questions	Tips and pearls
Substance history – What was/were the substance(s) to which the child was exposed? – How much of the substance was the child exposed to? (e.g., 1 pill, 50 mg, 30 mL) – When was the exposure? – How was the child exposed? (e.g., inhaled, ingested, splashed)	*Tip*: Parents may not know the exposure substance or when it occurred. If this is the case, refer to the "Exposure Risks" section *Tip:* Ask, "when did you last see your child acting normally?" This can help determine approximately when an exposure occurred
Exposure risks – What medications does the child take? – What over-the-counter and/or prescription medications are in the home? – Where are medications stored in the home? Are they secured or locked? – Are there any other household chemicals or toxins in the home? (e.g., household cleaners, plants, pets, pet supplies) – Have there been any visitors or changes to the household environment?	*Tip*: These questions help you create a list of all possible exposure substances. This is very helpful in unknown exposures *Pearl:* A child may be exposed to more than one substance or may be exposed to a different substance than that reported by caregivers

1. What symptoms have caregivers noticed, and when did they start?
2. If there are multiple symptoms, what was the order and timing of those symptoms relative to one another?
3. What has been the trajectory of the child's symptoms? Have any symptoms improved or worsened?

These questions are important because certain substances cause a very specific set of symptoms. Other substances present with a set of initial symptoms that gradually evolve over time. For example, patients with iron poisoning may initially present with abdominal pain, vomiting, and diarrhea in the first several hours after ingestion. These patients may subsequently appear to improve but can develop signs and symptoms of acute liver failure several days after the initial exposure.

Involvement of Poison Control

Poison control is a 24-h national hotline (1-800-222-1222) available both to the public and to healthcare professionals for advice on poisonings. The hotline is staffed by medical professionals—including physicians, pharmacists, and nurses—with advanced training in toxicology. Because families may have contacted Poison Control prior to presenting to care, be sure to ask the following as part of your history:

1. Did caregivers contact Poison Control prior to presenting to care?
2. If so:
   (a) When did the family contact Poison Control?
   (b) What did Poison Control recommend to the family?

You can also call the Poison Control hotline to see if there is information available from the caregiver's call and to receive management recommendations.

Prior Therapies

Questions to ask about prior therapies given or tried include:

1. Did caregivers try any treatments or therapies at home prior to presenting to care?
2. Were any of these therapies recommended by Poison Control (if contacted)?
3. Was there any change in the child's symptoms after receiving the therapies?

Table 32.3 Poisoning social history questions

Questions	Tips and pearls
Social history – Are the circumstances of the exposure plausible given the child's developmental age? – Was the child supervised at the time of the incident? – How many people are in frequent contact with the child or live in the child's care environment? – Does anyone in the child's care environment have a substance use disorder or are they undergoing treatment for one?	*Pearl*: If the history of poisoning does not seem plausible relative to the child's developmental capabilities (e.g., a 2-month-old infant self-administering an oral medication capsule), it should raise suspicion for possible malicious intent or non-accidental poisoning *Pearl:* These questions help characterize a child's environment. Unsafe environments may require further evaluation or support by a social worker or child protection agency
Behavioral and Mental Health – Was the poisoning an attempt at self-harm? – Is there a history of substance use disorders in the patient? – Is there a history of mental health disorders in the patient? – Is there a past or active history of suicidal or homicidal ideation?	*Pearl*: These questions typically apply to older children and adolescents *Tip:* Use the HEADSSS history framework with empathy and sensitivity when reviewing these questions. Refer to Chap. 37 for more information

Social History

An important and sometimes overlooked part of a poisoning-oriented history is a thorough social history. The information obtained can identify risks to a child that may require additional social support. Table 32.3 summarizes several questions to review with the child and their caregivers.

Physical Exam

Vitals

Pay close attention to all vital signs—temperature, heart rate, respiratory rate, blood pressure, and pulse oximetry—in a suspected poisoning, as many substances have effects on the autonomic nervous system. Abnormal vital signs are not only important to inform management but may also serve as clues to the causative poison or agent (see Toxidromes).

Exam

A thorough head-to-toe exam is important for any poisoned patient. Several key systems to focus on are highlighted in Table 32.4.

Table 32.4 Pediatric poisoning selected physical exam elements

System	Exam elements	Tips and pearls
General	Well or ill appearing?	*Pearl:* Determining "sick or not sick" is important, regardless of the exposure
Eyes	Pupil size and reactivity? Presence of nystagmus?	*Pearl:* Substances that affect the autonomic nervous system can affect pupil size and reactivity[a] *Pearl:* Nystagmus may be vertical, horizontal, or rotary. Anticonvulsants, ethanol, lithium, phencyclidine, and ketamine are common causes of nystagmus
Mucous membranes	Level of secretion? Mucosal injury or erosions?	*Pearl:* Dry versus moist mucous membranes may suggest a toxidrome[a] *Tip:* Look carefully for ocular or oral burns caused by caustic substances
Cardiovascular	Rate and rhythm? Perfusion?	*Pearl:* Tachycardia can be caused by sympathomimetics or anticholinergics[a] *Pearl:* Bradycardia or hypotension may suggest exposure to blood pressure medications, antiarrhythmics, or organophosphates[a]
Respiratory	Rate and respiratory effort? Lung sounds clear? If not, what is heard?	*Tip:* Listen carefully. Excessive wheezes or other lung sounds may support a "wet" picture of excess secretions[a]
Gastrointestinal (GI)	Abdominal tenderness? Hepatosplenomegaly? Hyper- or hypoactive bowel sounds?	*Tip:* Listen carefully. Peristalsis can be slowed by substances such as opioids or increased by cholinergic agents[a]
Neuro	Mental status? GCS? Strength and tone? Tremors or clonus? Reflexes?	*Pearl:* A thorough neurologic exam is important, as many substances affect the central and peripheral nervous systems.[a] For example, findings such as hyperreflexia or clonus may suggest selective serotonin reuptake inhibitor overdose
Skin	Rashes, blisters, or burns? Color and temperature? Especially moist or dry?	*Tip:* Look carefully at the skin for any burns from splash injuries, especially in cases of caustic substance exposure *Pearl:* Diaphoretic versus dry skin may suggest a toxidrome[a]

[a]Refer to the Toxidromes section for further information on how to integrate different exam findings into a cohesive clinical picture

Detection of a distinct smell on the patient, on their clothing, or on their belongings may suggest exposure to a specific type of poison and is a unique aspect of the toxicology physical exam (Table 32.5). Odors, however, should not be used by themselves to diagnose a patient. They should be integrated with the other history and physical exam elements to determine or confirm the exposure substance.

Table 32.5 Odors and associated substances

Odor	Associated substance(s)
Bitter almond	Cyanide
Mothballs	Camphor
Garlic	Arsenic, organophosphates, thallium
Rotten eggs	Sulfur dioxide, hydrogen sulfide
Fruit	Isopropyl alcohol
Alcohol	Alcoholic beverages
Gasoline	Hydrocarbons
Wintergreen	Methyl salicylate

Toxidromes

Determining the actual substances involved in a poisoning is helpful in informing management. Sometimes, the history alone is sufficient to determine the exposure. In other cases, you may need to look for patterns in symptoms, vital signs, and exam findings to identify the poison. These patterns—referred to as *toxidromes*—are related to specific substances or to classes of substances. Common pediatric toxidromes are summarized in Table 32.6.

Though toxidromes can be helpful in identifying substances, they should be interpreted carefully. Other illnesses (e.g., sepsis) can mimic toxidromes, and in cases of polysubstance exposure, symptoms of multiple possible toxidromes can become difficult to interpret.

Electrocardiograms

Electrocardiograms (EKGs) are a convenient and valuable tool in evaluating a poisoned patient. They can provide clues to the identity of an exposure substance and can aid in the assessment of exposure complications and complication severity. EKGs also can be used to inform both management and disposition decisions. Numerous substances affect the cardiac action potential and thus affect the morphology of EKG tracings. It can be helpful to conceptualize EKG changes into five major categories (Table 32.7). Be aware that some substances can cause multiple types of EKG changes and that other changes to EKG tracing exist other than what are summarized here.

Table 32.6 Common pediatric toxidromes

Toxidrome	Example substances	Vital signs	Clinical findings
Anticholinergic	Antihistamines, atropine, tricyclic antidepressants	T: ↑ HR: ↑ RR: ↔ BP: ↑	*Mental status/neuro*: agitation, delirium; seizures *Pupils*: dilated *Bowel sounds*: decreased *Skin*: red, flushed, dry *Other*: urinary retention
Cholinergic	Organophosphate pesticides, physostigmine	T: ↔ HR: ↑↓ RR: ↑ BP: ↔	*Mental status/neuro*: confusion, somnolence; seizures *Pupils*: constricted *Bowel sounds*: increased *Skin*: diaphoretic *Other*: SLUDGE mnemonic (salivation, lacrimation, urination, defecation, emesis)
Opioid	Fentanyl, methadone, morphine	T: ↓ HR: ↓ RR: ↓ BP: ↓	*Mental status/neuro*: euphoria, somnolence, coma; hyporeflexia *Pupils*: constricted to pinpoint *Bowel sounds*: decreased *Skin*: no specific change
Salicylate	Aspirin	T: ↑ HR: ↔ RR: ↑ BP: ↔	*Mental status/neuro*: agitation, lethargy *Pupils*: no specific change *Bowel sounds*: no specific change *Skin*: no specific change *Other*: emesis
Sedative-hypnotic	Barbiturates, benzodiazepines, ethanol	T: ↓ HR: ↔ RR: ↓ BP: ↓	*Mental status/neuro*: agitation, somnolence, coma *Pupils*: no specific change *Bowel sounds*: no specific change *Skin*: no specific change
Sympathomimetic	Amphetamines, cocaine	T: ↑ HR: ↑ RR: ↑ BP: ↑	*Mental status/neuro*: euphoria, agitation, delirium, psychosis; tremors, myoclonus *Pupils*: dilated *Bowel sounds*: increased *Skin*: diaphoretic

↑ increased, ↓ decreased, ↔ equivocal

Table 32.7 EKG changes and selected associated substances

EKG change	Substances
Tachycardia	Amphetamines, anticholinergics, antihistamines, beta-agonists, caffeine, carbon monoxide (CO), cocaine, nicotine, selective serotonin reuptake inhibitors, tricyclic antidepressants
Bradycardia	Alpha-agonists, beta-blockers, calcium channel blockers, digoxin, opioids, organophosphates
Prolonged QRS	Chloroquine, carbamazepine, hydroxychloroquine, class IA and IC antiarrhythmic drugs, tricyclic antidepressants
Prolonged QTc	Antihistamines (e.g., diphenhydramine), antipsychotics (e.g., haloperidol), chloroquine, hydroxychloroquine, class IA, IC, and III antiarrhythmics, macrolides, tricyclic antidepressants
ST elevation or depression	CO, cocaine, digoxin

Laboratory Assessment

Conventional Testing

Conventional laboratory studies are not used to definitively identify a substance. Instead, they are helpful in assessing acid-base status, metabolic derangements, and other changes to blood counts and chemistries associated with a toxic exposure. Testing is individualized based on the suspected type and magnitude of exposure and on the symptoms observed (Table 32.8). In mild exposures, laboratory testing may not be necessary.

Toxicology Testing

Toxicology testing is generally divided into studies of the serum and of the urine. Common toxicologic serum tests include quantitative acetaminophen, salicylate, and ethanol levels. These levels are often ordered in cases of polysubstance exposures, in instances of intentional or self-harm ingestions, or if there is suspicion of exposure to one of the tested substances. Other serum toxicology studies exist (e.g., for antiepileptic drugs, digoxin, lead) though the availability of these tests is often institution dependent.

Table 32.8 Laboratory tests to consider for poisonings

Lab test	Purpose
Point-of-care blood glucose	Evaluate for hypoglycemia, which can be caused by substances such as ethanol or diabetes medications
Basic metabolic panel	Identify electrolyte derangements as a complication of poisoning (e.g., vomiting) and for anion gap calculation. Anion gap acidosis can be associated with several substances (e.g., acetaminophen, iron, isoniazid, toxic alcohols, salicylates)
Hepatic function panel	Identify signs of liver damage related to exposure to hepatotoxic substances (e.g., acetaminophen)
Complete blood count	Evaluate for changes in cell counts; anemia is often seen in metal poisonings (e.g., arsenic, lead)
Coagulation studies	Elevations can be seen due to impaired liver function or liver failure from poisonings or due to exposure to an anticoagulant (e.g., warfarin, rat poison)
Blood gas (arterial or venous)	Determine acid-base status to characterize poisoning complications (e.g., respiratory failure) or raise suspicion for a substance (e.g., respiratory alkalosis and metabolic acidosis in salicylate toxicity)
Serum osmolality	Elevated values are seen in cases of alcohol toxicity (e.g., ethanol, methanol, ethylene glycol)
Co-oximetry	Detect elevated levels of carboxyhemoglobin (from CO poisoning) and of methemoglobin (from benzocaine, nitrite, or chloroquine poisoning)

Many institutions have a urine screen to identify common drugs of abuse. These are often sent in cases of polysubstance ingestion, in instances of intentional or self-harm ingestions, or if suspicion exists for a substance use disorder. Comprehensive urine toxicology testing, which can identify an additional array of prescription and over-the-counter drugs or environmental chemicals, may also be available at some institutions. These may require special approval to order or may require delivery to a reference laboratory for analysis.

Toxicology testing can take hours to days to result, limiting its utility in time-sensitive situations. Furthermore, the care of most poisoned patients is supportive in nature (see Management), limiting the extent to which such tests change clinical management in the acute setting. Toxicology testing, however, can be useful in the following situations:

- Evidence for medicolegal cases
- Evaluation for child abuse or neglect
- Informing further mental health assessments or substance use disorder therapy
- If determination of a causative substance is desired or necessary

False positives and negatives can occur on toxicology testing, and not every possible substance can be identified with testing, even on comprehensive toxicology panels. Discussing toxicology testing with a poison specialist or with a toxicologist can be helpful to interpret results accurately.

Imaging

Imaging tests are individualized based on the type and magnitude of exposure and are often used to characterize complications of poisoning rather than for substance identification (Table 32.9).

Table 32.9 Imaging tests to consider for poisonings

Imaging test	Purpose
Airway radiograph	Evaluate for presence of radiopaque foreign bodies or for airway edema from caustic exposures
Abdominal radiograph	Identify presence of radiopaque substances (e.g., iron, lead, metallic foreign bodies) in acute ingestions. Evaluate for abdominal complications from exposures (e.g., ileus, bowel perforation)
Chest radiograph	Evaluate for pulmonary edema or for signs of aspiration related to exposure to certain substances (e.g., salicylates, hydrocarbons, irritant gases)
Cross-sectional imaging (e.g., CT, MRI)	Selectively used to evaluate for complications of poisonings (e.g., head CT for altered mental status)

Management

Supportive Care

Supportive care is the mainstay of poisoning management and includes several components:

- Addressing life-threatening conditions (e.g., intubation for airway protection)
- Reducing harmful effects related to the poisoning (e.g., dextrose-containing fluids for hypoglycemia)
- Addressing pain or discomfort (e.g., ondansetron to reduce nausea and emesis)
- Providing medical observation and monitoring (e.g., admission for observation, for trending laboratory studies, or for telemetry)

Supportive care is tailored to the suspected or confirmed exposure substance(s) and to the child's clinical status. Poison control can provide consultation to healthcare providers to help determine appropriate next steps in management. For critically ill patients, a rapid initial assessment followed by timely focused management may be required (refer to Chap. 42 for more information regarding an emergency department initial assessment).

Specific Therapies

In addition to supportive care, there may be cases where specific, poisoning-focused therapies are warranted. These therapies center on accomplishing one key task—reducing the bioavailability of a substance—that is, the proportion of the substance able to have an active clinical effect on the body. There are three main types of poisoning-focused therapies—decontamination, enhanced elimination, and antidotes. Often, such therapies are administered with consultation from a Poison Control Center or from a medical toxicologist.

Decontamination focuses on removing a poison from the body before it is absorbed and becomes bioavailable (Table 32.10).

Enhanced elimination is the concept of reducing bioavailability by increasing the rate that the substance is removed from the body (Table 32.11).

Antidotes work through a variety of mechanisms to counteract or to prevent the effects of a poison (Table 32.12). Contrary to popular belief, they are not used in the management of every poisoning due to their lack of universal availability and their potential risks.

Table 32.10 Decontamination therapies for poisonings

	Target substances	How it is performed	Considerations
Topical decontamination	Residual substance on skin and eyes (e.g., laundry detergent packet, household cleaner)	Generous irrigation with water or normal saline	Risk of aspiration if irrigating near the oropharynx
Activated charcoal	Nonpolar, water-soluble organic substances (e.g., digoxin, salicylates, phenothiazines)	Single dose of activated charcoal administered by mouth (PO) or by nasogastric tube (NG) to bind the substance of concern	Not effective for alcohols, metals, or polarized substances Most effective within 1 h of ingestion Aspiration and emesis risk
Whole bowel irrigation	Ingested substance for which activated charcoal is ineffective (e.g., iron, lithium)	High volume of polyethylene glycol or balanced electrolyte solution PO or NG to flush the substance from the GI tract	Aspiration and emesis risk May require electrolyte monitoring Ineffective if peristalsis compromised

Table 32.11 Enhanced elimination therapies for poisonings

	Target substances	How it is performed	Considerations
Urinary alkalinization	Weak acids (e.g., salicylates, phenobarbital)	Administration of intravenous (IV) sodium bicarbonate to ionize the substance, leading to its excretion in urine	May require electrolyte monitoring
Multiple dose-activated charcoal	Drugs that bind to charcoal and that have enterohepatic recirculation (e.g., carbamazepine, phenobarbital)	Multiple doses of charcoal PO or NG to interrupt enterohepatic circulation of the substance	Aspiration and emesis risk Ineffective if peristalsis compromised
Hemodialysis	Small, non-protein-bound molecular weight compounds (e.g., lithium, salicylates, theophylline)	Renal replacement therapy to remove the substance	Reserved for life-threatening poisonings Requires intensive medical monitoring

Table 32.12 Selected toxic substances and associated antidotes

Substance	Antidote(s)
Acetaminophen	N-acetylcysteine (NAC)
Anticholinergic agents	Physostigmine
Benzodiazepine	Flumazenil
Beta-blockers	Glucagon
Carbon monoxide	Oxygen
Cholinergic agents (organophosphates, carbamates)	Atropine, pralidoxime
Cyanide	Amyl nitrite, sodium nitrite, sodium thiosulfate, hydroxocobalamin
Digoxin	Digoxin-specific antibodies
Ethylene glycol, methanol	Ethanol, fomepizole
Iron	Deferoxamine
Isoniazid	Pyridoxine
Lead	Succimer, calcium disodium ethylenediamine tetraacetic acid, dimercaprol
Opioids	Naloxone
Sodium channel blockers	Sodium bicarbonate
Warfarin	Vitamin K

Summary of Selected Poisonings

Table 32.13 explores the clinical features and basic approach to managing several types of poisonings seen in the pediatric population.

Anticipatory Guidance

Anticipatory guidance for poisonings centers around prevention. Important concepts to share with a family either during a well-child check or as part of inpatient discharge counseling are summarized below:

- Store medications and potentially hazardous household consumer products out of reach and out of sight of children
- Keep medications and products in their original containers
- Install safety latches on cabinets that contain dangerous products
- Purchase products that come with child-resistant packaging or safety caps
- Be aware of potentially hazardous substances stored in common places, such as in a purse or backpack

Families should be encouraged to contact the Poison Control hotline at 1-800-222-1222 for help if their child is exposed to a potentially toxic substance.

Table 32.13 Summary of the clinical features and management for selected poisonings

Substance or substance class	Pathophysiology	Signs and symptoms	Management considerations
Acetaminophen	– Depletion of glutathione – Buildup of toxic metabolite N-acetyl-*p*-benzoquinoneimine in the liver	– 0–24 h: asymptomatic, nausea, vomiting, abdominal pain – 24–72 h: improved symptoms but rising liver transaminases – 72–96 h: liver failure, encephalopathy – >96 h: death or resolution of symptoms, possible permanent liver damage or failure	– Determine if NAC should be administered using Rumack-Matthew nomogram. The nomogram is most appropriate for use in one-time, single-substance acetaminophen ingestions within 24 h of presentation. – Monitor liver enzymes and liver function – Supportive care for symptoms
Blood pressure medication (e.g., angiotensin-converting enzyme inhibitor, beta-blocker)	– Multiple mechanisms—vasodilation, blood volume reduction, reduced cardiac output—depending on drug	– Decreased measured BP, poor peripheral perfusion, altered mental status	– IV crystalloid fluids – Vasopressors in cases refractory to IV fluids – Some substances may warrant additional therapies (e.g., calcium or insulin for calcium channel blockers) – Some blood pressure medications may cause hypoglycemia (e.g., beta-blockers)
Carbon monoxide	– CO tightly binds to hemoglobin and displaces oxygen – Interferes with oxygen-carrying capacity, delivery, and utilization	– At low levels: headaches, shortness of breath, dizziness – At high levels: hallucinations, confusion, coma, death	– Co-oximetry measurement to measure hemoglobin-bound CO – Provide 100% oxygen to displace CO – Hyperbaric oxygen is considered in severe poisonings to enhance CO displacement

Table 32.13 (continued)

Substance or substance class	Pathophysiology	Signs and symptoms	Management considerations
Caustic agents (e.g., acids, alkalis including laundry detergent packets)	– Acids cause coagulation necrosis – Bases cause liquefactive necrosis, which are deeper burns	– Pain, burning, and tissue damage – If ingested or aspirated, can cause vomiting, airway edema, or esophageal perforation	– Removal of any external caustic agent by rinsing with sterile water or normal saline – Supportive care for symptoms
Diabetes medication (e.g., sulfonylureas, insulin)	– Multiple mechanisms—including actions on beta cells or mimicking endogenous insulin—depending on drug	– May present with symptoms of hypoglycemia of varying severity, including tachycardia, nausea, vomiting, weakness, somnolence, coma, or seizure	– Provide dextrose and support with dextrose-containing fluids – Supportive care for symptoms
Iron	– Combination of direct damage to GI tract and systemic cellular toxic effects	– 0–6 h: abdominal pain, vomiting, diarrhea, GI bleeding – 6–12 h: Paradoxical resolution of symptoms – 12–48 h: Circulatory collapse, hepatorenal failure, acidosis – >48 h: Hepatic failure leading to death or resolution of symptoms with permanent liver damage or failure	– Potential whole bowel irrigation or gastric lavage in acute ingestions – Monitor iron level, liver enzymes, and liver function – IV deferoxamine for severe poisonings – Supportive care for symptoms

(continued)

Table 32.13 (continued)

Substance or substance class	Pathophysiology	Signs and symptoms	Management considerations
Lead	– Broad effects on cellular metabolism and on enzymatic function	– Anemia, abdominal pain, constipation, behavioral concerns – Lead poisoning often presents as a chronic, rather than an acute exposure	– Obtain lead level – Management of severe poisonings may include chelation agents (e.g., succimer, calcium disodium ethylenediamine tetraacetic acid)
Opioids	– Binding at opioid receptors to produce primarily inhibitory-type effects	– Opioid toxidrome (see Toxidromes)	– Naloxone is an effective antidote to opioid overdose; may require more than one administration depending on severity and type of opioid ingestion – Supportive care and respiratory support
Salicylates	– Stimulate respiratory center and uncouples oxidative phosphorylation	– Vomiting, tinnitus, tachypnea, agitation, delirium – Mixed respiratory alkalosis and metabolic acidosis	– Obtain serum salicylate level – Potential gastric lavage or activated charcoal administration in acute ingestions – Urinary alkalinization with IV sodium bicarbonate to enhance drug elimination – Dialysis in life-threatening poisonings

Application Exercises

1. A 16-year-old female presents to the ED after taking "a lot" of acetaminophen in an attempt at self-harm. She states that she took multiple pills 6 h ago but cannot recall the number and denies taking any other medications or substances. On exam, the patient has unremarkable vital signs and is tearful but well-appearing. A serum acetaminophen level is 175 μg/mL.

   A. What signs and symptoms of acetaminophen toxicity could this patient develop?

   B. Based on this patient's serum acetaminophen level and timing of ingestion, she is eligible for medical therapy. What is the appropriate antidote to administer in this situation?

C. Are there additional studies that may be helpful in the management of this patient?

Answers:

A. Patients experiencing acetaminophen toxicity may be asymptomatic. However, some can develop nausea, vomiting, or abdominal pain in the first 24 h of ingestion. In cases of severe toxicity, liver transaminases will begin to rise 1–3 days after ingestion and a subset of patients may progress to liver failure.

B. The Rumack-Matthew nomogram is used to determine if patients are eligible for antidote use for acetaminophen toxicity. Based on the patient's serum acetaminophen level of 175 μg/mL at 6 h post-ingestion, she is eligible for treatment. The appropriate antidote for acetaminophen toxicity is N-acetylcysteine (NAC). NAC therapy is most effective if given within the first 8 h of exposure though it may still reduce hepatic damage if administered beyond that timeframe.

C. Laboratory studies that evaluate for liver function and hepatotoxicity can be useful in acetaminophen ingestions. These include a basic metabolic panel, hepatic function panel, and coagulation studies. Given the patient's intent at self-harm, obtaining serum salicylate and ethanol levels as well as a urine drug screen would be justified.

2. A 3-year-old male is found on the kitchen floor unresponsive and is brought to the ED by family. On initial assessment, his vitals are heart rate 85, respiratory rate 11, blood pressure 86/43, temperature 98.3 °F and oxygen saturation 93% on room air. His exam is notable for bilateral pinpoint pupils, decreased bowel sounds, and movement to painful stimuli.
   A. Which toxidrome best fits with the patient's vital signs and exam?
   B. What is the appropriate antidote to administer in this situation?

Answers:

A. The patient is presenting with a classic opioid toxidrome, which is characterized by bradycardia, bradypnea, hypotension, pinpoint pupils, and decreased bowel sounds.

B. Naloxone should be administered to this patient to reverse the effects of a presumed opioid overdose. This can be administered intravenously, but also intramuscularly or intranasally, depending on the type of device and equipment available.

Further Reading

Calello DP, Henretig FM. Pediatric toxicology: specialized approach to the poisoned child. Emerg Med Clin North Am. 2014;32(1):29–51.

National Capital Poison Center. webPOISONCONTROL. Washington (DC): National Capital Poison Center; 2022 (updated 2022; cited 2022 Mar 14). Available from: https://www.webpoisoncontrol.org/

Renny MH, O'Donnell KA, Calello DP. Toxicologic emergencies. In: Shaw KN, Bachur RG, editors. Fleisher & Ludwig's textbook of pediatric emergency medicine. 8th ed. Philadelphia, PA: Wolters Kluwer; 2021. p. 1029–83.

Toce MS, Burns MM. The poisoned pediatric patient. Pediatr Rev. 2017;38(5):207–20.

Chapter 33
Seizures and Status Epilepticus

Maysa Hamade and Lisa Matlen

Background

Many seizure classifications exist: sorting by location (focal, generalized, or unknown), presence or absence of retained awareness, and motor or non-motor presentations. Examples can include tonic (stiffening), clonic (shaking), tonic-clonic (stiffening followed by convulsions), atonic (loss of muscle tone or "drop attacks"), absence (staring spells, behavioral arrest), myoclonic (brief sudden jerks), or epileptic spasms (infantile spasms—brief arm extension with head drop movements associated with developmental regression), among others. Focal onset seizures that start in one part of the brain may generalize and look like a typical tonic-clonic seizure or can appear like a staring spell. Seizures can be provoked by illness or injury to the brain or can be considered unprovoked. Epilepsy is defined by two or more unprovoked seizures occurring at least 24 h apart, or at least one seizure and additional estimated risk of recurrent unprovoked seizures exceeding 60% over the following 10 years.

Epidemiology

Approximately 1% of children will have at least one unprovoked seizure by age 14 with highest incidence within the first few months of life. While typically self-limited to a few minutes or less, sometimes seizures can be abnormally long. Status epilepticus is a term for seizures that do not self-abate and is classically defined as convulsive seizures lasting more than 5 min OR a series of seizures over the course

M. Hamade (✉) · L. Matlen
Department of Pediatrics, University of Michigan Medical School, Ann Arbor, MI, USA
e-mail: hamadem@med.umich.edu; lmatlen@med.umich.edu

N. Liao et al. (eds.), *Pediatric Rotations*,
https://doi.org/10.1007/978-3-031-59873-9_33

of 30 min between which there is no return to normal function. For non-convulsive seizures, prolonged is defined as longer than 10 min. The timepoint at which seizures are estimated to cause irreversible neuronal injury is 30 min for convulsive seizures. Status epilepticus occurs in approximately 10–20% of children with epilepsy.

Pathophysiology

Seizures can occur from a heterogenous group of etiologies including infectious, immune/autoimmune, metabolic, structural and genetic causes. Many genetic etiologies underlie epilepsy syndromes of childhood and tend to begin during specific ages in development (e.g., absence seizures in school-age children, juvenile myoclonic epilepsy in adolescence) although a specific gene has not been isolated for many of these syndromes. Known genetic syndromes are commonly caused by an ion channel abnormality. Structural etiologies are also frequent etiologies, with a wide range of possibilities including perinatal stroke or migration abnormalities (e.g., focal cortical dysplasia or heterotopia). Metabolic etiologies may include glucose transporter deficiency and mitochondrial disorders. Autoimmune causes are rare, yet serious, and may include anti-*N*-methyl-D-aspartate (NMDA) receptor encephalitis or Rasmussen encephalitis. Finally, infectious causes may include any number of central nervous system (CNS) infections including meningitis, encephalitis, and neurocysticercosis, among others.

Status epilepticus is caused by dysfunction of neurotransmitter systems such that there is excessive activation and insufficient inhibition. In a simple sense, glutamate (the major excitatory neurotransmitter in the brain) may be overactivated while gamma-aminobutyric acid (GABA, the primary inhibitory neurotransmitter in the brain) may function insufficiently. If status epilepticus is prolonged, cell death may occur.

History

The most important aspect of seizure evaluations is obtaining a detailed history of the nature and sequence of events surrounding the seizure. This will help classify the type and etiology of the seizure, predict risk for recurrence, and tailor treatment options. The primary points to gather are why the patient had a seizure (provoked or not; known history or not), the semiology (a description of what the seizure looked and felt like), the duration of the seizure, and information to distinguish the seizure from other diagnoses on the differential diagnosis.

Physical Exam

On arrival, a patient's vital signs as well as the basic ABCs (airway, breathing, circulation) should be assessed. The child may have already stopped seizing by the time they arrive to the hospital, but if they are still seizing, appropriate treatment should be provided. The physical exam during any witnessed seizure should include observations as listed in Table 33.1. If the seizure has stopped, perform a detailed neurologic exam as able, starting with a mental status assessment. In a first-time seizure, a newly discovered asymmetric exam, particularly with upper motor neuron signs (e.g., hyperreflexia) may confer a need for head imaging. An abnormal fundoscopic exam with papilledema would similarly compel urgent head imaging.

It is not uncommon for young children to have post-ictal drowsiness following a seizure. If they have a fever, they may also act more somnolent due to a febrile illness. However, patients with a febrile seizure should wake up rather easily. If a patient does not arouse with stimulation in the context of febrile seizure, this should raise suspicion for a potential CNS infection or ongoing subclinical seizure. Assessing for signs of meningismus is important as well; this includes nuchal rigidity (neck stiffness), positive Kernig's sign (the patient is laying supine with a thigh flexed at the hip and the knee flexed at 90 degrees; further extension of the knee is met with resistance), or positive Brudzinski's sign (when a patient is laying supine, the neck is forced into flexion and this causes the patient to flex at the hips). These signs are not very sensitive, and the lack of their presence does not rule out meningitis. Another important component of the neurologic exam is focal weakness, which would suggest that the seizure was focal rather than generalized.

Neurologic exam:

- Vital signs
- Mental status: level of alertness, speech, ability to answer questions and follow commands
- Cranial nerves including fundoscopic exam
- Motor strength, tone, and bulk
- Sensation
- Reflexes
- Coordination
- Gait

General exam: perform a detailed assessment to evaluate for etiologies of seizure (e.g., trauma, or evaluate further for causes of fever when present)

Table 33.1 Detailed history questions in pediatric patient presenting with seizure

Seizure phase	Question	Reasoning
Prodrome (prior to the seizure)	Does the child have any prior history of seizures? If so, did the child have fever with the seizures (i.e., were these febrile or afebrile seizures)?	Knowing about a prior diagnosis of epilepsy or febrile seizures will guide the framework for the rest of the interview. Afebrile seizures are managed differently given a higher risk for repeat afebrile seizures
	If the child has a history of epilepsy, what medications were they prescribed, what were their doses, and have they been taking their medications regularly?	Missed doses of medications are among the most common reasons for breakthrough seizures
	Was there any known ingestion of substances or medications?	Overdoses or inappropriately taken substances or medications can cause a seizure
	Is there a known family history of afebrile or febrile seizures?	A positive family history of seizures increases the likelihood of a diagnosis of epilepsy
	Was the child ill or have they developed signs of illness such as a fever?	Illness or fever will help formulate whether the seizure is considered provoked (or febrile) vs. unprovoked. This will determine whether it is necessary to treat with anti-seizure medications
	Was the child recently sleep-deprived?	Sleep deprivation is a common seizure trigger
	Has there been any recent head trauma?	Consider trauma in the differential. Don't forget to consider non-accidental trauma/child abuse
	Did the child experience any symptoms/signs (behavioral changes, difficulty staying focused, mood changes) or auras (numbness, headache, panic, odd smells or tastes, vision difficulties, déjà vu) before the seizure?	Some children experience early symptoms/signs or auras before a seizure. Characterizing these can help patients and caregivers anticipate possible seizures
Ictal stage (during the seizure)	Ask the witness to describe in detail the sequence of events surrounding the seizure from start to finish	If possible, have the witness demonstrate the types of movements observed. Ask for a video if available
	Was the child sleeping at the onset of the seizure?	This helps to guide risk of sudden unexplained death in epilepsy. The risk is higher when the patient has seizures during sleep
	How long was the seizure?	Duration will help inform if this was considered status epilepticus and inform treatment decisions about providing rescue medications

Table 33.1 (continued)

Seizure phase	Question	Reasoning
	Was the child conscious during the seizure?	Retained awareness could clue toward a focal-onset seizure or non-epileptic event
	Describe the face: were eyes open or closed? Deviated left, right, upward, or straight?	Closed eyes points toward non-epileptic event. Lateral gaze deviation can clue toward a focal seizure
	Describe the limbs: was there shaking, stiffening, limpness of one or more extremities? Did both sides move symmetrically? What was the amplitude and nature of any shaking or tremulous movements?	These questions best guide toward formulation of the type of seizure (e.g., tonic, tonic-clonic, atonic). Arrhythmic movements can guide toward non-epileptic event
	Were there any vocalizations?	Some seizures include an "ictal cry" or guttural throat noises
	Were there any repetitive or automatic movements (chewing, lip-smacking, or picking behaviors)?	Automatisms are a feature of some seizure types
	Was there loss of bowel or bladder control?	If present, can guide toward seizure and away from non-epileptic event
	Were there any oral injuries (tongue or cheek biting, bleeding from the mouth)	If present, can guide toward seizure and away from non-epileptic event
	Was a rescue medication provided? How long did it take after the medication was administered for the seizure to stop?	This information can be helpful in formulating future rescue medication plans
Post-ictal stage (after the seizure)	Was the child confused? Tired?	These are common features of a post-ictal state, particularly after generalized seizures
	Was there any weakness or paralysis on one side of the body after the seizure?	Some focal-onset seizures can result in a brief period of hemi-paralysis ("Todd's paralysis")
	How long did it take to regain full alertness?	A prolonged post-ictal state would guide more toward seizure and away from syncope

Laboratory Assessment/Imaging

The appropriate degree of imaging and laboratory investigation is tailored to the expected etiology. Electrolytes and blood glucose should be obtained; hyponatremia, hypernatremia, hypoglycemia, hypocalcemia, and severe diabetic ketoacidosis can cause a seizure. If an infectious etiology is present or suspected, appropriate infectious workup should be pursued. This may include a lumbar puncture in the appropriate clinical context (e.g., meningismus or other concern for intracranial infection). If ingestion is suspected, a toxicology panel should be performed. If significant head trauma was present, including signs suspicious for non-accidental trauma/child abuse, a non-contrast head computed tomography (CT) scan (and other evaluation for abuse, where applicable) should be performed. If syncope is on the differential, an electrocardiogram should be performed.

A routine electroencephalogram (EEG) is part of the standard workup for new-onset afebrile seizures, and long-term EEG monitoring may be incorporated for events of clinical uncertainty or suspected subclinical status epilepticus (e.g., prolonged post-ictal state or persistently altered mental status). EEGs are not typically useful for patients who solely have febrile seizures. In this situation, EEG may show abnormal slowing, but this does not typically have any bearing on the risk of future epilepsy. Additional workup for epilepsy includes a brain magnetic resonance imaging (MRI), particularly if there was a focal seizure or if the EEG demonstrates focal abnormalities. Additionally, epilepsy genetic testing should be offered to people with a diagnosis of epilepsy.

Studies:

- Point-of-care glucose
- Basic metabolic panel and magnesium
- Routine EEG ± long-term video EEG monitoring
- Anti-seizure medication trough levels when appropriate
- ± infectious studies
- ± toxicology panel
- ± non-contrast head CT scan

Outpatient (non-urgent) workup:

- Routine EEG (if not already performed)
- Genetic epilepsy panel (if the patient meets criteria for epilepsy)
- Brain MRI (for any focal-onset seizure or focally abnormal EEG)

Key Differential Diagnosis

Seizures can present a long differential diagnosis (Table 33.2), which can commonly be narrowed by a careful, detailed history.

Management

The treatment of seizures can be targeted to the etiology and usually includes anti-seizure medications, but may also incorporate epilepsy surgery and treatment of an underlying metabolic, autoimmune, or infectious disorder.

A daily anti-seizure medication should be initiated for any child who meets criteria for epilepsy. This is typically after two or more unprovoked seizures but may also be met if a child has at least one unprovoked seizure and additional risk factors such as epileptiform features on an EEG.

Table 33.2 Differential diagnosis: seizure mimics

Mimic	Similarities	Differences	Notes
Syncope	Loss of consciousness, may have convulsive-looking movements	Stereotypical prodrome, triggers	*Prodrome:* tinnitus, tunnel vision, vertigo, lightheadedness, palpitations, diaphoresis, pallor *Triggers:* dehydration, fasting, positional changes, prolonged standing
Staring spells (non-seizure)	May not respond to verbal and visual stimuli	Should respond to vigorous physical stimuli (tickling, pinching, picking up the child)	Common in children with attention deficit hyperactivity disorder
Motor stereotypies	May appear repetitively/ rhythmically	Retains full awareness, increase with excitement, distractible	E.g., hand flapping, rocking; often in young children
Motor tics	Some movements may look similar (e.g., upward gaze deviation)	Premonitory urge, suppressible, vary in semiology over time, increase with stress/ excitement	E.g., repetitive eye blinking, eye rolling, head tilting, but also more complex movements
Non-epileptic events	May look similar to epileptic seizures (e.g., apparent convulsions, episodes of loss of consciousness)	Closed eyes, irregular (arrhythmic) movements, pelvic thrusting, retained awareness despite bilateral movements, distractibility	Synonyms: psychogenic non-epileptic seizures, functional neurologic symptom disorder

The choice of an anti-seizure medication should be tailored to the type of epilepsy, administration route, and side effect profile. Certain medications only cover some seizure types: for example, ethosuximide is a first-line treatment for absence epilepsy, but is not effective in treating convulsions. Some medications are "broad spectrum" (e.g., levetiracetam) which may cover more than one epilepsy type, and others are intended for certain kinds of epilepsies such as focal-onset epilepsy (e.g., oxcarbazepine, carbamazepine, phenytoin, fosphenytoin). Broad spectrum medications can typically be chosen without negative consequences for any seizure type, but many medications for a focal epilepsy can provoke seizures in generalized epilepsies. However, targeted focal medications may be more effective for some focal epilepsies than broader spectrum medications.

If a child presents in status epilepticus using the practical definition of seizure > 5 min, rescue medications should be provided. If the patient is in a medical setting, a high-dose benzodiazepine (typically lorazepam, midazolam, or diazepam) intravenous (IV) should be administered. Most centers have a status epilepticus protocol; if the child is still seizing, they typically progress to a second dose of benzodiazepine, followed by a second-line agent: one of high-dose IV levetiracetam, fosphenytoin, or valproate. If these fail to stop the seizure, the child's status would be classified as refractory status epilepticus. At this point, if the child is not already intubated, they would undergo such at this point, while administering IV infusions midazolam or pentobarbital.

Any child who has a history of prolonged seizures or clusters of seizures should be provided a rescue medication for home. This may include rectal diazepam, intranasal diazepam or midazolam, or oral disintegrating tablets of clonazepam. Note that oral medications should not be given for convulsive status epilepticus both because administration through a clenched jaw would be practically difficult and absorption is not as fast through the oral route; however, oral medications are helpful for clusters of seizures. An exception is absence seizures; the child's baseline seizure frequency may be 100s per day, but these are typically not treated with rescue medications.

Anticipatory Guidance

For children with seizures, providing the caregiver and child appropriate first-aid measures is critical, as reviewed below. Most pediatric neurologists make seizure action plans for caregivers to give to the school and other caretakers. Rescue medications should be prescribed when indicated for both home and school, and instructions should be adequately discussed. For children with convulsive seizures, particularly those occurring at night or out of sleep, there is a small yet present risk of sudden unexplained death in epilepsy (SUDEP), and this should be gently discussed with families of children with epilepsy. Protective factors against SUDEP include treating epilepsy to reduce seizure frequency. Reviewing medications, doses, side effects, and evaluating medication compliance are all important upon follow-up evaluations. Children with seizures can participate in most activities including school and social events, but the most caution should be exercised around swimming/bathing and driving. Individuals with epilepsy should never bathe unattended or swim alone and should only swim in environments where they have 1:1 supervision by someone who can save them from drowning if the circumstance were to arise. There are also driving laws in many states such that individuals who have seizures must not drive for a particular period of time after a seizure or other impairment of awareness; check state laws.

Seizure first aid:

- Make sure the child is in a safe space (e.g., away from the top of a staircase or sharp objects)
- Put something soft such as a rolled-up shirt or blanket under his/her head
- Turn the child on his/her side
- Do not put anything in his/her mouth
- Do not restrain the movements
- Time the seizure
- Provide a rescue medication as prescribed (such as for seizure > 5 min)

– Call Emergency Medical Services for a seizure > 5 min, new onset seizure, cluster of seizures, or signs of difficulty breathing

Febrile Seizures: Simple and Complex

Background

A febrile seizure is defined as a seizure that occurs in a child aged 6 months to 5 years without history of afebrile seizures, in association with a fever (greater than 38 °C) and without an associated CNS infection. Febrile seizures are typically considered a benign condition but one that does carry a slightly higher risk for epilepsy than in the general population. Febrile seizures are relatively common, impacting anywhere from 2% to 10% of children. The peak age for occurrence is 18–24 months; most affected patients have their first febrile seizure before the age of 3 years.

Pathophysiology

It is important to distinguish between a seizure provoked by fever and that which is unprovoked because the evaluation, management, and prognosis of the patient is different between the two. Children with epilepsy are also more likely to have a seizure when ill with a fever because fever reduces the seizure threshold, but their management is different precisely because of their tendency toward unprovoked seizures.

There seems to be a genetic predisposition to febrile seizures; 25–40% of children with febrile seizures have a family history of febrile seizures. In most cases, there is no need for genetic testing and no described genetic variant or syndrome. A small fraction of patients who present with febrile seizures go on to develop atypical features such as febrile seizures occurring past the typical limit of 5 years of age or developing afebrile seizures as well. In these cases, genetic testing may be warranted.

There are other risk factors that have been studied as possible triggers for febrile seizures, such as infection with particular viruses including influenza A and human herpes virus type 6. Further possible associations that have been proposed include post-vaccination fevers, high peak temperature of fever, rate of rise of temperature, and low birth weight. However, none of these potential precipitants affect management in any meaningful way.

Simple and complex febrile seizures are differentiated by factors in Table 33.3. Simple febrile seizures are most common. Complex febrile seizures carry a higher risk of developing epilepsy compared to simple febrile seizures. This may relate to the higher likelihood of complex febrile seizures in neurologically abnormal

Table 33.3 Features consistent with simple febrile seizures vs. complex febrile seizures

	Simple	Complex
Only one "complex" feature is required in order to qualify as a complex febrile seizure		
Focality	Generalized	Focal
Length of seizure	<15 min	≥15 min
Number of seizures in 24 h	1	>1

children. Although workup is typically not required for either type of febrile seizure, some complex febrile seizures with higher risk features may prompt some additional evaluation at the discretion of the neurologist.

History

The most important part of an evaluation of a febrile seizure is the history provided by the caregiver. The history will help differentiate a provoked seizure from an unprovoked seizure and a simple febrile seizure from a complex febrile seizure, as well as determine any risk factors for epilepsy which may warrant further investigation or closer monitoring.

The most common history provided is that a child was ill with either a respiratory or gastrointestinal infection and either felt very warm to touch or had a documented fever. The caregiver will most often report stiffening of the child's extremities and possibly posturing or stiffening of his or her body. They will often report jerking or tremulousness of the child's extremities, either bilaterally or unilaterally.

It is important to ask approximately how long the seizure lasted. However, if it was the child's first seizure, caregivers may not know to keep track of the time and may give a rough estimate of the length of the seizure. It is also important to ask whether the seizure appeared to be generalized, which means involving both sides of the body equally and with altered awareness or loss of consciousness, or focal with stiffening or jerking of only one side of the body and possibly with eye or head deviation to the left or right. The number of seizures in a 24-h period is important information as well.

These specific questions are important to ask because they help to differentiate between a simple febrile seizure and a complex febrile seizure which has implications regarding future risk of epilepsy.

Physical Exam

See the above section

Laboratory Assessment/Imaging

Points of differentiation from afebrile seizures include not routinely obtaining EEG, brain MRI, and epilepsy genetic testing for simple febrile and most complex febrile seizures. EEG and/or MRI may be considered in some cases, particularly extraordinary complex febrile seizure cases, at the discretion of the neurologist or as indicated by institutional protocol.

Key Differential Diagnosis

In patients presenting with fever and a seizure, a CNS infection such as meningitis or encephalitis is an important possibility to consider, as discussed above. Patients with epilepsy can have seizures while febrile as well. In fact, the threshold to have seizures is lowered with illness and fevers as well as with sleep deprivation. It is possible that a child with an underlying epilepsy will have their first seizure during a febrile illness. In a child who is typically developing, without risk factors for epilepsy (family history of epilepsy or personal history of CNS infection, structural brain abnormality, or prematurity), and presenting within the typical age range for febrile seizures, there is no need for further evaluation for possible epilepsy.

Febrile myoclonus in infants can present as myoclonic jerks of the extremities and can be mistaken for seizure. If the history suggests that the child became limp rather than stiff, syncope is another consideration. The syncope may be due to dehydration or for another unknown reason.

Management

If a patient presents in febrile status epilepticus, as stated above, emergent treatment with IV anti-seizure medications should be initiated to abort the seizure. In cases where a CNS infection is highly suspected, the patient should be promptly treated with an appropriate IV antibiotic course. If the patient has returned to their baseline mental status or has only mild post-ictal drowsiness or malaise from a febrile illness, reassurance and anticipatory guidance is the only necessary management. Antipyretics such as acetaminophen or ibuprofen may be administered for the comfort of the child but there has not been good evidence to suggest that this helps prevent recurrence of febrile seizures.

It is reasonable to provide a rescue medication, such as rectal diazepam or intranasal midazolam, to caregivers of children who have had a prolonged febrile seizure (>5 min) as they are at a higher risk of having further prolonged febrile seizures. In patients who have recurrent febrile seizures that cause them to present frequently to the emergency department, intermittent benzodiazepines prescribed to be taken during a febrile illness can sometimes be useful at preventing febrile seizures. However, the sedating side effects of benzodiazepines must be taken into consideration. Pediatric neurologists rarely ever prescribe daily anti-seizure medications for patients with febrile seizures. There is no good evidence that this changes prognosis and is typically only used in a very small fraction of children with frequent febrile seizures, febrile status epilepticus, or other risk factors for epilepsy.

Anticipatory Guidance

Once other more dangerous diagnoses are ruled out and it is established that the patient has had a febrile seizure, counseling caregivers regarding what to expect and how to manage future febrile seizures is arguably the most important aspect of care. Pediatric neurologists sometimes see patients with febrile seizures either in the emergency department or as an outpatient consultation in clinic. Very often, emergency department physicians or primary care physicians provide anticipatory guidance to families whose child had a febrile seizure.

It is important to explain to families that when a child has a febrile seizure, they have a 20–40% risk of having further febrile seizures. Because of this risk, seizure safety precautions must be explained (seizure first aid). In addition, the child's overall lifetime risk of developing epilepsy slightly increases. The lifetime risk of epilepsy in the general population is approximately 1%. Simple febrile seizures increase this risk to approximately 2–3% and complex febrile seizures increase this risk to approximately 4–15%.

Parents may be worried that the febrile seizure has caused damage to their child's brain. Thankfully, febrile seizures do not cause any damage to the brain and do not seem to have any effect on development. However, there can rarely be long-term neurologic consequences in some patients with prolonged febrile seizures.

Application Exercises

1. A four-year-old child presents with a new onset seizure. Which of the following is anticipatory guidance that you should tell the child's parents?

   A. Turn the child on his/her side
   B. Hold the limbs down to prevent injury
   C. Secure the tongue to prevent the child from choking on it
   D. Give rescue medication at first sign of seizure

   Answer A: The child should be turned on his/her side because people can vomit when they seize and in such a case, the lateral position will help reduce the risk of aspiration. Restraining the child's limbs while they are seizing may cause injury to the child or the caregiver. One should not stick anything in a child's mouth while having a seizure: this can cause harm to the parent's hands or object that is inserted into the mouth. Furthermore, whatever is placed in the mouth could be bit off and choked upon. A person having a seizure cannot choke on or swallow their tongue; this is an old myth and untrue. A rescue medication should be given for seizures >5 min because this meets functional criteria for status epilepticus and represents a timepoint at which seizures would not be expected to self-abate.

2. An 8-month-old infant presents to the emergency department after his parents say he had one 3-min episode of whole-body stiffening and bilateral limb jerking while at home. This is the first time anything like this happened and his temperature is 39.2 °C. He is back to his baseline mental status and activity level with congestion and rhinorrhea that his parents say he picked up at daycare. He has a normal neurological exam for his age. What is the appropriate next step?

   A. Brain MRI
   B. EEG
   C. Lumbar puncture
   D. Reassurance and anticipatory guidance regarding seizure safety precautions

   Answer D: Reassurance and anticipatory guidance regarding seizure safety precautions. The description of this patient's febrile seizure is consistent with a simple febrile seizure since it involved generalized shaking and stiffening, was less than 15 min long, and only occurred once. Since he is back to his baseline neurologic status, there is no need for a lumbar puncture to assess for a central nervous system infection such as meningitis or encephalitis. He has a normal neurologic exam and had no focal features during his seizure, so a brain MRI is not necessary. An EEG is also not necessary for a simple febrile seizure.

Further Reading

Dang LT, Silverstein FS. Drug treatment of seizures and epilepsy in newborns and children. Pediatr Clin North Am. 2017;64(6):1291–308.

Fine A, Wirrell EC. Seizures in children. Pediatr Rev. 2020;41(7):321–47.

Seinfeld S, Shinnar S. Febrile seizures. In: Swaiman KF, Ferriero DM, Schor NF, Finkel RS, Gropman AL, Pearl PL, Shevell MI, editors. Swaiman's pediatric neurology. 6th ed. Elsevier; 2017. p. e1250–e6.

Chapter 34
Sepsis

Julia Lloyd and Maegan Reynolds

Background

Sepsis is a clinical diagnosis resulting from a body's response to an infection. The necessary components include a bacterial infection and an inflammatory response, which often leads to end organ damage and shock. Shock is characterized by any condition that leads to inadequate oxygen delivery to the tissues. Inadequate oxygen delivery may result from a decrease in the amount of blood delivered to the tissues, the oxygen content of the blood, or the cardiac output.

Pathophysiology

Shock is characterized by any condition that leads to inadequate oxygen delivery to the tissues. Clinical evidence of shock typically occurs as an end-stage of four possible processes: inadequate circulating volume of blood (preload), inappropriate distribution of intravascular volume (afterload), poor cardiac contractility, or obstruction to blood flow. The most common types of shock seen in pediatrics include hypovolemic shock, hemorrhagic shock, and distributive shock. Less common types are cardiogenic shock and obstructive shock (Table 34.1).

The most common etiology of shock in pediatric patients is sepsis. Sepsis is the body's overwhelming and potentially life-threatening response to infection. It can occur with any type of infection (bacterial, viral, fungal, etc.) and is mediated by various pro- and anti-inflammatory cytokines, resulting in an inappropriate response to infection by the body itself. Sepsis may encompass several of the different types

J. Lloyd (✉) · M. Reynolds
Department of Pediatrics, Nationwide Childrens Hospital/The Ohio State University College of Medicine, Columbus, OH, USA
e-mail: julia.lloyd@nationwidechildrens.org; maegan.reynolds@nationwidechildrens.org

N. Liao et al. (eds.), *Pediatric Rotations*,
https://doi.org/10.1007/978-3-031-59873-9_34

Table 34.1 Differentiation of different types of shock in pediatrics

Types of shock	Preload	Afterload (systemic vascular resistance)	Cardiac contractility	Perfusion (capillary refill)	Clinical examples
Hypovolemic	Low	High	Low	Long	Gastroenteritis, hemorrhage
Cardiogenic	High	High	Low	Long	Myocarditis, cardiomyopathy
Distributive	Low	Low	High	Short	Anaphylaxis
Obstructive	High	High	Low	Long	Tension pneumothorax, pulmonary embolism

of shock described above. Septic shock may have features similar to hypovolemic, cardiogenic, and/or distributive shock and cannot be put into a single category.

Sepsis exists along a continuum from mild to severe to shock. Sepsis can be conceptualized as the presence of infection plus organ dysfunction. New pediatric sepsis definitions no longer incorporate the Systemic Inflammatory Response Syndrome (SIRS) criteria.

Definitions:

- Infection can be defined as any suspected or proven infection - viral, bacterial, or fungal, as well as any clinical findings pathognomonic for infection.
- Sepsis is the presence of infection plus organ dysfunction.
- Septic shock is the presence of sepsis with cardiovascular dysfunction.
- Organ dysfunction associated with increased mortality includes:
  - Cardiovascular dysfunction includes age-based hypotension, the need for vasoactive medications, and impaired perfusion as measured by lactate levels.
  - Respiratory dysfunction is a spectrum from need for oxygen support up to and including invasive ventilation.
  - Hematologic dysfunction includes coagulopathy, including low platelets, prolonged International normalized ratio (INR), elevated D-dimer levels, or low fibrinogen levels.
  - Neurologic dysfunction includes an abnormal Glasgow Coma Scale (GCS) and pupil evaluation.

History

Taking a history in patients with sepsis can be difficult, as symptoms are often nonspecific and variable because sepsis may be caused by any type of infection. Fever or concerns for active infection should raise the question of sepsis in all patients.

Beyond that, patients may present with a wide variety of symptoms including vomiting and diarrhea, cough, congestion, sore throat, abdominal pain, respiratory distress, or malodorous urine. The initial complaints by patients/caretakers are frequently nonspecific, so it is imperative to maintain a high level of suspicion for sepsis.

There are many conditions that can predispose a patient to sepsis. In general, these are conditions that increase risk of infection or an inappropriate immune response. These include immunodeficiency (acquired or congenital), immunosuppression, some hematologic conditions, solid organ or bone marrow transplants, asplenia, or recent or ongoing chemotherapy. Additional risk factors include congenital or acquired chronic conditions such as cerebral palsy, sickle cell disease, cystic fibrosis, anatomic urinary tract abnormalities with frequent infections, or indwelling medical devices such as tracheostomy, ventriculoperitoneal shunts, or indwelling catheters or central lines. Neonates are also a special population at higher risk for sepsis.

There may be historical information shared by parents or caregivers that raise concern for end organ dysfunction or shock due to the decreased tissue perfusion with decreased oxygen delivery. Common signs include tachycardia and skin changes (i.e., delayed capillary refill, color change in the skin including red or purple patches, also known as mottling), decreased urine output, or declining mental status. The clinical history can help to rule out other etiologies of vital sign abnormalities or symptoms and determine the type of shock involved. It is important to ask about history of trauma, fluid losses (can be from multiple sources, such as vomiting, diarrhea, polyuria, hematemesis), fever or concern for infection, known immunosuppression, exposures to allergens, or known ingestions.

Physical Exam

The physical examination of children with sepsis can be challenging. Adding to the already challenging task of the basic pediatric physical exam, ill children can be difficult to distinguish from fussy or tired children. First and foremost, vital signs are critically important and may give you the first suggestion of sepsis. Next, the clinician should evaluate for presence of end organ dysfunction or shock (see Table 34.2).

Other than fever, tachycardia and tachypnea are often the first sign of sepsis seen in pediatric patients. Tachycardia is often noted in febrile children, so it is important to distinguish between the child who is simply febrile and the child who is tachycardic in an attempt to maintain their cardiac output in a shock state. The heart rate in a child with a fever can be elevated, but in general, tachycardia out of proportion to the degree of fever is concerning for the presence of a more significant process. Tachypnea may also be seen due to fever alone. Treating fever to see how the heart rate and respiratory rate change may help you distinguish between vital sign abnormalities due to fever vs. presence of shock, yet the time spent allowing for an antipyretic to take effect may lead to detrimental delays in treatment for sepsis patients. Therefore, in pediatric patients with fever and tachycardia/tachypnea, further careful review of the vital signs and exam findings is necessary.

Septic patients may present with shock. Tachycardia alone can be a sign of "compensated shock," where the body is successfully keeping up with metabolic demand by increasing the heart rate and therefore the cardiac output. Hypotension is a sign of advancing disease, and a late finding in pediatric patients, indicating significant decompensation, specifically "uncompensated shock." Pediatric patients are better able to compensate for cardiovascular dysfunction than adults and for longer periods of time. Children have better peripheral vascular resistance than adults and are better able to compensate for decreases in cardiac output using vasoconstriction. However, when this compensation is no longer adequate to keep up with the metabolic demand, the patient transitions into uncompensated shock manifested by hypotension. Uncompensated shock requires rapid recognition and treatment.

Septic shock is particularly confusing in pediatric patients. Most etiologies of shock present with exam findings due to peripheral vasoconstriction as the body attempts to increase afterload and preserve cardiopulmonary tissue perfusion. Skin perfusion may be altered as a result of vasoconstriction, so patients may be quite cold to the touch, particularly in the extremities. If this has occurred, capillary refill will often be delayed, and the patient may appear pale, mottled, or even cyanotic/blue. However, in pediatric septic shock, inappropriate vasodilation may occur. Some patients may present with bounding pulses, brisk/flash capillary refill, and diffuse erythema over their skin. As shock progresses, mental status changes occur. See Table 34.3 for physical exam findings associated with sepsis.

Table 34.2 Vital signs and physical exam findings of patients with sepsis

Vital sign changes	Fever Tachycardia Tachypnea Hypotension
Signs of peripheral vasoconstriction	Poor perfusion Delayed capillary refill Pallor, mottled skin appearance, or cyanosis
Signs of peripheral vasodilation	Bounding pulses Flash capillary refill Diffuse erythema

Table 34.3 Additional physical findings associated with sepsis

General physical findings associated with sepsis	• Ill or toxic appearance • Signs of dehydration: dry mucus membranes, decreased urine output, delayed capillary refill time, decreased skin turgor • Rigors/chills • Altered mental status can be seen with fussiness or irritability, or with decreased level of consciousness/arousal • Poor tone: seen more in infants • Peripheral edema due to capillary leak • Respiratory depression or failure
Specific exam findings which may indicate the source of infection in septic patients	• Seizures or meningismus from encephalitis or meningitis • Lung crackles or decreased breath sounds such as with pneumonia • Abdominal tenderness, distention, or rebound • Costovertebral angle or suprapubic tenderness such as with a UTI or pyelonephritis • Diffuse erythema or erythroderma such as with toxic shock syndrome or staph scaled skin syndrome • Petechiae or purpura, which may be specifically associated with pathogens or disseminated intravascular coagulopathy • Localized cellulitis or abscess

Key Differential Diagnosis

The differential diagnosis of sepsis can be extensive (Table 34.4).

Initial Evaluation of Shock

The mainstays of treatment for shock rely on the rapid identification of the source of shock and appropriate treatment (Table 34.5). For example, a patient with shock following a car accident is more likely to have hemorrhagic shock and would need initial resuscitation with infusion of intravenous fluids, followed by blood administration. Patients with obstructive shock would need treatment for the source of obstruction, such as a pneumothorax or a pulmonary embolus. Many types of shock respond well to fluid resuscitation, and a single crystalloid fluid bolus (20 mL/kg) should be initiated for patients with hypotension and other signs of shock. Cardiogenic shock is important to recognize quickly, as patients with cardiogenic shock may become fluid overloaded in a brief period of time. Patients with a high concern for cardiogenic shock should receive minimal fluids (initial bolus 10 mL/kg) and consider early pressor treatment.

Table 34.4 Differential diagnosis of sepsis

Neonates and young infants	Older children and adolescents
• Child abuse (abusive head trauma) • Hypoglycemia • Exogenous hyperthermia • Seizures • Congenital heart disease • Cardiac arrhythmias • Myocarditis or primary cardiomyopathy • Inborn errors of metabolism • Congenital adrenal hyperplasia • Malrotation with volvulus • Intussusception • Pyloric stenosis • Posterior urethral valves (or other obstructive uropathy) leading to urinary infections/urosepsis • Necrotizing enterocolitis • Severe dehydration • Water intoxication (improper mixing of formula) • Toxic exposures • Acute bilirubin encephalopathy • Viral hemorrhagic fever	• Anaphylaxis • Myocarditis or cardiomyopathy • Malrotation with volvulus • Diabetic ketoacidosis • Heat stroke • Serotonin syndrome • Neuroleptic malignant syndrome • Malignant hyperthermia • Toxic overdose or ingestion • Kawasaki's disease • Multisystem Inflammatory Syndrome in Children (MIS-C) • Baclofen withdrawal

Table 34.5 The initial management of a patient presenting with shock

Evaluation for patients presenting with signs of sepsis and/or shock	
Dedicated history and physical exam	• Dedicated questions and exam to identify the source of infection • Consider cardiogenic shock if new murmur, crackles on lung exam, hepatomegaly, splenomegaly
IV access	• IV fluid or blood resuscitation • Broad-spectrum antibiotics • Vasoactive medications
Laboratory evaluation	• Blood cultures • Complete Blood Count (CBC) • Basic metabolic panel • Liver function tests • Consider inflammatory markers: Procalcitonin, Erythrocyte Sedimentation Rate (ESR), C-reactive protein (CRP), and lactate
Imaging studies	Consider based on history and physical exam • Chest X-ray to evaluate for pneumonia • Ultrasound for cellulitis or abscess • CT or ultrasound for abdominal pain
Additional testing guided by history and physical examination results	Consider urine testing, lumbar puncture, respiratory viral panel, etc.

The evaluation for sepsis is relatively standardized. Basic laboratory samples and imaging studies targeted to the source of infection, and signs/degree of inflammation should be done. Procalcitonin levels are emerging as a useful tool in the diagnosis of sepsis. Additional labs may be indicated based on the patient's medical history and symptoms. For example, a patient with notable diarrhea may warrant a stool culture or gastrointestinal pathogen polymerase chain reaction (PCR) panel. Imaging studies are ordered based on patient symptoms/complaints. For instance, chest X-rays can be utilized both to evaluate for pneumonia or other respiratory infections and evaluate cardiac size and shape to better distinguish the possible etiology. Identifying a source for infection can be crucial to treatment of sepsis, so all attempts with laboratory or imaging studies to find the source should be pursued.

Sepsis is caused from many types of infection so, identifying the involved system (i.e., respiratory, renal, GI) from the history, exam, and lab results can help guide the development of a differential diagnosis. For example, a patient presenting with primarily gastrointestinal symptoms may have a differential of appendicitis, small bowel obstruction, intestinal perforation, gastroenteritis, or enterocolitis. A patient presenting with primarily respiratory symptoms may have pneumonia, a viral infection, bronchiolitis, or wheezing/asthma exacerbation. When the only presenting symptoms are fever and abnormal vital signs, the source of the infection and thus the differential can be more difficult to delineate. Casting a broad net is valuable in searching for a source of infection and may involve additional laboratory evaluation and imaging. Given the nonspecific vital sign changes and exam findings seen in sepsis, many children may have noninfectious sources of shock. Keeping a broad differential while simultaneously providing initial stabilization and often empiric treatment for the most life-threatening causes is key.

Management of Shock

The first hour of treatment for patients with sepsis is sometimes known as "the golden hour," as rapid initiation of treatment is associated with better outcomes. Significant work has been done in standardizing treatment for sepsis, and many institutions have protocols or bundles in place to increase the standardization of care. The basic components of a sepsis treatment bundle include obtaining a blood culture and administering IV fluids and broad-spectrum antibiotics (Table 34.6). Rapid fluid resuscitation includes rapidly infused boluses of crystalloid fluids at 20 mL/kg, up to and over 60 mL/kg until perfusion improves or signs of fluid overload appear (except in patient with cardiogenic shock). Lactated Ringers' solution and normal saline solution are both acceptable and frequently utilized.

Table 34.6 Recommended broad-spectrum antibiotics for patients with sepsis

Patient category	Recommended antimicrobials
Neonates 0–28 days	Ampicillin Gentamicin ± Cefixime, Acyclovir
Neonates 29–60 days	Ampicillin Ceftriaxone ± Vancomycin, Acyclovir
Infants and children >60 days	Ceftriaxone ± Vancomycin
Patients with high-risk conditions	Cefepime or Zosyn Vancomycin Amikacin
Febrile neutropenia	Cefepime ± Vancomycin
Sickle cell anemia + fever	Ceftriaxone ± Vancomycin

Blood cultures should ideally be obtained prior to initiation of antibiotics, but the provider should not delay antibiotic administer to obtain blood cultures. In children with concerns for septic shock, every attempt should be made to start antibiotics within 1 h of recognition. Empiric broad-spectrum therapy should be utilized initially, and antibiotic coverage can then be narrowed once appropriate identification of the bacterial source has been made.

After initial resuscitation with IV fluids and treatment with broad-spectrum antibiotics, if shock symptoms are not yet reversed, consideration of vasoactive agents should be undertaken. Epinephrine and norepinephrine are the most commonly used vasoactive agents. Epinephrine is more commonly used in pediatric patients when treating cardiac dysfunction or when there are signs of low cardiac output or "cold shock" with mottling, cool extremities, and delayed capillary refill. Norepinephrine is used more frequently in patients who need an increased systemic vascular resistance or peripheral vasoconstriction to respond to shock. If an additional vasoactive medication is needed, for children who require high-dose catecholamines (epinephrine, norepinephrine), the recommended second-line agent is vasopressin. In patients who may have adrenal insufficiency (i.e., patients on chronic steroids, patients on chemotherapy or other immunosuppressive medications) or patients with fluid-refractory shock, it may be reasonable to administer IV steroids such as hydrocortisone.

Finally, additional ventilatory support should be considered in patients with sepsis. In patients who present with vital sign abnormalities, hypotension, altered mental status, or other signs of end organ dysfunction, early intubation should be considered to decrease metabolic demand. Although there are no direct recommendations for intubation, many providers will choose to proceed with intubation in patients with fluid-refractory, catecholamine-resistant septic shock, regardless of whether they have signs of respiratory failure.

Special Considerations

Neonates

Neonates represent a special population in the evaluation for sepsis. Historically, infants less than 90 days have an increased risk for a serious bacterial illness (SBI). Approximately 8–12% of infants who present with fever (temperature ≥ 100.4 °F or 38 °C) are found to have an SBI, defined as bacterial meningitis, bacteremia, urinary tract infection (UTI), or pneumonia. We distinguish between SBI (serious bacterial illness) and IBI (invasive bacterial infection) with IBI only representing meningitis or bacteremia. IBI represents less than 1–2% of all SBI in the United States. Approximately, 90% of infants with fever will have a viral infection, but they are at a significantly higher risk for complications and long-term sequalae of missed bacterial infections. Neonates have higher rates of morbidity and mortality from sepsis due to decreased immune response and lack of immunizations compared with older infants and children.

Over the past 40 years, the epidemiology of neonatal SBI has changed significantly. Specifically, the recommended vaccination series against *Haemophilus influenzae* type B (HiB) and *Streptococcus pneumoniae (*Pneumococcus) in neonates at 2 months of age have played a role in that change. Additionally, *Streptococcus agalactiae* or Group B *Streptococcus* (GBS) screening in pregnant patients and treatment during delivery of mothers with positive GBS screens has significantly reduced the incidence of GBS infection in neonates. The most common bacteria found in SBIs currently are *Escherichia coli (E. coli), Staphylococcus aureus,* viridans streptococci, and gram-negative bacilli.

Neonates also represent a special population regarding a high risk for vertical transmission of herpes simplex virus (HSV) during vaginal delivery. Previously, disseminated HSV in neonates had a high mortality of up to 80–90%, and HSV meningitis had a mortality of 50%. This has improved with the use of acyclovir, but the infection still represents up to a 30% mortality risk and concern for long-term developmental delays. To reduce the risk of HSV infection in infants, pregnant females with either historical or new HSV lesions are started on empiric anti-viral medications during the third trimester and have elective caesarean sections to prevent vertical transmission.

The clinical features of sepsis in infants can be vague. All infants who present with a fever (measured temperature ≥ 100.4 °F or 38 °C) should be evaluated for sepsis or SBI. Providers should obtain rectal temperatures in all infants less than 3 months, and caregivers are encouraged to use rectal thermometers for accurate measurement. However, infants can also present with surrogate markers for infection including hypothermia (literature varies regarding specific temperature but usually ≤36 °C or 96 °F), hypoglycemia, lethargy, decreased feeding, or other changes in behavior. The clinical assessment of an infant before 6–8 weeks of age when they are able to give a social smile can be challenging. Thus, providers are encouraged to have a high index of suspicion for sepsis or occult infection in infants presenting with any changes in behavior in addition to fever.

The care and evaluation of febrile infants have changed significantly in the past 40–50 years. Historically, all infants less than 90 days presenting with fever had blood, urine, and cerebral spinal fluid studies and were admitted on empiric antibiotics for minimum 48 hours. This presented a significant emotional and financial burden to families and hospitals. Gradually, clinical decision rules have decreased the number of infants undergoing lumbar puncture, empiric antibiotics, and admission. Newer tools incorporate the use of inflammatory markers, specifically procalcitonin and C-reactive protein (CRP) in addition to white blood cell count (WBC), absolute neutrophil count (ANC), and urinalysis (UA) for risk stratification. Laboratory advances have allowed for the detection of a viral source of infection through tools such as rapid antigen testing for influenza, respiratory syncytial virus (RSV) and Covid-19, or rapid PCR respiratory viral panels. Additionally, rapid blood and cerebral spinal fluid (CSF) testing with PCR panels for viral and bacterial sources has significantly speed up the time to rule out a bacterial source of sepsis in infants, leading to significant decreases in antibiotic use and duration of hospitalization.

A landmark clinical practice guideline was published in 2021 by the American Academy of Pediatrics (AAP) regarding the evaluation of febrile infants and is significantly changing the way providers approach neonatal sepsis. These guidelines separated infants into 3 groups based on their days of life, 0–21 days, 22–28 days, and 29–60 days. A full sepsis work-up (blood, urine, CSF), admission, and empiric antibiotics are only recommended for infants 0–21 days. The decision-making for the 22–28 day group and 29–60 day group factors in inflammatory markers, specifically CRP, procalcitonin, and ANC to determine which infants would be at higher risk and would thus need a lumbar puncture, antibiotics, and/or admission. The AAP guidelines also lay out inclusion and exclusion criteria including special considerations for infants at high risk for HSV (Table 34.7). The role of positive viral testing remains controversial, but the AAP does note this is an ongoing area of research focus and providers are encouraged to use results in addition to clinical appearance, individual and community health resources, and shared decision-making when determining patient management.

Unfortunately, while the 2021 AAP febrile infant guidelines were the first unified position statement for the risk stratification and management of febrile infants, there

Table 34.7 Symptoms frequently seen in neonates with high risk for HSV infection

Neonates at high risk for herpes simplex virus (HSV) often exhibit these symptoms
• Known exposure to HSV (i.e., maternal genitourinary infection)
• Hypothermia (temperature <36 °C (96 °F)
• Toxic appearance or hemodynamic instability
• Severe respiratory distress or apnea
• Abnormal neurologic exam or seizure-like activity
• Vesicular or petechial rash
• Conjunctivitis
• Abnormal labs: CSF WBC >14, low platelets, elevated alanine aminotransferase (ALT)

are several limitations and nuances with these guidelines. First, there are several inclusion and exclusion criteria including recommending exclusion of infants with bronchiolitis or recent immunizations. The guidelines only address infants with fever, they do not provide recommendations for infants presenting with other clinical concerns for sepsis including hypothermia, lethargy, etc. The guidelines also advocate for the use of CRP and procalcitonin for risk stratification, though many clinical practice environments still do not have rapidly available access to these tests, in particular procalcitonin. Additionally, there are many places in the published clinical guideline that use vague language such as "may perform lumbar puncture" or "may observe at home." As such, a high degree of variability in interpretation and implementation may occur. The guidelines also factor in social situations such as limiting discharges in infants 22–28 days and 29–60 days who live far from pediatric care, have no access to primary care follow-up, or parental (dis) comfort with at home observation. The significant advances in care include: (1) risk stratification with inflammatory markers, (2) separating infants 22–28 days into a separate risk stratification algorithm, (3) overall decrease in recommendations for lumbar punctures, admissions, and empiric antibiotics. Notably, for all infants 0–60 days, AAP recommends that if a source of infection is identified at 24–36 h, narrow to targeted treatment, consideration of discontinuing antibiotics if a viral source identified, and consideration of discharge if the infant is well appearing.

Overall, providers must keep a high index of suspicion for sepsis and occult infection in infants less than 60 days. Multiple newer algorithms and the 2021 AAP guidelines provide improving guidance on the work-up and treatment for this special population. Risk stratification and management of febrile infants remain an active area of research, and the literature will likely continue to be updated and modified at a rapid pace.

Meningitis/Encephalitis

Meningitis/Encephalitis is the presence of a bacterial or viral pathogen within the cerebrospinal fluid (CSF). Similar to other infections, with the availability of the HiB, pneumococcal and meningococcal vaccines, the incidence of bacterial meningitis/encephalitis has declined significantly in children except for infants <60 days. Meningitis can now be more often found in adults than children over 2 years of age. The most common pathogen in infants remains *E.coli* and Group B Strep, in contrast to adolescents, who have higher rates of *Neisseria meningitides*. The most common viral pathogens include enterovirus and parechovirus, with a high incidence of HSV in infants and adolescent/young adults.

A CSF infection may present with different symptoms based on the area of inflammation and type of pathogen. Meningitis, when compared to encephalitis, is more commonly bacterial and diagnosed more often in unimmunized children or those with predisposing conditions such as indwelling medical devices (VP shunts, cochlear implants) or primary or secondary immunodeficiency. It can also be seen following trauma or recent infections with hematologic spread such as sinusitis or mastoiditis. Meningitis causes inflammation of the meninges, and children often present with fever, headache, lethargy, vomiting, and neck stiffness. Nuchal rigidity or the inability to flex the neck is seen in 60–80% of pediatric patients with meningitis, though classic meningeal signs are more easily elicited in older children and teens. Nuchal rigidity can also be present with other conditions such as a retropharyngeal abscess.

Encephalitis is primarily from viral pathogens and causes brain parenchyma inflammation. The clinical presentation is often vague with fever plus more neurologic symptoms, such as confusion, behavior or personality changes, seizures, movement disorders, or neurologic deficits including weakness, numbness, or vertigo. Focal neurologic symptoms such as focal weakness, numbness, or bowel/bladder dysfunction are rare, but may be seen with encephalitis. Since fever, lethargy, and headache are common clinical signs in all types of sepsis, the provider must be vigilant to consider meningitis or encephalitis. If key signs are present such as nuchal rigidity or focal weakness, meningitis and encephalitis must be ruled out.

Meningitis and encephalitis are diagnosed through testing of the CSF, so all patients with clinical suspicion for meningitis/encephalitis must undergo a lumbar puncture for diagnosis. The rates of morbidity and mortality associated with bacterial meningitis rise with delays in treatment. Because of this, the lumbar puncture (LP) should be performed as early as possible to facilitate treatment. If there is consideration for increased intracranial pressure (ICP), providers should also consider obtaining head imaging such as a head CT prior to performing an LP. Generally, infants with open fontanelles should not require head imaging as they are at lower risk for herniation. If there is evidence for cerebral edema on imaging, the LP should not be performed due to the risk of herniation. Once obtained, CSF should be sent for gram stain and bacterial culture, cell count with differential, glucose, and protein, and PCR studies as available. Table 34.8 outlines CSF results in patients with meningitis. Readily available tests for viral sources include HSV, enterovirus, or

Table 34.8 Cerebrospinal Fluid (CSF) results in patients with meningitis

	Normal	Bacterial meningitis	Viral meningitis	Fungal/TB
Appearance	Clear	Turbid/cloudy	Clear	Clear/fibrin web
Opening pressure (cm H2O)	<20	>30	Normal	Slightly elevated
Protein (mg/dL)	15–45	>100–200	<200	50–500
Glucose (mg/dL)	50–80	<45	Normal	<80
White blood cell count (mm^3)	<5	>500–1000	<1000	100–500
Cell differential		>80% neutrophils	Lymphocytes	Lymphocytes/ monocytes
Gram stain/Alt test	Normal	50–90% positive	Normal HSV, Entero, PCR panel positive	Fungal wet prep, alternate antigens

parechovirus. However, broader PCR panels testing for bacterial and viral pathogens are commercially available and expanding at a rapid pace. PCR panels can identify bacterial pathogens within hours rather than waiting 24–48 h for positive bacterial cultures. Distinguishing between viral or bacterial meningitis/encephalitis can be challenging especially if it was a traumatic LP, i.e., the CSF sample contains a large amount of blood and red blood cells (RBCs).

Meningitis/encephalitis treatment is based on the pathogen identified and severity of illness. As noted, the primary consideration is initial resuscitation and stabilization of shock symptoms. While ideally an LP should be obtained prior to starting antibiotics to assist with later interpretation of CSF cultures to guide the antimicrobial treatment plan, resuscitation of an unstable patient takes priority. If there is a high index of suspicion for bacterial meningitis, antibiotics should be given as soon as possible and not delayed to perform an LP. Broad-spectrum antibiotics such as ceftriaxone, cefepime, or vancomycin are some of the most common empiric antibiotics administered. If there is a high suspicion for HSV based on age (infants < 60 days or teens), clinical scenario, or lab testing, treatment with acyclovir should be started in addition to the antibiotics. Steroids, specifically dexamethasone, were previously advocated for administration prior to antibiotics for children with high concern for meningitis as it was shown to decrease the long-term rates of hearing loss. Given the declining rates of *Haemophilus influenzae* infections with the introduction of the HiB vaccines, this is no longer general practice though can be considered on a case-by-case basis. Duration of antimicrobial therapy is based on the pathogen identified, but ranges from 10 to 21 days. Pediatric patients with meningitis/encephalitis should be monitored long term for sequela. Though mortality rates have been reduced to less than 5–10%, children remain at high risk for hearing loss, seizures, spasticity, or developmental delay. Thus, all children treated for meningitis and/or encephalitis, in particular bacterial meningitis, should have a hearing screen following discharge, regular developmental screening, and additional evaluation as indicated.

Bacteremia

Bacteremia is defined as the presence of bacteria in the bloodstream. Rates of bacteremia are lower than previously seen as a result of widespread vaccination efforts. Historically, more than 70% of occult bacteremia was related to *Streptococcus pneumonia* but since the introduction of the pneumococcal vaccine, cases of occult bacteremia have dropped significantly. Similarly, cases of *Haemophilus influenzae* type B have dropped following introduction of the HiB vaccine.

Clinical findings of bacteremia can vary from the absence of any signs/symptoms beyond fever (known as occult bacteremia), through the spectrum of sepsis to manifestations of septic shock. Typically, bacteremic patients present with fever and nonspecific symptoms such as malaise. In the absence of laboratory evaluation, it is very difficult to ascertain which pediatric patient with a fever has bacteremia versus which patient has a viral infection. Current research is exploring the utilization of inflammatory markers such as procalcitonin in distinguishing patients with a bacterial infection from other causes of fever.

Management of bacteremia should follow the pathways described below. Children who are unimmunized or have not yet completed the recommended immunization series against *Streptococcus pneumoniae* and *Haemophilus influenzae* type B are at increased risk of bacteremia, as are those patients with high-risk conditions. In patients who are unimmunized or incompletely immunized, providers should consider a broader work-up for presentation with fever without a source, which may include complete blood count, blood cultures, and inflammatory markers. If the inflammatory markers or white blood cell count are elevated, consideration should be given to empiric administration of parenteral antibiotics such as ceftriaxone which will provide 24 h of coverage to allow additional laboratory testing to result. These patients require follow-up within 24 h for reevaluation and adjustment of treatment based on clinical status and any new test results. If the inflammatory markers and white blood cell count are normal, antibiotics may be held with continued outpatient monitoring.

Patients who are completely immunized may require additional testing such as urine analysis and cultures, chest radiographs to evaluate for pneumonia, or other viral testing to evaluate for a source. However, if the patient remains well appearing with no symptoms beyond fever, it is reasonable to discharge these patients home with detailed instructions, including asking the family to return if the child appears sicker, develops any signs of dehydration, further symptoms emerge, or the fever is still present after 48 h. Completely immunized, immunocompetent patients with a fever do not necessarily need a blood count or culture obtained unless they have additional signs/symptoms of sepsis.

Pyelonephritis

Pyelonephritis is the more severe version of a urinary tract infection which can occur when bacteria spreads upwards from the bladder, into the ureters and kidneys. It can be very difficult to differentiate cystitis, or infection of the lower urinary tract, from pyelonephritis, which is infection of the upper urinary tract. Particularly in children under the age of 2 years, symptoms can be nearly identical. In older children, fever may be present in both cystitis and pyelonephritis, but is more commonly present in pyelonephritis. The general term urinary tract infection (UTI) may be used to encompass both cystitis and pyelonephritis.

When obtaining the history of a patient with sepsis, it is important to ask about risk factors for and prior history of UTI. Risk factors include any bowel/bladder dysfunction, vesicoureteral reflux (VUR), renal or bladder structural abnormalities, or family history of frequent UTI, VUR, or other abnormalities. Infants and toddlers will often present with nonspecific signs and symptoms similar to many reviewed earlier in this chapter. Often, fever and fussiness are present. Family members may report additional symptoms such as foul-smelling urine or other non-urinary complaints such as vomiting or diarrhea, but these complaints have not been shown to correlate with the presence of bacteria in the urine. Older patients may share more specific signs and symptoms, including abdominal pain, back or flank pain, urinary frequency or dysuria, and occasionally urinary incontinence. The constellation of fever, chills, and flank pain is highly suggestive of pyelonephritis in older children.

A high index of suspicion should be maintained for a urinary source of infection in patients presenting with sepsis or shock. Urosepsis is a commonly seen phenomenon, and the threshold for obtaining a urine analysis and culture should be low. The presence of leukocyte esterase and/or nitrites in a urinalysis can be indicative of a urinary tract infection, although leukocyte esterase is a nonspecific finding that may be seen in many other conditions. The presence of nitrites indicates that UTI is likely. A patient with sepsis who is found to have nitrites on urine analysis should be treated for a urinary source. Providers should send the urine for culture to ensure appropriate antibiotic treatment, but fluid resuscitation and empiric antibiotics coverage should not be held if the patient presents with sepsis.

Conclusion and Key Points

- Sepsis is a common cause of shock in pediatrics, and it is important to consider sepsis in any patients presenting with infectious symptoms.
- Classic physical exam findings of sepsis include vital sign abnormalities, as well as abnormalities of perfusion and capillary refill.
- Remember that early recognition and treatment improve outcomes.
- It can be hard to anticipate the clinical course of any type of shock, particularly sepsis, until response to initial resuscitation and identification of etiology is made.
- Early recognition and treatment of sepsis is typically achieved through rapid fluid resuscitation and IV antibiotic administration.

Application Exercises

1. A 2-year-old female presents with fever. Which of the following findings are most concerning for septic shock?

   A. Fussy with exam but consoles with mother, doesn't want you to examine her
   B. Flushed, tachycardic, and whiny
   C. Frequent urination with large wet diapers and recent weight loss
   D. Difficult to arouse with mottled extremities and capillary refill 4–5 s

   Answer D: Answer choice A might be seen in any developmentally appropriate 2-year-old. Choice B could be concerning; however, these symptoms can also often be seen in any patient with a fever, and these symptoms are not necessarily concerning for septic shock. Choice C is more concerning for high blood sugar and concerns for diabetes mellitus. The physical findings described in choice D would be highly concerning for the presence end organ dysfunction (decreased perfusion) and uncompensated shock, specifically septic shock in a patient with a chief complaint of fever.

2. An 8-year-old boy presents with fever to 103 °F, cough, decreased urine output, and rapid breathing. He is sleepy on exam with cool, mottled extremities. Your initial management should include:

   A. CBC, type and screen, and blood transfusion for hemoglobin <8
   B. Epinephrine IM, steroids, and albuterol
   C. Labs including blood cultures, empiric antibiotics, chest X-ray, and rapid boluses of crystalloid fluids
   D. Chest X-ray, bedside echocardiogram, and cardiology consult

   Answer C: This patient is presenting with symptoms concerning for septic shock. The appropriate first treatment includes obtaining blood cultures, giving empiric antibiotics, and give boluses of crystalloid fluids (20 mL/kg at a time) with frequent re-assessment. Answer A would not address the patient's fever or exam findings and is not traditionally be used for patients with sepsis. Choice B is appropriate for a patient presenting in distress related to status asthmaticus. Epinephrine is the most important treatment for anaphylaxis, and other symptomatic treatments may include antihistamines and albuterol. Choice D would be appropriate if your primary concern was cardiogenic shock.

Further Reading

Fleischer & Ludwig Textbook of Pediatric Emergency Medicine. Chapters on infectious disease emergencies and shock; n.d.

Gomez B, Mintegi S, Bressan S, et al. Validation of the "step-by-step" approach in the management of young febrile infants. Pediatrics. 2016;138(2):e20154381.

Pantell RH, Roberts KB, Adams WG, Dreyer BP, Kuppermann N, O'Leary ST, Okechukwu K, Woods CR Jr. Subcommittee on febrile infants. Evaluation and management of well-appearing febrile infants 8–60 days old. Pediatrics. 2021;148(2):e2021052228. https://doi.org/10.1542/peds.2021-052228.

Weiss, et al. Surviving sepsis campaign international guidelines for the management of septic shock and sepsis-associated organ dysfunction in children. Intensive Care Med. 2020;46:510–67.

Chapter 35
Social Determinants of Health

Padma Swamy and Julie Krueger

What Are Social Determinants of Health (SDOH)?

Social determinants of Health (SDOH) as defined by Healthy People 2030 are "conditions in the environments where people are born, live, learn, work, play, worship and age that affect a wide range of health, functioning, and quality-of-life outcomes and risks." *Have you ever wondered how these types of conditions alter how a child grows and learns?* It is different for every child and every situation, but research has shown that these determinants alter a child's long-term health outcomes. To break down these determinants further, SDOH are often grouped into five domains including: (1) economic stability, (2) education access and quality, (3) health care access and quality, (4) neighborhood and built environment, and (5) social and community context. Sometimes these broad groupings make these issues challenging to understand, but specific examples can make it more comprehensible. For example, having local job opportunities, safe housing, clean water, access to education, and safe neighborhoods; as well as living in a place without inequities, racism, and violence are all considered SDOH. SDOH are often driven by a wide set of forces such as economics, social policies, and both local and national politics and need to be considered on how they affect not only a single individual, but also an entire community. The five major SDOH domains listed above can be broken down into more specific areas of focus as shown in Table 35.1.

P. Swamy (✉) · J. Krueger
Goldberg Center for Community Pediatric Health, Children's National Hospital, Washington, DC, USA
e-mail: pswamy@childrensnational.org; jkrueger@childrensnational.org

N. Liao et al. (eds.), *Pediatric Rotations*,
https://doi.org/10.1007/978-3-031-59873-9_35

Table 35.1 Five major SDOH domains

Economic stability	Education access and quality	Health access and healthcare quality	Neighborhood and built environment	Social and community context
Poverty	High school graduation	General access to health care	Access to healthy foods	Social cohesion
Employment	Higher education	Access to primary care	Quality of housing	Civic participation
Food insecurity	Language and literacy	Access to dental care	Crime and violence	Discrimination
Housing instability	Early childhood education	Health literacy	Environmental conditions	Incarceration

Adapted from: Healthy People 2030 [1]

How Do These Factors Impact Children?

SDOH impact children in a variety of different manners, some effects are similar to how they impact adults, and others are more explicit, especially in areas such as development, education, and childhood maltreatment. A prime example of an SDOH that has a known major connection to a child's growth and success is food insecurity. Food insecurity has been connected directly to both poor growth and obesity. Food insecurity can also detrimentally impact other areas such as school performance as a child has a hard time focusing and learning when hungry. Certain pediatric medical conditions are severely impacted by social determinants of health including pediatric asthma, obesity, sickle cell disease, and mental health. *Consider why these specific diagnoses would be altered by SDOH.* For example, it is easy to understand how limited or no access to quality primary or specialty health care can greatly affect a child's trajectory of growth. This concept is especially relevant in areas such as delayed access to dental care and identification of developmental delays.

Certain populations of children and adolescents such as LGBTQ+ youth, American Indian/Alaska Native Tribal populations, immigrant and migrant populations, populations with disabilities, racial and ethnic minority populations, and those with limited English proficiency are more affected by SDOH. For these populations, it is even more important for providers and the general healthcare field to find ways to reach out to them and address the effects of high rates of challenging SDOH that can be very difficult to overcome on one's own. In addition, working to establish better policies at local, state, and national levels to help address SDOH that greatly affect these populations is an important step that we can help support as health care professionals.

What Can Be Done?

Now that we have discussed examples of social determinants of health and how SDOH impact child health, *what can you do as a medical student?* This next section provides guidance for medical students in the clinical setting to address pediatric SDOH. The first section addresses SDOH screening and practical pearls for the clinical setting, and the second section addresses next steps after receiving screening results and highlights programs across the nation that are addressing SDOH.

SDOH Screening

There are existing SDOH tools for the pediatric setting. In choosing and evaluating the appropriateness of the tool, it is important to consider: (1) the purpose of the screening tool: food insecurity versus mental health concerns versus child abuse, (2) the age of the child: using a screening tool for a child less than 5 is not appropriate for a teenager, (3) who is to complete or respond to the survey: child versus caregiver, and (4) how the tool is to be administered: verbal screening tool versus a paper screening tool versus online form. Note that low literacy can impact results when using a paper or online screening tool. Please see Table 35.2 for common pediatric SDOH screening tools.

What Are Some Factors to Consider Before Starting SDOH Screening?

When determining the appropriateness of SDOH screening in a patient encounter, it is important to consider the patient's/caregiver's thoughts and feelings regarding the screening as well as your own comfort with and perspectives of screening (Fig. 35.1). If you are uncomfortable with screening, patients and caregivers can sense it. It is understandable to feel uncomfortable with these topics as they are not part of our daily social communication and can be incredibly personal and private. Here are some of the possible concerns from the patient and provider perspective.

How Do You Screen for SDOH?

Like the HEADDS exam, screening for SDOH can be awkward at first. There are available techniques to create a trusting environment for screening:

Table 35.2 Common pediatric SDOH screening tools

Tool	Setting*	Age	Person screened	Screening method	Domain
SEEK PSQ	Clinic	0–5 years	Caregiver	Paper, tablet, computer	Economic stability, health and health care, family context
iScreen	Hospital	0–18 years	Caregiver	Computer, tablet, phone interview, face-to-face interview	Economic stability, education, health and health care, neighborhood and built environment, social and community context, family context
HealthBegins Upstream Risks Screening Tool	Clinic	N/A	Caregiver	Face-to-face interview	Economic stability, education, health and health care, neighborhood and built environment, social and community context, family context
FMI	Home	0–5 years	Caregiver or social worker	Face-to-face interview	Economic stability, family context
ASK Tool	Clinic	0–18 years	Caregiver	Paper	Economic stability, education, neighborhood and built environment, family context
IHELP	Hospital	N/A	Caregiver	Face-to-face interview	Economic stability, education, health and health care, neighborhood and built environment, family context
WE CARE	Clinic	0–10 years	Caregiver	Paper	Economic stability, education, family context
FAMNEEDS	Clinic	0–18 years	Caregiver	Paper	Economic stability, education, health and health care, neighborhood and built environment, social and community context, family context
Child ACE Tool	Clinic	0–5 years	Caregiver or physician	Paper	Education, family context
Social history of Standard Well Child Care template in HER	Clinic	0–5 years	Caregiver	Face-to-face interview	Economic stability, neighborhood and built environment, family context
Health related social screening social problems screener	Clinic	0–6 years	Caregiver	Computer, tablet	Economic stability, health and health care, neighborhood and built environment, family context

Adapted from: Screening Children for Social Determinants of Health: A Systematic Review published in the journal of Pediatrics [2]

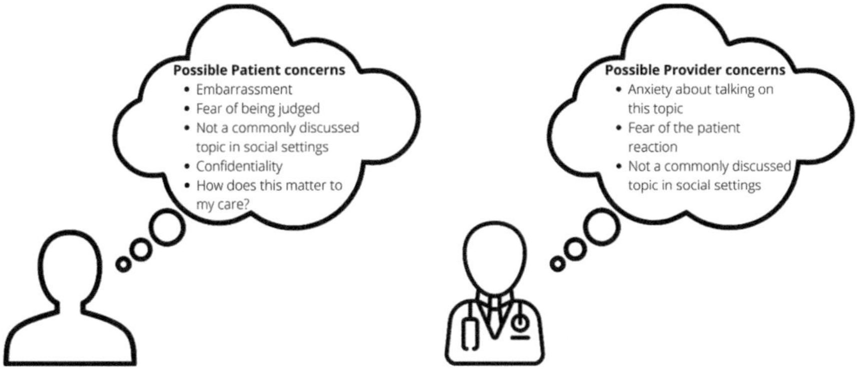
Possible Patient concerns
• Embarrassment
• Fear of being judged
• Not a commonly discussed topic in social settings
• Confidentiality
• How does this matter to my care?
Possible Provider concerns
• Anxiety about talking on this topic
• Fear of the patient reaction
• Not a commonly discussed topic in social settings

Fig. 35.1 Patient and provider concerns to consider prior to SDOH screening. Adapted information from curriculum in MedEdPORTAL Portal [3] with figure designed by P. Swamy using Canva

Table 35.3 Examples of verbiage to use when screening for a sensitive topic

Technique	Example language
Normalizing	"Our clinic cares for many immigrant families. We ask all our families questions about their immigration history."
Transparency	"The journey of immigration can impact a child's health which is why we are asking you these questions. We will not be asking about your immigration status and nor we will put that into the medical record. The information that will be discussed will be private."
Permission	"I understand that these questions may make people feel uncomfortable. If you do not feel comfortable, you do not have to answer the question. Is it okay if I ask you these questions?"

1. *Normalizing* helps frame the screening for the patient (2)
2. *Transparency* allows the patient to understand why you are screening (you may include types of questions to be asked and what you will do with the information) (2)
3. *Permission* which is most important for creating a trusting environment (allowing caregivers to not respond is key in preserving patient autonomy and building trust) (2).

Table 35.3 shows examples of verbiage that can be used when screening for a sensitive topic such as immigrant health.

In addition to these techniques, sometimes utilizing close-ended questions may help the patient when discussing sensitive topics. For example, if we look at the questions "Do you feel safe at home?" vs "Has anyone hit, punched or you at home?" The first question is vague, and if you intend to screen for intimate partner violence, the first option may not result in the answer you need. You may elicit that the neighborhood is unsafe, and that may be all you want to discuss in this clinic visit. It is important to also recognize what is within our scope as health care professionals and when something is better addressed by other experts.

Referral to Programs

As health care providers, we do not practice alone but rather within systems and teams. It is important to be aware of various resources within your community that can help address the needs of your patients. In the United States, we operate with the idea of a medical home which is a central place to receive all your medical care. However, children live in neighborhoods and partnerships with co-located non-medical organizations can better address SDOH. It takes time to build rapport with various agencies/organizations. But as a student, you can start by connecting with the social worker on your team to learn about community organizations. Social workers have a wealth of knowledge on available community organizations, services, and resources. Another way to learn about various resources in the community is by volunteering in organizations like the food bank or with a group that has a mission about which you are passionate.

What Are the Ethics of SDOH Screening?

Like anything we do in medicine, it is important to understand and evaluate how SDOH screening impacts our patients, the patient–provider relationship, and the provider/healthcare team. Utilizing the 4 principles of medical ethics, consider the impact of SDOH screening.

Beneficence

Beneficence, which means, "to do good." As healthcare providers, we have an ethical duty to ensure that interventions, including SDOH screening, are of benefit to the patient. *How do you think SDOH screening benefits the patient?*

1. *Addressing external factors*: A population's health is impacted to a greater extent by social factors than medical care. A patient may spend 30 minutes in a visit with you or the health care team, but in every other moment of their life, their health is influenced by factors outside of the clinic. By considering external factors, you can better address the health of the patient.
2. *Barriers to treatment*: As you read about your patient's condition(s), sincerely consider factors that may impact their ability to comply with a treatment regimen. As you work closely with your patient with mutual goals, your satisfaction in seeing progress can help lower your risk for burnout.
3. *Trusting patient–provider relationship*. Through discussion of these important issues, you can build a stronger patient–provider relationship which benefits the patient's care.

See Table 35.4 for case example below of how learning about the SDOH screening can benefit families.

Table 35.4 Case example of SDOH screening benefits

Case #1: You are in clinic caring for a 13-year-old girl who has history of asthma and poor symptom control despite your best efforts. You have sent her medications to the pharmacy for pick up. At the follow up, you notice that her asthma is still not under good control, and she has not followed the recommendations that you set. What factors may have impacted her compliance?	
Medical cost	Her family may have financial issues impacting their ability to afford the medication. Mother may have 2 jobs making it difficult for her to go to the pharmacy and pick up the medications
Health literacy	Mother may not understand the importance of the medication and/or how to use the inhaler. In addition, this patient may be on 2 inhalers which can be confusing for mother to know when to use which inhaler
Poor living environment	She may live in a house with mold, cockroaches, and other infestations which all negatively impact her asthma symptoms
Case #1 Continued: What can you do to better address her asthma? Through learning about what impacts her compliance you can make some specific, tailored recommendations	
Medical cost	You may utilize the discount pharmacy program to send the medication, and mother can use a coupon to lower the cost of the medication. You may look into a pharmacy that does home deliveries
Health literacy	You may utilize a program like the IMPACT DC clinic at Children's National. This clinic focuses on asthma education and provides information to families on their medications and how to take them. The longer visits allow patients to be better able to learn about asthma/triggers/management
Poor living environment	You may refer the child to a medico-legal partner to address the home situation. Modifying the home situation may have a larger impact on the child's health than increasing asthma medications

Non-malfeasance

Non-malfeasance means that our interventions should not cause harm to the patient. As healthcare providers, it is important that we are aware of how SDOH screening can unintentionally cause harm (Fig. 35.2). *What are some potential negative consequences of SDOH screening?*

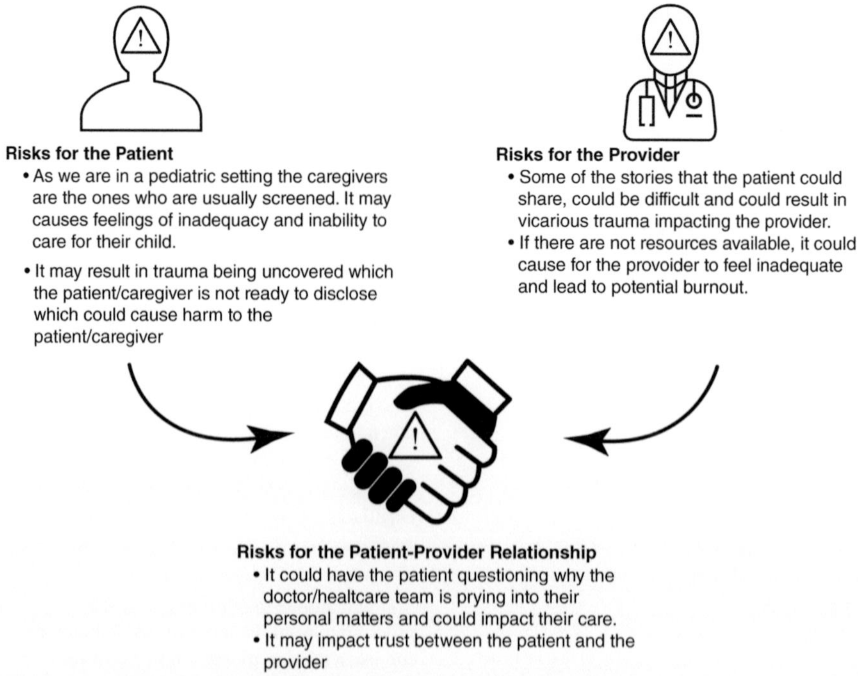

Fig. 35.2 Potential risks of SDOH screening. Figure designed by P. Swamy using Canva

Autonomy/Resilience/Permission

Autonomy is an important concept in medical ethics and one that is especially key to SDOH screening. Autonomy is the recognition of the patient/caregiver as an individual who is capable of making their own decisions. For many of us in health care, we pursued this career to be able to help others. Sometimes this idea of altruism can conflict with the principle of autonomy. It is important to recognize that it is the patient's decision if they would like help or not. By asking patients if they would like a resource, you are empowering the patient to make decisions about their health.

As health care professionals, we are often evaluated by our thoroughness in taking a medical history. However, some questions may cause harm. By giving patients/caregivers the permission to not answer a question, we are preserving the idea that the person is an individual. While counter-intuitive to allow them to not answer a question, this process can build trust, and in a future encounter, a patient may feel comfortable sharing.

Justice

Justice is this principle of health equity that all people are receiving the resources they need for equitable health(5). SDOH screening is a key in achieving health equity by directly addressing the health inequities that exist in our communities. To ensure equity, it is important to evaluate the tools that we are using for SDOH. Ensuring that the screening tools are meeting the needs of a population is key. Equity also includes that a tool is available to different people of different backgrounds. Having tools translated in a culturally sensitive manner and having options for those that have limited literacy are ways to preserve justice. Many of the current tools ask the patient/caregiver if they want assistance with a certain need. In addition to preserving autonomy, this question is important as it also preserves equity, builds trust, and decreases the power dynamics that can occur between the patient and provider.

Defining Adverse Childhood Experiences (ACEs)

Adverse Childhood Experiences, often referred to as ACEs, are defined as "traumatic events or occurrences that children experience before the age of 18 that can have lasting impacts on their mental health, physical health and general well-being." Many ACEs are reflected by SDOH, but ACEs also include individual traumatic events such as losing a family member, having a mentally ill parent or an incarcerated parent, or surviving a stressful life experience. SDOH are not usually random events but are related to the child's surrounding community and economic status of the family. There is notable clinical research that connects the topics of SDOH, ACEs, and health outcomes. ACEs research focuses on how stress affects a person both in a moment and long term, but this can vary greatly from one individual to another. *Have you ever wondered if stress can be a positive influence?* Well, in certain situations it can be. The body's adrenaline response can put a person on high alert to perform (at a performance or during a big test), and if focused correctly, can help one be at their best. However, there is a continuum of stress. Figure 35.3

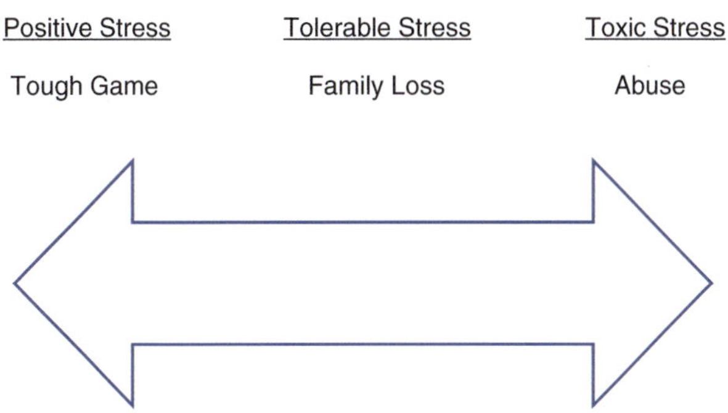

Fig. 35.3 Continuum of stress

demonstrates the range of positive to toxic stress. And again, this may be different for different people. In the middle of the continuum, "tolerable stress" includes stressors that are only manageable if one has supports and resilience measures in place.

Exposure to toxic stress can have serious impacts on the developing bodies and minds of children. Toxic stress on the nervous system can lead to changes in the brain which increases risk of attention deficits, challenges with self-regulation and hyperactivity, intellectual disabilities, anxiety, and poor memory. The cardiovascular system under long-term toxic stress can lead to elevated blood pressure and inflammation which can result in cardiovascular damage and increased risk of future heart disease and stroke. Toxic stress also has been shown to weaken our immune system leading to higher rates of infection and autoimmune disease. Finally, toxic stress effects on the endocrine system can impact growth and development. Examples include increased risk of obesity and changes in timing of puberty. As demonstrated by research and published by the CDC, if ACEs are addressed effectively there can be reduction of negative outcomes in adulthood. The CDC has research that shows certain health conditions such as depression are lessened, health risk behaviors such as smoking and heavy drinking are lowered and socioeconomic challenges such as unemployment are shown to be lessened.

Research on ACEs is relatively new and limited. In 1998, the Centers for Disease Control and Prevention (CDC) in conjunction with Kaiser Permanente published the first landmark ACEs study of 17,000 adults that demonstrated a connection between childhood traumatic events and adult health outcomes. Using a survey method, researchers assigned an "ACE score" by summing the number of adversities each participant reported (Table 35.5) [4].

Table 35.5 Original 10 categories of ACEs

	Category	Description
1	Physical abuse	Non-accidental harm
2	Sexual abuse	Sexual exploitation
3	Emotional abuse	Verbal, mental, and psychological maltreatment
4	Physical neglect	Failing to provide for a child's basic needs
5	Emotional neglect	Failing to provide social support or ignoring a child
6	Mental illness	Living with a relative with mental health
7	Incarcerated relative	A child grows up with an incarcerated parent
8	Mother treated violently	Witnessing domestic violence
9	Substance abuse	Living in a home with substance users can be unsafe
10	Divorce	Growing up with parents that are divorced or divorce leading to custody battles

Adapted from Felitti VJ, Anda RF, Nordenberg D, Williamson DF, Spitz AM, Edwards V, et al. Relationship of childhood abuse and household dysfunction to many of the leading causes of death in adults. The Adverse Childhood Experiences (ACE) Study. Am J Prev Med. 1998;14(4):245–58

The original 10 categories of ACEs included:

In the study, over two-thirds of responders had experienced at least one ACE and almost 20% had experienced four or more. The researcher's noted that a higher ACE score was a risk factor for chronic disease as an adult (10). These chronic diseases included both higher rates of behavioral and mental health problems as well as higher rates of morbidity and mortality from physical health problems such as heart disease and cancer. This was one of the first formal studies that connected stressful life events to future poorer health, and truly broke open a new field in medicine. This study had limitations. First, it only looked at 10 ACEs in adults, and these were limited to occurrences in one's own home. The researchers did not consider the possible impact of social and community factors such as violence, discrimination, poverty, or bullying on these health and mental health outcomes. The study was also deficit-based and did not investigate resiliency factors that can combat the stress response and make certain toxic stress more tolerable for certain individuals. This is an area in which a lot of recent research has been focused. Despite having some limitations, this study propelled a wide variety of research studies focused on stress response and building resiliency. This truly groundbreaking study brought to the public a concept that many health care providers recognized already but didn't have research or data to back up their theories.

Most ACEs research since that time has utilized this 10-category ACE questionnaire, but some have been modified for specific populations. For example, the Pediatric ACEs and Related Life-events Screener (PEARLS) has been adapted for children and adolescents and includes screening for ACEs and additional adversities.

The more recent ACEs research has had a relatively positive spin regarding children and adults being able to overcome past experiences if provided the correct tools to build resiliency. It has also been noted that although the specific number of ACEs may be directly graphed to match with long-term challenges, at an individual patient level, the number of ACEs is less relevant when compared to how that individual is supported to overcome the ACE. For example, one ACE such as parent divorce can lead to many challenges for one person, but for another, this major life change can cause a minimal effect on their life if they have coping skills and support to overcome this stressor. It can even have a positive effect on the child, for example, if a parent was abusive to their partner and now the child is removed from this exposure. Despite these findings at an individual level, large studies have shown consistently that (1) ACEs are universal, (2) ACEs often occur together, and (3) there is often a dose–response relationship to number of ACEs and health problems.

Screening for ACEs

Screening for ACEs can help clinicians assess risk of stress to their patients, but more importantly, it can help guide supportive responses and allow a clinician to provide resources, if available. Identifying specific ACEs should not be the final outcome of interest, but rather a method to build an ACE score that can act as a proxy of toxic stress. Based on the appropriateness for the situation, ACEs screening data can be collected in a de-identified or an identified manner. In de-identified screening, the patient views a list of ACE categories/questions and gives their provider a total score, but they don't identify specify which ACEs they or their child have experienced. Identified screening is the opposite, where a patient checks off the actual ACE(s) they or their child have experienced. Identified screening can initially seem more useful to the provider as more focused strategies can be applied; however, it has been found that de-identified screening has often facilitated higher rates of disclosure and higher patient comfort with the process. Screening for ACEs is similar to SDOH screening as discussed above, as it needs to be transparent regarding the goal and framed correctly for patients. The questions asked are very personal, and it can be traumatizing to a patient/caregiver to see a long list of challenges they have lived through. Screening should never add to the trauma and stress a patient has already experienced. To avoid any re-traumatization, the purpose of screening must be framed in a culturally sensitive and transparent manner. Parents/caregivers should understand that by gathering this information, the provider hopes to help recognize resilience factors that can be used or augmented in the patient to combat the negative effects of ACEs.

An example of an ACEs screener that was built by the California Surgeon General's Clinical Advisory Committee is shown in Fig. 35.4.

Advocacy

Parents, communities, physicians, and policy makers can all help prevent ACEs and improve SDOH for families and communities. We can protect children from SDOH and ACEs by providing support to build resiliency in their communities. Advocacy focused on decreasing the effects of SDOH and ACEs should be performed at the individual, community, and national level. Many physicians believe that being an advocate at the individual level can be the most rewarding because of the personal connections made and helping a family into a more positive situation can show immediate benefit. One example of this is a healthcare provider helping a family into a safer and healthier housing situation by writing letters to landlords and the local housing board outlining the negative environmental effects of the current home on the child. Although we need advocacy at the individual level, addressing these issues on a broader scale with policy changes and community programming is often more effective, as it improves lives for larger numbers of individuals. *Can you think of ways you can advocate for your patients to address SDOH or ACEs?* Advocating for better education options, more parks, and healthy food options that are lower priced or free from taxes are initiatives that have been successful in many communities at the national level.

It is important to consider how you want to advocate for your patients. You can focus on the patient in front of you, and in reality, all physicians in all specialties do this to some extent. You can also get involved in the local chapters of your

Our relationships and experiences—even those in childhood—can affect our health and well-being. Difficult childhood experiences are very common. Please tell us whether you have had any of the experiences listed below, as they may be affecting your health today or may affect your health in the future. This information will help you and your provider better understand how to work together to support your health and well-being.

Instructions: Below is a list of 10 categories of Adverse Childhood Experiences (ACEs). From the list below, please place a checkmark next to each ACE category that you experienced prior to your 18th birthday. Then, please add up the number of categories of ACEs you experienced and put the *total number* at the bottom.	
1. Did you feel that you didn't have enough to eat, had to wear dirty clothes, or had no one to protect or take care of you?	☐
2. Did you lose a parent through divorce, abandonment, death, or other reason?	☐
3. Did you live with anyone who was depressed, mentally ill, or attempted suicide?	☐
4. Did you live with anyone who had a problem with drinking or using drugs, including prescription drugs?	☐
5. Did your perents or adults in your home ever hit, punch, beat, or threaten to harm each other?	☐
6. Did you live with anyone who went to jail or prison?	☐
7. Did a parent or adult in your home ever swear at you, insult you, or put you down?	☐
8. Did a parent or adult in your home ever hit, beat, kick, or physically hurt you in any way?	☐
9. Did you feel that no one in your family loved you or thought you were special?	☐
10. Did you experience unwanted sexual contact (such as fondling or oral/anal/vaginal intercourse/penetration)?	☐
Your ACE score is the total number of checked responses	

Do you believe that these experiences have affected your health? ○ Not Much ○ Some ○ A Lot

Experiences in childhood are just one part of a person's life story.
There are many ways to heal throughout one's life.

Please let us know if you have questions about privacy or confidentiality.

5/5/20

Fig. 35.4 California Surgeon General's Clinical Advisory Committee ACEs screener [5]

specialty-specific medical organizations, and this can lead to your involvement with national organizations. Other methods such as writing Op-Eds in local and national papers, voting to support politicians that support views that promote healthy living, and building relationships with these politicians once they are elected are all ways to advocate for your patients by addressing SDOH and ACEs.

Dr. Mona Hanna-Attisha is a pediatrician who noticed that her patients were having elevated lead levels in the community and increased behavioral issues. She then took that data and published it; however, she did not stop there. She disseminated her data at the state and national level. She showed that a change in the water source in Flint, MI had resulted in an increase in lead levels for her patients. She advocated and used different strategies including meeting with state representatives, op-eds, and publishing data in an academic journal to make the change for this community. You can also similarly impact the population with whom you are working. As a physician, your views, opinions, and experiences carry significant weight within the medical and lay community. It is your opportunity to use this weight to improve the lives of your patients.

References

1. Office of Disease Prevention and Health. Social Determinants of Health. United States of America: Healthy People 2030. Office of Disease Prevention and Health Promotion (US); (reviewed 2023; cited 2023 Aug. 31). Available from: https://health.gov/healthypeople/priority-areas/social-determinants-health
2. Sokol R, Austin A, Chandler C, Byrum E, Bousquette J, Lancaster C, et al. Screening children for social determinants of health: a systematic review. Pediatrics. 2019;144(4):e20191622.
3. McBride R. Talking to patients about sensitive topics: communication and screening techniques for increasing the reliability of patient self-report. MedEdPORTAL. 8:9089.
4. Felitti VJ, Anda RF, Nordenberg D, Williamson DF, Spitz AM, Edwards V, et al. Relationship of childhood abuse and household dysfunction to many of the leading causes of death in adults. The Adverse Childhood Experiences (ACE) Study. Am J Prev Med. 1998;14(4):245–58.
5. California Surgeon General's Clinical Advisory Committee. Adverse childhood experience questionnaire for adults. California: California Surgeon General's Clinical Advisory Committee. (updated 2020 May 5; cited 2023 Aug 31. Available from: https://www.acesaware.org/wp-content/uploads/2022/07/ACE-Questionnaire-for-Adults-De-identified-English-rev.7.26.22.pdf)

Chapter 36
Trauma Injuries

Kristin Stukus, Morgan Wurtz, and Daniel Scherzer

Injury remains the most common cause of death and disability in childhood. Morbidity and mortality from injury surpasses all major diseases in children and young adults, making trauma the most serious public health and healthcare problem in this population. A general understanding of the mechanisms and patterns of injury in pediatric patients is essential to provide best care for affected children.

Anatomic, physiologic, and social factors contribute to a child's vulnerability to trauma. Anatomic factors include small size and mass, large head relative to body, compliant chest wall and relatively unprotected abdominal organs. Physiologic factors include increased metabolic rate, more insensible losses of water and heat, and less water and energy reserves. Socially, children are particularly vulnerable to child abuse (non-accidental trauma) because of their dependence on others, reduced ability to communicate and diminished capacity to protect themselves relative to the adults around them.

Major/Multisystem Trauma Overview: Initial Assessment

Most injuries involve one system or one body region. For injuries that are severe or involve multiple regions or systems, a systematic trauma approach is used, defined below.

For major or multisystem trauma, the initial assessment begins with primary and secondary surveys. Though the focus of this chapter is on trauma, the components

K. Stukus (✉) · M. Wurtz · D. Scherzer
Division of Emergency Medicine, Department of Pediatrics, Nationwide Children's Hospital, The Ohio State University, Columbus, OH, USA
e-mail: Kristin.Stukus@nationwidechildrens.org; Morgan.Wurtz@nationwidechildrens.org; Daniel.Scherzer@nationwidechildrens.org

N. Liao et al. (eds.), *Pediatric Rotations*,
https://doi.org/10.1007/978-3-031-59873-9_36

of this initial assessment are applicable to a broad range of clinical problems. The primary and secondary surveys encompass a rapid physical exam to screen for systemic compromise and multiple injuries. The primary survey consists of a rapid assessment of airway, breathing, circulation, and disability. During the primary survey, the patient is fully exposed and then recovered for privacy and warmth. The mnemonic ABCDEF (airway, breathing, circulation, disability/dextrose, exposure/environment, family presence) is used to guide the sequence. The secondary survey is a rapid head-to-toe exam in which every observable and readily palpable body part is examined. In a stable patient, the initial assessment usually takes less than 3 min. In an unstable patient, the primary survey may reveal a problem requiring immediate intervention, and the secondary survey may be temporarily deferred.

The *primary survey*, commonly referred to as the "ABC's," starts with the airway, which is the most important part of the initial assessment and deserves the most attention. The airway assessment consists of three components: maintainability (function), patency (structure), and risk. Airway assessment begins with evaluation of alertness. A patient who is alert and can talk probably has a stable airway, at least for the moment.

Airway maintainability, or function, is the ability to use the airway as demonstrated by normal breathing, vocalizing, clearing secretions, and maintaining airway positioning including positioning of the tongue, jaw, and neck. Even though " normal breathing" sounds like it belongs in "B," it actually is part of "A." ABC is a convenient mnemonic, but what it really represents is a sequence of lethality—hypoxia (airway), hypoventilation (breathing), hypoperfusion (circulation). Without a functioning airway, hypoxia will rapidly ensue. The ability to titrate respiratory drive to maintain oxygenation and ventilation is a CNS function, which is why airway assessment begins with alertness. The ability to clear secretions and optimize airway positioning are also CNS functions. Problems with airway function are addressed by administering oxygen, providing suction and supporting positioning. A person who is maintaining her/his airway easily is said to "have a spontaneous airway."

The assessment of airway patency is primarily visual. Are there obvious injuries to the face or neck? Are there congenital anomalies of the face or neck? Is there apparent blood in the mouth or nose, or swelling of oral or nasal tissues? Is there swelling or other injury of the neck? Are there foreign bodies in the mouth or nose, or are there missing or broken teeth? Is the patient actively vomiting? Obstructions and potential obstructions must be cleared through suctioning or extraction and, in some cases, can be mitigated by repositioning the patient such as turning the patient to the side if there is vomiting or profuse bleeding.

After assessing airway function and patency, assessing airway risk includes anticipating the patient's clinical course. Examples of risks to consider are mental status deterioration, repetitive vomiting, or airway swelling from smoke inhalation or angioedema. These considerations are why we sometimes intubate patients who are oxygenating and ventilating adequately but in whom we anticipate deterioration. It is safer and easier to intubate the patient during a period of relative physiologic stability than to wait for further deterioration. We also consider the venue—it is safer to intubate a patient in a fully staffed trauma bay than in a computed tomography (CT) scanner, elevator, or transport vehicle.

If we determine problems with function or patency, or if we anticipate impending risks, then we support the airway in a stepwise fashion. In the patient with compromised alertness, the first step is ensuring the airway is open. This is done by using both hands to provide an upward jaw thrust while simultaneously keeping the head and neck midline. This position can also hold an oxygen or ventilation mask in place. Suction should be turned on and ready to use. We usually start with a nonrebreather mask which can provide >90% FiO_2. If the patient is breathing inadequately, we will provide oxygen and ventilation via a bag-mask device. If bag-mask ventilation is difficult or if prolonged ventilation is anticipated, then intubation or other steps will be considered and planned as needed. Intubation planning might begin immediately, but the intubation itself will typically not occur until after a few minutes or more of preoxygenation and after the patient is deemed hemodynamically stable enough to tolerate intubation.

After the immediate needs of oxygenation, ventilation, positioning, and suctioning are met, "B" or breathing can be assessed. This may occur while preparing for intubation, if it is indicated. Whereas "A" focuses more on assessing hypoxia risk, "B" focuses more on hypoventilation risk. This involves primarily an observational exam of chest rise, symmetry of movements, respiratory rate, and effort. Auscultation is done to assess air movement and breath sounds, though this may be difficult in a noisy trauma bay. As with the airway, pulse oximetry and capnography, if available, contribute to this assessment. The breathing assessment informs those managing the airway as to whether more needs to be done to support ventilation.

The circulation or "C" assessment focuses on hypoperfusion risk. As with A and B, the patient's mental status and overall appearance contribute to this assessment. The two specific core components of assessing perfusion in the primary survey are pulse quality and capillary refill. These are checked centrally and peripherally. Proximal and distal pulses are compared on all four extremities and are described as 2+, 1+ or absent. Truncal or proximal capillary refill is compared to that of the distal extremities. Skin color, dampness, and tactile coolness or warmth can also be noted. Features of inadequate circulation include prolonged cap refill (>3 s in children), weak or absent pulses, pale skin color, and cool/damp skin.

The disability assessment in the primary survey is a rapid assessment of level of consciousness. A quick mnemonic for assessing and reporting responsiveness is AVPU.

- A is for alert—the patient is spontaneously paying attention and responding as expected.
- V is for verbal stimulation—the patient does not seem to be spontaneously alert but clearly responds when you talk to him or her.
- P is for painful or tactile stimulation—the patient is not responding directly to talking but does respond in an obvious and specific way to tactile stimulation such as nail bed pressure, trapezius pinch, or the placement of an IV.

– U is for unresponsive—the patient is notably lethargic, persistently and nonspecifically irritable, or is silent and motionless.

A more detailed, yet rapid, disability assessment is the Glasgow Coma Scale (GCS), which was designed for adults and entails scoring of eye opening, verbal responsiveness, and motor function. You can learn more about GCS on the website https://www.glasgowcomascale.org/ where you will find an 8-min video and a 14-question quiz. There are infant and pediatric GCS tools which tend to be institution-specific and can be useful if done the same way each time and if the findings are described clearly. For infants, toddlers and preschoolers, you will assess them by how vigorous they are and how appropriately interactive they are for age and circumstance. This requires a degree of familiarity with development. If a child has abnormal mental status, check pupil symmetry and responsiveness to light as part of the primary survey's disability assessment.

In pediatrics, "D" is also a reminder to think about dextrose. Because of smaller reserves and faster metabolic rates, young children are at increased risk for hypoglycemia when stressed. Initial glucose checks may reveal a high serum glucose during acute stress, but as time goes on, particularly if the child is nil per os, it is important to recheck the serum glucose periodically.

"E" for exposure/environment is a reminder to fully uncover the patient, but to do so incrementally and to replace sheets or blankets as the exam progresses. This is to reduce psychological stress and to help maintain normothermia. Hypothermia, even mild, can change the shapes of proteins and have adverse effects on hemoglobin function and coagulation.

Finally, "F" for family presence should not be underestimated. This is not only important for the patient, but also enables the family to see how much is being done and helps them feel included in decisions. We bring parents to the bedside when feasible. Family members may need to sit down or have a staff member with them. Contrary to some concerns, family presence does not interfere with care quality.

Proceed to the *secondary survey* after the primary survey has been completed and immediate threats have been stabilized.

1. Head—examine the head and face for any tenderness or swelling, pupillary response, extraocular movements, inside the nose for septal hematoma, dental alignment and jaw opening, and tympanic membranes bilaterally for hemotympanum.
2. Neck—check the cervical spine for pain by palpating each vertebra one at a time—look for discomfort or ask the patient. Examine the anterior neck for swelling, bruising, crepitus, or asymmetry. Carefully open the cervical collar while maintaining manual C-spine alignment and then resecure after performing the exam.
3. Chest—look at chest rise, effort, and symmetry; palpate chest wall for tenderness, crepitus, ecchymosis, or wounds; auscultate heart and lungs.
4. Abdomen—look at the shape of the abdomen and for ecchymosis; listen for bowel sounds; palpate each quadrant for tenderness.

5. Pelvis—palpate bony symmetry and stability, assess tenderness with gradual bilateral pressure on the anterior iliac crests.
6. GU (external only)—look for ecchymosis, lacerations, abrasions, blood at the urethral meatus, blood from the vagina.
7. Back exam—palpate all thoracic and lumbar vertebrae for tenderness and anatomic alignment, check for costo-vertebral angle tenderness; look for abrasions, lacerations, bruises, and penetrating wounds.
8. Rectal exam—look for blood, digital exam for tone (remember to replace gloves after the GU or rectal exam).
9. Extremities—look at and palpate all bones and joints, assess passive and active range of motion in all joints and evaluate for joint pain. It may not need to happen at the initial examination, but prior to discharge, ensure that the patient is able to ambulate.
10. Recheck pulses and capillary refill.
11. Recheck mental status and quick neuro exam—able to state name and age, follow commands to squeeze hands, wiggle toes (if appropriate for developmental level).

Special Considerations in Pediatric Trauma

Non-accidental Trauma (Child Abuse)

Evaluation for child abuse is of critical importance when evaluating a patient with an injury. True incidence is difficult to determine, due to reporting and investigative differences. The recognition, documentation, and reporting of physical abuse by the medical community represents a fraction of those children experiencing maltreatment. History and physical exams are critically important to detecting inflicted injuries. Both patients and parents may not be forthcoming regarding history of inflicted injury, so it is incumbent on the practitioner to have a high index of suspicion with every pediatric physical exam. Children of all ages, ethnicities, and socioeconomic groups are at risk for child abuse. However, the risk of death is highest for those under the age of 3. Some children are at increased risk of experiencing physical abuse, with boys being at slightly higher risk than girls. Other risk factors include those with medical or behavioral disabilities, having two or more siblings, and low infant birth weight. Inconsistency between the history of injury and exam (or the lack of any injury reported) should raise concerns for inflicted trauma, or child abuse. There are a number of findings on physical exam that should raise concerns about child abuse.

The use of the "TEN-4" rule provides a good guideline for determining whether bruising is normal or potentially inflicted injury. It refers to any bruising in a child under the age of 4 months, or bruising to the torso, ears or neck in a child younger than 4 years. Injuries that seem inconsistent with developmental stage (i.e., not yet rolling over, not pulling up to a stand) should raise concerns about inflicted trauma. In addition, subconjunctival hemorrhages in infants (after the immediate newborn period), bruising to the external ears, damage to the upper or lower lip frenulum, or bruising to the hard palate can all be signs of inflicted injury. There may be specific patterns of bruising if a child is struck with an object or is bitten. Children less than a year old should have a complete skin exam at every provider visit to help identify any signs of inflicted trauma. Symptoms of inflicted head trauma in infants and young children may be non-specific. In cases of abuse, when no trauma is reported, patients may present with fussiness, vomiting, increased sleepiness or lethargy, or seizures. Symptoms are sometimes subtle and may not be detected until increased head circumference is noted at well-child visits.

Investigation into inflicted injuries differs depending on the patient's age. Bruising in any non-ambulatory patient should prompt further investigation. Findings of injuries more severe than the defined mechanism given should also prompt investigation. For children under the age of two, radiologic tests should include a head CT to evaluate for occult head injury and a skeletal survey, which involves X-rays of all the long bones of the body to evaluate for occult or healing fractures. Children with concerns for abusive head trauma should have consultation with a pediatric neurosurgeon and ophthalmologist for a dilated fundoscopic exam to evaluate for retinal hemorrhages. Retinal hemorrhages are frequently found in cases of abusive head trauma. They are typically numerous in number and distributed through multiple levels of the retina. Laboratory investigation should include electrolytes, including calcium and phosphorus to detect congenital or acquired anomalies of bone mineralization, leading to easy fracture; and complete blood count and coagulation labs to detect underlying coagulopathies which may result in easy bruising. Empiric testing can be deferred in an ambulatory, verbal child, who can describe their mechanism of injury in detail. In these cases of suspected physical abuse, social work and law enforcement should be involved early in the evaluation, in order to minimize repeated and sometimes leading questioning.

Head Injuries

Head injuries are a very frequent occurrence in the pediatric population. Relative to their bodies, children's heads are larger and heavier compared with adults. Children learning to pull to a stand and walk often experience numerous falls and often strike their forehead or other parts of their head. There are several criteria that may be indicative of more significant head injury and may require a head imaging for further evaluation.

- In any child presenting with a head injury and who has a GCS of 14 or less, is showing signs of altered mental status, or has signs of a skull fracture, the risk of significant traumatic brain injury is about 4%. In these cases, CT scan is recommended.

- In children who do not fit these criteria, risk factors help to stratify the risk of significant head injury and help with decision-making.
- In children under the age of two, with a non-frontal hematoma (occurring in the occipital, parietal, or temporal scalp), loss of consciousness, not acting normally per parent, or falls over 3 ft. (as well as other severe mechanisms of injury), current recommendations are to either observe the child for a period of time for worsening symptoms or perform a CT scan.
- In children over the age of two, similar risk stratification occurs. Higher risk factors for children over two are history of loss of consciousness, history of vomiting, falls over 5 ft. (and other severe mechanisms of injury), and severe headache. If one or more of these factors are present, observation or CT scan may occur based on physician preference, multiple vs one risk factor, parental comfort level, and the ability to observe the patient.

For children at very high risk for clinically significant head injury, head CT or magnetic resonance imaging may be required to exclude intracranial bleeding. For those at lower risk, shared decision-making with the family is recommended. Depending on the family, a period of observation may be preferable to the risk of radiation from head CT.

Concussions may occur even without the high-impact injuries discussed above. A concussion is a brain injury that alters brain function and can include dysregulation in cognition, vision changes, irritability, sleep disturbance, balance issues, and headaches. There are several tools to evaluate symptoms of concussion immediately after the injury and as the child or adolescent recovers. The CDC Heads Up includes scoring tools and informative materials for medical providers, athletic trainers, and caregivers. Concussion care includes gradual return to activities after a period of 24–48 h of rest. Patients with concussion are encouraged to have good sleep hygiene, adequate hydration, and decreased screen time. Return to exercise and sports should be supervised by a healthcare provider.

Cervical Spine Injuries

For the most part, cervical spine (c-spine) injuries can be adequately assessed by obtaining a history of the mechanism of injury, how the child was moving (or not) immediately after the injury and how the child has been doing in the interim, combined with the physical exam. Imaging is not usually necessary though there are certain risk factors to keep in mind. If the mechanism was high-force (e.g., motor vehicle crash without proper restraint, car versus pedestrian or bicycle, fall from an elevation, high-impact sports collision), or if there was a concomitant head, face or chest injury, or if there is altered mental status, then the c-spine cannot be cleared without serial exam or without radiologic imaging. In those cases, the c-spine will be protected with an appropriately sized collar as well as appropriate supervision from a healthcare provider or parent.

Even very young children can be cleared clinically. For instance, the infant who rolls off a changing table, or a toddler who tumbles down the stairs, may arrive to the emergency department with a cervical collar in place. If the parents tell you that the child was active at the scene, and you can see that the child is clearly awake and unhappy about being restrained, it is reasonable to release the child from the restraints and take a moment to watch their comfort level and spontaneous movements. If the child is moving everything and reaching for their parent, it's ok to let the parent pick the child up. Allow the child to be comfortable and reassess.

Dental

In addition to head trauma, teeth are particularly at risk of injury from falls or sports-related injury. Tooth eruption typically begins around age 6–12 months and continues until age 3. Around age 5–6, children will begin shedding their primary teeth and may have a mixed dentition picture, consisting of both primary and permanent teeth at the same time. When evaluating a dental injury, it is very important to determine whether the affected teeth were primary or permanent, as the care plan will vary greatly.

Examination of a patient with dental trauma should include careful examination of the entire head and neck area. Any trauma to the mouth area could also result in concussion or other head or neck injury. The ears should be examined to make sure there is no injury to the auditory canal or hemotympanum. The facial bones should be palpated to evaluate for facial fracture. Dental occlusion, bite strength, and jaw opening should all be tested to evaluate for mandibular fracture or temporomandibular joint injury. Dental injuries should then be assessed, with photo-documentation if possible, in order to accurately communicate with a dentist.

Primary teeth are lettered, beginning in the upper right maxillary side with the second molar (typically erupting around age 2–3). There are a total of 20 primary teeth. Exfoliation of these begins around school age, typically starting with the lower central incisors, followed by the upper central incisors. Secondary teeth are named by a numbering system, also starting in the upper right side. Teenagers and adults have up to 32 secondary teeth, including the 4 wisdom teeth (Fig. 36.1).

During falls or direct trauma, teeth may be completely avulsed (removed from the socket), luxated (moved in the anterior/posterior or lateral planes), intruded (driven into the alveolar ridge), or extruded (partially out of the socket). Teeth may also be subluxed, meaning that there is mobility to the tooth, without displacement. Dental concussion occurs with trauma to the tooth or teeth without mobility or malposition of the teeth. In these cases, the family should be advised to monitor for discoloration, as necrosis of the pulp can occur, but no intervention is needed in the acute setting. Complete intrusion and avulsion may be hard to distinguish and require radiographic imaging if no tooth is found at the time of injury. Injury to a primary tooth (i.e., avulsion, luxation, fracture or significant laxity) is typically managed by extraction of the tooth, so the subsequent management discussion

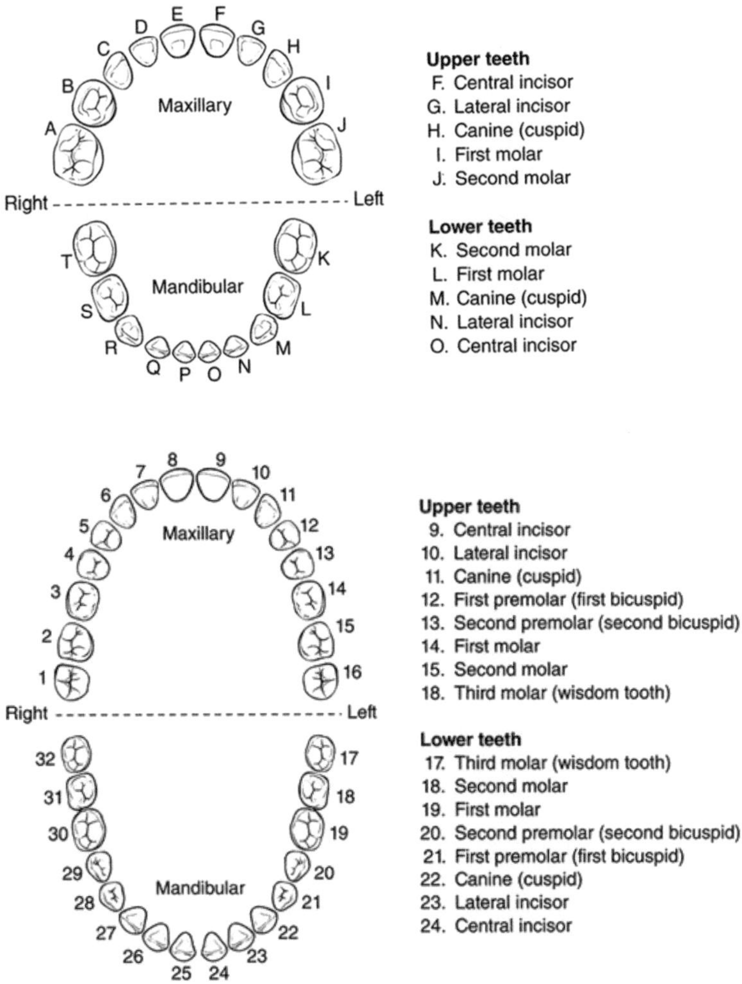

Fig. 36.1 The upper image show the lettered primary teeth, while the lower image shows the numbered secondary teeth

involves secondary teeth. The exception to this is an intruded primary tooth. An intruded primary tooth risks damage to the underlying secondary tooth, so needs to be evaluated urgently by a dentist. These teeth are sometimes allowed to re-erupt on their own and sometimes require extraction. An avulsed secondary tooth, if it can be located and is intact, should be placed back into the socket as quickly as possible. If there is visible soil, the tooth should be gently rinsed in saline or water, but the tooth root should never be scrubbed. Ideally, the tooth root is gently inserted into the open socket, then the patient puts pressure by biting on folded gauze to keep the tooth in place until they can be seen by a dentist. If the tooth is unable to be placed into the socket, having the patient hold the tooth in their mouth between the teeth and the buccal mucosa is the next best way to keep the root cells alive. The tooth can also be placed in milk while a dental provider is contacted. Dental laxity should also be seen urgently by a dentist in order to brace the teeth and limit permanent damage to the teeth.

Teeth may also suffer fracture, with loss of part of the tooth. Management of these types of fractures also varies, depending on how much of the tooth is lost. Patients with fractures through the dentin or pulp should have urgent dental consultation for both pain control and to ensure optimum tooth survival.

Long Bone Injuries

Relative to adults, children's bones are more flexible, with relative strength of the ligaments and tendons. As a result, with any mechanism of injury, children are more likely to sustain a fracture, rather than sprain. As a result, the provider must have a high suspicion for fracture with any injury.

In assessing a patient with suspected fracture, several portions of the physical exam are of vital importance. The fracture site must be assessed visually to determine if the fracture is open or closed. If there is any tenting of the skin or obvious deformity, urgent reduction of the fracture is indicated. The extremity distal to the fracture must also be examined, to determine that the pulses and capillary refill are normal, and that there is no nerve injury from the fracture.

When plain-film radiographs are obtained, there are several fracture types that may be seen, which are unique to the pediatric bone structure. A greenstick fracture is fracture of only one portion of the cortex but is incomplete to the other aspect of the bone (Fig. 36.2). A bowing fracture may also occur, with bending of the flexible bone without clear fracture on X-ray. A Torus, or buckle fracture, occurs with axial loading of the extremity, and results in buckling or protuberance of the bone cortex (Fig. 36.3). A fracture with multiple pieces of bone is described as comminuted or compound.

In discussing a fracture and planning its management, it is also important to discuss displacement and angulation. Displacement is how much the distal portion of the bone aligns with the proximal portion and is expressed as a percentage. If there is 100% displacement, the fracture segments will often overlap, due to muscle contracture force on the distal fragment. Angulation is the amount the distal fragment angles away from the fracture and is expressed in degrees, with 0 ° being no

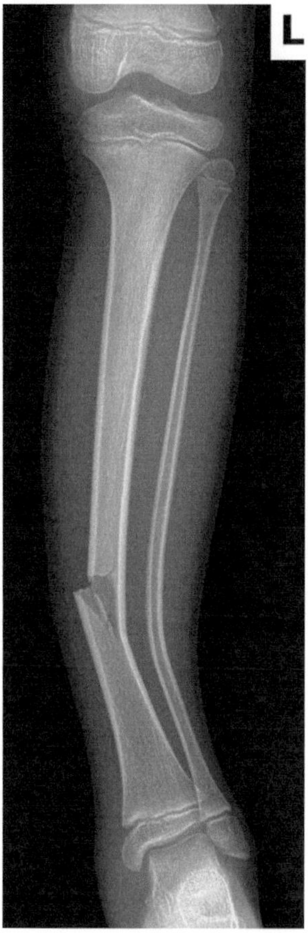

Fig. 36.2 Greenstick fracture of the left tibia. You can see fracture and deformity of the bone, with intact lateral cortex opposite the fracture site. There is also a bowing deformity to the fibula

angulation. The amount of angulation acceptable varies depending on the age of the patient and the amount of bony remodeling still to take place before they reach skeletal maturity. Hence, younger patients have a higher threshold for angulation before closed reduction of the fracture is required. The fracture in Fig. 36.2 would be described as a greenstick fracture to the mid-shaft of the tibia, with 20 ° of angulation, apex medial, with a bowing fracture of the fibula.

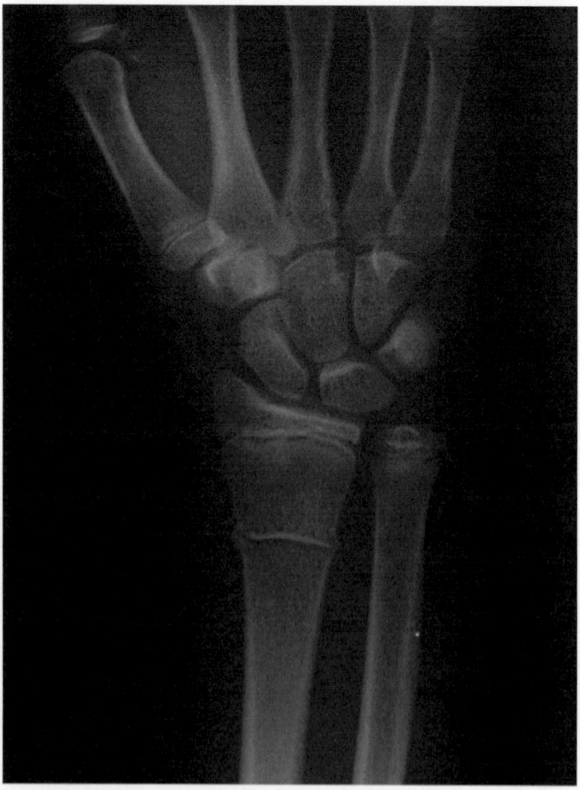

Fig. 36.3 Buckle fracture of the right radius

Prior to skeletal maturity, the area of cartilaginous growth leads to injuries which are classified using the Salter-Harris classification system. Numbered I–V: they increase in severity and higher numbers have increased likelihood for long-term ramifications.

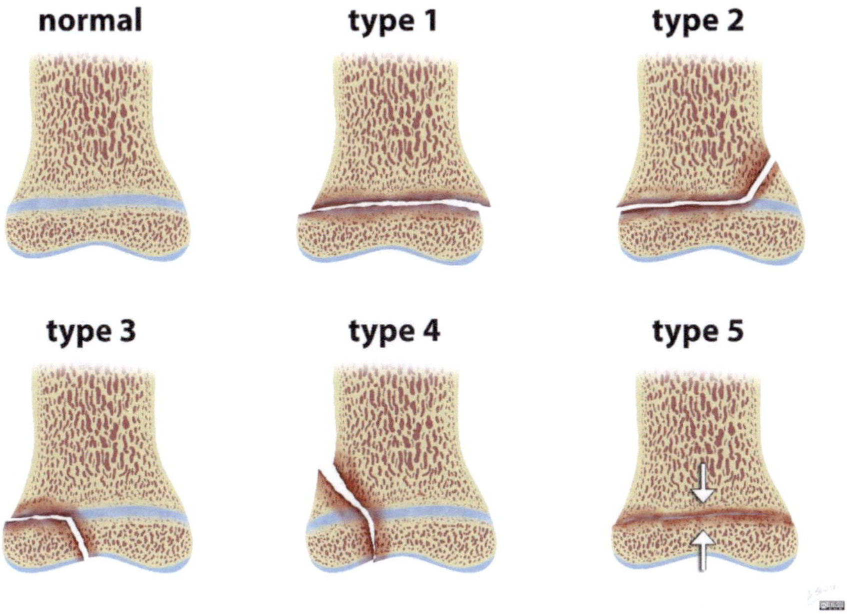

SH-I—fracture through the growth plate only. These injuries may not be visible on initial X-rays. Should have a high index of suspicion and immobilize if there is tenderness over the growth plate.

SH-II—fracture involving the growth plate and the metaphysis of the bone.

SH-III—fracture involving the growth plate and the epiphysis of the bone.

SH-IV—fracture of the metaphysis and epiphysis extending though the growth plate.

SH-V—compression of the growth plate. These fractures have the highest risk of limitation of long bone growth and limb-length discrepancies due to growth plate injury.

Children's bones are growing and have an area of cartilage called the growth plate. Because these areas are radio-lucent on X-rays, fractures through the growth plate may not be visible at the initial injury. These injuries should be treated as a suspected fracture and immobilized, with repeat evaluation in 7–10 days. Families should also be instructed to follow up for persistent pain and repeat X-ray imaging 7–10 days after injury if pain persists. Repeat imaging may show signs of a healing fracture.

Radiation Risk

Evaluation of traumatic injuries often requires some form of radiographic imaging, most commonly plain radiographs or CT scans. CT images are obtained by emission of X-rays, exposing the patient to ionizing radiation. Radiation exposure can be limited by focusing on specific body parts (i.e., obtaining a pelvic CT rather than a CT of the abdomen and pelvis), adjusting various parameters of the CT machine for pediatric size and weight, or performing helical CTs, which rotate faster and thus emit lower radiation doses. Without adjusting for the size of the patient, a newborn will receive approximately twice the amount of radiation as an adult patient receiving the same test.

There has been a remarkable increase in the use of radiographic tests over the past few decades, leading to efforts for radiation reduction and judicious testing. Because they are actively growing, the tissues of children are more radiosensitive than those of adults, putting them at higher risk of injury from radiation exposure. In addition, children have a longer lifespan than an adult exposed to the same radiation, leading to increased chance of malignancy from the radiation exposure. Radiation damages cells by directly damaging DNA, or by causing free radical formation that subsequently interacts with DNA. Cells that are rapidly growing and undergoing mitosis at a higher rate may be more susceptible to radiation effects. In addition, the risk of radiation exposure is higher in girls than in boys, due to the risk of developing breast cancer. The estimated lifetime risk of cancer from adult-radiation dose head CT and abdominal CT is 1-in-700 for a newborn, and 1-in-1000 for a 10-year-old.

The "Image Gently" Campaign (www.imagegently.org) provides education for parents and providers about medical imaging and reducing radiation risk. In discussing the risks of radiation exposure with patients and parents, it is very helpful to be aware of the specific tests ordered, and the amount of radiation from those tests at your institution. Background radiation exposure from the environment is approximately 2.5–3 mSv per year. For comparison, an airplane flight from the East Coast to the West Coast exposes one to approximately 0.035 mSv. Adult level exposure from a two-view chest X-ray is approximately 0.1 mSv, whereas a head CT is approximately 2 mSv and an abdominal CT scan is approximately 8 mSv.

Application Exercises

1. For all fractures, displacement and angulation impact immediate management strategies. An additional factor to consider in pediatric long bone injuries is that particularly affects growing children is

   A. History of past fractures
   B. Mechanism of injury
   C. Past radiation exposure
   D. Growth plate injuries

Answer D: Growth plate injuries are described using the Salter-Harris classification.

2. In addition to head trauma, teeth are particularly at risk of injury from falls or sports-related injury. Dental injuries should be assessed carefully, with photo-documentation if possible, in order to accurately communicate with a dentist. For children, it is important to remember that tooth eruption typically begins around age 6–12 months and continues until age 3. Primary teeth begin to be normally shed at around

   A. 3–4 years of age
   B. 5–6 years of age
   C. 8–9 years of age
   D. After 10 years of age.

Answer B: Normal age for primary tooth shedding is typically between 5 and 6 years of age although a year earlier or later should not be considered abnormal. The first baby teeth to fall out are typically the two bottom front teeth (lower central incisors) and the two top front teeth (upper central incisors), followed by the lateral incisors, first molars, canines, and second molars.

Further Reading

Christian CW, Committee on Child Abuse and Neglect, American Academy of Pediatrics. The evaluation of suspected child physical abuse. Pediatrics. 2015;135(5):e1337–54.

Fahey FH, Treves ST, Adelstein SJ. Minimizing and communicating radiation risk in pediatric nuclear medicine. J Nucl Med. 2011;52(8):1240–51.

Leonard JR, et al. Cervical spine injury patterns in children. Pediatrics. 2014;133(5):e1179–88.

Narang SK, et al. Abusive head trauma in infants and children. Pediatrics. 2020;145(4):e20200203.

O'Connell KJ, Carter EA, Fritzeen JL, Waterhouse LJ, Burd RS. Effect of Family Presence on Advanced Trauma Life Support Task Performance during pediatric trauma team evaluation. Pediatr Emerg Care. 2021;37(12):e905–9.

Chapter 37
Approach to Well Child Checks (WCC)

Betty Del Rio Rodriguez and Ana C. Monterrey

Well child visits are a critical component of outpatient pediatric primary care. A well child check (WCC) targets specific areas of growth and development and provides the opportunity for health surveillance and screening for disorders and diseases affecting children and adolescents. These visits also focus on providing age-specific anticipatory guidance emphasizing health promotion and disease prevention. The American Academy of Pediatrics *Bright Futures: Guidelines for Health Supervision of Infants, Children, and Adolescents* (https://brightfutures.aap.org) is a comprehensive resource for pediatric health care providers with updated recommendations to follow in conducting these visits by age. Routine well child visits are recommended as indicated in Table 37.1 and are typically scheduled for a longer amount of time than a sick visit. It is important to note that while many elements must be included as part of these visits, providers must also balance the needs of families presenting for care and be adaptable to address family concerns.

Before you go into the room and start the visit, you should take time to prepare for the encounter. Think about what you know about the patient and identify what you need to know. This will keep your encounter organized and help you cover all the critical areas of the well child exam.

B. D. R. Rodriguez (✉) · A. C. Monterrey
Division of Academic General Pediatrics, Department of Pediatrics, Baylor College of Medicine, Houston, TX, USA
e-mail: betty.delriorodriguez@bcm.edu; monterre@bcm.edu

N. Liao et al. (eds.), *Pediatric Rotations*,
https://doi.org/10.1007/978-3-031-59873-9_37

Table 37.1 Schedule of well child care visits

Newborns	3–5 days and 2 weeks
Infants	1, 2, 4, 6, 9, and 12 months
Young children	15, 18, 24, and 30 months
Older children	3–18 years of age (1 visit annually)

Presentation to the Clinic

Children presenting for a well child visit may be established or new patients. For new patients, more time is needed to obtain prior medical history such as birth history, hospitalizations, medications, surgeries, and any significant disease history such as asthma, allergies, prematurity, and developmental delay. For well newborn visits, details such as prenatal care, complications during pregnancy and during or after delivery are important to know. It is also important to know if the mother has any significant medical history that could present a risk of present or future medical problems for the child.

Before Going into the Room

- Review available prior medical history, medications, and concerns addressed during the last visit.
- Review vital signs, growth charts, and screening questionnaires (Table 37.5) recommended for specific ages.
- For children 3 years or older, check for vision screening results, and ≥4 years old, check for hearing screening results.
- Review immunizations and be ready to discuss those that are due for the visit.
- Check if there is any laboratory screening recommended for the child's age (Table 37.5).

Preparation before entering the room will prepare you for the interview and help you conduct a focused history appropriate for the age of the child and guide you on the main topics to cover when talking to parents about preventive care and anticipatory guidance.

The Sick Child Presenting for a WCC

Sometimes when children come for a WCC, they might be sick, or the parent may have an acute concern that they want to address. Depending on the complexity of the complaint or how sick the child is, a well child visit may or may not be appropriate. For the outpatient sick encounter, it is still important to review any prior medical history, medications, and vital signs before going into the patient's room.

In the Patient Room

Once in the room and after a proper introduction, ask about the visit's purpose to help set the stage. Ask who accompanies the child and document in the chart, as children may come to clinic with a person other than a parent like a legal guardian, grandparent, sibling, or another relative. After the parent confirms the reason for the visit, follow by asking if they have any concerns they would like to discuss before asking questions related to the well child visit. As you would with any complaint, ask about timing, location, quality, and duration, etc. gathering all the information you think is pertinent based on the complaint.

Growth and Nutrition

Monitoring Growth Parameters

Each well child visit includes monitoring of a child's growth parameters and overall trends in growth. Be sure to review these on the appropriate growth chart CDC (Centers for Disease Control) and World Health Organization (WHO).

- Weight
- Length/height
- Weight for length (<2 years old)
- Head circumference (≤2 years old)
- Body-Mass-Index (BMI) (≥2 years old)

Abnormal growth patterns in weight gain, length/height, and head circumference (less than or greater than two standard deviations from the mean) should be correlated with elements of the history and physical exam as this may signify underlying disease, illness, or poor nutritional habits. Weight for length or BMI <5th percentile or ≥95th percentile warrant further nutritional history and/or counseling on appropriate nutrition for age.

Of note, infants born prematurely are not expected to follow the same growth parameters as full-term infants and should be monitored using growth curves appropriate for their gestational age.

Nutrition

Assessing nutrition is an essential element of every WCC, and your history should include reviewing feeding and nutritional habits with children and adolescents of all ages. How you assess nutrition will vary by age as per Tables 37.2 and 37.3 below. Additionally, keep in mind that cultural practices and the families' social context such as the presence of food insecurity can affect how feeding recommendations are implemented. Remember to ask about and connect families, as needed, to nutrition resources like the Supplemental Nutrition Assistance Program (SNAP), Special Supplemental Nutrition Program for Women, Infants, and Children (WIC), and School Lunch and Breakfast programs as these can improve access to high quality nutritious foods.

Table 37.2 Newborns and Infants Nutritional Assessment

	Sample questions	Tips
Breast feeding	How long does baby feed on each breast and how often (including overnight feedings)? Are there any difficulties with latching or milk supply? How is your milk supply? Does the baby still seem hungry after breastfeeding?	Place baby to the breast with each feeding—this increases milk supply Consider referral to lactation support for parents with difficulty or concerns about breast feeding
Formula feeding	How many ounces of formula does the baby take and how often (including overnight feedings)? What type of formula is the baby taking? How do you prepare the formula?	Correct mixing is 1 unpacked, level scoop of formula in 2 oz. of water (always check the can for directions and use the scoop that comes with the can as not all scoops are the same size)
Vitamin supplementation	Is your baby taking any vitamins like vitamin D or iron?	Give vitamin D to babies who are feeding <33 oz. of formula per day Give iron to exclusively breastfeed infants at 4 months of age unless iron-rich foods are introduced
Complementary feeding	What type of solid foods does your baby eat? (e.g., iron fortified baby cereals, meat, vegetables, or fruits) How often does your baby eat solids and what texture (e.g., pureed, mashed, small chunks)? Have you introduced any allergenic foods yet? (e.g., peanuts, eggs, fish, and seafood)	Start with solid foods between 4 and 6 months of age. Give a variety of foods from all food groups in a healthy and safe manner (e.g., avoid choking hazards, offer appropriate texture foods for oral motor skills) Allergenic foods should be introduced at 4–6 months No juice in the first year of life unless recommended by the pediatrician

Table 37.3 Children and Adolescents Nutritional Assessment

	Questions	Tips
Foods	Tell me about your child's nutrition What type of food groups do you eat and how many servings per day? Does the child follow any special diet? Are there any food groups or types you or the child restrict or do not eat?	Children should eat 3 meals and 1–2 snacks per day with appropriate portion sizes for age based on their activity level. They should eat a varied diet of fruits, vegetables, whole grains, and protein. Avoid calorically dense, low nutrient foods. Limit sodium.
Beverages	How many cups of milk per day and what type (milk % or milk alternatives)? How many cups per day of water? Juice? Other sugary drinks?	Children should transition to cow's milk starting at 12 months of age Children should drink plain, unflavored water and avoid sugar sweetened beverages including juice, soda, and sports drinks
Considerations for toddlers and young children	Does your child have any picky eating habits?	Picky eating is common in young children. Remind parents it can take as many as 8–10 exposures for a child to accept a food
Considerations for teens	Do you skip any meals? How often do you eat meals outside of home or school? Are you following any special diets?	Energy needs will vary based on activity level and timing of puberty and physical growth Teens tend to skip meals frequently, especially breakfast and may start to eat out more (e.g., fast food) Teens may follow fad diets placing them at risk for nutritional deficiencies

Obesity Prevention and Treatment

With rising rates of overweight and obesity in children of all ages, pediatricians play a significant role in preventing and managing obesity in children of all ages. Obesity in pediatrics is defined as BMI ≥95th percentile (Overweight ≥85th to 94th percentile). Any counseling on obesity should be done in a sensitive manner with a focus on improving health and health behaviors, promoting positive body image, and avoiding weight stigma. Using neutral terms like "weight" or "unhealthy weight" is preferred by families and teens while terms like "fat" and "obese" are considered less desirable and unmotivating. Using motivational interviewing techniques to help families make behavior change goals is ideal. Any changes or goals should be focused on what is important and feasible for families (see Table 37.4). Using online resources like MyPlate.gov and Let's Go (5-2-1-0) can help with counseling recommendations and can provide education on healthy nutrition and lifestyle habits. Close follow-up is recommended at 1–3-month intervals to support motivated families as they work towards changing and building healthier lifestyles.

Table 37.4 Talking about obesity

Tips	Talk about nutrition not diets Avoid terms like obesity Focus on health, not weight loss Encourage change for the whole family Celebrate all accomplishments however small
Sample phrases and approaches	*"I am concerned about your child's/your health today. We know increased weight can lead to health problems like high blood pressure, diabetes, and heart problems. Would it be ok if we talked about some ways, we could improve your child's/your health so we can prevent these problems?"* *"Our first goal is to get you healthier! Not to lose weight. This is about your health and not how you look."* *"What changes do you think you and your family would be interested in working on? How easy or challenging do you think it will be to make these changes and why?"* *"Remember these changes can take time. We will start with small changes and build over time. It is ok if things don't always go the way we planned. We will keep working together as a team"*
Resources for families	**MyPlate** graphics (½ plate fruit or veggies, ¼ grains, ¼ protein) and other handouts with healthy nutrition and lifestyle information https://www.myplate.gov/ **Let's Go** (5-2-1-0). The 5-2-1-0 message is easy to remember, and highlights health behaviors recommended for all children 5 or more fruits and vegetables 2 h or less recreational screen time 1 h or more of physical activity 0 sugary drinks, more water https://www.mainehealth.org/Lets-Go **Healthy Children** from the *American Academy of Pediatrics* has nutrition and exercise information and parent handouts for children of all ages https://healthychildren.org/

Developmental Milestones

Screening and surveillance of developmental milestones are key to ensure the child's optimal growth and development. Child development is evaluated in four developmental domains: social emotional, language/communication, cognitive, and motor. While screening is done with the use of a screening questionnaire, developmental surveillance consists of evaluating the growth and development of the child by conducting a thorough physical exam and eliciting any parental concerns regarding the way their child is developing and behaving and should happen at every encounter.

To evaluate development on each visit:

- Ask the parent if the infant or child is attaining the milestone, e.g., "*Does your infant smile when you talk or smile at him?*"
- Observe the milestone, e.g., place infant on her belly to assess if able to lift head to 45° (2-month gross motor milestone), observe the child walking or cruising.

Table 37.5 Components of the Well Child Visits by Age

Age	Developmental assessment	Questionnaire	Laboratory screening
Newborn	Surveillance		Newborn screening
2–6 months	Surveillance	Edinburgh	
9 months	Screening and surveillance	PEDS or ASQ	
12 months	Surveillance		Hgb, Hct, Lead
15 months	Surveillance		
18 months	Screening and surveillance	PEDS or ASQ, MCHAT-R	
24 months	Screening and Surveillance	PEDS or ASQ, MCHAT-R	Lead
30 months	Screening	PEDS or ASQ	
3 years	Surveillance		
4 years	Surveillance		
5 years	Surveillance		
6–8 years	Home and School performance	ASQ, PSC	
9–11 years	Home and School performance	PSC	Lipid screening

PEDS parent's evaluation of developmental status, *ASQ* age and stages questionnaire, *MCHAT* modified checklist for autism in toddlers-revised, *PSC* pediatric symptom checklist, *Hgb* hemoglobin, *Hct* hematocrit

- Interact with the child, e.g., ask the child about the colors in a book, shapes, or words.

Evaluating milestones during the WCC can be highly informative and fun. To learn about what to ask at each WCC visit go to: https://www.cdc.gov/ncbddd/actearly/milestones/index.html.

Table 37.5 is a summary of the WCC components. For complete guidance of what to perform at a WCC refer to the AAP WCC Periodicity Schedule.

Developmental Delays

If a child is found to be developmentally delayed, further evaluation is warranted. When an infant's delay is mild and only involves one domain of development, the pediatrician may opt to provide specific guidance to parents on how to help the child progress in his/her development and follow up. If the developmental delay is significant or there are two or more areas of delay, the patient should be referred for evaluation by a specialist. Children younger than 3 years can be referred to the state program for early childhood development for evaluation and treatment, provided usually in the child's home. Children 3 years and older can be referred to local schools for evaluation and treatment. If available, a child of any age may be referred to private developmental clinics or therapy centers to undergo evaluation and treatment with therapies such as speech therapy (ST), occupational therapy (OT), or physical therapy (PT).

School Age Children

Although developmental milestones can be assessed for children aged up to 6 years old, developmental screeners are not usually recommended unless not previously done. The best way to assess the development of a school age child is to ask about how the child is doing in school and at home. There are also other questionnaires that can be incorporated during the visit that facilitate eliciting concerns for developmental or behavioral problems https://publications.aap.org/toolkits/resources/15625/.

Tips to assess development in older children:

- Ask parents if they are concerned about how their child is learning.
- Ask parents if they have heard any concerns from teachers about their child's development or behavior.
- Ask parents about concerns for inattention or hyperactivity, if so, the child can be evaluated for conditions such as attention deficit hyperactive disorder (ADHD).
- Ask the child what their favorite subject in school is, what their least favorite subject is, and whether they are struggling or failing in any class.

If there are concerns with the child's learning, parents can request the child to be evaluated by the school. They should also talk to the school and find out what resources like tutoring might be available for their child.

Social History

For children to develop and grow to their best potential, having a stable home and strong support system increases their chances to reach that potential. When obtaining the social history, you should ask the following in a compassionate manner:

- Who lives in the home with the child?
- Where does the child go to school?
- Do they participate in any afterschool activities?
- Who takes care of the child when the parents are not home?
- Any problems with accessing food or basic needs?

For more guidance on how to ask questions regarding social determinants of health and what questionnaires, you could refer to: AAP Poverty and Child Health: Practice Tips

The Adolescent Well Visit

Adolescent well visit components are based on risk factors that usually affect children older than 12 years of age. The HEADSS assessment is an essential component of the adolescent interview and can be supplemented with the use of questionnaires that target-specific risk factors (Table 37.6). These questionnaires, if administered and reviewed ahead of the interview, can help facilitate the interview with the adolescent.

Table 37.6 How to Conduct the HEADSS Exam

		What to ask	How to ask	Helpful questionnaires
H	Home	Where and with whom they live, house vs apartment vs trailer Ask about safety at home	Where do you live? Who lives at home with you? Do you feel safe at home? Can you confide in family members when needed?	
E	Education	Their grade and school Any recent changes in school. Any change in grades. Their favorite/least favorite class	What grade are you? What is the name of your school? What is your favorite or least favorite class? Are you passing all your classes? Do you ever get bullied at school?	
A	Activities/ employment	Afterschool activities, sports participation, school or church clubs Work while in school	Do you participate in any extracurricular activity, sport or club in or outside school? Do you have a job?	
D	Drugs	Drug or alcohol use, smoking or vaping	It may be easier to start asking about known friends who use drugs: "Do your friends smoke or vape?" "Do any of your friends use drugs?" "Have you used drugs?" But can be more direct when appropriate: "How often do you smoke or vape?" "Which drugs have you tried?"	CRAFFT
S	Sex	Sexual activity, number of partners, sex and age of the partner, type of sex, condom use, contraception, STI testing in the past	Are you dating someone? How did you meet your partner? Do you like girls, boys, or both? Have you had sex? What is the age of your partner? How many partners have you had? Do you always use contraception?	
S	Suicidality	Symptoms of depression, anxiety, difficulties coping, sudden change in school performance	Have you been feeling sad or anxious? Have you thought about harming yourself? If so, how?	PHQ-A, C-SSRS

PHQ-A patient health questionnaire 9-adolescent, screening for depression, *C-SSRS* Columbia suicide severity scale

Table 37.7 The Adolescent Well Visit Components (ages 12–19 years old)

Age		Screening questionnaire	Laboratory screening
12–15 years	HEADSS assessment	PSC-Y, PSC-17-Y, PHQ-9	STI if applicable
16 years old	HEADSS assessment	PSC-Y, PSC-17-Y, PHQ-9	HIV, lipid screening
18 years old	HEADSS assessment	PSC-Y, PSC-17-Y, PHQ-9	Hep. C screening

Setting the stage for the HEADSS exam:

- Inform the adolescent and parent that you will be conducting a private interview with the adolescent.
- Normalize the private interview: "with all our adolescents, we like to talk to them in private."
- Request the parent to step out of the room and let them know that the information shared by the adolescent will be kept confidential unless there is a risk or safety concern.
- Start the conversation with the adolescent by stating the privacy of your conversation, and that you will not share the information with his parents unless you feel that there is risk or concerns for anyone's safety.

For more guidance on how to conduct the HEADSS examination, you can refer to the following resources:

- HEADSS: The "Review of Systems" for Adolescents [1].
- http://www.bcchildrens.ca/Youth-Health-Clinic-site/Documents/headss20assessment20guide1.pdf.

Other psychosocial screeners that can be used at the well adolescent visits are the Pediatric Symptom Checklist-Youth which is administered to the adolescent at the start of the visit. This should be answered by the adolescent only and it screens for attention problems, internalizing and externalizing symptoms. A briefer version is available, and it comes in several languages. For more information on commonly used screening tools during the WCC visit: https://publications.aap.org/toolkits/resources/15625/.

Other screening recommendations for adolescents are related to risk for sexually transmitted illnesses (STIs) including chlamydia, gonorrhea, syphilis, and HIV. Hepatitis C screening is also recommended starting at age 18 years. The components of the adolescent well visits are outlined in Table 37.7.

Well Child Physical Exam

Conducting a complete and thorough physical exam is an essential part of the well child visit. To best conduct the complete physical exam, children should be undressed and in a gown. Keeping diapers or underwear beneath the gown can make the child more comfortable, and these can be removed briefly only for the sensitive

Table 37.8 Tips for Examining Children

- Stand or sit close to the child before starting your exam so they can become more comfortable with you
- Keep young or fearful children in their parent's lap for as much of the exam as possible
- Save any uncomfortable or difficult portions of the exam until the end for younger children (e.g., ear and throat exam). Reviewing proper holding techniques with parents can help make your exam easier
- Small toys, books, or large stickers may help calm and distract children
- Remember certain exam techniques easily conducted in adults and older children may not be possible with younger children due to normal limitations in comprehension and their developmental stage (e.g., breathing deeply, cranial nerve evaluation, heel-to-toe walking)
- Asking the child to breathe like they are "blowing out the candles" or blow on a tissue or paper towel can help get deep breaths on the lung exam

Table 37.9 Physical Exam Elements Specific to Age

Vitals	Head circumference - birth to 2 years Weight for length - birth to 2 years BMI - starting at 2 years of age Blood pressure - starting at 3 years of age
Newborns	Fontanelles, hip clicks/clunks (Barlow and Ortolani maneuver up to 4–6 months), Moro reflex, suck reflex, inspection of external genitalia and patent anus, sacral dimples, skin changes such as jaundice or dermal melano-cytosis
All infants	Head shape or signs of plagiocephaly, red reflex, symmetric corneal light reflex, cover uncover test of eyes (starting at 6–9 months), any cardiac murmurs, testes descended (males), muscle tone
Teens	Scoliosis evaluation, breast exam (female), external genital exam, testicular and hernia exam (males), more thorough musculoskeletal and cardiac exam for pre-sports participation

portions of the exam. Table 37.8 includes some general tips on how to approach examining children keeping in mind that they may be fearful and uncooperative during certain portions of the physical exam. Table 37.9 reviews some elements of the physical exam that differ for children of certain ages.

Conducting a Genital and Breast Exam in Children and Adolescents

Examining the external genitalia and breasts (females) is an important part of the well child exam. The purpose of this exam is to note variations of normal, any abnormalities, and to determine appropriate progression of puberty. A sexual maturity rating (1–5) should be documented for each child as part of the annual well child exam (Table 37.10). Prior to conducting sensitive exams, you should obtain consent from the parent and ascent from the child or adolescent. Parents should remain in the room and be present for this portion of the exam for children <12 years of age. Adolescents may prefer to have this portion of the exam done privately by

Table 37.10 Sexual Maturity Rating[a]

Boys	Genital development	Pubic hair growth
1	Pre-pubertal, no change in size of testes or penis	No pubic hair
2	Enlargement testes with some change in texture of scrotum, little or no penis enlargement	Fine, sparse hair at base of penis
3	Increase penile length and growth of testes	Courser, dark hair, curling and with increased amount
4	Further enlargement of penis and growth of testes with darkening of scrotal skin	Hair resembles adult type, but does not spread to medial thighs
5	Adult size and shape genitalia	Adult type and quantity with spread to medial thighs
Girls	**Breast development**	**Pubic hair growth**
1	Pre-pubertal, nipple only elevated	No pubic hair
2	Small, raised breast bud	Fine, sparse hair on labia
3	Enlargement of breast beyond areola	Courser, dark hair, curling and with increased amount
4	Further enlargement of breast, areola, and nipple as secondary mound	Hair resembles adult type, but does not spread to medial thighs
5	Mature breast with areola in same contour as breast, only nipple projecting	Adult type and quantity with spread to medial thighs

[a] Adapted from Kleinman RE, Greer FR, editors. Pediatric Nutrition [Internet]. American Academy of Pediatrics; [cited 2022 May 27]. Available from: https://doi.org/10.1542/9781610024181

the provider with a chaperone (another member of the health care team). After discussing with parents and patients what the exam will entail, adolescents should be offered the opportunity to have their parents present or not. Female patients can be examined supine with appropriate gown and draping, while older male patients should be examined standing.

Preventative Care and Anticipatory Guidance

Preventative care refers to what we can do to keep children healthy and safe. For example, to prevent disease, we recommend a healthy nutrient rich diet from the first days of life, we recommend physical activity, and we encourage healthy and age-appropriate guidance feeding practices. Preventive care also includes immunizations to prevent severe disease and death. Dental care is recommended as well. Another important aspect is how we keep our children and adolescents safe. Unfortunately, unintentional injuries are the leading cause of death among children and teenagers in the USA. For this, we provide anticipatory guidance based on the age of the child and some of the most common causes of injury or death by age (Table 37.11).

Table 37.11 Anticipatory Guidance Focused on Most Common Causes of Death in Children and Teens

Ages	Type of injury	Anticipatory guidance
Infants	Suffocation injuries	Counsel about bedding, discourage co-sleeping
Ages 1–4 years	Drowning	Counsel on water safety practices, swimming lessons
Ages 5–19 years	Motor vehicle accidents	Counsel on proper use of car seats, boosters, and seat belts
Ages 10–14 years	Suicide	Counsel on access to guns, mental health resources, and how to get help

Other common causes of injuries in children are burns, falls, poisoning, or drug overdose. For more information on what topic should be covered when providing anticipatory guidance to parents, visit https://www.healthychildren.org/English/health-issues/conditions/COVID-19/Pages/default.aspx.

Immunizations

Immunizations are another essential part of a WCC. They prevent serious illnesses and diseases and are safe and effective. Vaccine administration follows the Centers for Disease Control and Prevention (CDC) Vaccine Schedule and provides protection at just the right time for each child. You should review or have available to reference the Child and Adolescent Vaccine schedule from the CDC to determine what vaccines are needed at each visit. Children should receive vaccines around the following ages, coinciding with well child visits:

- Birth.
- 2, 4, 6, 12, and 15–18 months
- 4, 11, and 16 years.

Most children do well after receiving vaccines; however, you should provide parents some basic counseling on what to expect post-vaccination including minor side effects. Infants and young children may have low-grade fever and fussiness after receiving vaccines. Redness and soreness at the injection site is common. These side effects are signs that the child's immune system is responding to the vaccine and should last only a few days at most. Children who are experiencing discomfort post-vaccination can be treated with appropriate medications for pain relief or a cool washcloth can be applied to the site.

Vaccine Hesitancy

Over the last few decades, an increasing number of parents are requesting alternate vaccine schedules, postponing, or declining vaccines. All members of the health care team can play an important role in ensuring children receive the recommended vaccinations at the appropriate time. The recommendation and guidance of a health care provider is the most crucial factor influencing parents' decision to vaccinate [2].

Tips for talking to parents about vaccines:

- Use a presumptive approach, assuming parents have the intention to vaccinate.
- *DO SAY: Your child is due for ____ vaccines today.*
- *DON'T SAY: What would you like to do about your child's vaccines today?*
- Provide a strong recommendation for vaccines even when parents hesitate or express concerns.
- *I strongly recommend your child receive all recommended vaccines today to protect him/her from serious diseases.*
- If parents still decline, ask them to share their concerns. You should listen and validate their concerns. If you feel comfortable, share what you know. If you do not feel confident in counseling the family, let them know you will share their concerns with your attending and continue the conversation later.
- *"Can you tell me more about why you do not want your child to get the___ shot?"*
- *"Thank you for sharing this with me. Lots of parents have questions or concerns like this. I will talk with my attending so we can be sure to discuss your concerns further."*

You can learn more about how to talk with parents about vaccines by reviewing the CDC website's section titled: Talking to Parents about Vaccines. There you can find more tips, sample phrases, and how to prepare for common questions about vaccines.

Special Populations

Many children who are seen for well child visits are healthy and may have only minor medical illnesses or complaints. However, certain populations of children who present to well child visits may warrant special attention or screening.

Children with Chronic Disease

Children with chronic diseases should also receive routine WCC. Pediatricians can serve as an important liaison for coordination of care between the family and pediatric subspecialists. While the pediatrician may not necessarily be managing the chronic disease (such as severe asthma or a seizure disorder), it is important to ensure that the child's disease is well controlled, any medications are accessible and being taken as prescribed, and that routine follow-up is occurring with the appropriate subspecialist.

Sample questions to ask during the well child visit HPI:

- How is your child doing regarding his/her diagnosis of _____?
- What medications is your child taking to treat this problem? Are you having any difficulty getting these medications?
- When was the last time you saw the pediatric [subspecialist] and when is your next appointment?
- Do you have any questions about the care your child is receiving for this problem?

Children with Medical Complexity

Children with medical complexity or children and youth with special health care needs (CYSHCN) have multiple significant chronic health problems affecting multiple organ systems, with high health care needs. These children frequently have functional limitations and may have the need for medical technology or devices (such as gastrostomy tubes or respiratory support). They also frequently require a multidisciplinary approach with care provided by multiple pediatric subspecialists, nutritionists, therapists (physical, occupational, speech, etc.), and more. CYSHCN are also at risk for unmet health care and social needs such as poor dental care, lack of mental/behavioral health services, and food insecurity. Screening families as needed and connecting them to other health services and community resources is also important when caring for this population.

One subset of CYSHCN is those children with Trisomy 21 (Down Syndrome). The American Academy of Pediatrics' Clinical Report on *Health Supervision for Children and Adolescents with Down Syndrome* can be referenced when caring for this population. Down Syndrome-specific growth charts should also be used, and the supplemental age-specific guidance reviewed at each WCC.

Children in Immigrant Families

Children in immigrant families (CIF) are those who are foreign born or have at least 1 parent who is foreign born. This group of children is considered together since some US born children with foreign-born parents share the same vulnerabilities as those who are foreign born themselves. CIF are at high risk for lack of or inconsistent health insurance coverage (even when eligible), a variety or social and psychosocial needs and cultural barriers such as limited English proficiency. Newly arrived children and youth including refugee children should be screened for medical needs, mental health or trauma needs, and developmental or educational needs. The AAP's *Immigrant Child Health Toolkit* a helpful resource for clinicians and includes specific considerations that can be incorporated into the WCC like screening for trauma, social determinants of health, and targeted labs (e.g., tuberculosis screening).

Be sure to use a certified medical interpreter for all encounters with families who have limited English proficiency, even when adolescent patients may prefer speaking in English. Also, remember to be thoughtful when asking immigration-related questions as many families will need to build trust before sharing sensitive information like trauma or may have immigration status-related fears. Lastly, be sure to never document a patient's or caregiver's immigration status in the medical record.

Sample framing and questions to ask during the well child visit HPI:

- *I am asking these questions because it will help me better understand your child's health needs and provide your family with support. I will not be sharing this information with anyone other than the medical team.*
- Can you tell me about your journey to the USA? Did the family come together or separately?
- Did your child receive any medical care on the journey or since arrival to the USA?
- How is your child or family adjusting to life in the USA?

LGBTQ and Gender Diverse Youth

Children and adolescents who identify as lesbian, gay, bisexual, transgender, or questioning (LGBTQ) of their sexual or gender identity are likely to be a part of the population you will be caring for during well child visits. Creating safe, open, and welcoming environments for these adolescents regardless of their gender identity or sexual orientation is vital for building trust and rapport. You should remember to always use inclusive language (e.g., avoid assumptions about boyfriends/girlfriends) and respect gender preferences (e.g., ask what pronouns or name they prefer) when communicating with all adolescents. Additionally, LGBTQ youth are at increased risk for mental health concerns such a depression, suicidality, and bullying, substance abuse and sexually transmitted infections [3]. Therefore, mental health screening at WCCs is even more important. Counseling should also be provided on safe sexual practices and STI prevention. Adolescents should be referred as needed to appropriate subspecialty care (such as gender medicine specialists) and mental and behavioral health services. Pediatricians can also play an important role in supporting families and youth as they navigate this process and find acceptance.

References

1. Katzenellenbogen R. HEADSS: the "review of systems" for adolescents. Virtual Mentor. 2005;7(3):231–3.
2. Edwards KM, Hackell JM. The committee on infectious diseases, the committee on practice and ambulatory medicine. Countering vaccine hesitancy. Pediatrics. 2016;138(3):e20162146.
3. Levine DA, the COA, Braverman PK, Adelman WP, Breuner CC, Levine DA, et al. Office-based care for lesbian, gay, bisexual, transgender, and questioning youth. Pediatrics. 2013;132(1):e297–313.

Chapter 38
Newborn Care

Roshni Sambasivan and Tracy Thomas

Introduction

This chapter will review how to complete a thorough assessment of the newborn and the expected management in the newborn period. It is important to be able to differentiate normal versus abnormal findings in the neonatal period to allow the clinician to address concerning medical conditions promptly.

Newborn Transitional Period

After delivery, immediate care of the newborn includes drying, clearing the airway of secretions, and providing warmth. If the newborn is full term, has good muscle tone, and is breathing or crying, they should remain with the mother and be placed skin-to-skin to promote infant-maternal bonding and early initiation of breastfeeding.

The Apgar scores at 1 and 5 minutes after birth provide an accepted, universally used method to assess the status of the newborn infant immediately after birth. The Apgar score should not be used to predict individual neonatal outcome as it is not an accurate prognostic tool. Five objective signs are evaluated and given values of 0, 1, or 2 at 1 and 5 minutes of life and are added to compute the Apgar score (Table 38.1).

R. Sambasivan (✉)
General Pediatrics, PurePediatrics, Bellaire, TX, USA
e-mail: dr.sam@purepediatrics.com

T. Thomas
Division of Neonatology, Department of Pediatrics, Baylor College of Medicine, Houston, TX, USA
e-mail: Tracy.Thomas@bcm.edu

N. Liao et al. (eds.), *Pediatric Rotations*,
https://doi.org/10.1007/978-3-031-59873-9_38

Table 38.1 APGAR scoring [1]

Sign	0	1	2
Heart rate	Absent	Below 100	Over 100
Respiratory effort	Absent	Slow, irregular, weak cry	Good, crying
Muscle tone	Limp	Some flexion of extremities	Active motion
Reflex	No response	Grimace	Cry or active withdrawal
Color	Blue, pale	Body pink, extremities blue	Completely pink

Adapted from *The APGAR Score*, American Academy of Pediatrics Policy Statement 2006

Infants undergo a complex sequence of physiologic changes as they make the transition from intrauterine to extrauterine life. This transition is successful in almost all infants although some may have cardiopulmonary abnormalities that require intervention. Observation of healthy infants during the transitional period should occur in the mother's room with intermittent assessment by nursing personnel. Physiological changes that occur during the transitional period include decreasing pulmonary vascular resistance with increased blood flow to the lungs, lung expansion with clearance of alveolar fluid, and closure of the ductus arteriosus.

Newborn History

A newborn history includes maternal chart review for relevant information. This comprises review of the current pregnancy including prenatal testing and fetal ultrasounds, prenatal labs including maternal blood type and maternal serologies for human immunodeficiency virus (HIV), syphilis, hepatitis B, and hepatitis C, rubella status, as well as group B streptococcal (GBS) colonization testing. Screening for these conditions help to evaluate risk for perinatal infections (Table 38.2). Other tests that may be performed include *Neisseria gonorrhoeae*, *Chlamydia trachomatis*, and/or urine drug screen.

Perinatal Infections

Review of the maternal history includes relevant medical and family history, maternal medications, review of past pregnancies, history of congenital anomalies, still births, or genetic conditions. Risk factors including history of domestic violence, child abuse/neglect, homelessness, substance abuse should also be reviewed.

The events of labor and delivery should be reviewed for any complications including risk factors for sepsis, for example, maternal intrapartum fever, prolonged rupture of membranes ≥18 hours, premature delivery, GBS colonization without adequate intrapartum antibiotic prophylaxis, and/or maternal chorioamnionitis.

Table 38.2 Perinatal infections

Perinatal infection	Clinical manifestation	Diagnosis
Cytomegalovirus	Intrauterine growth restriction, microcephaly, periventricular calcifications, hepatosplenomegaly, persistent jaundice, chorioretinitis	Urine or saliva culture, early antigen detection
HIV	Typically, asymptomatic at birth, persistent thrush, lymphadenopathy, hepatosplenomegaly	HIV DNA PCR
HSV	Fever, poor feeding, vesicular lesions, conjunctivitis, hepatosplenomegaly, seizures	Viral cultures of skin lesions, conjunctiva, mouth or nasopharynx, rectum; PCR of CSF
Rubella	Heart defects (PDA, PPS, VSD, ASD), microphthalmia, cataracts, sensorineural deafness, microcephaly, "blueberry muffin" rash	IgM antibody or persistently IgG positive
Syphilis	Anemia, thrombocytopenia, leukopenia, hepatitis, osteochondritis, maculopapular rash, persistent rhinitis	Nontreponemal test: RPR or VDRL Confirm with treponemal test (after 12–15 months of age): FTA-ABS, TP-PA
Toxoplasmosis	Microcephaly, hydrocephalus, intracranial calcifications, microphthalmia, chorioretinitis	Serologic testing

Abbreviations: *HIV* human immunodeficiency virus, *DNA* deoxyribonucleic acid, *PCR* polymerase chain reaction, *HSV* herpes simplex virus, *CSF* cerebrospinal fluid, *PDA* patent ductus arteriosus, *PPS* peripheral pulmonary stenosis, *VSD* ventral septal defect, *ASD* atrial septal defect, *IgG* immunoglobulin G, *IgM* immunoglobulin M, *RPR* rapid plasma reagin, *VDRL* venereal disease research laboratory, *FTA-ABS* fluorescent treponemal antibody absorption, *TP-PA* treponema pallidum particle agglutination

Newborn Physical Examination

The newborn physical exam should be performed in a systematic manner to ensure a complete examination. While the exact order of the exam is not important, the exam can be optimized by beginning with observation of the general appearance, then auscultation of the lungs and heart while the newborn is quiet. Then a head-to-toe approach allows for consistency and completeness.

Standard measurements obtained on newborns include the head circumference (frontal-occipital circumference (FOC)) and length measured in centimeters and the birth weight measured in grams. The weight, length, and FOC are plotted on curves to determine the percentile of intrauterine growth according to gestational age.

Normal vital signs in the newborn include an axillary temperature of 36.5–37.5 °C (97.7–99.5 °F), respiratory rate of 40–60 breaths per minute counted over a full minute and a heart rate of 120–160 beats per minute.

General appearance: The newborn should be observed undressed in a resting, non-stimulated state. General inspection includes sex determination, identification of any gross anomalies, respiratory effort, activity, position, movement, and color assessment.

Head: Size and shape of the head should be noted. Immediately after birth, passage through the birth canal may result in cranial molding, temporary asymmetry of the skull due to overlapping or overriding of the sutures. Within a few days, the distortion caused by cranial molding disappears, and one can better estimate the shape of the head and the suture lines. Fontanelles should be palpated; they are normally soft and flat. The anterior fontanelle is located where the metopic, sagittal, and lamboid sutures meet and can vary in size. The posterior fontanelle is located where the sagittal and lamboid sutures meet and are usually smaller than 1 cm in diameter. A bulging fontanelle may be an indication of increased intracranial pressure. A depressed fontanel may be normal or may be early evidence of dehydration.

Eyes: Initially after birth, the eyes can be difficult to examine as they are often edematous. Note the spacing and symmetry of the eyes, width of palpebral fissures, appearance of the sclera and conjunctiva, pupillary size and shape, red reflex, and eye movement. Subconjunctival hemorrhage may be present, usually as a consequence of delivery. All neonates require an ophthalmoscopic examination to visualize the red reflex which is seen if the lens and underlying structures are clear. A normal red reflex should emanate from both eyes symmetrically without opacities or white spots. Abnormalities of the red reflex including dark spots, diminished reflex, or white pupil are an indication for a referral to an ophthalmologist.

Ears: Note the position, size, and appearance of the ears. Normal position of the ear is when the helix is intersected by a horizontal line drawn from the outer canthus of the eye to the occiput. If the helix falls below this line, the ears are considered low set. The ears should also be inspected for any external abnormalities such as pits or tags.

Nose: Patency of the nasal canals may be tested by noting the movement of a piece of cotton placed before the infant's nose. Note presence of nasal discharge, breathing through the mouth, and flaring of nares.

Mouth: Assessment of the mouth includes the gingiva, tongue, palate, and uvula. Epstein pearls are benign whitish-yellow inclusion cysts commonly visualized at the midpoint of the junction between the soft and hard palate.

Neck: The neck should be assessed for mobility, masses, and excess skin. The clavicles should also be palpated for evidence of fracture manifesting as a step-off, crepitus, or swelling.

Chest: The chest should be examined with the head midline for size, symmetry, and movement. Intercostal, subcostal, and supraclavicular retractions can indicate signs of respiratory distress.

Lungs: Breathing rate and pattern should be observed for one full minute to account for variations in rate. Normal respirations are 40–60 times per minute. The lungs should be auscultated while the newborn is quiet (ideally earlier in the assessment) and should be assessed for quality and symmetry. In addition to retractions, other signs of respiratory distress include tachypnea, nasal flaring, grunting, and oxygen saturations below 90% on room air.

Heart: The baby must be quiet for an adequate exam. Palpate the apical impulse to locate the position of the heart. Observe for cardiac activity and palpate for thrill. Newborn babies are right heart dominant; thus, the PMI is displaced medially compared to an adult. The heart rate at birth varies from 100 to 200 but stabilizes shortly after birth to 120–160 beats/min. Auscultate for a regular rate and rhythm. Arrhythmias or tachycardia are abnormal. Poor or distant heart sounds occur with pneumothorax, pneumomediastinum, cardiac failure, or diaphragmatic hernia. Cardiac murmurs should be described as to location, quality of sound, where they occur in the cardiac cycle, whether they are transmitted, and intensity. In the first few days of life, a transient and benign murmur can be present. A murmur caused by a patent ductus arteriosus (PDA), is continuous harsh in quality or "machine-like" and is loudest in the second left intercostal space. A majority of PDAs close by 48 h of life. Femoral and brachial pulses should be palpated bilaterally and the force and timing should be noted. Blood pressure is not usually measured in a well newborn unless there is concern for congenital heart disease.

Abdomen: Abdominal examination should include an overall evaluation of the size and appearance and presence of bowel sounds. If the abdomen is distended, one should consider intestinal obstruction, organomegaly, and tumors. If the abdomen is flat or scaphoid, one should consider a diaphragmatic hernia. Diastasis recti or a wide separation of the abdominal muscles is a normal finding in newborns. Palpation of abdomen is easier if the newborn is not crying. Relaxation of the abdominal muscles may be facilitated by holding the legs in a flex position or having the newborn suck on a pacifier or the examiner's gloved finger. The liver edge can be palpated 1–3 cm below the right costal margin and the spleen is usually not palpable, but the tip may be felt in normal infants. The lower pole of the right and left kidneys may be palpated. The bladder can be palpated or percussed 1–4 cm above the symphysis when bladder is full. Any other masses palpable in the abdomen must be identified and described. The umbilical cord can be inspected shortly after birth for general appearance and the presence of two arteries and one vein.

Male Genitalia: The presence of testes, size of the penis, and appearance of the scrotum should be noted. Physiologic phimosis is expected in newborn males, but in some, the foreskin may be retracted sufficiently to reveal the urethral meatus. A ventrally displaced urethral meatus indicates the presence of hypospadias. The testes should be noted for size and location (canal, scrotum, or if undescended). Hydroceles may be present but disappear over the first months of life. Masses should be transilluminated and discoloration of the scrotum noted.

Female Genitalia: The size and location of the labia, clitoris, and vaginal opening should be noted. The labia minora can be more prominent than the labia majora in the premature female. The vaginal opening should be visible; many female newborns have hymenal skin tags which are slight protrusion of the vaginal epithelium. Presence of any discharge from the vagina (white, blood-tinged or frankly bloody) should be noted—milky white or blood-tinged physiologic discharge may be present due to withdrawal from maternal hormones.

Anus: Note the location and presence of an anus, patency is verified when meconium is seen at the anal opening. Routine rectal examination in the neonatal period is not done.

Trunk and spine: Note any obvious deformity of the trunk or spine. Run a hand along the vertebrae to determine overt deformities of the vertebrae. The gluteal folds should be separated to inspect for a sacral dimple. In general, a sacral or lower back dimple is benign and not representative of occult spina bifida if all of the following are noted: solitary lesions, located within the gluteal cleft, less than 2.5 cm above the anus, less than 0.5 cm in width and completely covered by skin.

Extremities: Check for polydactyly and syndactyly, abnormal palmar creases, fractures, paralyses, and dislocations. Fractures may not be obvious early but are brought to your attention by the newborn not moving the extremity or crying when the extremity is moved.

Hips: The hips are examined to detect developmental dysplasia of the hip (DDH). The examination for hip instability should be performed gently, but firmly, and with the infant quiet and relaxed. Techniques to detect hip instability use adduction and posterior pressure to feel for dislocation (Barlow maneuver) and abduction and elevation to feel for reduction (Ortolani maneuver). The sensation of dislocation or reduction is distinct and best described as a "clunk" and differs from that of benign joint popping or tendon snapping. Risk factors for DDH include female gender, in utero breech position, and positive family history.

Skin: Skin should be inspected for abnormalities that may warrant further evaluation or indicate an underlying disorder including color, consistency, hydration, rashes, abrasions, bruises, petechiae, abnormal pigmentation, congenital nevi, or hemangiomas. Various benign and transient findings can be found in normal newborns, these are outlined in Table 38.3. Acrocyanosis (cyanosis of hands and feet) can be normal in a newborn up to 48 h of age. Full-term newborns have a hemoglobin of 17–20 g/dL, which may cause the baby to appear plethoric. Jaundice can first be noted on the face and areas of bony prominence. Clinical jaundice is first obvious at bilirubin levels of 5 mg/dL; however, this varies by skin tone and can be missed in infants with darker skin tone.

Neuromuscular Status: Level of alertness should be observed, keep in mind the level of alertness in a newborn can depend on the state of hunger, sleep, and time after delivery. The nervous system of the neonate is immature which is demonstrated in many primitive reflexes, outlined in Table 38.4. Tone should be noted and varies depending on gestation; flexor tone is greater in newborns. A full term and older premature infant should be able to bear weight on the lower extremities. Tremulousness or jitteriness may indicate hypoglycemia or drug withdrawal, or may be an exaggerated startle reflex (more common in preterm infants). Irritability should be noted and if the infant is consolable.

Table 38.3 Common newborn skin findings

	Finding	Characteristics	Location
Birthmarks	Nevus simplex	Most common vascular malformation, of capillary origin Macular pink-red capillary dilations Typically fade by 18 months of age without need for intervention	Forehead, upper eyelids, nose, upper lip, or nape of the neck
	Congenital dermal melanocytosis	Most common form of cutaneous hyperpigmentation Grayish blue patch Most commonly in children with darker skin pigmentation Due to pigment cells in the deep layers of the skin Usually fade by 1 year of age	Most often in the sacral region, can be present on trunk and extremities
	Infantile hemangioma	Benign vascular tumor Caused by increased growth of endothelial cells on blood vessels Often benign and self-involutes Further work-up depends on size and location	Nonspecific
	Café au lait spots	Light brown macule Often seen in healthy children Six or more spots greater than 0.5 cm in diameter warrant further investigation for neurofibromatosis	Nonspecific
	Nevus-flammeus ("port-wine stain")	Large dark purple or red capillary malformation Generally, does not fade	Nonspecific
	Melanocytic nevus	Benign proliferations of cutaneous melanocytes If large (>9 cm on the head or >6 cm on the body), refer to dermatology due to the risk of malignant transformation	Nonspecific
	Sebaceous nevi	Isolated smooth plaques Hairless, round or linear Slightly raised Range from pink to yellow, orange, or tan	Typically located on the scalp or face

(continued)

Table 38.3 (continued)

	Finding	Characteristics	Location
Rashes	Erythema toxicum	Most common rash in newborns Flesh or red macules or pustules with an erythematous base Self-limiting and benign Biopsy or stain of the material in the lesion reveals eosinophils	Diffuse
	Neonatal pustular melanosis	Vesiculopustules and pigmented macules Self-limited, benign condition More common in darkly skinned infants	Diffuse
	Milia	Small 1–2 mm smooth, white papules without associated erythema Spontaneously resolves within the first month of life	Forehead, cheeks, chin, nose
	Sebaceous hyperplasia	Tiny, smooth, yellow-white papules Spontaneously diminish in size and disappear within the first few weeks of life	On or around the nose

Table 38.4 Primitive reflexes

Reflex	Initiate	Response	Duration
Babinski	Stroke lateral sole of foot upwards	Toes fan out	Disappears by 6–9 months of age
Grasp	Palms of hands are touched	Hands tightly grasp stimulus	Disappears by 4–6 months of age
Moro	Extension of neck, sudden movement, or loud noise	Extends arms and legs and then brings arms in	Disappears by 2 months of age
Rooting	Touch cheek or corner of mouth	Turns head toward stimulus	Disappears by 3–4 months of age
Stepping	Hold infant upright and allow feet to touch flat surface	Places one foot in front of the other and "walks"	Disappears by 2 months of age
Suck	Touch the roof of the mouth	Sucks rhythmically	Disappears by 4 months of age
Tonic neck	Turn head to one side	Corresponding extremities extend and opposite extremities bend	Disappears by 5–7 months of age

Ballard Scale

The Ballard score helps determine the gestational age of a newborn within a 2 week range by assessing the neuromuscular and physical maturity of the baby. The scoring is most accurate when done in the first 12 hours of life. Figure 38.1 illustrates

Neuromuscular Maturity

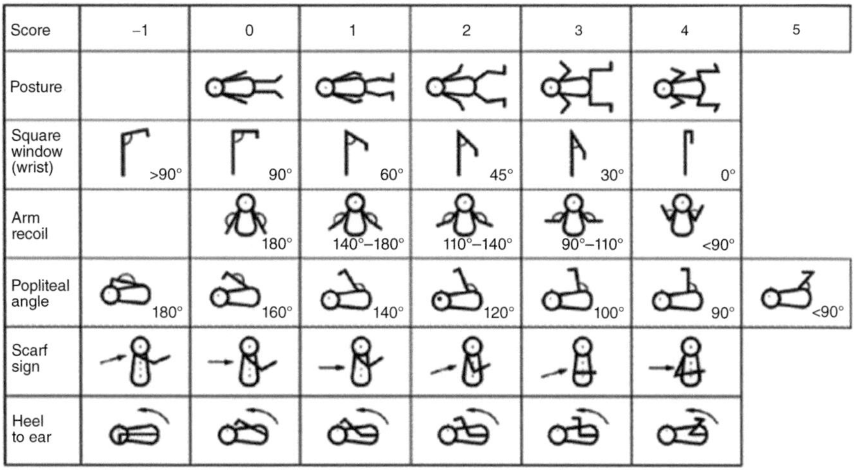

Physical Maturity

Skin	Sticky, friable, transparent	Gelatinous, red, translucent	Smooth, pink; visible veins	Superficial peeling and/or rash; few veins	Cracking, pale areas; rare veins	Parchment, deep cracking; no vessels	Leathery, cracked wrinkled
Lanugo	None	Sparse	Abundant	Thinning	Bald areas	Mostly bald	
Plantar surface	Heel-toe 40-50 mm: –1 <40 mm: –2	>50 mm, no crease	Faint red marks	Anterior transverse crease only	Creases anterior ⅔	Creases over entire sole	
Breast	Imperceptible	Barely perceptible	Flat areola, no bud	Stippled areola, 1–2 mm bud	Raised areola, 3–4 mm bud	Full areola, 5–10 mm bud	
Eye/Ear	Lids fused loosely: –1 tightly: –2	Lids open; pinna flat; stays folded	Slightly curved pinna; soft; slow recoil	Well curved pinna; soft but ready recoil	Formed and firm, instant recoil	Thick cartilage, ear stiff	
Genitals (male)	Scrotum flat, smooth	Scrotum empty faint rugae	Testes in upper canal, rare rugae	Testes descending, few rugae	Testes down, good rugae	Testes pendulous, deep rugae	
Genitals (female)	Clitoris prominent, labia flat	Clitoris prominent, small labia minora	Clitoris prominent, enlarging minora	Majora and minora equally prominent	Majora large, minora small	Majora cover clitoris and minora	

Maturity Rating

Score	Weeks
–10	20
–5	22
0	24
5	26
10	28
15	30
20	32
25	34
30	36
35	38
40	40
45	42
50	44

Fig. 38.1 Ballard scale. (With permissions from Elsevier)

scoring of the Ballard scale and each of the different neuromuscular and physical components is explained in detail below.

Neuromuscular maturity:

- Posture: How are the arms and legs positioned at rest?
- Square window (wrist): How far can a hand be flexed toward the wrist?
- Arm Recoil: When the forearm is extended at the elbow, how far does the arm return back into the flexed position when released?

- Popliteal angle: How far does the lower leg extend from the knee from a bent position?
- Scarf sign: How far can the newborn's elbow be brought across the chest?
- Heel to ear: How close can the foot be brought to the ear?

Physical maturity:

- Skin: Is the skin sticky, smooth, or cracked and leathery?
- Lanugo: Is there abundant soft, fine hair on the newborn? Are there areas of thinning or is it mostly bald?
- Plantar surface: Are the soles of the feet smooth or are there creases? How far do the creases cover the sole of the feet?
- Breast: How developed are the breast tissue and areola?
- Eye/Ear: Are the eyelids fused or open? How does the ear curve and how stiff is the ear?
- Genitals (male): Are the testes descended? Is the scrotum smooth or wrinkled?
- Genitals (female): How prominent is the clitoris? Are the labia majora small, equal or larger than labia minora?

Common Newborn Skin Findings

Birth Sequelae and Injuries

Three different types of birth sequelae involving the head include caput succedaneum, cephalohematoma, and subgaleal hemorrhage. Each of these types of birth sequelae can be differentiated on physical examination. Caput succedaneum is a boggy, vaguely demarcated area of edema and bruising of the presenting portion of the scalp during a vertex delivery. The soft tissue swelling crosses suture lines and may be associated with petechiae and ecchymosis. Usually, no specific treatment is indicated and resolution occurs within 48 hours.

Cephalohematoma is a subperiosteal collection of blood usually affecting the parietal and temporal bones. The bleeding occurs during labor or delivery and is caused by rupture of diploic blood vessels and separation of periosteum from the bone. Cephalohematomas are more common in prolonged labors and vacuum or forceps-assisted deliveries. They present as a sharply demarcated swelling that does not cross suture lines. Generally, cephalohematomas are benign; however, they can be associated with hyperbilirubinemia and, less commonly, an underlying skull fracture. Cephalohematomas typically do not require intervention and spontaneously reabsorb by 2 weeks to 3 months of age. Calcification can occur resulting in bony swelling that may persist for several months.

Subgaleal hemorrhage is an accumulation of blood in the space between the epicranial aponeurosis and the periosteum. It is caused by rupture of emissary veins. This potential space is so large that this type of extracranial bleeding may become massive and life-threatening. Subgaleal hemorrhages are most common with vacuum extraction deliveries but can also occur in spontaneous vaginal deliveries. This type of hemorrhage presents with rapidly progressing diffuse cranial swelling with ill-defined borders and fluctuant consistency possibly with a fluid wave. Extracranial symptoms include signs of hypovolemia (pallor, tachycardia, shock) and central nervous system (CNS) injury (lethargy, hypotonia, seizures). When suspected, the infant must be monitored closely in the Neonatal Intensive Care Unit (NICU) with frequent vital signs, serial head circumference measurements, serial hematocrits, and close observation for signs of hypovolemia.

Other types of birth injuries can occur when instruments such as a vacuum or forceps are used at the time of delivery. When the use of these instruments is necessary, marks may occur where instruments were applied and may be associated with nerve, soft tissue, or bony injury. Lacerations can occur during cesarean delivery and commonly affect the scalp, buttocks, and thighs. Superficial wounds can be treated with wound closure adhesive strips; however, deeper wounds may require sutures. Electrode marks result from direct monitoring of the fetal heart rate during labor. They may lead to lacerations, hematomas, or superficial abrasions at the site of application. Only local treatment is typically required; however, if an abscess develops, evaluation for infection may be necessary.

Newborns are also at risk of fractures during the delivery process. The clavicle is the most frequently fractured bone in newborns. Most clavicle fractures are unilateral, non-displaced, and asymptomatic. Physical examination may be notable for tenderness, localized crepitus, asymmetric Moro reflex, a palpable step-off, or swelling. An X-ray can be obtained to document the fracture. Education for parents with strategies for supportive care to minimize movement of the affected side is provided, and immobilization is not necessary. Humerus and femur fractures are less common in newborns. If suspected due to pain with palpation, an obvious deformity, or swelling, plain radiographs should be obtained.

Lastly, brachial plexus injuries typically occur when the cervical nerve roots are stretched or severed during delivery. Depending on the extent of injury and progression through the hospital stay, referral for specialty services for management and/or therapy may be beneficial.

Routine Prophylaxis in the Newborn

Routine prophylaxis in the newborn period includes erythromycin eye prophylaxis, intramuscular (IM) Vitamin K administration, and hepatitis B vaccination.

Erythromycin eye prophylaxis is given to prevent vision-threatening gonococcal ophthalmia neonatorum. Ocular prophylaxis is recommended for all newborns by the United States Preventive Services Task Force and is safe, easy to administer, and inexpensive. Appropriate prophylaxis includes the application of a 1–2 cm ribbon of 0.5% erythromycin ophthalmic ointment to the eyes within 2 hours of birth. Erythromycin ophthalmic ointment is not effective in preventing neonatal chlamydial conjunctivitis. The most effective measure to prevent neonatal chlamydial conjunctivitis is the diagnosis and treatment of chlamydial infections during pregnancy.

All newborns are given prophylactic Vitamin K, also known as phytonadione, as an IM dose of 1 mg within the first 6 hours of life to prevent vitamin K deficient bleeding (VKDB). Vitamin K is essential for the formation of clotting factors II, VII, IX, and X. Fetal vitamin K is derived from the mother; however, placental transfer of the vitamin is poor. A newborn obtains vitamin K from the diet and putrefactive bacteria in the gut. Therefore, production of vitamin K is dependent on initiation of feeding. VKDB is classified according to when it presents:

- Early VKDB: occurs within 24 hours of birth. Primarily in newborns whose mothers took vitamin K inhibiting drugs during pregnancy.
- Classic VKDB: 24 hours– 7 days of age.
- Late VKDB: 1–24 weeks of age.

VKDB in the newborn can manifest as bleeding from various sites such as needle puncture sites, circumcision site, umbilical stump, GI tract, and the brain. 30% to 60% of babies with late onset VKDB will have intracranial bleeding which can result in long-term neurological sequelae and possibly death. Oral forms of Vitamin K for the prevention of VKDB have not been approved for use in the United States and do not prevent late onset VKDB. If a parent refuses Vitamin K administration, a discussion should ensue about the role of IM Vitamin K for the prevention of VKDB and the potential devastating consequences of vitamin K refusal including intestinal hemorrhage, intracranial hemorrhage with subsequent neurodevelopmental impairment and possible death.

Universal vaccination regardless of maternal hepatitis B virus surface antigen (HBsAg) status is recommended. All babies with a birth weight greater than or equal to 2 kg born to Hepatitis B-negative mothers should receive the first Hepatitis B vaccine (HBV) by 24 hours of age. Infants with a birth weight <2 kg should receive the first HBV at 1 month of age, or at hospital discharge, whichever occurs first. Newborns of HBsAg-positive mothers should receive HBV in addition to hepatitis B immunoglobulin (HBIG) within 12 hours of age.

Routine Newborn Care

Bathing: A newborn's first bath is usually given when stability through the transitional period has been demonstrated. This includes effective thermoregulation and normal blood glucose values, for babies at risk for hypoglycemia. Before the umbilical cord falls off, a newborn should have sponge baths only. Thereafter, infants can be placed directly into warm water (warm to touch on the inside of one's wrist) using mild, non-perfumed soaps.

Cord Care: Keeping the umbilical cord clean and dry is as effective and safe as using antiseptics, and it shortens the time to cord separation. Alcohol application is not needed for routine cord care. The normal process of cord separation, including appearance and possible odor, should be explained to caregivers. Caregivers should be instructed to keep the umbilical cord open to air for natural drying and to use water at the base of the cord to remove any discharge that may develop. The umbilical cord usually separates from the abdomen 6–14 days after birth.

Nails: Newborn fingernails are small and grow quickly. Fingernails should be kept short and smooth to prevent scratching. They can be trimmed as needed using an emery board or nail clippers made specifically for babies.

Sleep position: Healthy infants should be placed in a supine position for sleep. A supine position confers lowest risk for sudden infant death syndrome (SIDS). The side position is not recommended. Soft surfaces, such as pillows, soft mattresses, stuffed animals, or crib bumpers should not be placed under or around infants. Nighttime sleeping in car seats, baby swings, or co-sleeping is not recommended. The use of pacifiers during sleep throughout the first year of life has been associated with a reduced risk of SIDS.

Feeding

Newborns should be fed early and frequently to prevent hypoglycemia. The frequency, duration, and volume of feeds will be dependent upon whether the newborn is breastfed or formula feeding. Each feeding length and/or volume should be recorded.

Breastfeeding has been recognized as the preferred form of nutrition during the first year of life because of its direct benefits of improved nutrition, gastrointestinal function, host defense, and psychological well-being. The American Academy of Pediatrics (AAP) recommends exclusive breastfeeding for the first 6 months of life followed by continued breastfeeding with the introduction of appropriate complementary solid foods for the 2 years of life as mutually desired by mother and child. Human milk contains macro- and micronutrients as well as living cells, growth factors, and immunoprotective substances. Short-term benefits include prevention of illnesses including gastroenteritis, respiratory disease, otitis media, urinary tract infections, sepsis, as well as prevention of SIDS.

Breastfeeding should be initiated within the first hour after birth and with baby hunger cues at a frequency of 8–12 times a day and lasting until the infant is satisfied, which is usually for a duration of at least 10–15 minutes on each breast.

Absolute contraindications to breastfeeding include (1) infants of mothers with HIV or human T-cell lymphotrophic virus type I or II, (2) active herpes lesions on the breasts, (3) infants with classic galactosemia, (4) active untreated maternal tuberculosis, and (5) active maternal substance use disorder.

Healthy newborns who are fed formula should be offered standard infant formula (19–20 kcal/oz.). They should also feed on demand and duration between feeds should not exceed 3–4 hours. Volume of feeds in the first few days of life will range from 10 mL/feed to 30 mL/feed.

Most infants will urinate within the first 30 hours of life. Any infant with suspicion of failure to void within the first 30 h of life requires a thorough examination with focus on palpable, enlarged kidneys, a distended bladder, as well as a careful neurological examination of the lower extremities.

Meconium, a thick, dark, tar-like substance, is usually passed within the first 48 hours of life. An infant who does not pass stool in the first 48 hours of life requires further evaluation. Over several days, the stool transitions to a yellow-green color and looser consistency. Bowel movement frequency varies. Many infants will stool after each feeding (due to gastrocolic reflex) and others only stool once every several days. In general, formula-fed infants have at least one bowel movement a day (more formed, green/brown), while breast-fed infants usually stool more frequently (yellow, seedy, loose consistency).

In general, babies should have at least 1 wet diaper daily from birth up to day 6 of life at which time the expectation is at least 6 wet diapers daily. Weight loss during the first several days of birth is generally physiologic. Term newborns may lose up to 10% of their birth weight in the first few days of life and regain birth weight by 10–14 days of life.

Newborn Screenings

In the United States, screening for metabolic and genetic disorders, critical congenital heart disease, and congenital hearing loss are routinely performed on all neonates.

State Newborn Screening: Each state requires newborn blood spot screening for multiple genetic disorders and congenital conditions that are threatening to life or long-term health and for which early intervention is expected to improve outcomes. Disorders screened include cystic fibrosis, congenital hypothyroidism, galactosemia, hemoglobinopathies, congenital adrenal hyperplasia, biotinidase deficiency, and inborn errors of metabolism (amino acid disorders, organic acid disorders, and disorders of fatty oxidation). The screen is obtained by analyzing drops of blood on a special paper and depending on each state's testing requirements, one or two specimens are collected.

Hearing Screening: The prevalence of newborn hearing loss is approximately 1–2 per 1000 live births. Newborn hearing screening using a physiologic assessment tool is required by law. Babies are screened with otoacoustic emissions (OAE) or an automated auditory brainstem response (AABR). Newborns who fail the hospital hearing screen will require a full audiologic diagnostic evaluation after discharge. Some institutions consider cytomegalovirus evaluation in infants who fail their newborn hearing screen.

Critical Congenital Heart Disease (CCHD) Screening: Congenital heart defects are the most common birth defects. Some of these defects are critical, requiring early intervention and management to save the life of a baby. Early diagnosis and timely intervention of CCHD can significantly reduce morbidity and mortality and lead to better outcomes. Newborn screening with pulse oximetry has been shown to be useful for the detection of severe primary targets of CCHD including hypoplastic left heart syndrome, pulmonary atresia (with intact atrial septum), tetralogy of fallot, total anomalous pulmonary venous return, transposition of the great arteries, tricuspid atresia, and truncus arteriosus. Screening should occur after 24 hours of age and is performed by obtaining and comparing pre-ductal and post-ductal oxygen saturations via pulse oximetry.

Bilirubin Screening: Screening for hyperbilirubinemia via collection of a serum bilirubin or transcutaneous bilirubin typically occurs at 24–48 hours of age. If neonate appears jaundiced before 24 hours of life or there are risk factors for hyperbilirubinemia, a bilirubin should be obtained sooner. For management of elevated total bilirubin levels refer to Chap. 23 in this book.

Risk-Based Screening: Glucose screening is indicated for babies at risk for hypoglycemia including those who are large for gestational age (>90th percentile), small for gestational age (<10th percentile), preterm (<37 weeks), infants of diabetic mothers, and infants of mothers with no prenatal care. Babies who fall into one or more of these categories should have an initial glucose screen at 30 minutes to 2 hours of life, and at regular intervals during the first 12–24 hours of life to ensure euglycemia.

Hospital Discharge

The hospital stay of a mother and her infant should be long enough to identify early problems and ensure adequate maternal recovery and readiness for discharge. Infant should have a normal physical examination and uncomplicated perinatal course that has not identified any abnormalities requiring continued hospitalization. The infant should have stable vital signs including temperature stability in an open crib and have completed two successful consecutive feedings, urinated adequately, and have passed stool at least once.

In breastfed infants, the successful latch, swallow, and satiety of the breastfed infant should be documented by a caregiver knowledgeable in breastfeeding. In formula-fed infants, the ability to coordinate sucking, swallowing, and breathing should be documented.

Newborn metabolic, hearing, CCHD, and bilirubin screening should be performed. Clinical risk for subsequent hyperbilirubinemia should be assessed and follow-up arranged. If a circumcision is performed, there should be no evidence of excessive bleeding from circumcision site for at least 2 hours after the procedure.

Caregivers should receive education and demonstrate understanding of the following infant care tasks: frequency and length (volume if bottle feeding) of feeds; appropriate frequency of urination and stooling; umbilical cord, skin, and genital care; proper infant safety including supine sleeping position on a firm mattress, use of a rear-facing car seat and hand hygiene; and recognition of signs of common neonatal illnesses for which to seek care immediately.

Reference

1. American Academy of Pediatrics, Committee on Fetus and Newborn, American College of Obstetricians and Gynecologists, Committee on Obstetric Practice. The Apgar Score. Pediatrics. 2006;117(4):1444–7. https://doi.org/10.1542/peds.2006-0325.

Suggested Readings

Warren JB, Phillipi CA. Care of the well newborn. Pediatr Rev. 2012;33(1):4–18. https://doi.org/10.1542/pir.2022-005511.

McInerny TK, Adam HM, Campbell DE, DeWitt TG, Foy JM, Kamat DM, editors. American academy of pediatrics textbook of pediatric care. 2nd ed. American Academy of Pediatrics: Elk Grove Village, IL; 2017.

Chapter 39
Neonatal Intensive Care

Ganga Gokulakrishnan and Davlyn Tillman

Classification of Neonates According to Birth Weight and Gestational Age

Understanding the classification of premature neonates is crucial in understanding the morbidities and outcomes of prematurity associated with each category (Tables 39.1 and 39.2). It also allows providers to institute best practices in the management of preterm infants.

The Late Preterm Infant

In the United States, the incidence of preterm births is approximately 10%. Out of this fraction, late preterm infants roughly comprise 70% of all preterm births in the United States. The reasons for increase in the incidence of late preterm birth are multifactorial in nature. Increased obstetrical surveillance has led to an increase in medically indicated late preterm births. The increasing occurrence of multiple births by assisted reproductive technologies and maternal factors such as advanced maternal age and maternal obesity also contribute to late preterm births. Late preterm infants are at risk for numerous complications listed in Table 39.3.

Feeding difficulties in late preterm infants place such infants at risk for failure to thrive. This is secondary to several factors which influence their caloric intake and feeding intolerance which are outlined in Table 39.4.

G. Gokulakrishnan (✉) · D. Tillman
Division of Neonatology, Department of Pediatrics, Baylor College of Medicine, Houston, TX, USA
e-mail: gokulakr@bcm.edu; davlyn.tillman@bcm.edu

N. Liao et al. (eds.), *Pediatric Rotations*,
https://doi.org/10.1007/978-3-031-59873-9_39

Table 39.1 Classification of neonates based on birth weight

Classification based on birth weight	
Low birth weight (LBW)	<2500 g
Very low birth weight (VLBW)	<1500 g
Extremely low birth weight (ELBW)	<1000 g

Table 39.2 Classification of neonates based on gestational age

Classification based on gestational age	
Post term	>42 0/7 weeks and beyond
Late term	41 0/7–41 6/7 weeks
Full term	39 0/7–40 6/7 weeks
Early term	37 0/7–38 6/7 weeks
Preterm infant	**<37 weeks**
Late preterm	34–36 6/7 weeks
Moderately preterm	32–34 weeks
Very preterm	28–32 weeks
Extremely preterm	Less than 28 weeks

Table 39.3 Morbidities associated with late preterm infants

Morbidities associated with late preterm infants
• Great need for resuscitation • Respiratory distress • Hypothermia • Hypoglycemia • Feeding difficulties • Hyperbilirubinemia • Apnea • Sepsis • Increased risk for admission to NICU after birth and readmission after discharge

Table 39.4 Nutrition complications seen in late preterm infants

Nutrition complications in late preterm infants

• Inadequate caloric intake
  – Poor suck/swallow coordination
  – Fatigue
• Feeding intolerance
  – Delayed stooling
  – Feeding residuals
• Exaggerated physiologic jaundice
• Increased need for parenteral nutrition
• Dehydration, hypernatremia
• Failure to thrive

Nutritional Needs of Late Preterm Infants

Breastfeeding and human milk remain the preferred method of feeding for late preterm infants. However, given their relative immature feeding skills, they often need assistance in meeting their caloric needs. Late preterm infants often take only ~5–10 mL per feed on day #1 of life. Their intake and hydration status can be monitored using their daily weights and urine output, in addition to the physical exam. If weight loss in 24 h is greater than 3% or total weight loss >7%, supplementation is necessary and can be provided with expressed breast milk or donor breast milk, if available. Otherwise, a term 20 kcal/oz. formula is generally sufficient. Supplementation can be provided by numerous methods depending on the clinical situation and parent's preference—gavage feeds, cup, syringe, supplemental device, or bottle.

You should look for signs of severe dehydration if intake is inadequate. Such signs include weight loss greater than 10%, inadequate urine output, hypernatremia, and lethargy.

Fortification of breast milk is not usually indicated unless infants are severely growth restricted.

As late preterm infants are at higher risk for morbidities and readmission following discharge, it is extremely important that parents of such infants are educated about risks associated with late preterm infants, given anticipatory guidance, and counseled on the importance of close follow-up with a pediatrician after discharge. In addition to routine discharge criteria recommended for healthy term infants, Table 39.5 outlines several additional criteria outlined by the AAP [1].

Table 39.5 Additional criteria to consider when discharging a late preterm infant

Criteria for discharging a late preterm infant
• Vitals signs are stable—respiratory rate <60, heart rate 100–160/min and axillary temperature 36.5–37.4 with infant in open crib and appropriate clothing • 24 h of successful feeding has been documented • A breastfeeding and supplementation feeding plan has been developed and shared with family • If weight loss is >2% to 3% of birth weight per day or a maximum of 7% of birth weight during hospitalization, assess for dehydration prior to discharge • A risk assessment and follow-up for hyperbilirubinemia has been performed • Medical home has been established and a follow-up appointment in arranged for 24–48 h after discharge • A car safety seat study has been performed observing for apnea, bradycardia, or desaturations

Neonatal Thermoregulation

Newborn infants, particularly preterm infants, often experience hypothermia after birth. The recognition and management of hypothermia is crucial as hypothermia increases risk for morbidity and mortality in the preterm population. The recommended range of normal newborn body temperature is 36.5–37.5 C (97.7–99.5 F) with neonatal hypothermia defined as an axillary temperature less than 36.5 C. Several factors predispose neonates to hypothermia: (1) higher body surface area to weight ratio, (2) less subcutaneous fat, and (3) relatively thin permeable dermal layer resulting in trans-epidermal water loss. Body temperature is a balance between heat production and heat loss; and neonates lose significant heat through radiation, conduction, convection, and evaporation. Table 39.6 includes means to minimize heat loss in neonates.

Upon admission, all vital signs should be recorded including axillary temperature. In the neonatal intensive care unit (NICU), thermal stability is maintained using radiant warmers and double-walled incubators. Radiant warmers minimize heat loss from radiation and conduction by keeping objects in direct contact with the infant warm. Unfortunately, radiant warmers permit large amounts of evaporative and convective heat loss given their open design. For extremely preterm infants, it is advised to place them in double-walled incubators as early as possible given the advantages over radiant warmers. In a double-walled incubator, the inner wall can be kept warm when compared to the outer wall and this minimizes radiation losses. Port holes in the incubator allow nursing cares to occur with minimal convective heat loss since nurses are not opening up the incubator entirely. The humidity maintained within the incubator also aids in minimizing evaporative losses.

Once hypothermia is established and heat losses continue to exceed the infant's ability to generate heat, infants can develop acidosis, increased oxygen consumption, apnea, hypoglycemia, poor growth and rarely, pulmonary hypertension and

Table 39.6 Modes of heat loss and measures to prevent heat loss

Mode of heat loss	Definition	Measures to prevent heat loss
Evaporation	Heat loss when water evaporates from skin and respiratory tract; of significance in extremely preterm infants	Drying infant immediately after birth Use of hats and occlusive plastic wrap Use of humidity in incubators
Radiation	Heat lost by radiation of infrared energy to cooler walls and objects	Prewarm operating and labor rooms to 25 °C
Conduction	Direct heat transfer from skin to a cooler object in direct contact with infant	Use of prewarmed towels and equipment using radiant warmer Exothermic chemical mattresses Skin to skin contact with parent
Convection	Heat loss due to flow of heat from infant's body surface to cooler surrounding air	Minimize opening incubator and avoid drafts Prewarm operating and labor rooms to 25 °C to keep ambient temperature warm

death. In the event of clinical instability, hypothermia should always be suspected, monitored, and treated.

Neonatal Hypoglycemia

In neonates, blood glucose decreases after birth and subsequently reaches the "normal range" in the first few hours of life. Available evidence however does not identify a specific glucose value below which neurologic injury has been associated. The most common cause of neonatal hypoglycemia is transient neonatal hypoglycemia which usually resolves 48–72 h after birth. Transient neonatal hypoglycemia is thought to be due to dysfunctional insulin regulation as the infant transitions from the intrauterine to extrauterine environment; glucose levels fall immediately after birth; instead of the normal transition of a decrease in insulin levels, insulin levels remain "normal"; resulting in suppression of ketone and fatty acid fuels. Infants who are at most risk for transient neonatal hypoglycemia include:

- Infants of diabetic mother (IDM).
- Large for gestational age infants (LGA).
- Small for gestational age (SGA) infants or intrauterine growth restriction (IUGR)/growth-restricted infants.
- Preterm infants <37 weeks.

Clinical Signs and Symptoms of Neonatal Hypoglycemia

- Seizures
- Hypotonia
- Temperature instability
- Respiratory distress
- Lethargy
- Cyanosis
- Apnea
- Poor feeding
- Irritability, tremors
- Jitteriness
- Tachypnea

The AAP guidelines provide guidance for screening and management of transient neonatal hypoglycemia for at risk infants [2] (Fig. 39.1).

Equation to Calculate Glucose Infusion Rate

$$\textbf{Glucose infusion rate}\ (\text{GIR})\ mg\ glucose/kg/\text{min} = \frac{[\%\ \text{dextrose} \times \text{fluid goal}\ (mL/kg/day)]}{144}$$

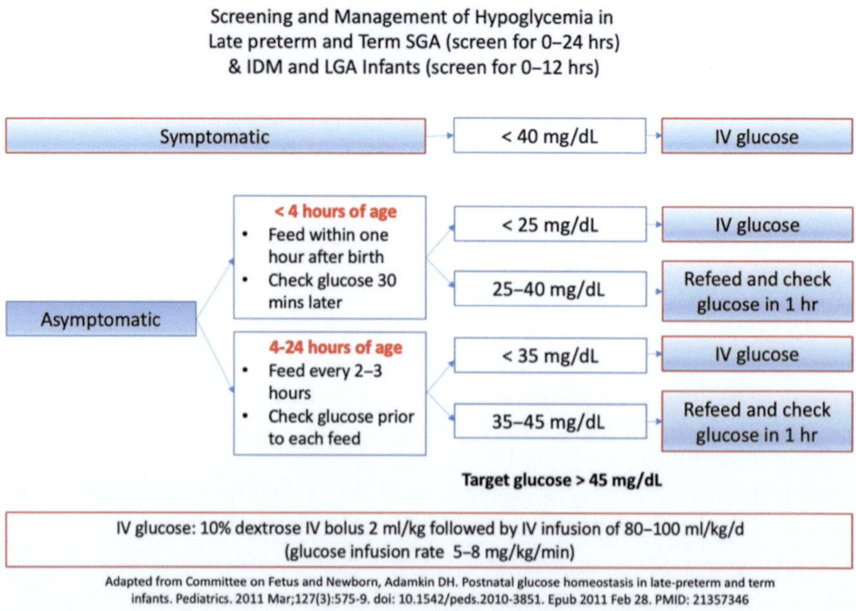

Fig. 39.1 Screening and management of hypoglycemia in infants at risk

Need for screening and intervention will usually involve one of the following clinical scenarios [3]:

Symptomatic infants with blood glucose (BG) value of <40 mg/dL should immediately be given a bolus of 2 mL/kg of 10% dextrose followed by a continuous glucose infusion of 5–8 mg/kg/min, titrated to maintain BG >60 mg/dL. One should not wait for the results of laboratory plasma glucose levels to initiate management of symptomatic infants.

Late preterm (34–36 6/7 weeks) infants and term IDM, SGA, or LGA infants who are stable and asymptomatic should be offered feeds within 1 h after birth (breastfeeding, oral, or gavage feeding with human milk or formula) and have BG tested 30 min after the feed. Frequent feeding should continue every 2–3 h with BG monitoring prior to each feed. The initial treatment target is a progressive rise in BG value to >45 mg/dL in the first 4 h of life. Monitoring of BG values should continue for 12–24 h. If BG values >45 mg/dL cannot be achieved with frequent feedings, supplementation with IV dextrose is necessary.

When BG values are stable >60 mg/dL and oral feeding is established, weaning of dextrose-containing IV fluids can be attempted with BG checks after each wean.

Fluid Management in Neonates

At birth, full-term infants have total body water comprising 75% of their body weight whereas preterm infants can have total body water up to 80–90% of their body weight. In comparison, in adults, this fraction is around 60%. After birth, as part of a normal physiologic transition during the first few days of life, neonates can lose up to 10% of birth weight secondary to reduction in extracellular water by diuresis.

Preterm neonates are at a further disadvantage in terms of fluid balance: (1) sub-optimal capacity to concentrate urine resulting in physiologic limitations to respond when they experience disturbances in fluid homeostasis, (2) immature epithelial skin layer, and (3) increase in body surface area to body weight ratio which contributes to increased trans-epidermal losses. Preterm neonates can lose up to 15% of their birth weight and are at a higher risk of morbidity due to disturbances in fluid homeostasis. As a result, increasing prematurity is associated with higher fluid requirements.

Given all the above factors, neonatal fluid requirements vary widely based on birth weight, gestation, and the neonate's environment. Daily fluid requirement calculations must also take into account insensible losses, urinary losses, and gastrointestinal losses such as losses from nasogastric tube or from an ostomy. Two-thirds of insensible losses are evaporative losses from the skin and one-third are evaporative losses from the respiratory tract.

At the bedside, you need to determine fluid status using clinical signs and all available data points. Clinical signs such as tachycardia, hypotension, decreased skin turgor, prolonged capillary refill, dry oral mucosa, and sunken fontanelle point towards dehydration and need for increased fluid input. Other data points to consider include any significant weight loss or gain, urine and stool output, net fluid balance and electrolytes. Note that *hypernatremia* may indicate dehydration whereas *hyponatremia* may be dilutional in nature indicating the need to restrict fluid intake.

Table 39.7 below provides guidelines for managing fluids in neonates. Fluid requirements often need to be individualized based on clinical circumstances. Maintenance fluid requirements are inversely proportional to birth weight and gestational age. As trans-epidermal losses are significant in neonates, extensive skin breakdown in ELBW infants or congenital abdominal wall defects such as gastroschisis can significantly increase daily fluid requirements. Increase in environmental temperatures, elevated body temperature, and placing infants under phototherapy or a radiant warmer can all increase their fluid requirements. Infants who are on a ventilator have increased respiratory insensible losses. Conversely, the use of a double-walled incubator in ELBW infants with 60–70% humidity can decrease fluid requirements. It is important to pay close attention to such details when prescribing fluids, particularly to critically ill infants.

Table 39.7 Fluid requirements in term and preterm infants (Gokulakrishnan, Gollins, July 2021)

Fluid requirements in stable term and late preterm infants who can be exclusively enterally fed			
	Day 0–1	**Day 2–3**	**Day 4 and beyond**
Minimum suggested fluid intake (mL/kg/d)[a]	30–40	30–40	>50
Suggested fluid requirement in critically ill infants who require intravenous support ± enteral nutrition (mL/kg/d)[b]			
Birth weight (g)	**Day 0–1**	**Day 2–3**	**Day 4 and beyond**
<750	130	140	150
751–1000	110	130	150
1001–1250	80–110	120	150
1251–1500	80	100–120	150
1501–2000	65–80	100	150
2000[b]	65–80	100	150

[a] Neonatal fluid requirements vary widely depending on environmental conditions, body weight, and gestation

[b] Neonatal fluid requirements vary widely depending on environmental conditions, body weight, and gestation

Adapted with permission from: Gokulakrishnan G, Gollins G. Fluid and Electrolyte Therapy. In: Metabolic Management: Guidelines for Acute Care of the Neonate 29th edition (2021–2022), Fernandes CJ, Pammi M, Katakam L, et al. (Eds), Baylor College of Medicine, Section of Neonatology, Department of Pediatrics. Copyright © 2021 Baylor College of Medicine

Bronchopulmonary Dysplasia

Bronchopulmonary Dysplasia (BPD) is a significant morbidity which preterm infants, particularly ELBW infants, may experience. BPD results from an alteration in lung development secondary to prematurity, with a disruption in the balance between lung injury and repair mechanisms. Risk factors for BPD include severe growth restriction, surfactant deficiency, mechanical ventilation, and infection. While various classifications exist, for clinical purposes, the diagnosis of BPD is generally based upon the need for oxygen therapy at 36 weeks post-menstrual age. The most commonly used classification from the National Institute of Child Health and Human Development [4] defines BPD as infants who have required oxygen treatment for at least the first 28 days after birth. Infants with BPD may be weaned to room air prior to discharge or may continue to require nasal cannula, noninvasive respiratory support, or mechanical ventilation after discharge, depending on the severity of lung disease.

BPD is a chronic lung disease, and its management requires a multifaceted approach consisting of optimizing respiratory support by minimizing ventilator-induced lung injury, optimizing neonatal nutrition and growth, fluid restriction, neurodevelopmental care, and avoidance of infections.

Various medications are used for moderate and severe forms of BPD which include diuretics, inhaled bronchodilators, and inhaled corticosteroids. The complications which arise secondary to BPD are listed below.

Complications of BPD

- Growth failure
- Tracheobronchomalacia
- Neurodevelopmental delay
- Infections
- Pulmonary hypertension
- Cor pulmonale
- Reactive airway disease
- The need for a tracheostomy and long-term mechanical ventilation
- Increased risk for readmission

Respiratory Distress in the Neonate

Respiratory Distress Syndrome (RDS) is the most common cause of respiratory disease in preterm infants, with risk of RDS increasing as gestational age decreases. Additional risk factors include maternal diabetes, male sex, and perinatal asphyxia [5]. Maternal antenatal corticosteroids reduce the risk of RDS in premature infants.

The pathophysiology of RDS involves developmental deficiency of surfactant, a phospholipid and protein mixture that lowers alveolar surface tension. Alveoli deficient in surfactant are prone to collapse on expiration and require increased pressures to expand on inspiration [5].

Clinical symptoms include tachypnea, grunting, retractions, nasal flaring, and hypoxia. Symptoms typically present at birth and worsen over the first several hours of life as endogenous surfactant stores are depleted. Endogenous surfactant is produced by the third to fourth day of life [5]. Radiologic findings demonstrate low lung volumes and a diffuse, homogenous "ground glass" appearance (Fig. 39.2). Neonatal pneumonia, especially if caused by Group B Strep, may have a similar radiologic appearance to RDS. Evaluation of infants with symptoms of RDS may include a chest radiograph, blood gas, complete blood count, and blood cultures.

Treatment of RDS may require supplemental oxygen and positive pressure support via nasal continuous positive airway pressure (CPAP) or mechanical ventilation. Infants with moderate or severe RDS symptoms ($FiO_2 > 30–40\%$) may require tracheal administration of exogenous surfactant.

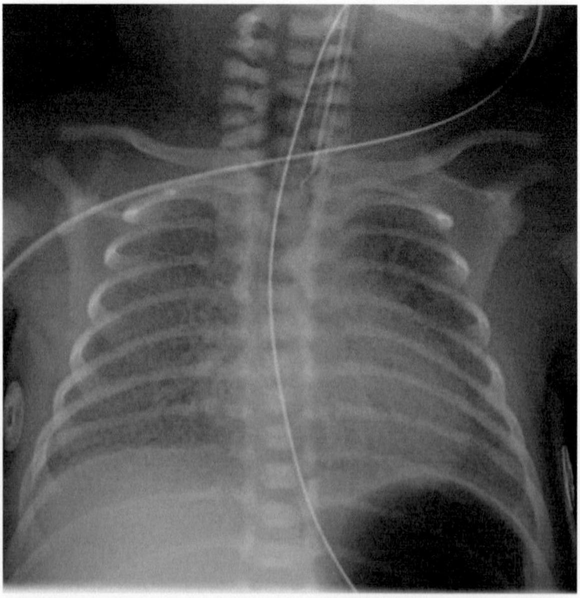

Fig. 39.2 Chest X-ray of neonate with respiratory distress syndrome

Transient Tachypnea of the Newborn: Transient tachypnea of the newborn (TTN) is a common cause of self-limited respiratory distress in term and late preterm newborns. Risk factors include cesarean delivery, precipitous delivery, fetal distress, and maternal diabetes. The pathophysiology of TTN involves delayed clearance of fetal lung fluid from alveolar airspaces, a process which occurs prior to, during, and after active labor.

Clinical symptoms include tachypnea, retractions, nasal flaring, and either normal or mildly decreased oxygen saturations. Symptoms may persist for 24–72 h. Improvement of symptoms with time distinguishes TTN from a diagnosis of RDS which worsens in severity with time. Classic radiologic findings demonstrate parenchymal infiltrates and "streaks" of fluid in the interstitium and interlobar fissures.

TTN requires supportive care with observation or supplemental oxygen support if hypoxia is present. Due to the risk for aspiration, infants with significant tachypnea may require nasogastric feeds or intravenous fluids.

Neonatal Resuscitation

The Neonatal Resuscitation Program (NRP) algorithm is a tool used by delivery room team members to respond to resuscitations in a standardized format. At birth, 4–10% of infants receive positive pressure ventilation (PPV), but less than 1% receive chest compressions [6].

Initial Questions at Delivery: When attending a delivery, the four questions to ask include:

1. Gestational Age?
2. Amniotic fluid clear?
3. Additional risk factors?
4. Umbilical cord management plan?

Ventilation: Effective ventilation is the most important step in newborn resuscitation. The indicators of effective ventilation are good chest rise and an increase in heart rate. Heart rate may be detected by auscultation or electrocardiogram (ECG) leads.

Continuous positive airway pressure (CPAP) is indicated if an infant is spontaneously breathing but showing signs of respiratory distress. CPAP is often the initial respiratory support for extremely preterm infants due to lung immaturity and need to establish lung volumes [3]. PPV should be started within 60 s of life if an infant is apneic, gasping, or heart rate is <100 bpm. If PPV does not result in effective ventilation, take corrective steps using the mnemonic MR. SOPA (Table 39.8). If there is still no adequate chest rise or increase in heart rate, an alternative airway such as an endotracheal tube should be placed.

Oxygenation: Resuscitation should begin with 21% FiO_2 in term infants and 21–30% FiO_2 in preterm infants [3, 6]. The oxygen level is titrated to maintain saturations in the minute-specific target range per NRP guidelines.

Circulation: If heart rate remains <60 bpm after an alternative airway is placed, chest compressions with 100% oxygen are initiated. The ratio of coordinated chest compressions to breaths is 3:1. If chest compressions do not result in heart rate increase >60 bpm after at least 1 min, epinephrine is given via intravenous route as the first-line medication [3, 6]. Volume expansion with normal saline or packed red blood cells are considered if there is a history of risk factors for hypovolemia or acute blood loss.

Enteral and Parenteral Nutrition

Development of Feeding Skills: The ability to feed orally requires an infant to safely synchronize sucking, swallowing, and breathing. Oral feeding skills can be achieved by most infants at 34–36 weeks of gestation [6]. Non-nutritive sucking

Table 39.8 MR. SOPA Mnemonic for ventilation corrective steps

Corrective step	Action
M	Mask adjustment
R	Reposition airway
S	Suction mouth and nose
O	Open mouth
P	Pressure increase
A	Alternate airway (ETT, LMA)

of a pacifier, breast, or syringe is used along with the infant's cues to assess oral feeding readiness.

Initiation of Enteral Feeds: Trophic Feeds: An important goal in the NICU is to provide premature infants with early nutritional support to promote growth and optimize neurodevelopment. Trophic feedings are low volume feedings that promote intestinal maturation and do not contain sufficient calories for growth [6]. Trophic feeding is defined as a volume of less than 20 mL/kg per day. Feeds are further advanced by a range of 15–30 mL/kg per day based on infant birth weight. Standardized feeding protocols are often used to decrease practice variation. Preterm infants require increased protein and electrolytes to promote growth comparable to in utero rates. As enteral feeds are advanced, preterm formula and breast milk are fortified to meet goal levels [7].

Gastric Tubes: Indications for nasogastric (NG) or orogastric (OG) tube include infants with immature suck and swallow ability, signs of respiratory distress, and gastric decompression of excess air. Possible complications include esophageal or gastric perforation and aspiration if tube is displaced.

Parenteral Nutrition: Preterm infants have decreased body stores of protein, fat, and glycogen, nutrients important for energy and metabolism. Preterm infants also have decreased stores of certain electrolytes and minerals (e.g., calcium, iron) that are accumulated in the third trimester [5]. Intravenous nutrition is initiated in preterm infants whose metabolic needs are not met by enteral feeds, as well as infants with gastrointestinal conditions resulting in decreased capacity for enteral feeds (e.g., congenital diaphragmatic hernia, gastroschisis). Total parenteral nutrition (TPN) is an intravenously administered combination of macronutrients, electrolytes, minerals, and vitamins.

Macronutrients Dextrose, protein, and lipids are the main macronutrient components of TPN. Table 39.9 lists the goal concentrations of macronutrients and electrolytes [3].

Electrolytes Electrolyte requirements (Na, K, Ca, Phos, Mg) are based on an infant's fluid status, urine output, and laboratory values. These salts provide a

Table 39.9 Total parenteral nutrition goals (Carter, Hair, Agnes, Rodman, July 2021)

	Units	Initial target goals	Goals for growth
Energy	kcal/kg	42–57	90–100
Protein	g/kg	2–3	3.5–4 (preterm), 2–3 (term)
Fat	g/kg	0.5–2	3
Glucose	mg/kg/min	5–7	11–12
Calcium	mmol/kg	1.0–1.2	1.5–2
Phosphorous	mmol/kg	1.0–1.2	1.5–2
Potassium	mEq/kg	0	2–4
Sodium	mEq/kg	0	2–4

Adapted with permission from: Carter A, Hair A, Agnes, M and Rodman E. Parenteral Nutrition. In: Nutrition: Guidelines for Acute Care of the Neonate 29th edition (2021–2022), Fernandes CJ, Pammi M, Katakam L, et al. (Eds), Baylor College of Medicine, Section of Neonatology, Department of Pediatrics. Copyright © 2021 Baylor College of Medicine

balance of acetate, chloride, and phosphorous [5]. During the first days of life, infants have low sodium needs due to expected free water diuresis. Adequate calcium and phosphorous levels are essential for prevention of osteopenia of prematurity, a disorder of bone mineralization.

Complications of TPN: Parenteral nutrition-associated liver disease (PNALD) is a complication that occurs most commonly in infants exposed to prolonged duration of parenteral nutrition. Laboratory markers of PNALD dysfunction include elevated direct bilirubin, GGT, and liver function tests. Infants diagnosed with PNALD may be switched to alternative forms of lipid emulsion. Manganese and copper should be discontinued as proper hepatic-biliary function is necessary for adequate excretion of these minerals. PNALD resolves with advancement of enteral feeds and decrease in TPN. In addition to hepatic complications, the use of indwelling venous catheters to provide TPN increases risk for central line-associated bloodstream infections.

Apnea, Bradycardia, and Desaturations

Physiology: Neonatal control of breathing involves the respiratory center, peripheral and central chemoreceptors, and respiratory muscles. Apnea of prematurity (AOP) is a developmental disorder that occurs due to immaturity of these components. This immaturity results in impaired ventilatory response to hypercapnia and hypoxia. It commonly occurs in infants born less than 34 weeks gestation, and incidence is inversely related to gestational age [3, 5].

Clinical Presentation: Apnea is defined as a cessation of breathing for greater than 20 s. Apnea may be associated with bradycardia and oxygen desaturation that requires sensory stimulation intervention. In contrast, periodic breathing is a pattern of regular breathing alternating with respiratory pauses of 3 s or more. Clinical symptoms appear within the first days of life and may persist for weeks to months and improve with advancing gestational age. Apnea is classified as central (no respiratory effort), obstructive (airflow obstruction), or most commonly, mixed (central and obstructive) [5]. It is important to consider alternative causes of apnea events including neurologic, pulmonary, infectious, metabolic, hematologic, and pharmacologic etiologies.

Treatment: Caffeine, a methylxanthine, is the first-line pharmacologic treatment for apnea of prematurity (AOP). Methylxanthines activate central respiratory centers, increase chemoreceptor sensitivity, and promote bronchodilation [5, 9]. Caffeine is started at birth for infants at risk for AOP and discontinued when symptoms resolve, typically at 34 weeks post-menstrual age. Infants are monitored for symptom recurrence for 5–7 days prior to consideration for discharge. Infants with persistent symptoms may require nasal cannula, CPAP or mechanical ventilation.

Necrotizing Enterocolitis

Clinical Presentation: Necrotizing Enterocolitis (NEC), commonly seen in premature infants, is a gastrointestinal emergency with significant risk of morbidity and mortality. The risk of developing NEC is inversely related to gestational age and birth weight. Term infants with intrauterine growth restriction, perinatal asphyxia, and congenital heart disease are also at risk for NEC. NEC presents with a variety of GI-specific and non-specific symptoms including abdominal distention, emesis, bloody stools, apnea, decreased perfusion, and lethargy [5, 8].

Imaging Findings and Diagnosis: Laboratory findings include metabolic acidosis, hyponatremia, hyperkalemia, neutropenia, and thrombocytopenia [5]. Diagnostic imaging findings of NEC include pneumatosis intestinalis (air in bowel walls), portal venous air and pneumoperitoneum suggestive of intestinal perforation (Fig. 39.3).

Treatment: NEC is treated supportively with medical or surgical interventions based on symptom severity and imaging findings. An infant with concern for NEC should have feeds withheld with gastric decompression. Medical treatment consists of fluid resuscitation, sepsis evaluation with antibiotic coverage of enteric pathogens, and respiratory support. A finding of pneumoperitoneum on abdominal X-ray is a surgical emergency requiring consultation of the Pediatric Surgical Service. Surgical management ranges from placement of a peritoneal drain if there is concern for intestinal perforation to exploratory laparotomy if concern for bowel necrosis.

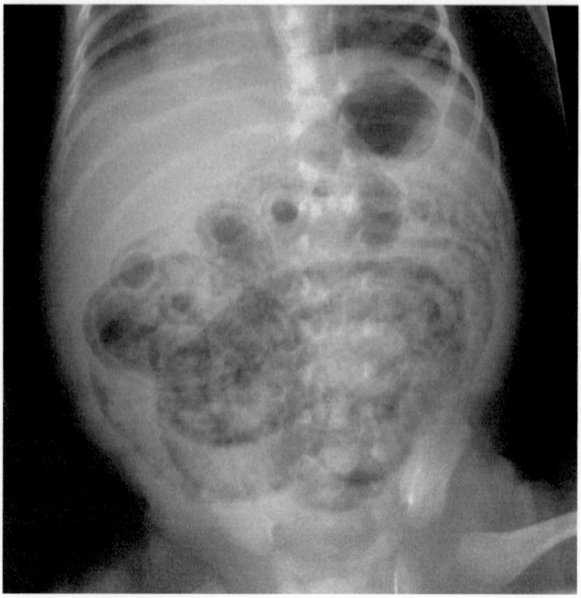

Fig. 39.3 Necrotizing Enterocolitis. Abdominal radiograph shows bowel distention and pneumatosis intestinalis (air in bowel walls)

NICU Procedures

Intubation: Indications for endotracheal intubation include respiratory failure or apnea, upper airway obstruction, congenital bowel anomalies (e.g., congenital diaphragmatic hernia), and administration of exogenous surfactant. Equipment includes an endotracheal tube, stylet, laryngoscope blade, suction catheter, bag and mask with oxygen source, and end tidal carbon dioxide detector. Table 39.10 provides guidelines on ETT size according to weight and gestational age [3]. Premedication is considered for non-emergent intubation and includes a vagolytic agent, analgesic, sedative, and neuromuscular blocker [9].

Umbilical Venous Catheter: Indications for Umbilical Venous Catheter (UVC) placement include administration of IV fluids, total parenteral nutrition, medications, blood products, and exchange transfusion. A UV line courses from the singular umbilical vein at the umbilicus, through the ductus venosus, to the inferior vena cava, with goal placement at the IVC and right atrial junction. A common equation used to calculate insertion length is length (cm) = [1.5 × birth weight (kg)] + 6. Chest X-ray is used to confirm placement, with goal thoracic level of T8–T10 [9]. Potential complications include infection, pericardial effusion, thrombosis, and hepatic injury.

Umbilical Arterial Catheter: Indications for Umbilical Arterial Catheter (UAC) placement include arterial access for labs (i.e., blood gases), continuous blood pressure monitoring, and exchange transfusion. A UA line courses from one of two umbilical arteries down into the internal iliac artery, into the common iliac, and into the aorta. A common equation used to calculate insertion length is length (cm) = is [3 × birth weight (kg)] + 9 cm. Chest X-ray is used to confirm placement, with goal thoracic level of T6–T9 [9]. Potential complications include infection and thrombosis.

Needle Thoracentesis: Needle aspiration is indicated for emergent evacuation of a pneumothorax. A pneumothorax is clinically suspected if an infant has acute hypoxia, hypercarbia, respiratory distress, or tachycardia and is confirmed with

Table 39.10 Endotracheal tube size selection

Weight or post-menstrual age	Tube size (mm)
<1 kg or 22–28 weeks	Size 2.5
1 to <2 kg or 29–34 weeks	Size 3.0
>/= 2 kg or 35+ weeks	Size 3.5
Post term or larger	Size 4.0

Adapted with permission from: Dinu D, Parmekar S, and N Sundgren. Airway Management. In: Respiratory Care: Guidelines for Acute Care of the Neonate 29th edition (2021–2022), Fernandes CJ, Pammi M, Katakam L, et al. (Eds), Baylor College of Medicine, Section of Neonatology, Department of Pediatrics. Copyright © 2021 Baylor College of Medicine

transillumination or chest radiograph. The site of needle puncture is the second intercostal space along the midclavicular line. An alternative site is the fourth intercostal space along the anterior axillary line. Care is taken to avoid damage to intercostal vessels which run immediately beneath each rib. A 23–25-gauge butterfly or venipuncture needle is inserted with an attached syringe to withdraw air.

Arterial Puncture: Arterial puncture is indicated for an arterial blood gas sample or additional labs requiring free-flowing arterial blood. The radial artery is the most common site, and alternative sites include the posterior tibial and dorsalis pedis arteries [9]. A 23–25-gauge butterfly or venipuncture needle is used with palpation or transillumination of the artery. Complications may include bleeding, hematoma, and transient thrombosis.

References

1. Engle WA, Tomashek KM, Wallman C, Committee on Fetus and Newborn, American Academy of Pediatrics. "Late-preterm" infants: a population at risk. Pediatrics. 2007;120(6):1390–401. https://doi.org/10.1542/peds.2007-2952. Erratum in: Pediatrics. 2008;121(2):451
2. Committee on Fetus and Newborn, Adamkin DH. Postnatal glucose homeostasis in late-preterm and term infants. Pediatrics. 2011;127(3):575–9. https://doi.org/10.1542/peds.2010-3851. Epub 2011 Feb 28
3. Fernandes CJ, Pammi M, Katakam L, et al, editors. Guidelines for Acute Care of the Neonate. 29th ed. Baylor College of Medicine, Section of Neonatology, Department of Pediatrics; 2021.
4. Weiner GM, Zaichkin J, editors. Textbook of neonatal resuscitation. 8th ed. Itasca, IL: American Academy of Pediatrics; 2021.
5. Gleason C, Juul S, editors. Avery's Diseases of the Newborn. 10th ed. St. Louis: Elsevier; 2017.
6. Weiner GM, Zaichkin J, editors. Textbook of Neonatal Resuscitation. 8th ed. American Academy of Pediatrics; 2021.
7. Kleinman RE, Greer FR, editors. Nutritional Needs of the Preterm Infant. In Pediatric Nutrition. 8th ed. American Academy of Pediatrics; 2020.
8. Jesse N, Neu J. Necrotizing Enterocolitis: Relationship to Innate Immunity, Clinical Features, and Strategies for Prevention. NeoReviews. 2006;7:e143–50. https://doi.org/10.1542/neo.7-3-e143.
9. Gomella T, Eval FG, Bany-Mohammed F, editors. Gomella's Neonatology: Management, Procedures, On-Call Problems, Diseases, and Drugs. 8th ed. McGraw Hill; 2020.

Chapter 40
Pediatric Critical Care

Sara Sanders, Jordan Lull, Megan Daniel, and Claire Stewart

Introduction

The Pediatric Intensive Care Unit (PICU) is where some of the sickest hospitalized pediatric patients receive necessary care. Patients of all ages and with a variety of conditions are admitted to the PICU, which makes each day and each patient in the PICU unique. The majority of learning in the PICU happens at the bedside, but this chapter will review several basic fundamentals of critical care management including systems-based presentations, sedation and analgesia, shock and vasoactive medications, and some common PICU procedures.

S. Sanders (✉)
Pediatric Critical Care Medicine, Department of Pediatrics, Connecticut Children's, University of Connecticut, Hartford, CT, USA
e-mail: SSanders@connecticutchildrens.org

J. Lull
Pediatric Critical Care Medicine, Department of Pediatrics, University of Virginia, Charlottesville, VA, USA
e-mail: Xkt6dp@uvahealth.org

M. Daniel · C. Stewart
Pediatric Critical Care Medicine, Department of Pediatrics, Nationwide Children's Hospital, The Ohio State University, Columbus, OH, USA
e-mail: Megan.Daniel@nationwidechildrens.org; Claire.Stewart@nationwidechildrens.org

N. Liao et al. (eds.), *Pediatric Rotations*,
https://doi.org/10.1007/978-3-031-59873-9_40

Epidemiology/Indications for PICU Admission

Epidemiology

Respiratory illnesses are the most common conditions in the PICU, with 40% of patients admitted to the PICU typically requiring mechanical ventilation. The length of stay is greater than 7 days for 40% of PICU patients, and the overall mortality rate ranges from 2% to 6%.

Within the PICU patient population, there is a subset of patients who are "high frequency PICU utilizers." These are children who are admitted to the PICU three or more times in a year. These are typically children who are younger, are technology dependent, and/or are publicly insured. In 2022, a large database study found that approximately 6% of all patients admitted to the PICU met criteria for being defined as high frequency PICU users, and they accounted for 24% of all PICU costs.

PICU Admission Criteria

PICU admission criteria are institution specific. For example, some institutions require all children on insulin infusions for diabetic ketoacidosis to be admitted to the PICU, but this is not universal. Other circumstances in which PICU admission requirements vary include the use of high flow nasal cannula, heparin infusions, patients with home tracheostomies and ventilators, continuous albuterol, or external ventricular drains (EVDs). Despite this heterogeneity, some conditions consistently require PICU admission across all institutions. These almost always include but are not limited to presence of an endotracheal tube and ventilator for respiratory support, vasoactive medications (for either hypertension or hypotension), and continuous renal replacement therapies or extracorporeal membrane oxygenation (ECMO).

Systems-Based Presentations

Introduction

Unlike many other rotations in pediatrics, where presentations and plans are organized by patient "problems," common practice in the PICU is to present in a systems-based manner (i.e., respiratory, cardiovascular, neurologic, etc...). PICU patients are often complex, with multiple problems and medications. Arranging each patient's data in a systems-based fashion allows the clinician to avoid missing important details and enables other team members to listen for key information (Table 40.1).

Table 40.1 Systems-based presentations

System/What to present	Example
One-liner	
A sentence/few sentences that concisely describes the patient, presenting illness, and current clinical status	A 7-year-male with a past medical history of cerebral palsy, baseline adrenal insufficiency and hypothyroidism, g-tube dependence, and epilepsy who is admitted with severe septic shock
Overnight events	
• Major overnight events • Do not need to go into every detail, you will do that in each system	Overnight a central line and arterial line were placed, an echo was done, and his epinephrine drip was able to be weaned
Respiratory	
• Exam: Respiratory rate, lung exam • Respiratory support: Nasal cannula, BiPap, ventilator, airway adjuncts, etc. • Ventilator settings • Airway clearance therapies and frequency • Systemic respiratory medications: e.g., steroids for asthma, glycopyrrolate for secretions • Inhaled respiratory medications: e.g., albuterol, mucolytics • Labs: Gas frequency • Images: Chest X-ray (CXR), chest CT scans, bronchoscopy, airway evaluations	Intubated shortly after admission by anesthesia due to known difficult airway On pressure control SIMV mode PSIMV: PIP 30, PEEP 10, pressure support 8, rate 20, Itime: 0.9, FiO_2 35% Patient breathing with the ventilator, no tachypnea, no nasal flaring, no retractions, no increased work of breathing no wheezing, lung sounds diffusely coarse Most recent blood gas: pH 7.26/PCO_2 55/PaO_2 80/ base deficit −4 Chest physiotherapy: Percussor Q4H with 3% NaCl nebs Q8H, albuterol Q4H PRN Arterial blood gasses q4H Daily CXR: AM CXR showed appropriate endotracheal tube (ETT) position and bilateral diffuse opacities consistent with acute respiratory distress syndrome (ARDS), improving from yesterday's film
Cardiovascular	
• Exam: Heart rate, blood pressure, perfusion • Vasoactives • Rhythms • Electrocardiogram (ECG or EKG) • Echo report • Cardiology consult recommendations • Labs: Lactate, mixed venous sat	HR: 120–140s, blood pressure: 80–90 s/50–60 s Tachycardic without murmurs; Extremities cool with capillary refill ~4–5 s Epi gtt at 0.08 mcg/kg/min weaning for MAPs > 60 EKG: Sinus tachycardia Echo: Moderate LV dysfunction, no effusion Labs: Lactate downtrending- started at 9 mmol/L, most recently 4 mmol/L
Fluids, electrolytes, nutrition (FEN), renal, gastrointestinal	
• Exam: Abdominal exam • PO vs. NPO • Feeds • Fluids/TPN/IL • Electrolyte replacements, supplements, bowel regimen • Diuretic regimen, fluid goals • Emesis, urine, and stools • NG/NJ/Gtube/GJtube/urinary catheter (Foley) • Labs/Imaging including electrolytes, renal function, and abdominal organs	Abdomen soft, mildly distended, bowel sounds present G-tube to drain NPO D5LR with 20 meq KCl running at MIVF of 65 mL/h Foley in place and UOP: 1–3 mL/kg/h; No emesis or stools Electrolytes unremarkable and stable this morning with baseline creatinine PRN calcium replacements to keep iCal >1.2 - received 3 in last 24 hours

(continued)

Table 40.1 (continued)

System/What to present	Example
Endocrinology	
• Exam: Thyroid exam • Thyroid medications • Vasopressin/DDAVP • Stress dose hydrocortisone • Insulin	On home synthroid - converted to IV while NPO Stress dose hydrocortisone IV
Hematology/oncology/ immunosuppression	
• Exam: Pallor, clinically significant bleeding or bruising • Labs: Complete blood count (CBC), coagulation labs • Recent transfusions • Transfusion thresholds • Immunosuppression medications: Chemo, steroids (for cancer)	AM CBC: WBC 25 with a left shift, Hgb 8.9, (baseline Hgb ~10), Plt 406
Neurology	
• Exam: Neurologic status • Pain and sedation medications • Delirium medications • Mood medications • Antiepileptic medications • Withdrawal assessment tool scores • Delirium scores • Neurologic monitoring: ICP, EEG • CT/MRI reports	Sedated, PERRL, +cough/gag, withdrawals to pain in all 4 extremities Fentanyl gtt at 1 mcg/kg/h, Dexmedetomidine gtt at 0.8 mcg/kg/h Home levetiracetam- converted to IV while NPO; No seizures noted since admission Head CT on admission showed stable chronic atrophy, no new area of concern
Infectious disease	
• Exam: Wounds, fever curve • Antibiotics, antifungals, antivirals • Labs/Imaging: Procalcitonin, erythrocyte sedimentation rate (ESR), c-reactive protein (CRP), blood culture, urine culture, tracheostomy or endotracheal tube (ETT) culture, cerebrospinal fluid (CSF) studies, viral respiratory panel, gastrointestinal pathogen panel, antibiotic levels, pertinent imaging including CXRs	Vancomycin 20 mg/kg Q6H Ceftriaxone 100 mg/kg Q24H Blood culture, urine culture, and ETT culture pending Elevated Procal/CRP on admission, trending down today Rhino/enterovirus + on viral pathogen panel Vancomycin level due tomorrow at 4 pm
Miscellaneous	
• Rheumatology, ophthalmology, orthopedics, gynecology, psych • Social concerns	Patient in custody of county social services Consent for procedures must be obtained from case worker
Lines/tubes	
• Endotracheal tube (ETT), chest tubes • Urinary catheter (Foley), feeding tubes (nasogastric or nasojejunal tube) • Central lines: Percutaneous, PICC, port • Arterial line	ETT placed by anesthesia CRITICAL AIRWAY Foley, percutaneous femoral CVL, and arterial line all needed for care
Lab schedule/imaging	
• Lab schedule • Ordered imaging	ABGs q4H Daily chemistries Daily chest X-ray

System-Based Presentation Basics

- Standard order of systems will vary by institution, but should be consistent from patient to patient.
- Start with a one-liner to describe the patient. This should be followed by a brief description of significant events of the last 12–24 h.
- Present subjective/objective information systematically, with pertinent physical exam findings, laboratory and imaging results, and medications in each section.
- Include an assessment to summarize the current status of the patient. Do not repeat the one-liner here.
- Many institutions formally incorporate nurses, respiratory therapists (RTs), and/or pharmacists during rounds/presentations. For example, the RT may present the majority of the respiratory system, including ventilator support and airway clearance therapies. Nurses may present overnight events or specific portions of a system (e.g., delirium scores or current IV access).

Tips for a Successful Presentation

- Present ranges of vital signs. PICU patients are dynamic, and a single blood pressure or heart rate is not nearly as representative as a range over time. Understanding vital sign trends is an important marker of clinical improvement or deterioration. Not only should trends in vital signs be described, but when presenting and interpreting lab findings, it is also important to identify and interpret those trends as well. For example: "the lactate has been decreasing after we gave 20 mL/kg of normal saline" or "the creatinine has doubled since yesterday when we added scheduled diuretics and IV vancomycin." Additionally, it might be helpful to state the patient's most recent vital signs.
- As part of pre-rounding, check in with the bedside nurse, RT, the parents/caregivers, and the patient when able, to include their questions and concerns in the presentation.
- The most important part of the presentation is the assessment. Do not simply repeat the one-liner or jump straight into the plan. The assessment helps the team understand your thought process and helps frame the patient's clinical trajectory. As part of pre-rounding, take a minute to determine your assessment of the patient that day and their active ICU problems. Writing it out prior to rounds can be useful to insure presenting a logical assessment.
- Expect interruptions. In the event of an interruption, remember that it does not necessarily mean that you are doing something wrong. Members of the team may have more recent information (patients in the PICU change quickly and

your exam from pre-rounding may no longer be the same), may have clarifying questions, or have a teaching point they do not want to miss. If interrupted, take a breath and regroup before continuing with the presentation.

Shock and Vasoactive Agents

Introduction

Shock is the state of inadequate tissue perfusion that occurs when oxygen delivery is not adequate to meet the body's oxygen demand. Classically, shock is broken down into four different categories: hypovolemic, cardiogenic, obstructive, and distributive (Table 40.2). Hypotension can be a late finding of shock, especially given the young child's ability to compensate to maintain cardiac output via tachycardia. Thus, a patient may be showing signs of impaired end organ perfusion with normal blood pressure for age.

It is imperative to frequently assess the patient with shock, paying attention not only to vital signs, but also the clinical exam, including central and peripheral pulses, capillary refill, mental status, and urine output, as well as lab markers of end organ dysfunction such as liver enzymes, creatinine, pH, mixed venous saturation (SvO2), and lactate. A patient's shock phenotype can change as the underlying disease state(s) evolves. Early recognition and appropriate treatment of shock, and specifically treating the underlying cause while providing appropriate supportive care, may prevent progression and lead to improved outcomes for the child. See Table 40.3 for receptors targeted by vasoactive medications and Table 40.4 for treatments for shock.

Table 40.2 Categories of shock

Types of shock	Primary physiologic disturbance	History clues	Clinical presentation	Drug of choice	Other treatment pearls
Hypovolemic – Hemorrhagic	Decreased preload	Decreased PO intake, excessive vomiting and/or diarrhea Trauma, or operative blood loss	Dry mucous membranes, tachycardia, weak and thready pulses, decreased capillary refill, narrow pulse pressure	Fluid, epinephrine Transfuse blood products	
Cardiogenic	Decreased cardiac contractility	History of congenital heart disease, cardiac arrest, or arrhythmias	Pulmonary edema, hepatomegaly, jugular venous distention (JVD), arrhythmias	Milrinone, dobutamine, or low dose epinephrine	
Obstructive – Cardiac tamponade – Tension pneumothorax – Large pulmonary embolism	Physical obstruction which prevents adequate cardiac output	Chest trauma, difficulty ventilating, recent surgery or hypercoaguable risk factors	Tracheal deviation, muffled heart sounds, absent breath sounds unilaterally, pulsus paradoxus	Treat underlying cause. Fluid administration while awaiting definitive treatment to help overcome obstruction (especially with tamponade and pneumothorax)	
Distributive – Septic – Anaphylactic – Neurogenic	Decreased vascular resistance in vasodilated shock ("warm" shock) or increased vascular resistance and poor cardiac output ("cold" shock)	– Fevers, chills, rigors, history, and lab abnormalities compatible with infection – Exposure to known or potential allergen – History of spinal cord injury	Vasodilation with warm shock or vasoconstriction with cold shock Signs of infection—fevers, chest X-ray abnormalities, rash/viral symptoms Stridor/wheezing, wide pulse pressure, hives, nausea/vomiting Bradycardia with hypotension	Norepinephrine for vasodilated shock Epinephrine for vasoconstricted shock or for anaphylaxis	Antibiotics and source control for septic shock Removing offending allergen for anaphylactic shock and other treatments including IM epinephrine, albuterol, h2 blockers, and steroids

[a] Any patient can present or develop a mixed picture of "warm" or "cold" shock due to presence of multiple different shock phenotypes at the same time

Table 40.3 Receptors targeted by vasoactive medications

Receptors	Location	Action
Adrenergic α_1	Vascular smooth muscle	Vasoconstriction
Adrenergic β_1	Cardiac muscle, sinus node, atrioventricular junction	Chronotropy (increased rate of contraction), inotropy (increased force of contraction)
Adrenergic β_2	Vascular smooth muscle, bronchial smooth muscle	Vasodilation, bronchodilation
Dopamine (D)	Kidney vasculature, heart	Splanchnic vasodilation, Chronotropy
Vasopressin (V1)	Vascular smooth muscle	Vasoconstriction

Table 40.4 Treatments for shock

Generic drug name	Mechanism of action	Starting doses*	Titration doses*	Side effects	Types of shock used for
Crystalloid (normal saline (NS), Plasmalyte, or Lactated Ringer's (LR))	Volume expansion	20 mL/kg push pull or smaller aliquots if concern for cardiogenic shock	Repeat up to 3 times with reassessment after each; may actually need more depending on the degree of hypovolemia	Electrolyte derangements depending on the type of fluid, specifically hyperchloremic metabolic acidosis with normal saline	All types initially; especially important for hypovolemic shock
pRBCs[a]	Volume expansion and increased oxygen carrying capacity	20 mL/kg or 1 U pRBCs With ongoing or massive blood loss, transfuse packed red blood cells: fresh frozen plasma: platelets as 2:1:1 or 1:1:1	Additional units as needed until bleeding is no longer life threatening	Risks of any blood transfusion including fluid overload, allergic reaction, infection	Hemorrhagic shock, septic shock (for deteriorating or unstable patients with anemia)
Epinephrine	β_2 at low doses (<0.04 mcg/kg/min); α_1, β_1, β_2 at higher doses	0.02–0.1 mcg/kg/min, or higher	0.02 mcg/kg/min	Tachycardia, lactic acidosis, hyperglycemia, skin necrosis if IV infiltrates	All types
Norepinephrine	$\alpha_1 >>> \beta_1 > \beta_2$	0.02–0.1 mcg/kg/min, or higher	0.02 mcg/kg/min	Skin necrosis if IV infiltrates	Septic shock/"warm shock" vasodilation with hypotension Refractory shock
Vasopressin	V1 receptors on smooth muscle cells	0.1–1 millunits/kg/min	0.5 milliunits/kg/min		Second line for shock (can be after epinephrine or norepinephrine)

Table 40.4 (continued)

Generic drug name	Mechanism of action	Starting doses*	Titration doses*	Side effects	Types of shock used for
Dopamine	Low doses (<5 mcg/kg/min) = D receptors Medium doses (5–10 mcg/kg/min) increasing $\beta_1 > \beta_2$ effect High doses (>15) increasing α_1, β_1	5 mcg/kg/min	5 mcg/kg/min	Suppression of hypothalamic–pituitary–adrenal axis The adrenal axis suppression can be severe; many institutions avoid dopamine, particularly in sepsis	All types; Stable medication so stocked in many code carts
Milrinone	Phosphodiesterase inhibitor	0.25 mcg/kg/min-1 mcg/kg/min	Not routinely titrated	Peripheral vasodilation can lower blood pressure Can accumulate in renal insufficiency	Cardiogenic shock
Dobutamine	β_1 receptors, β_2 receptors	0.5–1 mcg/kg/min	1 mcg/kg/min	Tachycardia, arrhythmias	Bradycardia
Hydrocortisone	Corticosteroid replacement	50–100 mg/m^2/day	Not routinely titrated		In children with known adrenal insufficiency, hydrocortisone needs to be given early, otherwise is given for vasoactive-refractory shock

[a] In some cases other than hemorrhagic, giving blood will be advisable *where to start depends largely on how ill the patient is; can be titrated every 3–5 min, or more aggressively if patient is unstable

Sedation and Analgesia

Introduction

Many patients in the PICU require sedation or analgesia for a variety of indications and for a variable length of time, ranging from a short procedure to a prolonged clinical course. For example, prolonged sedation is typically required to keep an endotracheal tube in place in a child. The medication(s) and dose(s) chosen depend upon a number of factors such as patient age, size, need for pain control, need for anxiolysis, duration of sedation, and side effect profile. See Table 40.5 for a list of medications for sedation and analgesia. In this section, we will discuss prolonged sedation and analgesia in the setting of maintaining respiratory support, but it is

Table 40.5 Medications for sedation and analgesia

Drug class	Mechanism	Provides	Side effects	Initial dosing* and titration
Opioids • Fentanyl • Morphine • Hydromorphone	Opioid receptor agonists	Analgesia, sedation	– Apnea – Itching (morphine especially) – Hypotension – Constipation – Rigid chest (fentanyl only - If given too quickly, the chest wall becomes very rigid and difficult to move even with high pressures)	Fentanyl 0.5–1 mcg/kg/h – Titrated by 0.5 mcg/kg/h Morphine 0.05–0.1 mg/kg/h – Titrated by 0.05 mg/kg/h Hydromorphone 0.025 mg/kg/h – Titrated by 0.005 mg/kg/h
Benzodiazepines • Midazolam (Versed) • Lorazepam (Ativan)	GABA receptor agonist	Anxiolysis, amnesia; No analgesia	– Delirium – Apnea – Hypotension	Midazolam 0.05–0.1 mg/kg/h –Titrated by 0.02–0.05 mg/kg/h Lorazepam- 0.01–0.1 mg/kg/h – Titrated by 0.02–0.05 mg/kg/h
Dexmedetomidine (Precedex)	Centrally acting alpha-2 agonist	Anxiolysis, mild analgesia, mild sedation	– Bradycardia – Sinus arrhythmia – Hypo/hypertension	0.4–0.6 mcg/kg/h – Titrated by 0.2 mcg/kg/h
Ketamine	NMDA antagonist - dissociative anesthetic	Analgesia, sedation Anxiolysis, amnesia, refractory status epilepticus and acute severe asthma (bronchodilation)	– Nystagmus – Hypertension/tachycardia – Sialorrhea – Laryngospasm – Nausea/vomiting – Emergence delirium	Initial bolus dose of 0.5–2 mg/kg Continuous infusion 0.5–1 mg/kg/h
Propofol	GABA receptor agonist	Anxiolysis, sedation; no analgesia	– Apnea – Hypotension (especially diastolic) – Propofol infusion syndrome: Metabolic acidosis, rhabdomyolysis, cardiac failure, renal failure	Initial bolus dose of 1–2 mg/kg Continuous infusion of 1–10 mg/kg/h
				**Starting doses are patient and institution specific* ***Weight base dosing provided; adult-sized patients should receive adult dosing, which is typically flat doses and not discussed here*

important to understand that these medications can also be used for short-term sedation and analgesia, such as for procedures.

In order to ensure that a patient is receiving the appropriate level of sedation and analgesia, there are several scoring systems used in PICUs. The most common scale for pain is the FLACC (Faces, Legs, Activity, Cry, Consolability), which is on a scale of 0–10, where 0 represents no pain and 10 represents uncontrolled pain.

To measure degree of sedation, there are several different standardized sedation scores including the Richmond Agitation Sedation Scale (RASS) and the State Behavior Scale (SBS). Both of these scales represent a range of degrees of sedation on a continuum of extremely agitated to alert and calm to unarousable. Provider teams choose the targeted level of sedation based on the clinical situation for an individual patient and sedation medications are titrated to achieve that level of sedation.

Discontinuing Sedation

Children requiring prolonged sedation or high doses of sedation medications may develop tolerance to these medications, especially opioids and benzodiazepines. In order to assess withdrawal, most PICUs use a Withdrawal Assessment Tool (WAT) score as a measure of withdrawal symptoms. WATs are specifically designed for opioid and benzodiazepine withdrawal; there are no standard withdrawal scores for dexmedetomidine or ketamine, thus close clinical monitoring must be used in these settings.

Clinicians may choose to either slowly wean a patient from sedation medications, reducing the dose of the continuous infusion in a standard way, or transition the continuous infusion into an enteral substitute given intermittently. For example, enteral methadone can be given in place of a fentanyl infusion or enteral lorazepam can be given in place of a midazolam infusion.

PICU Procedures

Introduction

In this section, we will discuss central lines, arterial lines, and chest tubes. Endotracheal intubation, another common ICU procedure, is discussed in Chap. 41.

Central Venous Lines

Central venous lines (CVLs) or central venous catheters (CVCs) are catheters that reside in a large central blood vessel such as the internal jugular or femoral vein. They are placed via the Seldinger technique, in which the vessel is accessed with a needle, a wire is inserted through the needle, the needle is removed, the catheter is placed over the wire, and the wire is withdrawn. Ultrasound guidance for vessel access is often used in children. After CVLs are placed into certain locations such as the internal jugular vein, a chest x-ray is obtained to confirm location placement.

CVLs are longer than peripheral IVs (PIVs) and have a larger lumen diameter. They often have multiple lumens and provide more stable access than a PIV. There are several reasons a patient might require a CVL. These include administration of medications with a high risk of significant injury in the event of infiltration, long-term access for administration of medications, exchange transfusion, plasmapheresis, dialysis, administration of parenteral nutrition, administration of multiple medications, or hemodynamic monitoring.

Due to the larger catheter size, CVLs are associated with the development of thrombi. Additionally, they are more likely to cause a serious blood stream infection (central line associated blood stream infection, i.e., CLABSI) than a PIV. To mitigate these risks, hospitals use CVL care bundles to ensure sterile placement and line care. When choosing the line size, providers should pick the smallest bore with the least number of lumens necessary for the patient. Providers should attempt to cluster the number of times the line is accessed in a day to minimize contamination. Additionally, whenever the patient no longer needs the CVL, it should be removed as soon as possible. Some patients who require central access for a long period of time (i.e., for chemotherapy) may have other types of central lines placed such as a peripherally inserted central catheter (PICC) or medication port. Discussion of these lines is beyond the scope of this chapter.

Arterial Lines

Arterial lines are small catheters (about the size of a peripheral IV) that are placed into an artery. Indications for arterial lines include need for hemodynamic monitoring, high frequency of lab draws, and/or need for arterial blood gas monitoring. Arterial lines are also placed over a wire, via Seldinger technique as described above. Risks associated with an arterial line are also infection and thrombosis, as well as injury to the artery affecting perfusion to the limb/organs that the artery supplies. Arterial lines are usually put in small, peripheral arteries (the radial artery being the most common), but can also be placed in larger, more central arteries such as the femoral artery.

Thoracostomy Tubes

A thoracostomy tube (also termed a "chest tube") is placed percutaneously in the pleural space to drain air (pneumothorax) or fluid (effusion) from the space. Fluid in the pleural space may represent simple transudative fluid, blood, infection, or malignancy. There are two different types of chest tubes: pigtail chest tubes and rigid, stiff chest tubes. Pigtail chest tubes are made of a softer plastic, and coil once placed inside the chest (like a pig's tail). Pigtail chest tubes are generally more comfortable, because the plastic is softer and causes less rib distension. They are ideal for evacuating air or simple fluid and are placed over a wire using the Seldinger technique as noted above. Rigid chest tubes or "surgical" chest tubes are stiffer with a larger lumen. Rigid chest tubes are less comfortable, but are better for evacuation of fluid that is prone to clogging or clotting (such as empyema or hemorrhage) and can be placed very quickly (which is especially helpful in a trauma situation). These chest tubes are inserted into the skin after making an incision, separating the subcutaneous tissue with forceps and puncturing the pleura. The chest tube is then guided into the pleural with forceps.

After either type of tube is placed, the tube is sutured to the skin, attached to an atrium with suction to facilitate evacuation of the space, and a chest x-ray is taken to confirm appropriate position before it is covered with an occlusive dressing.

Conclusion

The PICU rotation can be particularly challenging for several reasons. The acuity is high, patients can change and deteriorate quite quickly, and there is a new set of vocabulary, equipment, and perhaps even disease processes to learn. Additionally, it can be an emotionally taxing experience if there is a patient death or a complex ethical dilemma. For the same reasons, it can also be an incredibly educational and rewarding experience.

Application Exercises

1. Mix and match: Vasoactive and receptor site

A. Epinephrine	1. Phosphodiesterase inhibitor
B. Dopamine	2. V1 receptors
C. Norepinephrine	3. β_2 at low doses; α_1, β_1, β_2 at higher doses
D. Vasopressin	4. D receptors at low doses; β_1, β_2, α_1 at higher doses
E. Milrinone	5. $\alpha_1 >>> \beta_1 > \beta_2$

Answer: A3, B4, C5, D2, E1

2. Mix and match: Sedation medication and common side effects

A. Dexmedetomidine	1. Itching
B. Midazolam	2. Sialorrhea
C. Ketamine	3. Bradycardia
D. Propofol	4. Delirium
E. Morphine	5. Metabolic Acidosis

Answer: A3, B4, C2, D5, E1

Read this presentation. Underline three things you would do differently to create a better presentation for this patient the PICU on hospital day 3.

This is a 4-month-old, previously healthy male who is admitted with RSV bronchiolitis. He was admitted 3 days ago after having 2 days of runny nose, cough, and congestion at home. He was admitted to the PICU 3 days ago on HFNC, but then transitioned to BiPap, but continued to have work of breathing and needing more oxygen, and got intubated yesterday during rounds. Since then, he has been requiring escalating ventilator settings, an NG was placed overnight and feeds were started. He also has been having issues with sedation.

By systems:

Respiratory: Ventilator: Pressure- SIMV 26/8 PS 10 Rate 24 iTime 0.7. FiO_2 35%

Exam: breathing 70 times a minute, nasal flaring, poor aeration, and congestion

AM CXR showed ETT in good position, diffuse haziness. No pneumothorax

Chest physiotherapy scheduled every 4 h, we're getting thick secretions out

Cardiovascular: Warm, well perfused, heart rate 97, BP 93/47 mmHg

FEN/GI: Started on NG feeds of breastmilk goal feeds 28 mL/h; titrating up on feeds and down on D5 fluids

Neuro: Comfortably sedated after increasing sedation

Fentanyl drip at 1.5 mcg/kg/h, with boluses to match

Dexmedetomidine at 0.6 mcg/kg/h

Infectious disease: RSV+ on viral panel

ETT culture is growing methicillin-susceptible Staph aureus: Currently on amoxicillin

Blood culture and urine culture pending- no growth to date

Lines/tubes: ETT, PIVs × 2

Nursing/RT/family concerns: Mom says his breathing looks like it did yesterday when they intubated him. Nurse and RT both say that his secretions are clogging up the suction tubing, and that he starts to look worse about 3h after his chest physiotherapy.

Assessment/Plan: Overall, this patient is stable. We had to intubate for breathing problems, but I think he's better now. Plan for the day will be to keep increasing feeds, monitoring for sedation needs, and trying to turn down the ventilator.

Potential Answers

- Shorten the one-liner introduction. You only need a full history for the first time a patient is being presented on rounds. Since this patient was seen on rounds yesterday, you only need a true one-liner, and any major overnight events in your introduction. Instead, consider "4 month old, previously healthy male who is admitted with RSV bronchiolitis, who is intubated and required escalating ventilator settings and sedation overnight."
- Present vital sign *ranges*, not just single values.
- This patient is not stable. The presentation tells us this patient has required increased ventilator settings and the respiratory exam is concerning that the patient is under supported. A better assessment/plan would be "This patient has required escalating ventilator settings and on exam, I'm concerned that he still needs more support. The nurses and the RTs said that his secretions are thick and clogging the suction tubing and that at the 3-h mark, he starts to look worse. I would like to increase his chest physiotherapy to every 2 h and add a mucolytic treatment to help break up the mucus plugs".

Further Reading

Fuhrman BP, Zimmerman JJ. Pediatric critical care. 4th ed. Mosby; 2011.

Heneghan JA, Akande M, Goodman DM, Ramgopal S. High-frequency utilization of the PICU. Pediatr Crit Care Med. 2022;23(5):e230–9. https://doi.org/10.1097/PCC.0000000000002920. Epub 2022 Mar 4

Nichols DG, Shaffner DH, editors. Rogers' textbook of pediatric intensive care. 5th ed. Lippincott Williams and Wilkins (LWW); 2015.

Society of Critical Care Medicine; Critical-Care-Statistics [Internet]. [Cited 20 May, 2022]. www.sccm.org/communications/critical-care-statistics

Chapter 41
Respiratory Interventions in Emergent and ICU Settings

Claire Stewart, Megan Daniel, Olivia Ruth, and Elizabeth M. Bonachea

Introduction

Critically ill neonates and children frequently require supported respiration, either due to primary respiratory disease or as a sequela of systemic disease processes. Such support can be divided into non-invasive and invasive modalities. Non-invasive support is provided via the upper airway; invasive support involves bypassing the upper airway with a device such as an endotracheal tube. The core priorities of respiratory support are to achieve adequate gas exchange (oxygenation/ventilation) and reduce work of breathing while minimizing iatrogenic injury. This chapter will review the modalities, indications, and procedural and care considerations pertinent to the use of respiratory support in the Pediatric Intensive Care Unit (PICU) and Neonatal Intensive Care Unit (NICU). See Table 41.1 for common respiratory modalities and abbreviations in the PICU and NICU.

C. Stewart (✉) · M. Daniel
Division of Pediatric Critical Care Medicine, Department of Pediatrics, Nationwide Children's Hospital, The Ohio State University, Columbus, OH, USA
e-mail: claire.stewart@nationwidechildrens.org; megan.daniel@nationwidechildrens.org

O. Ruth
Division of Pediatric Critical Care Medicine, Department of Pediatrics, Nationwide Children's Hospital, The Ohio State University, Columbus, OH, USA

Division of Neonatal-Perinatal Medicine, C.S. Mott Children's Hospital at the University of Michigan, Ann Arbor, MI, USA
e-mail: oruth@med.umich.edu

E. M. Bonachea
Division of Neonatology, Department of Pediatrics, Nationwide Children's Hospital, The Ohio State University, Columbus, OH, USA
e-mail: elizabeth.bonachea@nationwidechildrens.org

N. Liao et al. (eds.), *Pediatric Rotations*,
https://doi.org/10.1007/978-3-031-59873-9_41

Table 41.1 Common respiratory modalities and abbreviations in the PICU and NICU

NIV	Non-invasive ventilation (ventilatory support via the upper airway)
IMV	Invasive mechanical ventilation (ventilatory support bypassing the upper airway)
HFNC	High flow nasal cannula
NIPPV	May refer to non-invasive positive pressure ventilation (such as CPAP) OR nasal intermittent positive pressure ventilation
CPAP	Continuous positive airway pressure
PEEP	Positive end expiratory pressure (the alveolar pressure above atmospheric pressure at expiration)
BiPAP	Bilevel positive airway pressure
IPAP	Inspiratory positive airway pressure (a BiPAP setting)
EPAP	Expiratory positive airway pressure (a BiPAP setting, equivalent to PEEP)
ETT	Endotracheal tube
CMV	Conventional mechanical ventilation (as opposed to high frequency ventilation)
HFOV	High frequency oscillatory ventilation
ECMO	Extracorporeal membrane oxygenation, include VV (veno-venous) ECMO for lung bypass and VA (veno-arterial) ECMO for heart-lung bypass

Respiratory Support in the PICU

Non-Invasive Respiratory Support

Introduction

Non-invasive (NIV) respiratory support is increasingly used in both pediatric and adult populations in patients with respiratory insufficiency or respiratory failure. Multiple studies cite a significant increase in NIV use and over a quarter of children admitted to PICUs internationally are treated with either high flow nasal cannula (HFNC) or non-invasive positive pressure ventilation (NIPPV). Endotracheal intubation and invasive mechanical ventilation can often be avoided through the use of NIV; NIV has a more favorable risk profile than invasive mechanical ventilation (IMV). It is important to note that in both these modalities (HFNC and NIPPV), the patient must initiate many or all of their own breaths, thus an adequate respiratory drive is needed for use of NIV.

High Flow Nasal Cannula

High flow nasal cannula is one of the more popular respiratory support modalities in the PICU. The majority of patients treated with HFNC in the PICU are those with bronchiolitis, although HFNC may also be employed for patients with such disease processes as pneumonia, post-extubation respiratory insufficiency, croup, and asthma exacerbations. Patients are provided with heated, humidified air through a non-occlusive cannula. Clinicians must set both a flow of oxygen (in liters per minute) and a fraction of inspired oxygen (21–100%). A typical starting flow rate ranges from 1 to 2 L/kg/min. There is limited evidence that flows above 2 L/kg/min are more effective so some clinicians will move to other modalities (NIPPV or IMV) if a patient is not improving on a flow of 2 L/kg/min. Teenage and adult patients tolerate flows of 40–60 L/min. High flow nasal cannula is thought to provide a small amount of positive pressure, though significantly less than true NIPPV, and helps to move oxygen-rich gas past nasopharyngeal and upper airway dead space or obstruction replacing carbon dioxide-rich gas, thereby improving ventilation and oxygenation potential. High flow nasal cannula also conveys the advantage that patients do not require sedation to tolerate the cannula. Additionally, patients may be fed either oro- or naso-gastrically. The decision of when to feed patients by mouth on HFNC varies by institution and provider preference.

Non-invasive Positive Pressure Ventilation

NIPPV encompasses both continuous positive airway pressure (CPAP) and bilevel positive airway pressure (BiPAP) and may be used as a both a short- and long-term modality in pediatric patients. CPAP provides one continuous airway pressure while BiPAP provides both an expiratory pressure (EPAP or positive end expiratory pressure—PEEP) and an inspiratory pressure (IPAP). CPAP (and additionally, the EPAP or PEEP component of BiPAP) helps to increase functional residual capacity, preventing alveolar collapse or atelectasis. The IPAP component of BiPAP supports the patient's breath and helps to increase tidal volumes (thereby often improving dyspnea/tachypnea) and decrease respiratory muscle work. Both elements help to improve gas exchange. There are several mask interfaces for patients on NIPPV ranging from a nasal cannula design to a full face "shield." Whatever modality is chosen, a well-fitting mask with a good seal is essential for efficacy. NIPPV may be used in a variety of respiratory pathologies ranging from bronchiolitis, pneumonia, and asthma to neuromuscular diseases and cystic fibrosis in both the acute and long-term settings. Usual settings range from an EPAP of 4–12 cm H_2O and an IPAP of 10–20 cm H_2O. NIPPV is usually well tolerated; however, younger children may require sedation to tolerate NIPPV. Dexmedetomidine is often the sedation medication of choice for these patients as it does not cause respiratory depression. Evidence is mixed regarding feeding while on NIPPV. Temporary enteric tubes and surgical ostomy tubes may be used to provide enteral nutrition but there is risk of emesis and aspiration with gastric feeding. Some patients on chronic NIPPV utilizing the nasal cannula interface may be able to feed by mouth.

Intubation and Invasive Mechanical Ventilation

Indications

There are several indications to intubate a patient's trachea for the provision of invasive mechanical ventilation (Table 41.2).

Table 41.2 Indications for intubation in the pediatric intensive care unit

Airway/respiratory indications	
Clinical condition	*Notes*
Upper airway obstruction	Examples: Croup, epiglottitis, severe mucositis, facial trauma
Oxygenation failure (despite non-invasive measures)	Examples: Bronchiolitis, pneumonia, pulmonary edema, severe asthma, others Signs: Inability to maintain appropriate saturations despite HFNC/NIPPV and >50–60% FiO_2
Ventilation failure (despite non-invasive measures)	Examples: Bronchiolitis, pneumonia, pulmonary edema, severe asthma, others Signs: Significant respiratory distress; carbon dioxide retention on blood gas
Compromise of oxygenation and/or ventilation, with contraindication to non-invasive support	Examples: Facial trauma, recent upper GI surgery, frequent emesis
Primarily non-airway/respiratory indications	
Clinical condition	*Notes*
Impaired respiratory drive	Examples: Ingestion of sedating substance, CNS disease (infectious, inflammatory, traumatic, or neoplastic), status epilepticus
Impaired airway protective reflexes	Examples: Ingestion of sedating substance, CNS disease (infectious, inflammatory, traumatic, or neoplastic), status epilepticus
Neuromuscular weakness	Examples: Guillain-Barre syndrome, myasthenia gravis, spinal muscular atrophy, botulism
Reduction of metabolic demand	Example: Septic shock
Need for procedures and/or imaging for which conscious sedation is contraindicated or would be inadequate	Surgery, MRI in uncooperative patient, renal or bone marrow biopsy, others

Complications may arise from the intubation procedure itself, or may occur later, due to the cumulative time spent with an endotracheal tube (ETT) in place. Complications of ETT placement may include oral or dental trauma, hemodynamic instability, and failure to intubate, which can lead to profound desaturations and ultimately cardiac arrest. Subacute complications of invasive mechanical ventilation include pressure injury to the trachea, which can cause edema or scar tissue formation; ventilator-associated tracheitis or pneumonia; ventilator-induced lung injury or pneumothorax; and sequelae of sedating medications needed to maintain the endotracheal tube, including hemodynamic compromise, delirium, sedative/narcotic tolerance, and prolonged weakness.

Procedural Considerations

Placing an endotracheal tube is a serious procedure, and thoughtful preparation is required. The patient should be NPO for 6–8 h if at all possible. If intubation is emergent, stomach contents can be evacuated via nasogastric tube, or rapid sequence intubation can be performed, in which medications are administered in immediate succession and the patient does not receive bag/mask ventilation prior to placement of the endotracheal tube.

There are a number of important differences between the pediatric and adult airway, which are especially accentuated in infancy. The large occiput relative to body size can pose challenges in achieving an appropriate "sniffing position," in which the oral, pharyngeal, and tracheal axes are optimally aligned. Young children have relatively large tongues, which can obstruct the airway and be challenging to stabilize during intubation. The pediatric epiglottis is also larger and less tethered to surrounding structures (i.e., "floppier") than in older patients, which may create difficulty in achieving an adequate view of the airway. The glottis itself is more superior and anterior in young children than in adolescents and adults. Finally, young children have lower metabolic reserve and often desaturate more quickly during laryngoscopy attempts.

The likelihood of a difficult airway should always be assessed before the procedure is performed. If the patient has been intubated before, prior records or caregiver report can be helpful. Certain anatomic features can also predict challenges, including small or recessed mandible, short or obese neck, limited mouth opening, and limited neck mobility (such as patients in a cervical collar after trauma). If a difficult airway is anticipated, only providers with extensive airway experience should attempt intubation. Video laryngoscopy should be strongly considered, and backup plans for airway management solidified.

A mnemonic used to recall equipment required for intubation is "SOAPME" (Table 41.3).

If difficulties are encountered with bag/mask ventilation, troubleshooting may include deepening sedation, repositioning the patient, employing two-person technique, or inserting an oropharyngeal airway. If intubation is challenging, ensuring optimal positioning, application of external cricoid pressure, or using a laryngoscope blade that is longer or of a different style may be helpful. The use of video laryngoscopy allows real-time coaching from more experienced providers. If these measures fail, a laryngeal mask airway (LMA) can generally secure the airway temporarily while an expert provider such as a pediatric anesthesiologist or otolaryngologist is contacted for assistance. Endotracheal tube placement should be confirmed in several ways, including colorimetric CO_2 detection or waveform capnography, auscultation of bilateral breath sounds, and chest radiography demonstrating proper ETT position.

Table 41.3 Equipment needed for endotracheal intubation ("SOAPME")

Item	Purpose/notes
Suction	Removal of airway secretions requires suction source, canister, and tubing, as well as suction catheters of various size and style
Oxygen	Patient should be pre-oxygenated for several minutes prior to intubation; 100% FiO_2 should then be connected to ventilation bag
Airway	• Appropriately sized ventilation bag/mask • Laryngoscope handle/blade: Both curved and straight blades are available; choice is based on provider preference with straight blades commonly used for infants. Both styles come in a variety of sizes • Cuffed endotracheal tubes are generally preferred. The size (internal diameter) of cuffed ETT for a given patient can be estimated by the formula (age in years/4) + 3.5 • Stylet if desired by intubator • In case of difficulty, smaller and larger ETTs should be immediately available, as should airway adjuncts (oropharyngeal, nasopharyngeal, and laryngeal mask airways)
Pharmacy	Medications needed for intubation, including choice of sedative/narcotic and neuromuscular blockade, as well as emergency medications such as atropine, epinephrine, and isotonic fluid
Monitoring	Pulse oximetry, cardiac leads for heart rate and rhythm monitoring, blood pressure cuff
Equipment	Carbon dioxide detection device (colorimetric or capnography), syringe to inflate ETT cuff, tape or tube holder device to secure ETT

Routine Care and Monitoring of the Intubated Patient

There are several strategies or "modes" of invasive mechanical ventilation, which are generally tailored to the patient's respiratory physiology and to clinician preference. There is no evidence to universally support one method over another. Initial settings are selected to maintain normal lung inflation, reduce work of breathing, provide adequate gas exchange, and limit lung injury. Settings may be titrated based on exhaled CO_2 detected via waveform capnography, capillary, venous, or arterial blood gases, information obtained from the ventilator such as gas flow waveforms and exhaled tidal volumes, chest X-ray findings, and the patient's appearance of dyspnea versus comfort.

In general, ventilator modes may be divided between pressure-controlled and volume-controlled modes. In pressure modes, the clinician chooses a set peak inspiratory pressure (PIP). The tidal volume of air the patient receives for the set pressure will change based on the patient's lung compliance. Starting PIPs range from 20 to 30 cm H_2O, with higher pressures needed if the patient has poor lung compliance due to respiratory disease. In volume modes, the clinician sets a tidal volume (for example 7 mL/kg); the ventilator delivers the amount of pressure that is required to achieve the goal volume. The pressure required to deliver the desired volume changes based on the patient's lung compliance. In both modes, the clinician will select the FiO_2, respiratory rate, and PEEP (usually starting between 6 and 10 cm H_2O with higher PEEPs needed for some disease processes). Additional ventilator settings may be chosen by the clinician and respiratory therapist but are beyond the scope of this chapter. In general, the respiratory rate and tidal volume affect ventilation while the PEEP and FiO_2 affect oxygenation.

Most pediatric patients will require continuous sedation to tolerate the endotracheal tube, and thus will need regular assistance with position changes, eye care, and pulmonary clearance. The endotracheal tube provides a direct route for therapeutic removal of secretions and for obtaining lower respiratory cultures and other laboratory studies. Aerosolized medications including bronchodilators, mucolytics, and antibiotics may be given directly via the ETT. Most intubated patients can be fed enterally via nasogastric or post-pyloric feeding tubes unless there is a specific contraindication inherent to their underlying clinical condition. Post-pyloric nutrition may be preferred for patients with uncuffed tubes to reduce the risk of aspiration.

Extubation Readiness

There are multiple important considerations when choosing an appropriate time for extubation. Primarily, the disease process which initially led to intubation should be resolved or substantially improved. The patient must have adequate respiratory drive and airway protective reflexes, based on their inherent neurologic status and also on the discontinuation or minimization of iatrogenic sedation. In patients who have been intubated for several days or longer, a careful sedative weaning plan is required in order to avoid withdrawal. Adequate gas exchange, lack of respiratory distress, and manageable secretion burden should be maintained despite weaning to minimal ventilator settings, typically including a trial period in a spontaneous mode of ventilation (spontaneous breathing trial or SBT). Although somewhat controversial, many providers will assess the degree of air leak around the patient's ETT; lack of an air leak may indicate localized edema and increased risk of post-extubation stridor. A short course of pre-emptive dexamethasone can be helpful in this instance.

Enteral feeds should be held several hours prior to extubation, in case of extubation failure and the need to provide NIPPV or to reintubate. For patients with residual lung disease, a prolonged course of intubation, or anticipated neuromuscular weakness, planned extubation to HFNC or NIPPV is often appropriate. Patients who fail multiple attempts at extubation, or who present ongoing contraindications to extubation, may ultimately require tracheostomy for ongoing mechanical ventilation.

Extracorporeal Membrane Oxygenation

Extracorporeal membrane oxygenation (ECMO) is a form of extracorporeal life support (ECLS) which serves as either a lung bypass or heart/lung bypass device reserved for the sickest of patients. Extracorporeal indicates that the oxygenation of blood occurs *outside* the body in an exterior membrane. Indications for ECMO differ between the neonatal intensive care unit and the pediatric intensive care unit. There are two main types of ECMO: veno-venous (VV) ECMO and veno-arterial (VA) ECMO. In VV ECMO, blood is removed from a venous site in the patient, carbon dioxide is removed, oxygen is infused, and blood is returned to a pre-cardiac vein. VV ECMO requires a functional heart to pump this newly oxygenated blood to the body, thus VV ECMO is used for purely respiratory indications such as severe pediatric acute respiratory distress syndrome, severe bronchiolitis or pneumonia, and acute severe asthma. In VA ECMO, a similar process occurs for the removal of blood; however, the blood is pumped back into the arterial side of the body, thus bypassing both the heart and the lungs. Thus, indications for VA ECMO tend to be more cardiac in nature including severe myocarditis/cardiomyopathy, post cardiac surgery, and severe septic shock with cardiac dysfunction. Blood is drawn from typically the inferior/superior vena cava (SVC) or the femoral vein. The blood then goes through a blood pump and membrane oxygenator which utilizes fresh gas flow (or "sweep" gas) to remove carbon dioxide before being returned to either the right internal jugular vein, SVC, or right atrium (VV ECMO) or the carotid artery (VA ECMO) (Fig. 41.1). Complications of ECMO are often related to both clotting and

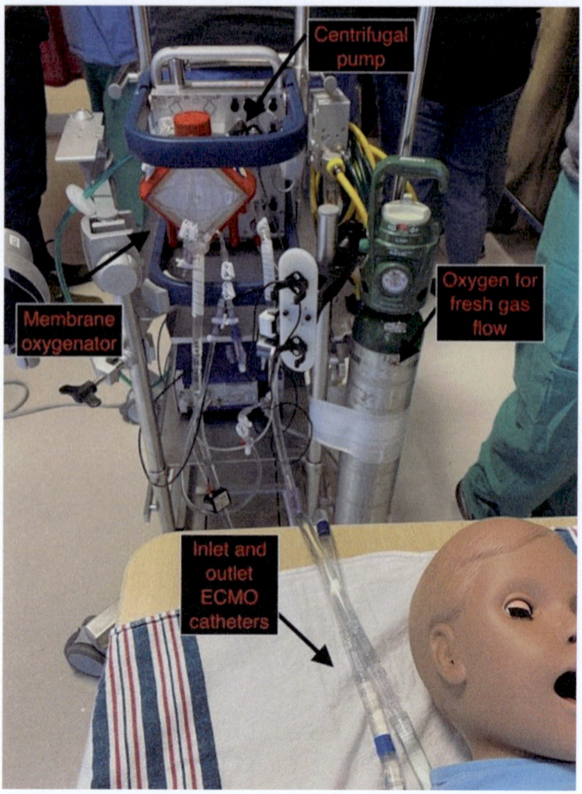

Fig. 41.1 Sample ECMO circuit in a simulated patient

bleeding as patients require systemic anti-coagulation to maintain patency of the circuit. The ECMO circuit must be monitored closely for clots. Infection and vascular injury are also of concern. Survival rates to decannulation (discontinuation of ECMO and removal of ECMO catheters) among pediatric patients hover around 65%.

Respiratory Support in the NICU

Introduction

Respiratory insufficiency is the most common disease in the NICU, with multiple underlying etiologies across disease processes and gestational ages. Premature lungs are susceptible to respiratory distress syndrome (RDS) and surfactant deficiency, with immature and poorly compliant lung tissue that may be difficult to ventilate and/or oxygenate. Lung disease of prematurity may progress to bronchopulmonary dysplasia (BPD), a chronic disease of abnormal, heterogeneous lung and airway development that may necessitate long-term respiratory support. Ill term newborns may also require respiratory support during critical illnesses such as meconium aspiration syndrome, neonatal encephalopathy, and sepsis, to name a few. Newborns with congenital lesions impacting the lungs may have hypoplasia/dysplasia of the parenchyma and vascular tissue of the lungs.

While the pathophysiology of neonatal respiratory failure is distinct from that seen in older children, many of the same modes of respiratory support seen in the PICU are also utilized in the NICU and can be broken down into the same broad categories.

Non-invasive Respiratory Support

Introduction

Though mechanical ventilation is a mainstay of therapy for respiratory failure in the NICU, it can contribute to lung injury, especially in an immature or hypoplastic lung that is particularly vulnerable to barotrauma (injury mediated by high ventilator pressures) and volutrauma (injury mediated by large tidal volumes). For this reason, non-invasive ventilation is commonly seen in the NICU, even in extremely preterm infants (<28 weeks gestational age).

Nasal Continuous Positive Airway Pressure

The most common form of non-invasive ventilatory support in the NICU is nasal CPAP, which can be delivered in two ways. The first is flow-driven or machine-derived CPAP, which delivers a constant PEEP (positive end expiratory pressure) via nasal prongs or a nasal mask. The second is bubble CPAP (BCPAP). This modality is unique to the NICU and delivers heated, humidified gas through nasal prongs or a nasal mask. PEEP is generated by submersing the expiratory tubing in water, causing the namesake "bubble" effect. It is theorized that the bubbling produces vibrations that transmit to the chest and aid in gas exchange. In both modalities, PEEP typically ranges between 4 and 8 cm H_2O.

Even if able to avoid mechanical ventilation, all extremely preterm infants will require non-invasive support for several weeks to months to maintain functional residual capacity, support immature respiratory drive, and promote lung development. Many ill term infants or infants with congenital anomalies may also be provided support with CPAP.

High Flow Nasal Cannula

HFNC is also utilized in the NICU, though less frequently than in the PICU. There are many practical benefits to the use of HFNC including a simpler and more well-tolerated interface and less nasal pressure injury. However, HFNC does not deliver a reliable PEEP, and the benefit of the washout of physiologic dead space (overcoming the parts of the respiratory tract that do not participate in gas exchange) may be less significant in preterm infants, who require PEEP to prevent atelectasis and maintain functional residual capacity. Flow rates of 2–8 L/min are typically used in the neonatal population. Use of HFNC may be more commonly seen in full-term infants, infants with congenital lung or airway anomalies, or in formerly preterm infants who continue to require respiratory support at term-corrected age.

Nasal Intermittent Positive Pressure Ventilation

In the PICU, NIPPV (non-invasive positive pressure ventilation) denotes CPAP and BiPAP, however, in the NICU, the term is generally used to refer to nasal intermittent positive pressure ventilation. In this modality, a PEEP, PIP, rate, and inspiratory time can all be controlled to achieve the desired effect in a manner more like mechanical ventilation, but delivered nasally rather than via endotracheal tube. The mechanism of action of NIPPV remains somewhat unclear and the use of NIPPV from institution to institution is highly variable. One potential benefit of NIPPV in neonates over CPAP is prevention of reintubation, though there are conflicting reports on this in the literature.

Intubation and Invasive Mechanical Ventilation

Introduction

There are several reasons that a neonate may require intubation, beginning at the time of birth. These are outlined below in Tables 41.4 and 41.5.

Surfactant Administration

A common indication for intubation in the NICU is administration of surfactant, a phospholipid and protein compound secreted by the lungs that is crucial for maintenance of alveolar surface tension. Preterm (<34 weeks) and low birth weight (<1500 g) infants are at risk for respiratory insufficiency, in large part due to surfactant deficiency. Without it, the lung is poorly compliant and prone to atelectasis. Preterm infants with surfactant deficiency commonly present with labored breathing, tachypnea, and an increased supplemental oxygen requirement. The lungs have a homogenous "ground glass" appearance on X-ray, indicative of microatelectasis and alveolar collapse. This disease process is referred to as RDS, or respiratory distress syndrome, and is classically seen in preterm infants. Other indications for surfactant administration include surfactant deactivation, such as in meconium aspiration and pneumonia.

Surfactant is administered directly into the trachea, traditionally via the endotracheal tube after intubation. Proper administration relies on a well-positioned endotracheal tube situated above the carina to ensure even distribution of surfactant to both lungs. If time allows, this should be confirmed with a chest X-ray. However, surfactant is often administered in the delivery room and/or in emergent situations where X-ray is not possible, so care must be given to auscultate both lung fields after intubation to ensure equal breath sounds. Once surfactant is given, there is a rapid change in lung compliance and infants may have a visible clinical

Table 41.4 Indications for intubation in the delivery room

Clinical scenario	Notes
Extreme prematurity	Infants <24 weeks often do not have the respiratory drive or lung maturity to sustain themselves without intubation and mechanical ventilation
Perinatal asphyxia	After delivery room emergencies such as cord prolapse, placental abruption, and shoulder dystocia, infants may be apneic with profound acidemia and hypoxemia
Meconium aspiration	Meconium aspiration leads to pneumonitis and small airway obstruction and can result in hypoxemia and respiratory failure
Congenital anomalies	Disorders that include airway anomalies or lung hypoplasia may require immediate intubation in the delivery room. A classic example of this is severe congenital diaphragmatic hernia (CDH)

Table 41.5 Indications for intubation in the NICU after delivery

Clinical scenario	Notes
Decreased respiratory drive	In preterm infants, respiratory drive is inherently impaired (apnea of prematurity). Other examples of decreased respiratory drive include sedation, seizure, and exposure to maternal medications like magnesium
Pulmonary hypertension/cardiac dysfunction	Pulmonary hypertension can lead to cardiac dysfunction. In severe cases, intubation may be necessary to optimize the infant's respiratory and acid/base status, deliver nitric oxide and other inhaled therapies, and ease cardiac strain
Septic shock	Infants with sepsis often become profoundly ill, with persistent apneas and significant acidosis requiring intubation
Surfactant administration	Many preterm infants will require surfactant administration to improve lung compliance and oxygenation. See further details below

Table 41.6 Size of equipment and insertion depth for endotracheal intubation in neonates

GA/weight	Endotracheal tube size	Laryngoscope blade size	Insertion depth (6 cm + weight in kg)
22–23 weeks/<500 g	2.0–2.5	000–00	~6 cm (or less)
24–28 weeks/500 g–<1 kg	2.5	00–0	~6–7 cm (or less)
29–32 weeks/1 kg–1.5 kg	2.5–3.0	00–0	~7–8 cm
33–35 weeks/1.5 kg–2 kg	3.0	00–0	~8–9 cm
36 weeks/2 kg and beyond	3.0–3.5	0–1	~8–10 cm

improvement in the minutes to hours following, with more comfortable breathing and a decreased supplemental oxygen requirement.

Extremely preterm or critically ill infants may require mechanical ventilation for other indications in addition to administration of surfactant (i.e., apnea, airway protection) and will be intubated, given surfactant, and placed on a ventilator. However, well appearing preterm infants may demonstrate enough stability to receive a dose of surfactant but avoid mechanical ventilation. This can be done via the INSURE (intubation, surfactant, extubation) method, or by less-invasive surfactant administration (LISA), where the infant's airway is viewed under direct laryngoscopy, a thin catheter is placed into the trachea, and surfactant is directly administered without ever placing an endotracheal tube. Procedural considerations involving endotracheal intubation are largely the same as those described above in the PICU. Endotracheal tube size and depth are based on patient weight and gestational age, and uncuffed tubes predominate in the NICU setting (Table 41.6). Blood sampling for assessing gas exchange is often less frequent in the NICU setting than in the PICU, owing to the remarkably low blood volumes of neonates, particularly those born preterm.

Types of Mechanical Ventilation

There are several modes of mechanical ventilation, all of which may be used in the NICU in the appropriate clinical setting. However, the two most common modes can be broadly defined as conventional mechanical ventilation (CMV) and high frequency oscillatory ventilation (HFOV). See Table 41.7 for a comparison of different modes of ventilation in neonates.

Just as in the PICU, CMV in the NICU can be further broken down into two categories: pressure-controlled or volume-controlled. In pressure-controlled ventilation, PIP generally ranges anywhere from 18 to 24 cm H_2O. In volume-controlled ventilation, goal tidal volume in neonates is typically 4–6 mL/kg. Other primary variables in both modes include PEEP, rate, and inspiratory time (*Ti*). Typical PEEP for a neonate on mechanical ventilation is 4–8 cm H_2O. Rate usually ranges from 30 to 50 breaths per minute.

The inspiratory time (*Ti*) refers to the amount of time spent in inhalation during one respiratory cycle and is closely related to the rate. The *Ti* can also be thought of as the time over which the ventilator will deliver the full tidal volume to the lung, and typically ranges between 0.25 and 0.5 s in neonates. In diseases of poor compliance like RDS, a high rate and short *Ti* are utilized to deliver more rapid, smaller volume breaths. Chronic diseases such as BPD may require a low rate and long *Ti*

Table 41.7 Comparison of modes of ventilation in neonates

Mode of ventilation	Clinical scenario
CMV-volume	Suitable for all neonates, particularly helpful when rapid changes in compliance are likely to occur (in the first days of life for preterm neonates or any patient receiving surfactant) as the pressure necessary to deliver a given volume will be autoregulated by the ventilator. Often the preferred mode of ventilation in many NICUs
CMV-pressure	Suitable for all neonates but may be more advantageous in older neonates with chronic lung disease or structural lung/airway anomalies who require high pressures to achieve adequate tidal volumes and maintain FRC
HFOV	Best for patients requiring "gentle ventilation," as in extreme prematurity, pulmonary hypoplasia of all causes, air leak syndromes, or as a mode of "rescue" in any patient failing CMV. Negative pressure facilitates active exhalation, which may be uncomfortable for the patient and cause need for sedation, particularly in term neonates who may be more alert at baseline
HFJV	May be used for all of the same indications as HFOV but may be better suited for non-homogenous lung disease such as severe BPD, as it allows for passive exhalation and adjustment of *Ti*. Use of HFOV or HFJV for HFV is generally based on institutional preference

due to the abnormal lung parenchyma that requires higher volumes and a longer time to complete a respiratory cycle.

High Frequency Ventilation

High frequency ventilation (HFV) is a mode of ventilation that is mostly used in the NICU, though may be seen in the PICU in rare cases. HFV is lung protective ventilation strategy that is often utilized in 22–24 week infants or in infants with pulmonary hypoplasia. This is because HFV utilizes a very rapid rate, low tidal volumes, and constant mean airway pressure, thereby minimizing barotrauma, volutrauma, and atelectotrauma (lung injury caused by the shearing force of repeated atelectasis and reinflation). This is particularly advantageous in infants who are more prone to lung injury or air leak. This includes not only extremely preterm infants with poor lung compliance, but also infants with other causes of pulmonary hypoplasia like CDH, diseases causing air trapping like MAS, and developmental disorders of the lung such as congenital lobar emphysema. In these conditions, uneven zones of alveolar overdistension result in tissue rupture, particularly when subjected to positive pressure ventilation. HFV can also be utilized as a rescue strategy in infants who are not improving on conventional mechanical ventilation.

High Frequency Oscillatory Ventilation (HFOV)

HFOV is one type of HFV. The relevant settings on HFOV are mean airway pressure (P_{aw}, cm H_2O), frequency (f, Hz), and amplitude (A, cm H_2O). P_{aw} typically ranges anywhere from 8 to 15 cm H_2O, though may be higher depending on the degree of parenchymal disease. When transitioning from CMV, P_{aw} is typically determined by starting 2–4 cm H_2O above the P_{aw} needed while on CMV. As in CMV, P_{aw} is a measure of lung inflation and oxygenation. Frequency ranges anywhere from 8 to 15 Hz and is usually determined by gestational age and size, with preterm infants requiring a higher frequency than a full-term infant. Frequency affects ventilation, with more frequent breaths delivering more rapid, smaller breaths leading to decreased gas exchange (i.e., increasing the Hz will increase the propensity for CO_2 retention). Amplitude typically ranges anywhere from 20 to 30 cm H_2O, though the starting amplitude is determined by degree of "wiggle," a rough clinical indication of appropriate ventilation. The goal is to have the infant's chest and abdomen visibly shaking, with the pelvis and legs mostly still. While both amplitude and frequency both affect ventilation, the amplitude is generally manipulated to achieve goal ventilation, while the frequency remains unchanged. This is because changes in frequency have a five-fold greater impact on ventilation than amplitude and may cause a very abrupt change.

High Frequency Jet Ventilation

Another form of HFV called High Frequency Jet Ventilation (HFJV) combines aspects of HFOV and CMV and requires that two ventilators be used in tandem—one to deliver pulses of a high-velocity "jet" of gas and one to deliver PEEP and PIP via CMV at a low rate. This leads to the delivery of rapid, small volume breaths with continuous passive exhalation and intermittent "sigh" breaths provided by the conventional ventilator.

Pulmonary Hypertension and Nitric Oxide

Neonates have unique cardiopulmonary physiology, largely owing to the transitions that must take place from fetal to extrauterine life. The fetus has fluid-filled lungs and is reliant on the placental circulation to supply oxygenated blood to fetal circulation. To achieve this, blood flow must be directed away from the lungs. This is accomplished in two major ways: by the presence of fetal cardiac shunts (foramen ovale and ductus arteriosus) that largely bypass the pulmonary circulation, and by maintenance of very high pulmonary vascular resistance (PVR). At the time of delivery, expansion of the lungs decreases PVR and clamping of the umbilical cord increases systemic vascular resistance (SVR) by removing the very low resistance placenta. These changes promote closure of the fetal cardiac shunts.

Many of the conditions mentioned previously (CDH, MAS, pneumonia, pulmonary hypoplasia, RDS, etc.) can impair this normal transition and cause persistent pulmonary hypertension (PPHN), previously called persistent fetal circulation (PFC). Clinically, this will manifest as cyanosis, respiratory distress, hypoxemia, and hypotension. If PPHN is suspected, an echocardiogram should be obtained and will demonstrate features such as elevated right ventricular pressure, tricuspid regurgitation, flattened intraventricular septum, and right to left shunts at the patent foramen ovale and ductus arteriosus. Over time, high PVR will lead to cardiac strain and decreased ventricular function.

Oxygen supplementation, surfactant administration, and gentle ventilation strategies are often utilized in the treatment of PPHN; however, these interventions may not provide significant pulmonary vascular relaxation. In these cases, additional pulmonary vasodilators can be provided. Inhaled nitric oxide (iNO) is the most common pulmonary vasodilator used in neonates. Continuous iNO can be administered through any respiratory interface, but is most often delivered through an endotracheal tube, as most infants with PPHN are already being supported with mechanical ventilation. Other pulmonary vasodilatory medications may be used in the NICU setting, but iNO is by far the most used and best studied. In the most severe cases of PPHN, none of the above measures are sufficient to decrease PVR, and life-threatening hypoxemia and hypotension may result. In this scenario, ECMO must be considered.

Neonatal ECMO

As described above, ECMO is the most extensive cardiorespiratory support that one can provide in the intensive care unit, with oxygenation of blood occurring outside of the body (VV ECMO) with the ability to offload the heart entirely if indicated (VA ECMO). As respiratory insufficiency and pulmonary hypertension are very prevalent in the NICU, it comes as no surprise that VV ECMO is the modality typically used in neonates. Historically, the most common diagnosis requiring ECMO was meconium aspiration syndrome (MAS), a complex disease characterized by surfactant inactivation, lung inflammation, and airway obstruction, leading to respiratory failure and superimposed pulmonary hypertension.

Advances in neonatal care have led to a decreased incidence and severity of disease like MAS while simultaneously improving our ability to manage infants with complex congenital abnormalities. Because of this, the most common indication for neonatal ECMO is now congenital diaphragmatic hernia (CDH). In CDH, the bowel and visceral organs herniate into the chest, leading to abnormal development of the lung parenchyma and vasculature. This results in a complex disorder at birth characterized by lung hypoplasia and severe pulmonary hypertension. Infants with CDH may require ECMO support in the first days to weeks of life before, and sometimes during, surgical repair. While many of these infants may be managed on VV ECMO, VA ECMO may be utilized in any disease process in the NICU that includes an element of cardiac dysfunction, including disease like MAS and CDH.

Further Reading

Alibrahim O, Slain KN. Noninvasive ventilation in the pediatric intensive care unit. In: Rotta AT, Zimmerman JJ, editors. Fuhrman and Zimmerman's pediatric critical care. 6th ed. Elsevier; 2022. p. 644–54.

Cave D, Duff JP, de Caen A, Hazinski MF. Airway management. In: Nichols DG, Shaffner DH, editors. Rogers' textbook of pediatric intensive care. 5th ed. Wolters Kluwer; 2016. p. 305–28.

Chahin N, Rozycki HJ. New modes of surfactant delivery. Paediatr Respir Rev. 2022;43:38–43. https://doi.org/10.1016/j.prrv.2021.10.002.

Lam R, et al. The effect of extended continuous positive airway pressure on changes in lung volumes in stable premature infants: a randomized controlled trial. J Pediatr. 2020;217:66–72. https://doi.org/10.1016/j.jpeds.2019.07.074.

Hong H, Li X, Li J, Zhang Z. High-flow nasal cannula versus nasal continuous positive airway pressure for respiratory support in preterm infants: a meta- analysis of randomized controlled trials. J Matern Fetal Neonatal Med. 2021;34(2):259–66. https://doi.org/10.1080/14767058.2019.1606193.

Maclaren G, Conrad SA, Dalton HJ. Extracorporeal Life Support. In: Nichols DG, Shaffner DH, editors. Rogers' Textbook of Pediatric Intensive Care. 5th ed. Wolters Kluwer; 2016. p. 581–620.

Martin RJ, Fanaroff AA, Walsh MC. Fanaroff and Martin's Neonatal-perinatal medicine: diseases of the fetus and infant. St. Louis, Mo: Mosby/Elsevier; 2020.

Masry A, et al. Reintubation rates after extubation to different non-invasive ventilation modes in preterm infants. BMC Pediatrics. 2021;21:281. https://doi.org/10.1186/s12887-021-02760-7.

Ramaswamy VV, Bandyopadhyay T, Nanda D, et al. Efficacy of noninvasive respiratory support modes as postextubation respiratory support in preterm neonates: a systematic review and network meta-analysis. Pediatr Pulmonol. 2020;55:2924–39. https://doi.org/10.1002/ppul.25007.

Wratney AT, Hamel DS, Cheifetz IM, Nichols DG. Inhaled gases and non-invasive ventilation. In: Nichols DG, Shaffner DH, editors. Rogers' textbook of pediatric intensive care. 5th ed. Wolters Kluwer; 2016. p. 565–80.

Chapter 42
Emergency Care

James Naprawa and J. Bryan Cooper-Sood

Introduction

The first shift in an emergency department can be overwhelming. It is common for there to be multiple patients waiting to be seen. The role of the medical student in this environment is to focus on the patient to which they have been assigned while being attentive to other patients being seen in the ED. On any given shift, there are incredible opportunities to learn from physical exam findings along with laboratory and imaging on your patients and those being seen by other providers. This chapter will clarify the roles and responsibilities of the new learner in the pediatric emergency department and provide tips and strategies for functioning in this environment.

General Strategies

First Shift

The student should introduce themselves to the attending(s) and resident/fellow(s) at the beginning of the shift and come prepared with goals to accomplish during each shift. Comfort and understanding of systems-based practice (i.e., how care of the patient fits into the larger context of the hospital and healthcare system) is an

J. Naprawa (✉)
Department of Emergency Medicine, UCSF Benioff Children's Hospital, Oakland, CA, USA
e-mail: James.naprawa@ucsf.edu

J. B. Cooper-Sood
Valley Children's Hospital, Madera, CA, USA
e-mail: jcoopersood1@valleychildrens.org

N. Liao et al. (eds.), *Pediatric Rotations*,
https://doi.org/10.1007/978-3-031-59873-9_42

Table 42.1 ED workflow

Patient flow through emergency department	• Ordering tests/imaging • Reviewing results • Admitting or discharging patients • Workflow for patients transferred from other hospitals
Location of supplies	• Splinting/suturing materials • Papoose boards (to secure young patients for procedures) • US machine • Popsicles (particularly important) • Food/beverages for patient/family (always ask if a patient is allowed to eat before providing) • Location of child-comfort items (blankets pillows, toys, books)
Consultation workflow	• Subspecialists, social work
Responsibilities of other members of the health-care team	• RN/LVN • Child-life specialist • Respiratory therapist • Splinting/suture tech

increasingly vital component of becoming a competent provider. As such, students should introduce themselves to other members of the healthcare team (nurses, ward clerks, etc.). Asking the attending and or resident/fellow if they could provide feedback at the end of the shift increases the likelihood that thoughtful feedback will be given. Letting residents and attendings know that, when possible, you would like to be involved in the care of any patient with interesting physical exam findings/labs/procedures is an effective way to increase exposure to different conditions.

Though details of each rotation are site dependent, the student is likely to be assigned a patient by the attending physician or a resident. Typically, medical students see patients with a resident. Depending on the circumstances (such as how busy the department is and the triage category of the patient), the student might see the patient at the same time as the resident or be allowed to assess the patient initially and then sign out to the resident and/or attending. As there may be more than one attending provider in the ED at the same time, the student should anticipate presenting to multiple providers.

Aspects of ED workflow that are important to learn during the rotation are listed in Table 42.1.

Preparing for the Patient-Encounter and Establishing Rapport

The medical student should review the chief complaint and patient age prior to evaluation. Brief chart review for pertinent medical history is important but should not significantly delay patient evaluation, particularly in potentially ill children (e.g., patients in respiratory distress). It is essential to review vital signs. The blood pressure can be high for age given patient anxiety and pain. Low blood pressures are uncommon and should be investigated (and repeated) immediately to verify accuracy. Abnormal respiratory rates and heart rates should be verified by the student on their exam. Highlighting abnormal vital signs when presenting should be standard practice. Respiratory rates for infants should be assessed for 30–60 s as recommended by the American Academy of Pediatrics' bronchiolitis guidelines.

Initial impressions go a long way in developing rapport with children and caregivers and can provide vital information regarding the patient's status ("sick" vs. "not sick"). Recommended steps include the following:

1. Introduce yourself to the family and patient and set expectations for the flow of the visit.
2. If possible, sit down on the other side of the room away from the infant/young child. Sitting down conveys to families that you are not in a hurry and allows the child to get used to your presence. Avoid examining the young child when you first enter the room (unless circumstances warrant it; e.g., a patient with respiratory distress). This is likely to lead to the patient crying which will increase patient, caregiver, and student anxiety.
3. Whenever possible, keep the child with the caregiver.
4. Consider playing age-appropriate games with the child (e.g., peak-a-boo) while taking the history.
5. Observe the child in the caregiver's arms. In general, children who appear well when afebrile are unlikely to have serious bacterial infection or SBI (UTI or pneumonia) or invasive bacterial infection or IBI (bacteremia or meningitis). Children with these conditions tend to appear ill whether they are febrile or afebrile.
6. As part of your initial assessment, evaluate respiratory rate, presence of retractions, level of alertness, and skin color. These aspects of the physical exam make up the components of the pediatric assessment triangle. This simple tool is used to quickly establish severity of illness in infants/children.

For patients with concerning findings, a supervising provider should be notified immediately to evaluate. Of note, it is very common to see young patients with fevers up to and above 105F. Typically, these patients look listless and unwell. When such a patient is encountered, attention should be given to level of alertness, presence/absence of nuchal rigidity, quality of pulses and cap refill, and vaccination status of the child (as vaccinated children are at very low risk of IBI). Most high fevers are due to viral illnesses. In the absence of nuchal rigidity or signs of shock, reassurance and administration of an antipyretic are appropriate first steps in management.

History of Present Illness (HPI)

History taking in the emergency department is based on chief complaint, age, and developmental status of the patient. It requires asking questions of two sources (child and caregiver) and determining which source is more reliable on a particular subject. Young children are suggestible, and their answers to review of systems questions may or may not be accurate. Asking the child questions followed by checking with the caregiver for their insights is recommended. For example, if you ask a 4 year old with a fever if they have a sore throat and they say "yes," check with the caregiver to confirm that they have had this complaint. Frequently a caregiver will say that that is the first they have heard of this complaint. If this is the case, the student should be suspicious of a sore throat as the source of the fever.

The interview should focus on the chief complaint. In general, tailoring questions to identify the location, quality, quantity, duration, associated symptoms, and mitigating factors of the chief complaint is the goal of the HPI in the ED. Detailed questions about the child's development are unnecessary unless the chief complaint warrants it (e.g., first-time seizure). However, there are times when detailed questioning is very important. For example, when asked how much a patient is vomiting and/or having diarrhea, a typical response is, "whenever I feed him/her." In such cases, it is useful to ask the caregiver to estimate the number of times the patient has vomited in the last 24 h. Providing the family with multiple choices (e.g., 5 times, 10 times, or 15 times in 24 h) is helpful.

Social History and Family History

As in other aspects of care in the emergency department, the social and family history should be appropriately concise and tailored to the presenting problem. Learning to tailor the information you collect, while not leaving out pertinent information, is paramount.

A thorough and confidential psychosocial history is indicated in all adolescents, especially those presenting with mental or reproductive health concerns (e.g., lower abdominal pain in an adolescent female; chest pain, chronic abdominal pain, or headaches which may have a psychiatric component; presentations for self-harm or suicidal ideation). Asking a caregiver to step out of the room for a few minutes can seem like a daunting task. However, an introduction such as, "I like to speak one-on-one with every adolescent patient I see for a few minutes" is almost always accepted by patients and caregivers. Using a screening tool such as the HEADDSS assessment (see Chap. 37) is standard practice in most pediatric emergency departments. Care should be taken to ensure confidentiality prior to starting this assessment unless the patient says they are going to hurt themselves or someone else.

In certain situations, it is important to ask about family history. Migraine headaches, for example, run in families. Migraine headaches tend to be moderate-severe, throbbing in quality, and associated with phono- and/or photophobia and nausea and vomiting. They are a common cause of pediatric headache and are most commonly encountered in adolescence. However, migraines can be seen in school-age and, rarely, preschool-age children. A family history of migraine in a patient with typical symptoms and a normal physical exam may obviate the need for imaging of the brain as well as guide medication decisions. Similarly, a family history of asthma, eczema, and/or seasonal allergies in first-degree relatives increases the pretest probability of asthma as the cause of respiratory distress in the young child. Care must be taken to contextualize questions. Explaining how you are thinking about a patient's symptoms can go a long way to improving the information obtained in the interview as well as creating a therapeutic alliance with the family. For example, it is not uncommon for a parent to deny family history of migraine only to endorse moderate-severe throbbing headaches associated with light/noise sensitivity and nausea/vomiting when asked more detailed questions. Similarly, a parent may deny a history of asthma, but indicate that they use an inhaler for recurrent coughing/wheezing or "bronchitis." An example of contextualizing your questions is:

"Cough and wheeze in young children are usually due to a viral infection. However, asthma is common in young children and there is often a parental history of asthma/eczema/allergic rhinitis as well as a history of respiratory distress and/or excessive coughing at night especially with colds. This is why I am asking these questions."

Review of Systems (ROS) and Physical Exam

As with the HPI, social, and family histories, the ROS and physical exam should be tailored to the chief complaint and developmental age of the child. A complete ROS is rarely necessary unless the patient is particularly medically complex or undifferentiated. Fever can cause tachycardia and tachypnea, particularly in young children. Persistent tachycardia, especially in ill-appearing and/or afebrile children, should prompt concern for serious pathologies and spur appropriate evaluation. Hypoglycemia, anemia, toxic ingestion, and myocarditis should be considered in persistently tachycardic children. Persistent tachypnea, specifically in the absence of abnormal lung findings, should raise the possibility of metabolic disturbance such as new onset DKA. Occult pneumonias can occur especially in younger children. These patients may present with high fevers, ill-appearance, and significant abdominal pain. Serial evaluation of children with abnormal vitals is essential.

The general appearance of the child provides important information as to the presence or absence of serious pathology. In general, if the child is well-appearing and interactive with parents and environment, the likelihood of serious illness and/or significant dehydration is low.

Medical students receive extensive instruction on a complete and thorough physical exam as part of their education. For more details on specific exam findings and techniques, see the appropriate chief complaint under "Specific Clinical Scenarios: HPI, Physical Exam, Diagnostics, and Treatment" as follows.

Presenting in the ED

The presentation of a patient in the ED is focused on the chief complaint. The student should begin with the age and gender of the child and any PMH that they feel is relevant to the chief complaint. For example, the student should point out in the initial statement that their patient with abdominal pain has a history of prior abdominal surgery. On the other hand, in a patient who presents with a laceration, there is no need to include prior surgeries in initial history. It is important to include CODIERS (Chronology, Onset, Description/Duration, Intensity, Exacerbating and Relieving factors, Symptoms associated) in descriptions of chief complaint. For instance, the student should report the presence or absence of phono- or photophobia and nature of pain (throbbing vs. dull, severity on scale of 1–10) in patients who present with headache. Prior history of similar symptoms is also important. If there is a prior history, quantification of frequency, impairment of child's daily activities, prior therapies should be obtained. Review of systems questions should focus on issues pertinent to the chief complaint. As an example, for a 15-year-old female with abdominal pain, the student might say "On my review of systems, there is no history of bloody diarrhea or weight loss to suggest inflammatory bowel disease (IBD). I also asked about joint pain/arthritis as I know IBD can have extra-intestinal symptoms but the patient denied." In this way, the student can convey to the attending why they asked for a particular ROS. It is unnecessary to include complete ROS in oral presentations.

The physical exam should follow the history beginning with vital signs and general appearance. Your general gestalt is important. How does the patient look to you? Is the infant playful and interacting with you, crying throughout the interview and exam or sicker appearing than you expected? The student should highlight abnormal vital signs and the student's own findings. For example, "The triage respiratory rate was 60 min. On my exam, the patient is breathing at 40 min." Reports of physical exam findings can, similarly, be focused on the patient's chief complaint. In an infant with fever, a thorough PE is important, whereas in an older child with abdominal pain, the exam can focus on the abdomen. Of note, it is critical to examine and report on testicular exam findings on any boy with abdominal pain.

In many pediatric EDs, it is common to care for patients who have been transferred from an outside hospital. In such patients, the student should review the records from the outside hospital and be prepared to report on lab and imaging results along with treatments given at the outside hospital. The student should ask the patient's nurse or ward clerk where these documents can be found.

Following HPI, PE, and report of labs/imaging already obtained, the student should give their assessment. It is recommended that the student begin with a summary statement that includes epidemiology, acuity of onset of symptoms, and cardinal features of the patient's symptoms. The summary statement can be thought of as the illness script for this patient (Table 42.2).

Table 42.2 Illness script

Epidemiology	Acuity of onset of symptoms	Cardinal features
Age/gender/pertinent HPI	Hyperacute/acute/subacute/chronic	Most important aspects of HPI/ROS/PE findings
Example summary statement/illness script		
"This is a 6-month-old male, no past medical or surgical history with acute onset of colicky intermittent abdominal pain with drawing of legs to chest and vomiting 6 times over past 24 h"		

The summary statement should be followed by a prioritized differential diagnosis with the student's most likely diagnosis stated first followed by other diagnoses considered and can't-miss diagnoses.

Example: My most likely diagnosis is intussusception because the patient is the right age (6–24 months), his symptoms are of acute onset, and he is vomiting. He does not have currant-jelly stool but this can be a late finding in this condition.

I also considered:

1. Acute gastroenteritis (AGE) because it is a very common condition that causes vomiting and abdominal pain. However, the patient has no fevers or diarrhea. It may be early AGE or a virus that causes vomiting only but, in this case, it would be a diagnosis of exclusion.
2. Constipation can cause intermittent abdominal pain but I don't think it should cause vomiting. Also, mom reports he typically has daily, soft bowel movements.
3. Appendicitis. We don't want to miss this diagnosis. I don't know how often it happens in this age-group, but I think the pain should be constant.

Committing to a diagnosis is important and encouraged. The student will remember a case better whether right or wrong if they have committed to a diagnosis and plan. It is ok for you to be wrong. You are here to learn. It is more important for you to explain your thinking to the best of your ability.

It is a common mistake for students to forget to mention a diagnosis that they considered and have already ruled out. It is important to mention such diagnoses in your presentation as well as in your written documentation. This will help the attending assess your reasoning and clinical knowledge and correct any errors in thinking. Furthermore, documenting your medical-decision making will help future providers understand your rationale and guide future care.

When discussing a differential diagnosis, the student should compare and contrast the summary statement for their patient with the illness script for that condition. For instance, "I considered intussusception in this 8-year-old patient with vomiting and abdominal pain but feel it is unlikely because intussusception is typically an acute onset of colicky abdominal pain and vomiting in a 6- month to 2-year-old child." This will allow the attending to correct misconceptions and add to the student's knowledge of conditions in the differential diagnosis. Furthermore, the student reinforces what they know and can identify knowledge deficits. Example: "This 15-year-old male has rectal bleeding. I considered Meckel's diverticulum. I think this condition typically presents as painless rectal bleeding in a 2-year-old. Can it happen in older patients? Perhaps I should read about it."

Plan: The presentation ends with the student's plan for the patient. Again, the student is encouraged to commit to a plan to the best of their ability which includes any testing, imaging, medications, and/or subspecialty consultations.

Making the Most of your Time in the ED

A medical student should always accompany the attending physician to see the patient after their presentation. This is an opportunity to see how an expert interacts with the patient and their guardians and performs a physical exam. Once a plan is formulated, the student can practice becoming efficient in the ED. Here are some suggestions:

1. If allowed, see a second patient.
2. After seeing the patient and before presenting this patient, reassess your first patient (assuming that your second patient is stable and does not require immediate attention). Did your patient with testicle pain get his ultrasound yet? Did your asthmatic patient receive their albuterol treatment? If so, how does the patient look and sound now? Did your patient with dehydration get their IV yet? By doing this, the student can make sure that tests and treatments are being done in a timely manner. This is also a time to ask the family if they have any additional questions or concerns. Families often feel ignored by their providers in the ED and appreciate reassessments and updates.
3. If a test/treatment/imaging study has not been performed, the student should let the resident or attending know that there is a delay. Another option is to politely ask the patient's nurse about the situation.
4. Remember to document any re-evaluation with a quick follow-up note in the patient chart (assuming, that is, that medical students are allowed to write notes at your institution). A good time to do this is when you are writing your second HPI.
5. At the time of your second presentation, let the attending know that you also have follow-up information on the first patient. This will advance the workup of the first patient and let the attending know that you are thinking ahead and acting in an organized manner.
6. If there are no new patients to be seen, the student has several options:
   (a) Are there other interesting patients in the ED? Ask if you can accompany the resident or attending to see patients with interesting exam findings.
   (b) Start working on disposition of your current patient(s). If discharge is anticipated, the student can begin working on discharge instructions.
   (c) If a patient requires a subspecialty consultation, ask if you can make the call. Speaking with a sub-specialist is covered elsewhere in this book. One tip is to practice the call with the resident or attending with whom you are working. Another suggestion is to pay attention when a resident is speaking with a sub-specialist to learn strategies for successful consultations.

(d) Assess/reassess your patient(s). This will help move patients through the ED and improve the family's experience.
(e) Update your notes as needed.
(f) Read about any knowledge gaps you have on any of your current patients.

Common Clinical Scenarios: HPI, Physical Exam, Diagnostics, and Treatment

Abdominal Pain

The differential diagnosis for abdominal pain is broad. It is important to take a thorough history to characterize the pain and help narrow the differential diagnosis, as well as to rule out surgical emergencies. See Table 42.3 for a key differential diagnosis and distinguishing characteristics and findings.

Table 42.3 Differential diagnosis and associated characteristics of abdominal pain and/or vomiting/diarrhea

Diarrhea/vomiting	Quantify frequency of each ("How many times has he vomited in last 24 h, 1×, 5×, 10×, more or less?") Giving multiple choice is helpful to parents. Usually due to viral infection. Bloody diarrhea strongly suggests bacterial etiology – Obtain stool culture – Empiric treatment with antibiotics is NOT indicated due to increased risk of hemolytic uremic syndromes in cases caused by *E. coli* 0157: H7.
Vomiting only?	Usually viral etiology. In young infants, physiologic GER is a common cause. Must consider: – Pyloric stenosis (3–5 week old, nonbilious, after every feed, weight loss) – Intussusception (6 months-2 years, intermittent, colicky pain, pulling legs to chest, currant-jelly stool is a late finding) – Occult pneumonia (child <5 years, high fever, lungs may be clear to auscultation, WBC >20; usually caused by strep pneumonia, rare since Prevnar) – Diabetic Ketoacidosis (25% of children have DKA as first presentation of diabetes; moderate-severe dehydration, obtunded) – Intracranial mass
Onset of symptoms:	**Hyperacute onset:** – Ovarian torsion – Ruptured ovarian cyst – Testicular torsion (always ask and examine testicles in any male with abdominal pain) **Acute (typically present within 24-48 h):** – Appendicitis – Intussusception **Chronic** – Functional abdominal pain/IBS – IBD

(continued)

Table 42.3 (continued)

Abdominal pain: Is pain constant or intermittent?	**Constant pain:** – Appendicitis – Pancreatitis (unusual in pediatric population) **Intermittent:** – Constipation – GERD (common in school age children/adolescents, rare in infants) – Intussusception – Mesenteric adenitis **Constant or intermittent:** – Ovarian torsion – Testicular torsion **Rare:** – Cholecystitis (rare in pediatrics; consider in adolescents and children with hemolytic anemias) – Nephrolithiasis – Ureteropelvic junction (UPJ) obstruction
Exacerbating features	**Worse with movement** (walking, ask patient to jump): appendicitis **Worse with eating:** Common: – Reflux Pain is epigastric Ask about sour/weird taste in mouth after eating – Constipation – Functional abdominal pain/IBS
Weight loss	IBD Celiac disease Malignancy
Hematochezia/ bloody diarrhea	**Common:** – Anal fissure secondary to constipation – Bacterial enteritis **Uncommon:** – IBD Intussusception Milk protein allergy (seen in young infants) **Rare:** – Meckel's diverticulum – Intestinal polyp – Intestinal hemorrhage secondary to vasculitis (e.g. IgA vasculitis) Intestinal ischemia secondary to volvulus

Constipation

"Any history of constipation?" is useful if the parent/child says yes but a "no" does not exclude constipation as a cause of the patient's symptoms. Up to 30% of American children are constipated. Constipation is a frequent cause of significant abdominal pain. After the age of 5–6 years, most children are independent enough to wipe their bottoms after a bowel movement. Parents are usually not involved in this process anymore and rely on the patient to report stooling problems. Children are unreliable historians so negative responses to "Are you constipated" should be followed up with detailed questions. For these reasons, when parents say there is no history of constipation it is wise to interpret this as "no history of constipation that I am aware of."

The diagnosis of constipation is based on the Rome IV criteria developed by the Rome Foundation (consensus recommendations from gastroenterologists on functional gastrointestinal disorders):

1. How often do you poop (every day, every other day)?
2. Is your poop ever hard?
3. Do you ever have to strain when having a bowel movement?
4. Does your poop ever plug up the toilet (i.e., large-caliber stools)?
5. Does the patient ever have stooling accidents (fecal incontinence)?

The last question is important because parents often do not volunteer that the child has fecal incontinence. They may assume that this is behavioral ("he doesn't stop playing to go to the bathroom") or that it is normal for children who have completed toilet training to have accidents. Parents often misconstrue fecal incontinence as diarrhea which further confuses the picture. If a patient is suspected of having significant constipation with fecal soiling (the preferred term over encopresis), consultation with a pediatric gastroenterologist is advised.

Another technique that can help elucidate consistency of stool is to use the Bristol stool chart. (Fig. 42.1).

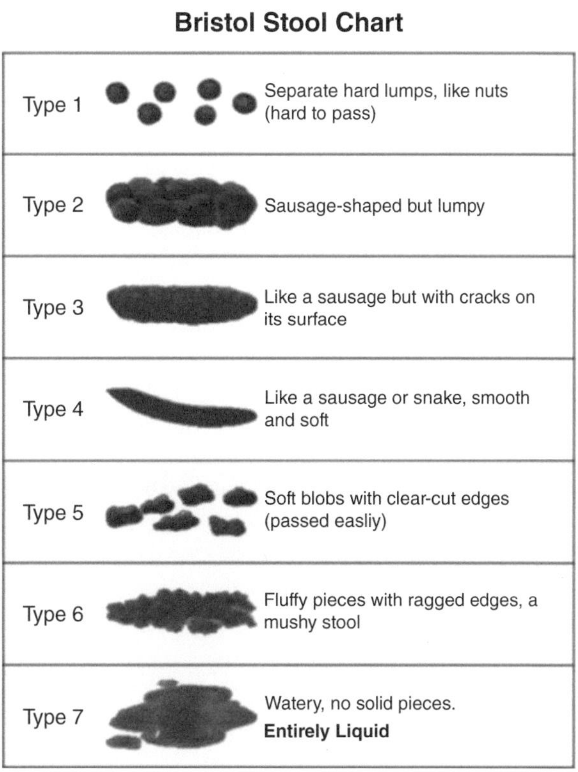

Fig. 42.1 Bristol stool chart

Constipation tends to cause intermittent, crampy pain which is often reported as moderate to severe (hence the frequency of emergency department visits). Because the history is often unclear and confusing in younger children, abdominal X-rays may be ordered. It should be kept in mind that constipation is a clinical diagnosis. X-rays are not reliable in ruling this diagnosis in or out. This discussion should be had with the caregiver as well. However, in a child with a benign abdominal exam, in whom constipation is being considered, an X-ray showing a large stool burden can help guide therapy (trial of MiraLAX, instructing parent to pay attention to stooling frequency, consistency, etc.).

Cough and URI Symptoms

The vast majority of cough in healthy vaccinated children is caused by viral illnesses and can be expected to last for 1–3 weeks.

Cough is a common source of parental anxiety leading to emergency department visits. Cough and fever raise parental concern for pneumonia and with good reason. Internationally, rates of pneumonia and burden of disease (i.e., ED visits, hospitalizations, deaths) are highest among children <5 years old. Chest X-rays and antibiotics are frequently employed in evaluation and treatment of young children with fever and difficulty breathing. However, vaccination against Haemophilus influenzae B (HIB) and, starting in 2006, streptococcus pneumoniae, have markedly decreased the incidence of bacterial pneumonia children. For this reason, the Infectious Disease Society of America recommends against routine testing and radiographic imaging in children <5 years of age with community-acquired pneumonia (CAP) who do not require hospitalization. Furthermore, antibiotics are not recommended in most cases because viral etiologies predominate.

Croup is common in young children and causes a barky cough, hoarse voice, and respiratory distress and stridor when more severe. Croup is a straightforward diagnosis when a patient has inspiratory stridor on exam in the appropriate context (typically fever, congestion, no history of choking episode). When mild, it can be more difficult to diagnose. One technique to help with the diagnosis when croup is being considered is to agitate the patient. Croup is worse with agitation and crying. If stridor is heard with agitation, croup is very likely.

While most cough/wheeze in preschool children is due to viral URI and/or bronchiolitis, it is very common for young children to present to the emergency department for recurrent episodes of cough/wheeze. Asthma is the most common chronic disease in childhood and should be considered in any patient who presents with a chief complaint of cough, especially if recurrent. Clues to the diagnosis are the following:

1. Cough worse at night that disrupts sleep.
2. Post-tussive emesis.
3. Recurrent cough that disrupts sleep when the child has a URI.

4. Persistent cough after a URI.
5. Coughing with exercise.
6. Recurrent healthcare visits (primary care provider, ED, admissions to the hospital) for similar symptoms.
7. Parental history of asthma or other atopy.
8. Patient history of atopic dermatitis/eczema.
9. Nighttime cough/cough with exertion when not ill.

Parents usually do not volunteer this information making detailed review of systems questioning essential in these cases. Care must be taken in making the diagnosis of asthma especially in younger children. However, the conventional wisdom that asthma cannot be diagnosed in children younger than 2 years is untrue. Diagnosis of asthma in young children is based on history of recurrent cough/respiratory distress, family/personal history of atopy, and response to typical asthma therapy. Pulmonary function tests cannot be performed until at least 5 years of age. In children with frequent and/or severe symptoms, consideration should be given to consultation with a pediatric pulmonologist.

While rare, pertussis should be considered in children with significant cough especially if there is no history of asthma/wheezing/recurrent episodes of cough. Pertussis cough tends to be paroxysmal and of prolonged duration (the "100-day cough"). The characteristic "whoop" is often not heard, especially in younger children. Immunity after pertussis vaccination tends to wane after a few years. Therefore, pertussis should be considered even in fully immunized school-aged children and adolescents with prolonged, significant cough.

Respiratory Distress

Respiratory distress is among the most common chief complaints encountered in the pediatric emergency department. It is most frequently seen in infants and preschool children. Older children and adolescents with this complaint usually have asthma. While most infants with respiratory distress have bronchiolitis, it is important to recognize those patients who are at higher risk of developing asthma. The author recommends that all children presenting to the emergency department with cough/respiratory distress be screened for asthma as discussed previously.

Assessing respiratory distress in preschool children requires patience and an organized approach. Observation of the young child from the other side of the room provides important information. Parents should be instructed to remove the young child's shirt/top or lift up their clothing. The student should observe for presence of retractions (intercostal, suprasternal, tracheal tugging, "belly breathing") and count respirations over 30-60 sec. Level of alertness and presence/absence of agitation should be noted. Attention should be paid to the pattern of breathing. Presence of head-bobbing and/or grunting is always concerning and should prompt the student to alert a supervisor. In young children, who are obligate nasal breathers, nasal suctioning with saline can provide relief of symptoms and help guide next steps in care. The student should pay attention to the presence of a prolonged expiratory phase (obstructive process) vs. inspiratory phase (upper airway process such as croup).

Pulmonary exams are notoriously difficult, subjective, and ever-changing in young children with respiratory distress. If possible, allow the patient to remain in the caregiver's arms. Sometimes, if the patient is allowed to turn away from the examiner and the stethoscope is left in one place on the chest or back, the patient may stop crying long enough to allow for auscultation. Pay attention to the quality of air movement (are good breath sounds heard or does the patient sound "tight"). It can be difficult to interpret lung findings in the young child. Expiratory wheezes may be heard but more commonly, coarser sounds are heard which are frequently misinterpreted as transmitted upper respiratory sounds or rhonchi. The commonly used term, "coarse breath sounds" should be avoided. If the patient is in respiratory distress and such sounds are heard on exhalation, the author prefers to use the term, "coarse wheeze." Lung exam findings change frequently so repeated evaluations are important.

In young children who are at increased risk of asthma (e.g., prior history of wheezing, history of asthma in a first-degree relative, patient with eczema), a trial of albuterol should be considered. However, bronchodilators are not indicated when viral bronchiolitis is prevalent in the community (RSV season, typically January–February) especially in young infants with first episode of wheezing. Inspiratory stridor at rest in a healthy, vaccinated child typically indicates croup. Racemic epinephrine and oral steroids, typically dexamethasone, are the standard of care. Stridor in croup can be subtle and intermittent. Presence of barky cough, hoarse voice, and worsening of symptoms at night and with agitation are typical in this condition. The student should listen for stridor when the patient cries to help make the diagnosis. Foreign body aspiration should be considered in an infant/toddler who is able to crawl or walk (and thus pick things up) who presents with sudden onset of cough, stridor, and/or wheeze. Epiglottitis is a much-feared cause of stridor which has become remarkably rare following the introduction of the HIB vaccine. It should be considered if a patient with stridor has any of the following:

1. Toxic appearance.
2. Drooling.
3. Tripoding respiration.

Fevers are common in viral croup and, by itself, do not increase concern for epiglottitis.

Fever

Fever is a very common presenting symptom in the ED. As a result of universal vaccination (against streptococcus pneumoniae and HIB, in particular), the risk of IBI in healthy, term children who have received at least two doses of these vaccines is so low that lab testing is not indicated. Exceptions:

1. Neonates.
2. Children who appear unwell or toxic.
3. Urinalysis and culture in the following febrile preverbal children:
   - Females <2 years old.
   - Uncircumcised males <6–12 months.
4. Children with underlying medical problems:
   - Chemotherapy patients.
   - Sickle cell disease.
   - Patients with primary immunodeficiencies.
   - Medically complex children.

Parents should be asked about vaccination status whenever a child presents for fever. In preschool children, parents are often unsure if immunizations are up to date. Most, however, will remember if their child received their 2, 4, and 6-month shots. Patients who have received these vaccinations have excellent immunity against HIB and streptococcus pneumoniae. High fevers remain a common cause of parental anxiety and ED presentations but are usually caused by viral infections.

Another commonly encountered scenario is an infant or young child presenting with prolonged fever. Most viral infections cause fevers that last 3–5 days. In patients with fevers longer than 5 days, possible etiologies include successive viral infections (one virus followed by another) and certain viral infections (particularly adenovirus and Epstein–Barr virus). Most children are infected with EBV early in life and have either nonspecific viral illness or asymptomatic infections. Occasionally, however, young children can develop mononucleosis.

While most children with high fevers (generally ≥102 F) daily for longer than 5 days have viral etiologies, there are many serious causes that require consideration.

1. Kawasaki Disease (KD).
2. Occult pneumonia.
3. Osteomyelitis.
4. Malignancy (particularly acute lymphoblastic anemia).
5. Rheumatologic conditions (e.g., systemic-onset juvenile idiopathic arthritis).

Kawasaki Disease (KD) must always be considered in any child with fever >5 days (Table 42.4). Most cases occur in children <5 years old. Older children and infants less than 6 months make up less than 10% of cases. As a result, younger and older patients often have a delay in diagnosis leading to increased risk of coronary artery disease in these populations.

Table 42.4 Kawasaki disease criteria and differential diagnosis

Kawasaki disease	Comments
Children <5 years old	Should consider in child of any age with fever >5 days.
Fever >5 days	Typically, more than 102 at least once every day
Clinical criteria	1. Bilateral, non-exudative conjunctivitis 2. Oral mucosal changes (cracked, red lips, strawberry tongue) 3. Truncal rash 4. Extremity changes (erythematous, edematous hands/feet) 5. One anterior cervical lymph node >1.5 cm
Typical laboratory findings	1. ESR >40 and/or CRP >3 mg/dL **Supplementary labs** (3/6 needed to diagnose incomplete KD) 2. WBC >15 3. Low hemoglobin for age 4. Platelets >450 (after 7 days of symptoms) 5. ALT >40 6. Albumin <3 7. Sterile pyuria, WBC >10/high-powered field
Signs/symptoms suggesting alternative diagnosis	– Exudative conjunctivitis (adenovirus) – Exudative tonsillitis (adenovirus, EBV) – Mouth ulcerations (Herpangina, HSV gingivostomatitis, Steven's Johnson syndrome (SJS)) – Bullous rash (SJS, staph scalded skin syndrome) – Sandpaper rash (scarlet fever due to group A streptococcus)

Signs of KD are very specific. It is recommended that the student commit these to memory given the morbidity associated with the diagnosis. Children with KD are admitted to the hospital for IVIG and aspirin to prevent coronary artery disease. Up to 25% of patients with KD meet only 2 or 3 of the criteria, a situation referred to as incomplete KD. These patients have the same risk for coronary artery disease (approximately 25% of untreated patients) as those with complete KD.

Children may have signs early in the course that resolve prior to presentation. Therefore, review of systems questions should include all of the signs of KD in patients with prolonged fever. It is important to discuss signs/symptoms of KD for anticipatory guidance purposes and signs of KD should be included in discharge instructions. Often, KD is a consideration in a child with fever for less than 5 days. In such cases, patients may be discharged home with instructions to return to ED if fever persists for longer than 5 days and/or more symptoms of KD develop. Strict return precautions are important because IVIG does not prevent coronary artery disease when fever has been present for >10 days.

Ear Pain

It is recommended that student ask attending provider to demonstrate techniques for examining the ear in young children.

Tips for examining the ear in young, uncooperative patients:

1. Place the child on the parent's lap, turned so that one arm is against the parent's chest. (An alternative method is to lie the patient on bed and have the caregiver hold arms and legs while the examiner holds the patient's head.)
2. Instruct the parent to then place their arm over the child's other arm and hug them closely to their body.
3. Instruct the parent to place their other hand on the child's head and bring it toward their chest as well.
4. Using your non-dominant hand, gently push against the child's temporal region while pulling the ear to be examined superiorly and posteriorly.
5. Look behind the ear and on the ear itself for signs of infection/inflammation prior to introducing the otoscope.
6. Using your dominant hand, carefully introduce the speculum and otoscope, evaluating the ear canal for signs of infection/inflammation/foreign body, and the tympanic membrane for signs of infection/effusion.

In general, otitis media is over-diagnosed and over-treated. It is not possible to distinguish bacterial from viral otitis media on clinical exam. Furthermore, bacterial otitis media often resolves spontaneously after a few days. For these reasons, pain control is the primary objective. Antibiotic stewardship along with side-effects of antibiotics has led to decreased use of antibiotics for this condition. For children with otitis media, Safety-Net-Antibiotic-Prescription (SNAP) is an evidence-based option that can reduce both unnecessary antibiotics and return visits to a health-care provider for persistent symptoms. Parents are given a prescription for antibiotics and told to fill it in 2–3 days if pain persists. As with all diagnoses, the appropriate context must be present for an accurate diagnosis. Otitis media is quite painful. Pulling at ears may be a clue to pain in preverbal children. On PE, erythema, purulent effusion (usually a yellowish color), AND bulging that obscures the ossicles should be present to make the diagnosis.

Otitis externa presents with purulent discharge and exquisite pain and tenderness with movement of the pinna and tragus. The application of topical antibiotics with steroids and pain control are the treatment of choice. Because the ear canal can become significantly narrowed, insertion of an ear wick may assist in delivery of topical medications to inflamed tissue.

Oropharyngeal Pain

Tips for examining the throat in young, uncooperative patients:

1. Ask the caregiver to sit the child in their lap facing you.
2. Have the caregiver carefully restrain the child using the following directions:

   (a) Put one arm around both of the patient's arms.
   (b) Put the other hand on the patient's forehead.

3. Ask the caregiver to extend the patient's neck and hold the child tightly.

4. Introduce tongue blade into patient's mouth (consider perpendicular introduction along the lateral aspect of the teeth in the child who is biting down). Most children will start crying at this time. When this occurs, press the tongue blade onto the back of the tongue. This will elevate the tonsils.

Assess for:

1. Soft palate vesicles (herpangina).
2. Tonsillar exudates (Adenovirus, EBV, Group A Strep).
3. Ulcers on tongue, lips, gingival swelling/friability (HSV).
4. Dental caries.
5. White plaques on tongue and buccal mucosa (thrush).

In young children, tonsillar exudates are usually due to a viral etiology such as adenovirus or EBV. Group A strep infection is an uncommon cause of pharyngitis in preschool children. Current recommendations state that rapid strep screens in children younger than 3 years old are unnecessary unless there is a family member with documented strep throat and the patient is symptomatic. Two other symptoms that suggest sore throat in preverbal children are drooling and refusal to drink. Parents often do not mention drooling so asking if parents have noticed this can be useful. Similarly, children with fevers usually have decreased appetites but continue to drink. Refusal to drink should prompt the provider to investigate for causes of throat pain in preverbal children. See Table 42.5 for a key differential diagnosis for sore throat and associated characteristics.

Head Injury

Head injuries are common in ambulatory children. The PECARN (Pediatric Emergency Care Applied Research Network- a federally funded, multi-institutional network for research in pediatric emergency medicine) Head Trauma rules were established to guide providers in the evaluation of head injuries in children. The rules provide evidence-based statistics on the likelihood of clinically significant traumatic brain injury (cTBI) based on the age of the patient, the mechanism of injury, symptoms, and physical exam findings. A cTBI is defined as a skull fracture or brain injury that requires medical intervention (e.g., surgery or hospitalization). These rules provide evidence-based guidance on children with closed head injuries who are at low risk for cTBI with the goal of decreasing unnecessary radiation exposure in this population. The specific rules are outside the scope of this manual and are easily accessible online.

In children who present with an acute head injury, applying a Glasgow Coma Scale (GCS) (Fig. 42.2) to the child can help guide management, particularly in the critically ill child who may require the establishment of a protective airway. The GCS is a score created by assessing a child's eye, verbal, and motor responses. Scores range from 3 (an obtunded, comatose child) to 15 (a normal child). A score of 8 or less in the setting of head trauma should prompt STRONG consideration of protective intubation in a critically injured child.

Table 42.5 Sore throat differential diagnosis

Condition	Epidemiology	Cardinal features	Physical exam	Evaluation	Comments
Group A strep	5–15 years	– Sore throat – Fever – Lack of URI symptoms	– Pharyngeal erythema – Palatal petechiae – Tonsillar exudates – Tender anterior cervical lymphadenopathy	Always obtain rapid strep antigen if symptoms suggest strep throat: – If positive, treat – If negative, send strep culture	– Treatment should not be based on CENTOR criteria alone in children – In patients with significant URI symptoms, likelihood of strep is low and testing is not recommended
Peritonsillar abscess	Adolescents most commonly affected	– Severe sore throat – Worse on side of abscess – Trismus – Inability to drink – Drooling – Hot-potato voice	– Unilateral tonsillar hypertrophy – Erythema extending onto soft palate – Trismus often limits ability of patient to open mouth	– Antibiotics (ampicillin-sulbactam, clindamycin) – Consider bedside I/D (may require ENT consultation)	School-aged children occasionally affected. Rare in young children
Retropharyngeal abscess	Preschool (peak 2–4 years) – Young children primarily affected because of lymph nodes in retropharyngeal space that tend to involute with age	– High fever – Drooling – Torticollis	– Throat exam usually normal – Pain with extension of neck – Neck swelling/cervical lymphadenopathy – Stridor (rare)	– Lateral neck X-ray (thickening of prevertebral soft tissue) – CT scan – ENT consultation	– If patient is stable, admit for IV antibiotics Due to radiation exposure, CT scan should be reserved for patients who: – Are septic-appearing – Have respiratory distress/stridor – Do not respond to antibiotics

(continued)

Table 42.5 (continued)

Condition	Epidemiology	Cardinal features	Physical exam	Evaluation	Comments
Mononucleosis	Adolescence (uncommon in young children but can occur)	– Fever – Sore throat – Hot potato voice – Fatigue – Excessive sleeping	– Exudative tonsillitis (often very impressive) – Anterior, posterior cervical lymph nodes – Bilateral upper eyelid swelling (Hoagland's sign)	If testing required: – CBC may show atypical lymphocytes – Monospot If negative, EBV titers	Monospot (i.e., heterophile agglutination test) is unreliable in young children. Obtain EBV titers in this age-group

Fig. 42.2 Glasgow coma score

GLASGOW COMA SCALE MODIFIED FOR INFANTS			
GLASGOW COMA SCALE		INFANT COMA SCALE	
RESPONSE	SCORE	RESPONSE	SCORE
Eye Opening		*Eye Opening*	
Spontaneous	4	Spontaneous	4
To speech	3	To speech	3
To pain	2	To pain	2
None	1	None	1
Best motor response		*Best motor response*	
Obeys verbal command	6	Normal spontaneous movements	6
Localizes pain	5	Withdraws to touch	5
Withdraws in response to pain	4	Withdraws to pain	4
Abnormal flexion	3	Abnormal flexion	3
Extension posturing	2	Extension posturing	2
None	1	None	1
Best verbal response		*Best verbal response*	
Oriented and converses	5	Coos, babbles, interacts	5
Confused	4	Irritable	4
Inappropriate words	4	Cries to pain	4
Incomprehensible Sounds	3	Moans to pain	3
None	1	None	1

Limp/Extremity Pain

Limping and/or refusal to walk is a common reason for an emergency department visit. Older children can provide history (e.g., recent injury, location, and quality of pain) making the diagnosis straightforward in most cases. Workup and diagnosis are challenging in preverbal children. The differential diagnosis for limp/lower extremity pain is broad in this age-group (Table 42.6). Particular attention should be paid to the hip as there are several "can't-miss" diagnoses that can present with limping.

In general, in non-injured children who cannot bear weight, admission to the hospital is indicated. In addition, unilateral limb pain without explanation should raise concern for bone tumors and leukemia.

Table 42.6 Limping-child differential diagnosis

Condition	Epidemiology	Cardinal features	Physical exam	Evaluation	Management
Toddler fracture	<2–3 years old	Refusal to bear weight Often no history of specific injury	Can be normal vs. pain with tibial torsion/ palpation	Two views of X-ray to evaluate—Spiral tibia fracture	Long leg splint and orthopedics referral
Transient synovitis	4–9 years old	Refusal to bear weight with recent or current URI	No hip swelling or redness (hip joint is deep compared to other joints) Pain with ROM of hip Hip may be held in antalgic position (flexed, abducted, externally rotated)	X-ray of hip and US of hip joint on all patients Obtain blood work (CBC, ESR/CRP, blood culture) if any of the following: 1. Refusal to bear weight 2. Fever 3. Ill-appearance	**Kocher Criteria**[a]: Rules OUT septic joint if ESR <40, WBC<12, no fever, and child is weight bearing If joint effusion on hip US AND negative Kocher criteria AND patient can ambulate, arthrocentesis of hip joint is unnecessary
Septic arthritis	Most common in <3 years old Can occur at any age	Fever with refusal to bear weight	Fever Ill-appearance Pain with ROM of hip Unable to bear weight Hip more likely to be held in antalgic position	– CBC – ESR/CRP – Blood culture – X-ray of hip – Ultrasound hip If joint effusion, arthrocentesis of hip joint is indicated	Orthopedics consult and IV antibiotics
Slipped capital femoral epiphysis	10–16 years old	Ipsilateral hip pain May present with knee pain	Usually seen in obese patients around time of puberty Pain with ROM of hip Limp and/or inability to bear weight	X-ray pelvis 2 VIEW: – AP – Frog-leg lateral	Immediate surgical management is recommended to avoid long-term complications

(continued)

Table 42.6 (continued)

Condition	Epidemiology	Cardinal features	Physical exam	Evaluation	Management
Avascular necrosis of femoral head	4–10 years old 4 times more common in boys	Leg pain and limp from knee or hip	Often normal Pain with ROM of affected hip Antalgic gait	X-ray pelvis 2 view: – AP – Frog-leg lateral	Orthopedics consultation Patient should be made non-weight bearing
Apophysitis – Osgood-Schlatter disease – Sever's disease (calcaneal apophysitis)	8–15 years old	Athletic, active child: Anterior knee pain Heel pain	Tenderness at the tendon insertion of: Tibial tubercle Achilles' tendon on calcaneus	Typically not indicated	Rest, ice, stretching, NSAIDS for both conditions Heel inserts for shoes

[a] Evidence-based guidelines that distinguish transient synovitis from septic arthritis of the hip

Further Reading

Dieckmann RA, et al. The pediatric assessment triangle: a novel approach for the rapid evaluation of children. Pediatr Emerg Care. 2010;26(4):312–5. https://doi.org/10.1097/PEC.0b013e3181d6db37.

Koppen I, et al. Using the Bristol stool scale and parental report of stool consistency as part of the Rome III criteria for functional constipation in infants and toddlers. J Pediatr. 2016;177:44–48.e1.

Ralston SL, et al. Clinical practice guideline: the diagnosis, management, and prevention of bronchiolitis. Pediatrics. 2014;134(5):e1474–502. https://doi.org/10.1542/peds.2014-2742.

Son MB, Newberger JW. Kawasaki disease. Pediatr Rev. 2018;39(2):78–90. https://doi.org/10.1542/pir.2016-0182.

Index

N. Liao et al. (eds.), *Pediatric Rotations*,
https://doi.org/10.1007/978-3-031-59873-9

MIX
Papier aus verantwortungsvollen Quellen
Paper from responsible sources
FSC® C105338

If you have any concerns about our products,
you can contact us on
ProductSafety@springernature.com

In case Publisher is established outside the EU,
the EU authorized representative is:
Springer Nature Customer Service Center GmbH
Europaplatz 3, 69115 Heidelberg, Germany

Printed by Libri Plureos GmbH
in Hamburg, Germany